Head and Neck Pathology

Head and Neck Pathology

A Volume in the Series
Foundations in Diagnostic Pathology

Edited by

Lester D. R. Thompson, MD, FASCP
Department of Pathology
Southern California Permanente Medical Group
Woodland Hills Medical Center
Woodland Hills, California

Series Editor

John R. Goldblum, MD, FCAP, FASCP, FACG
Chairman, Department of Anatomic Pathology
The Cleveland Clinic Foundation
Cleveland Clinic Lerner College of Medicine
Case Western Reserve University
Cleveland, Ohio

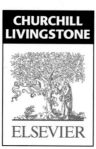

CHURCHILL
LIVINGSTONE

ELSEVIER

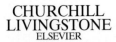

HEAD AND NECK PATHOLOGY (A VOLUME IN THE
FOUNDATIONS IN DIAGNOSTIC PATHOLOGY
SERIES, Series Edited by John R. Goldblum)
ISBN-13: 978-0-443-06960-4
ISBN-10: 0-443-06960-3

Copyright © 2006, Elsevier, Inc.

Library of Congress Cataloging-in-Publication Data
Thompson, Lester D. R.
    Head and neck pathology / Lester D. R. Thompson.—1st ed.
        p. ; cm.—(Foundations in diagnostic pathology)
    ISBN 0-443-06960-3
    1. Head—Pathophysiology.   2. Neck—Pathophysiology.   3. Head—Diseases—Diagnosis.
4. Neck—Diseases—Diagnosis.
    [DNLM: 1. Head and Neck Neoplasms.   2. Head—pathology.   3. Neck—pathology. WE 707
T473h 2006]   I. Title.   II. Series.
    RC936.T46 2006
    617.5′1—dc22   2005054931

Acquisition Editor: Belinda Kuhn
Developmental Editor: Karen Lynn Carter
Project Manager: Joan Sinclair
Cover Designer: Louis Forgione

Printed in China

Last digit is the print number: 9 8 7 6 5 4 3 2 1

*To all students
whose pursuit of knowledge
allows the achievement of wisdom.*

Contributors

Carol Adair, MD
Associate Clinical Professor
Department of Pathology
Uniformed Services University of Health Sciences
Bethesda, Maryland
Residency Program Director
Department of Pathology
Walter Reed Army Medical Center
Washington, D.C.
Non-Neoplastic Lesions of the Ear and Temporal Bone

Margaret Brandwein-Gensler, MD
Professor
Department of Pathology
Montefiore Medical Center
Albert Einstein School of Medicine
The Bronx, New York
Non-Neoplastic Lesions of the Nasal Cavity,
Paranasal Sinuses, and Nasopharynx

John W. Eveson, PhD, FDSRCS, FRCPath
Professor and Head of Division of Oral Medicine
Pathology and Microbiology
Department of Oral and Dental Science
University of Bristol
Honorary Consultant in Oral Medicine and Pathology
Bristol Royal Infirmary
United Bristol Healthcare NHS Trust
Bristol, United Kingdom
Malignant Neoplasms of the Salivary Glands

Jason C. Fowler, PA (ASCP)
Clinical Instructor
Department of Pathology
West Virginia University School of Medicine
Morgantown, West Virginia
Anatomy, Embryology, and Histology
Intraoperative Consultation and Grossing Techniques

Melissa H. Fowler, MD
Pathology Associates of Erie
Saint Vincent Health System
Erie, Pennsylvania
Intraoperative Consultation and Grossing Techniques

Nina Gale, MD, FRCP
Professor of Pathology and Director of Institute of
    Pathology
Institute of Pathology
Faculty of Medicine
University of Ljubljana
Ljubljana, Slovenia
Benign Neoplasms of the Larynx, Hypopharynx, and
Trachea

Jennifer L. Hunt, MD, MEd
Head, Section of Surgical Pathology
Director, Head and Neck/Endocrine Pathology
Director, AP Molecular Diagnostics Unit
Department of Pathology
The Cleveland Clinic
Cleveland, Ohio
Diseases of the Paraganglia System

Mario A. Luna, MD
Professor of Pathology
Department of Pathology
M.D. Anderson Cancer Center
Houston, Texas
Non-Neoplastic Lesions of the Neck
Benign Neoplasms of the Neck
Malignant Neoplasms of the Neck

Leslie Michaels, MD
Professor Emeritus
Histopathology
University College London
Honorary Consultant
Histopathology
Royal National Throat, Nose & Ear Hospital
London, United Kingdom
Malignant Neoplasms of the Ear and Temporal Bone

Susan Müller, DMD, MS
Associate Professor
Department of Pathology and Laboratory Medicine
Department of Otolaryngology–Head and Neck
    Surgery
Emory University School of Medicine
Atlanta, Georgia
Non-Neoplastic Lesions of the Oral Cavity and
Oropharynx

Brenda Nelson, DDS, LCDR, DC, USN
Department of Oral and Maxillofacial Pathology
Bethesda National Naval Dental Center
Naval Post-Graduate Dental School
Bethesda, Maryland
Benign Neoplasms of the Gnathic Bones

Bayardo Perez-Ordoñez, MD, FRCPC
Assistant Professor
Department of Pathology and Laboratory Medicine
Assistant Professor
Department of Otolaryngology–Head and Neck
    Surgery
University of Toronto
Staff Pathologist
Department of Pathology
University Health Network
Toronto, Ontario, Canada
Benign Neoplasms of the Nasal Cavity, Paranasal
Sinuses, and Nasopharynx

Mary S. Richardson, DDS, MD
Associate Professor
Director of Surgical Pathology
Department of Pathology and Laboratory Medicine
Medical University of South Carolina
Charleston, South Carolina
  Non-Neoplastic Lesions of the Salivary Glands

Pieter J. Slootweg, MD, DMD, PhD
Professor
Department of Pathology
University Medical Center St. Radboud
Nijmegen, The Netherlands
  Non-Neoplastic Lesions of the Gnathic Bones

Leslie H. Sobin, MD
Chief, Division of Gastrointestinal Pathology
Department of Gastrointestinal and Hepatic Pathology
Armed Forces Institute of Pathology
Washington, D.C.
  *TNM Classification and Consensus Reporting of Head
    and Neck and Endocrine Organ Tumors*

Lester D. R. Thompson, MD
Department of Pathology
Southern California Permanente Medical Group
Woodland Hills Medical Center
Woodland Hills, California
  *Non-Neoplastic Lesions of the Larynx, Hypopharynx,
    and Trachea*
  *Malignant Neoplasms of the Larynx, Hypopharynx,
    and Trachea*
  *Non-Neoplastic Lesions of the Nasal Cavity,
    Paranasal Sinuses, and Nasopharynx*
  *Benign Neoplasms of the Nasal Cavity, Paranasal
    Sinuses, and Nasopharynx*
  *Malignant Neoplasms of the Nasal Cavity, Paranasal
    Sinuses, and Nasopharynx*

  Benign Neoplasms of the Ear and Temporal Bone
  Malignant Neoplasms of the Ear and Temporal Bone
  Non-Neoplastic Lesions of the Neck
  Benign Neoplasms of the Neck
  Malignant Neoplasms of the Neck
  *TNM Classification and Consensus Reporting of Head
    and Neck Tumors*

Kevin Torske, DDS, MS, DABOMP
Oral and Maxillofacial Pathology and Forensic
  Odontology
Joint POW/MIA Accounting Command
Hickam Air Force Base
Waipahu, Hawaii
  Benign Neoplasms of the Salivary Glands

Gary Warnock, DDS, MS, MA
Associate Professor
Department of Dermatology
Johns Hopkins School of Medicine
Associate Staff
Departments of Dermatology and Pathology
The Johns Hopkins Hospital
Baltimore, Maryland
  Malignant Neoplasms of the Gnathic Bones

William Westra, MD
Professor
Department of Pathology
The Johns Hopkins Medical Institutions
Associate Director, Surgical Pathology
Department of Pathology
The Johns Hopkins Hospital
Baltimore, Maryland
  Benign Neoplasms of the Oral Cavity and Oropharynx
  *Malignant Neoplasms of the Oral Cavity and
    Oropharynx*

Foreword

The study and practice of anatomic pathology are both exciting and overwhelming. Surgical pathology, with all of the subspecialties it encompasses, and cytopathology have become increasingly complex and sophisticated, and it is not possible for any individual to master the skills and knowledge required to perform all of these tasks at the highest level. Simply being able to make a correct diagnosis is challenging enough, but the standard of care has far surpassed merely providing a diagnosis. Pathologists are now asked to provide large amounts of ancillary information, both diagnostic and prognostic, often on small amounts of tissue, a task that can be daunting even to the most experienced pathologist.

Although large general surgical pathology textbooks are useful resources, they by necessity could not possibly cover many of the aspects that pathologists need to know and include in their reports. As such, the concept behind *Foundations in Diagnostic Pathology* was born. This series is designed to cover the major areas of surgical pathology and cytopathology, and each volume is focused on one major topic. The goal of every book in this series is to provide the essential information that any pathologist, whether general or subspecialized, in training or in practice, would find useful in the evaluation of virtually any type of specimen encountered.

Dr. Lester Thompson, a renowned and prolific head and neck and endocrine pathologist, formerly of the Armed Forces Institute of Pathology and currently with the Southern California Permanente Medical Group, Woodland Hills, California, has edited an outstanding, comprehensive and state-of-the-art book on the essentials of head and neck pathology. This is one of those areas of surgical pathology that most surgical patholo-gists encounter with great frequency but in which few actually have formal training, and as such, a reference such as this has great practical value. The list of contributors includes some of the most renowned pathologists in this field, all of whom have significant expertise as practicing pathologists, researchers and educators. Each chapter is organized in an easy-to-follow manner; the writing is concise, tables are practical and easy to reference, and the photomicrographs are of uniformly high quality. There are thorough discussions pertaining to the handling of biopsy and resection specimens, as well as frozen sections.

This book is organized into 22 chapters and three appendices. There are separate chapters that provide thorough overviews of non-neoplastic, benign and malignant neoplasms of the larynx, hypopharynx, trachea, nasal cavity, nasopharynx, paranasal sinuses, oral cavity, oropharynx, salivary glands, ear, temporal bone, gnathic bones and the neck. There is a separate chapter dedicated to paragangliomas, since these lesions are frequently encountered by head and neck pathologists. The appendices are similarly comprehensive and include a thorough review of the anatomy, embryology and histology of structures of the head and neck, intra-operative consultation and grossing techniques and the most up-to-date TNM classification and recommendations for reporting of head and neck tumors.

I wish to extend my sincerest gratitude to Dr. Thompson, who poured his heart and soul into this book. I would also like to thank all of the authors who contributed to this outstanding volume in the *Foundations in Diagnostic Pathology* series.

JOHN R. GOLDBLUM, M.D.

Preface

During medical school, one of my best friends, Dr. Peter Bret Mitchell, said: "You see but you do not observe. The distinction is clear." This paraphrase, taken from "The Illustrated Sherlock Holmes Treasury" by Sir Arthur Conan Doyle, still rings clear in my head, as if he had said it yesterday. The precise scrutiny, the ability to memorize catalogues of information, and the mental facility to synthesize all one "sees," is what makes for an uncommonly superior pathologist.

The pages which follow will, through a highly templated format, allow for the acquisition of a compendium of knowledge as it relates to disease of the head and neck. Selected disorders of the larynx, sinonasal tract, ear and temporal bone, salivary gland, oral, gnathic, and neck regions will be presented in a fashion which allows for quick cross-referencing and comparison. *Pathology* is derived from the Greek meaning "a treatise of disease." As a branch of medicine, pathology is essentially a study of the elemental nature of disease. While pathologists are experts at microscopic interpre-

tation of diseases, they too must apply their knowledge to guide other clinicians and scientists in their management of the afflicted patient. Through a keen and discerning eye, the pathologist is able to amalgamate the clinical, radiographic, laboratory, macroscopic, microscopic, histochemical, immunohistochemical, ultrastructural, and molecular results into a cogent whole. This information can then be used to be a "physician's physician," ultimately leading to the correct patient management.

It is the intense aspiration of this editor that the information found within this treatise on pathology will provide the information necessary to achieve this goal.

LESTER D. R. THOMPSON, M.D.

Acknowledgments

How far does one throw the circle of acknowledgment and appreciation when so many people play various functions to bring this venture to publication? While independent, I have learned that interdependence yields a far better outcome. To that end, I would like to acknowledge a few of the most influential. My deep sense of gratitude goes to these people:

My parents, Dr. and Mrs. Ronald Thompson, who gave up their life in South Africa to allow my brother and I to fulfill our desires to be physicians in America;

My brother, Dr. Glynn M. Thompson, for his fierce loyalty and constantly competitive spirit which drove me to achieve more;

Dr. Douglas Wear, who, in college, first showed me what pathology was, double-heading over the microscope as he discovered the cause of cat-scratch disease;

Dr. Yao-Shi Fu, for his direction, guidance, and encouragement for going into Otorhinolaryngic-Head and Neck pathology;

Dr. Dorothy L. Rosenthal, who tempered my enthusiasm, guided my spirit, and taught me the finesse of diagnosis;

Dr. Dennis K. Heffner, for his encyclopedic erudition entirely emanated exclusively for eccentric me;

And for my wife, Pamela A. Thompson-Thompson, with whom everything is possible. Her love, devotion, support, and understanding gave me the time to make this happen. Oh yes; to say nothing of her computer programming expertise that organized the book, templated and structured the chapters, color-corrected the images, systematically arranged countless illustrations, scanned transparencies, backed up data, and helped with data management. She *always* makes life worth living to the fullest.

I also acknowledge the superb illustrations of Trisha Haszel. Many gave professional assistance at Elsevier, but I would like to specifically thank Karen Carter and Belinda Kuhn for their constant editorial assistance and guidance, and Natasha Andjelkovic for her original support. Thanks to Dr. John Goldblum for positing the original request.

Although axiomatic, the responsibility for any errors, omissions, or deviation from current orthodoxy is mine alone!

LESTER D. R. THOMPSON, M.D.

Contents

1 Non-Neoplastic Lesions of the Larynx, Hypopharynx, and Trachea

Lester D. R. Thompson

CONGENITAL AND DEVELOPMENTAL ABNORMALITIES

A number of congenital and developmental anomalies affect the larynx, including tracheopathia osteochondroplastica, laryngomalacia, subglottic stenosis, laryngeal webs, and laryngeal atresia. Many are clinical diagnoses for which a pathology sample is not obtained. For illustrative purposes, tracheopathia osteochondroplastica will be discussed here.

CLINICAL FEATURES

Tracheopathia osteochondroplastica (tracheobronchopathia osteochondroplastica) is a segmental degenerative disorder of the tracheobronchial tree characterized by multiple submucosal cartilaginous and osseous nodules of various sizes narrowing the upper respiratory tract. It is most common in elderly men, occasionally associated with chronic inflammation or with trauma. Tracheopathia osteoplastica can present clinically with nonspecific signs and symptoms, although stridor and dyspnea are common. Radiologic studies may suggest the diagnosis with scalloped nodular calcified opacities seen in the submucosa. The diagnosis is confirmed after endoscopic and pathologic examination.

PATHOLOGIC FEATURES

Histologically, metaplastic cartilage and bone are found in the submucosa, often in continuity with the inner surface of the tracheal cartilage (Fig. 1-1). The overlying mucosa is intact and may appear normal or metaplastic. There is an overall rigidity to the trachea. Heterotopic bone formation is seen in the soft tissue or stroma of the biopsy material (Fig. 1-2). The bony lamellae may protrude into the mucosa, thereby giving the characteristic appearance on bronchoscopy. The irregular bony spicules have thin walls surrounding fatty marrow. In children, there is often a limited degree of calcification. The histologic diagnosis is difficult only when the biopsy is small, from the periphery or only from the center (i.e., not from the whole lesion), or information about the radiographic studies is unknown.

DIFFERENTIAL DIAGNOSIS

The clinical differential diagnosis includes tracheobronchomegaly and tracheomalacia, both of which present with softening, flexibility or dilatation of the

CONGENITAL AND DEVELOPMENTAL ABNORMALITIES DISEASE FACT SHEET

Definition	Tracheopathia osteochondroplastica is a segmental degenerative disorder characterized by multiple submucosal cartilaginous/osseous nodules narrowing the upper respiratory tract
Incidence and location	Rare
Morbidity and mortality	May cause respiratory embarrassment
Gender, race, and age distribution	Male > Female Older patients (>60 yr)
Clinical features	Often associated with chronic inflammation or trauma Stridor and dyspnea
Radiographic findings	Scalloped nodular calcified opacities in the submucosa, seen most common on plain films
Prognosis and treatment	Excellent, but must have good tracheobronchial hygiene Laser removal or dilatation if significant narrowing

CONGENITAL AND DEVELOPMENTAL ABNORMALITIES PATHOLOGIC FEATURES

Gross findings	Submucosal, firm, nonmobile nodules within a rigid airway
Microscopic findings	Metaplastic or heterotopic bone or cartilage in the submucosa May be in continuity with the tracheal cartilages Bony lamellae may protrude into the mucosa
Pathologic differential diagnosis	Tracheomalacia, tracheobronchiomegaly, myositis ossificans, bony stenosis

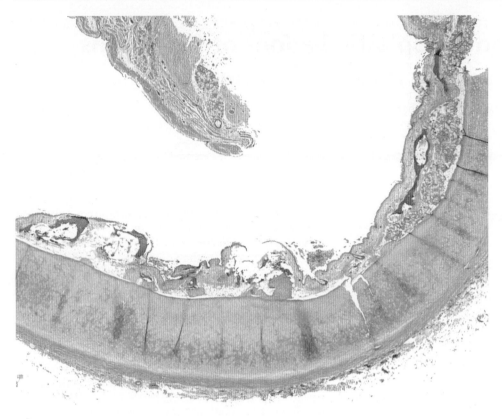

FIGURE 1-1

Submucosal bone deposition or metaplasia is found separated from the cartilage. This finding, combined with the clinical presentation, is distinctive for tracheopathia osteoplastica.

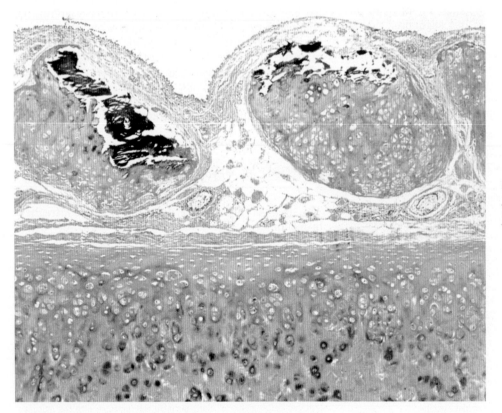

FIGURE 1-2

A spicule of metaplastic bone separated from the mucosa and cartilage in tracheopathia osteoplastica.

trachea, rather than the rigidity of tracheopathia osteoplastica. Tracheobronchiomegaly demonstrates absolute enlargement of the trachea and bronchi, with a histologic decrease in elastic longitudinal fibers and a thinning of the musculature of the tracheal wall. Laryngeal myositis ossificans has a zonal phenomenon with a highly cellular inner zone surrounded by bone in the outer zone. Bony stenosis is generally seen with polyps or papillomas and associated chronic inflammation.

PROGNOSIS AND THERAPY

Localized disease may not require treatment, but significant narrowing may require laser removal and dilatation. Meticulous tracheobronchial hygiene is imperative in long-term clinical management.

INFECTIONS

Both infectious and inflammatory conditions may result in laryngitis. Laryngitis is divided into acute and chronic forms, with age variability. Pharyngitis, laryngitis, "croup," epiglottitis, and laryngeotracheobronchitis, in either acute or chronic form, are all terms applied to infections or inflammations of the larynx, trachea, and hypopharynx. These terms have clinical implications based on anatomic location, but the diseases are caused by different etiologic agents. The antecedent events can be infectious, traumatic, neoplasms, surgical (vascular compromise), iatrogenic (feeding tubes or tracheostomy tubes), foreign bodies, or postradiation. A number of etiologies may be present synchronously, such that an infection may develop in association with radiation therapy. Therefore, multiple etiologies may need to be addressed. Many viruses, bacteria, fungi, and parasites are known to result in clinical laryngitis, but space considerations preclude an exhaustive discussion: herpes laryngitis will be the illustrative lesion.

CLINICAL FEATURES

Infections may manifest themselves in different clinical diseases depending on the age of the patient, with a single organism causing bronchiolitis in an infant, croup in an older child, pharyngitis in another patient, and a subclinical syndrome in an adult. With some exceptions, most of the histologic appearance is identical, as are the clinical manifestations, frequently dependent on the age, sex, and nutritional and immunity status. Cord function may be compromised. An extensive laboratory investigation to document the specific type of virus causing a "common cold" is probably not warranted except in extreme cases. Immunocompromised patients

INFECTIOUS DISEASE FACT SHEET	
Definition	An acute or chronic reaction to an infectious agent (laryngitis, pharyngitis, croup, epiglottitis)
Incidence and location	High frequency of "colds", but true laryngitis is less common
	Increased frequency in developing countries, low socioeconomic and poor hygiene patients
Morbidity and mortality	Limited, although sequelae of streptococcal infections may result in glomerulonephritis and acute rheumatic fever
Gender, race, and age distribution	Equal gender distribution
	All ages
Clinical features	Age, gender, nutritional and immunity status affect symptoms
	Cough, sore throat, difficulty swallowing, fever, chills
	Cord function may be compromised
Prognosis and treatment	Excellent with infectious agent specific therapy, although "supportive" care can be used for most viral infectious agents

are more likely to have herpes simplex laryngitis. Therefore, the index of suspicion for a herpes infection is higher in the very young, very old, pregnant, and immunocompromised patients.

PATHOLOGIC FEATURES

The mucus membranes are erythematous and swollen on gross examination, while the histologic findings are

INFECTIOUS PATHOLOGIC FEATURES	
Microscopic findings	Surface ulceration
	Acute and/or chronic inflammatory cells with necrosis
	Granulomatous inflammation may be present depending on agent
	Viral inclusions (multinucleated, ground-glass appearance, Cowdry A-type inclusions) may be noted
Special studies	Culture
	Various histologic stains (PAS, GMS, Brown-Hopps, AFB)
	Immunohistochemistry for specific organisms (HSV, CMV)
Pathologic differential diagnosis	Inflammatory conditions (Wegener's granulomatosis), environmental exposure, polyps

nonspecific inflammatory cells and edema fluid (Fig. 1-3), occasionally coupled with specific inclusions. Multinucleated giant cells with opacified, "ground glass" nuclei are characteristic (Fig. 1-4). Frequent secondary infections by bacterial agents can complicate the clinical and histologic appearance. Cultures and/or immunohistochemistry will help identify the organism(s).

DIFFERENTIAL DIAGNOSIS

The inflammatory infiltrate is frequently nonspecific and may be identified in association with infectious disease, inflammatory disease, allergies, trauma, and environmental exposures to noxious substances. Therefore, close correlation with the clinical setting in addition to serology, cytologic preparations, microbiologic cultures or tests, precipitant tests for fungi and other clinical studies (thyroid function tests, skin tests, etc.) are imperative to obtain a complete view of the disease process.

PROGNOSIS AND THERAPY

While slow to recover in some instances, antiviral therapy will usually result in complete resolution. Removal of the underlying abnormality may help to prevent a recurrent infection.

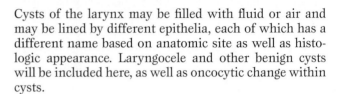

CYSTS OF THE LARYNX (INCLUDING LARYNGOCELE)

Cysts of the larynx may be filled with fluid or air and may be lined by different epithelia, each of which has a different name based on anatomic site as well as histologic appearance. Laryngocele and other benign cysts will be included here, as well as oncocytic change within cysts.

CLINICAL FEATURES

Outpouchings from the laryngeal ventricle and saccule of the normal laryngeal mucosa result in a laryngocele. Laryngoceles are divided clinically into internal (expansion into the false vocal fold) and external (extension through the thyrohyoid membrane into the soft tissues of the neck), with the vast majority presenting as internal unilateral masses. Symptoms are variable because the air may decompress spontaneously, removing the airway obstruction or hoarseness. Patients who repeatedly are subjected to increased pressure are more likely to have laryngoceles. In general, the symptoms for patients with cysts are nonspecific and heavily overlap those of laryngocele.

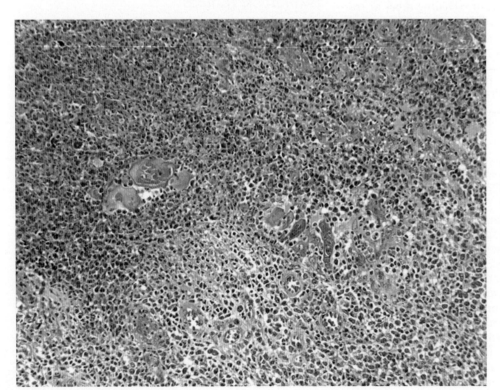

FIGURE 1-3

An intense acute inflammatory infiltrate with necrotic debris dominates the sample, although a few multinucleated giant cells with "ground glass" nuclei are characteristic for herpes simplex virus (HSV).

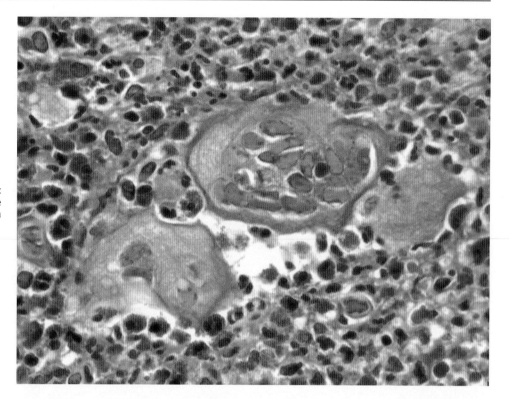

FIGURE 1-4
HSV will produce a characteristic "ground glass" appearance to the nuclei, especially when found in a multinucleated giant cell.

CYSTS OF THE LARYNX (INCLUDING LARYNGOCELE)
DISEASE FACT SHEET

Definition	Outpouchings of the laryngeal ventricle and saccule are called laryngocele
Incidence and location	Uncommon, although more frequent in younger patients
Gender, race, and age distribution	Equal gender distribution All ages
Clinical features	Variable and nonspecific with airway obstruction and hoarseness most common
Prognosis and treatment	Excellent Marsupialization or surgery

CYSTS OF THE LARYNX (INCLUDING LARYNGOCELE)
PATHOLOGIC FEATURES

Gross findings	Point of origin and type of cyst determines the macroscopic appearance Internal or external to the larynx Cysts do not generally communicate with the lumen Laryngocele is an air-filled herniation that does communicate with the interior of the larynx Saccular cysts affect false cord Retention cysts affect epiglottis Traumatic cysts affect the arytenoid region Size ranges from 0.5–8 cm
Microscopic findings	Cysts are surrounded by fibrous connective tissue Squamous or respiratory epithelium Vascular elements seen in vascular cysts Oncocytic epithelium may line the cysts
Pathologic differential diagnosis	External jugular phlebectasia, prolapse, branchial cleft cyst, thyroglossal duct cyst, dermoid cyst, teratoma, laryngeal webs

PATHOLOGIC FEATURES

GROSS FINDINGS

The gross appearance of laryngeal cysts is determined by the point of origin in the larynx and the type of cyst (saccular, retention/inclusion, ductal vascular, or traumatic). The cyst can be considered to be either external or internal to the larynx based on the degree of compression by the cyst and the extent of disease within the larynx. Cysts generally do not communicate with the interior of the larynx, while a laryngocele is an air filled herniation or dilatation of the saccule, either internal or external to the larynx, but communicating with the lumen (Fig. 1-5). Saccular cysts (anterior or lateral) are submucosal and do not communicate with the lumen, but are instead filled with mucus or acute inflammatory elements. As air and fluid is forced into a laryngocele, the distinction between a laryngocele and other laryn-

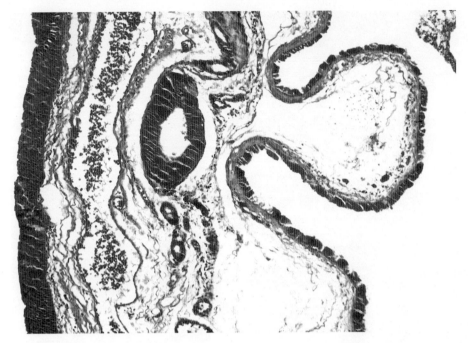

FIGURE 1-5
An intact mucosa is seen on the left, while an outpouching of oncocytic epithelium on the right is part of an external laryngocele.

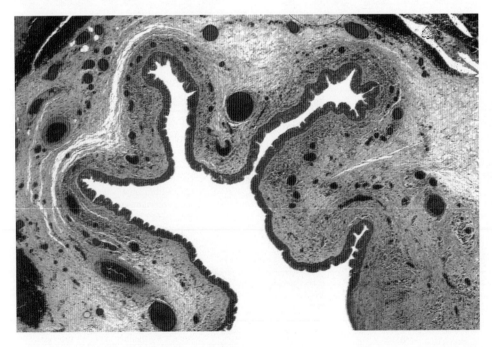

FIGURE 1-6
Air or fluid will sometimes fill a laryngocele, which is lost with processing, resulting in a smooth undulating periphery.

geal cysts may be impossible (Fig. 1-6). There are cysts of the all regions of the larynx, with retention types more frequent in the epiglottis, saccular cysts in the false cord, and traumatic type in the arytenoid region. The size of the cysts range from 0.5 to 8 cm, depending on the location, with small cysts on the vocal cords; larger cysts are found attached to the epiglottis, pushing the larynx to one side, or projecting into the hypopharynx. Eversion and prolapse occur, further complicating the classification of cysts of the larynx. The cysts are variably filled with thin serous fluid to tenacious, thick, mucinous, gelatinous, or bloody fluid.

MICROSCOPIC FINDINGS

Histologic examination is unnecessary for diagnosis of a laryngocele as radiographic studies are diagnostic. However, when removed, there is an epithelial lined cyst, containing respiratory or squamous mucosa.

Cysts have a variably thick surrounding wall of fibrous connective tissue. The lining of the cysts helps to differentiate them into a variety of subtypes. Most of the cysts are lined by squamous or respiratory epithelium (retention and saccular) (Fig. 1-7), while a few are lined by fibrous connective tissue. Cysts in which there

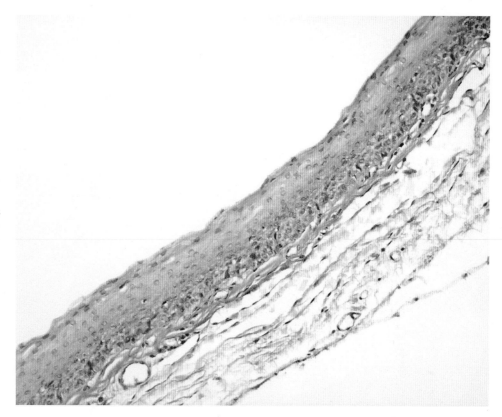

FIGURE 1-7

A metaplastic squamous mucosa is identified within this laryngeal cyst.

is an admixture of both mesodermal and endodermal layers qualifies the cyst as a congenital or embryonal cyst. This type of cyst contains squamous or respiratory epithelium along with some other mesodermal element, intimately associated with the epithelial component. The microscopic appearance of vascular cysts formed by a localized collection of lymph or blood vessels in a subepithelial tissue is very rare and may in fact be impossible to separate from a hemangioma or a lymphangioma. The traumatic cyst is not common, but is more frequently described as surgical intervention in the larynx has increased. Small islands of tissue are implanted deep into the stroma and undergo cystic degeneration. Any of the above cysts can become infected, and when infected, are referred to as a pyoceles, although still classified by the original cyst type. The larger the ventricular appendix, the more predisposed the individual is to infection or inflammation.

Oncocytes can be present within a wide variety of lesions in the larynx, including, but not limited to oncocytic papillary cystadenoma, oncocytic cyst (Fig. 1-8), oncocytoma, oxyphilic adenoma, eosinophilic papillary cystadenoma, and oncocytic hyperplasia. Oncocytic metaplasia and/or hyperplasia are most likely an aging phenomenon with an aggregation of mitochondria within the cytoplasm of the lesional cells. The separation from a cyst may be difficult, although oncocytic metaplasia and/or hyperplasia should be multifocal or diffusely present within the larynx. The cells

are polyhedral to round with distinct cell borders with cytoplasm surrounding small, round, centrally situated, pyknotic to vesicular nuclei (Fig. 1-9). Abundant cytoplasm containing a varying number of fine to coarse, eosinophilic granules is seen surrounding the nuclei.

DIFFERENTIAL DIAGNOSIS

External jugular phlebectasia (a congenital dilatation of the jugular vein) frequently presents as a neck mass, particularly during straining or crying (Valsalva maneuver) similar to a laryngocele. However, it does not require surgery, although surgery is often performed for cosmetic purposes. The histologic appearance is of a dilated vascular space and is different from laryngocele or other laryngeal cysts. The differential diagnosis is often limited histologically but may be rather involved from a clinical perspective. Therefore, histologic confirmation of the lesion is mandatory to help define the type of cyst. Prolapse of the ventricle can sometimes present a similar appearance to a cyst on the gross examination. However, prolapse can be restored, while cysts cannot be put back. Large branchial cleft cysts and thyroglossal duct cysts may push into the laryngeal spaces, thereby creating the illusion of a primary cyst of the larynx.

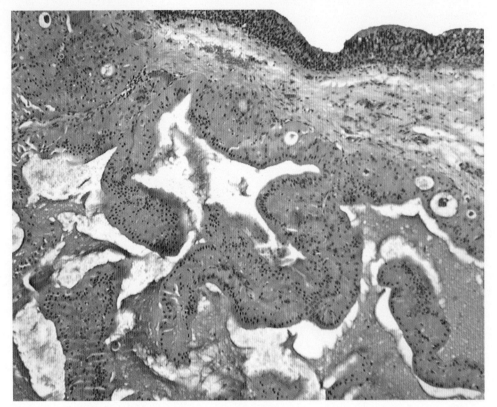

FIGURE 1-8

A papillary oncocytic proliferation within the larynx, composed of enlarged cells with abundant eosinophilic cytoplasm.

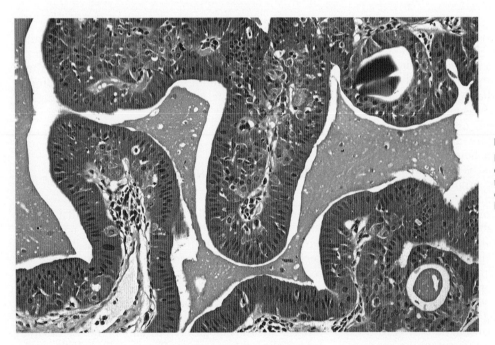

FIGURE 1-9

Large, polyhedral cells with abundant, opaque, oxyphilic cytoplasm are surrounding a cystic space in this oncocytic cyst. The nuclei are small and hyperchromatic.

Histologic examination, combined with clinical site of origin should help in distinguishing these other cysts of the region. A dermoid cyst generally contains two primordial cell types, with mesenchymal and ectodermal structures. This lesion is not a true teratoma as it lacks all three layers and is different from the development cysts of the larynx. Other clinical entities include laryngeal webs, vascular rings, hemangiomas, and foreign bodies. These entities can usually be excluded clinically or by biopsy. Squamous cell carcinoma (SCC), usually supraglottic, can be associated with laryngeal cysts, perhaps induced by the carcinoma.

PROGNOSIS AND THERAPY

Surgical marsupialization is the treatment of choice for a laryngocele; while benign cysts can be managed symptomatically, with surgery only as clinically necessary to maintain a patent airway.

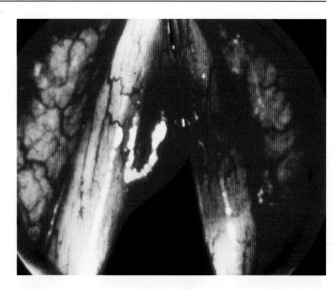

FIGURE 1-10
A bilaterally edematous nodule on opposing surface of the vocal cords.

VOCAL CORD POLYPS AND NODULES

CLINICAL FEATURES

A nodule and a polyp are not used synonymously clinically, although they frequently are interchangeable in the pathology community. A nodule is more frequent in young women associated with vocal abuse, while polyps occur in any age group associated with clinical hoarseness, infection, smoking, and hypothyroidism. Vocal changes and hoarseness is the most frequent presenting symptom.

PATHOLOGIC FEATURES

GROSS FINDINGS

Grossly, nodules are almost always bilateral, an edematous, gelatinous, or hemorrhagic mass involving opposing surfaces of the middle one-third of the vocal cord, typically a few millimeters in size (Fig. 1-10). In contrast, a polyp usually involves the ventricular space or Reinke's space of a single vocal cord, with a soft, rubbery, translucent to red mass (Fig. 1-11). A polyp can be sessile, raspberry-like to pedunculated, with a soft, rubbery or firm consistency, from translucent white to red, and up to a few centimeters.

VOCAL CORD POLYPS AND NODULES DISEASE FACT SHEET	
Definition	Reactive changes of the laryngeal mucosa and adjacent stroma which results in a benign polypoid or nodular growth
Incidence and location	Infrequent
Gender, race, and age distribution	Nodule is more common in young women
	Polyps occur at any age and in both genders equally
Clinical features	Vocal abuse and phonation changes, hoarseness
	Other causes include infection, smoking, and hypothyroidism
Prognosis and treatment	Excellent
	Treatment of underlying etiology with surgery as necessary

VOCAL CORD POLYPS AND NODULES PATHOLOGIC FEATURES	
Gross findings	Nodules are bilateral, edematous, on opposing surfaces usually in the middle third of vocal cord
	Polyps are single, involve ventricular or Reinke's space, and are a soft, rubbery translucent to red mass
Microscopic findings	Arc of development
	Edematous, vascular, myxoid, or hyaline (or fibrous)
	Dilated vessels and minimal inflammation
	Surface is usually unremarkable
Pathologic differential diagnosis	Amyloidosis, myxoma, granular cell tumor, spindle cell (sarcomatoid) squamous cell carcinoma

MICROSCOPIC FINDINGS

Nodules start out edematous with a myxoid matrix, but with time become fibrotic. Polyps can be divided into four main histologic subtypes: edematous (Fig. 1-12), vascular (Fig. 1-13), myxoid (Figs. 1-14, 1-15), hyaline or fibrous (Figs. 1-16, 1-17), often demonstrating all of these change in the same polyp. The dominant histo-

logic pattern determines the type. The edematous or myxoid type has a loose, myxoid, vascularized stroma admixed with a pale blue to pink matrix material (Fig. 1-12); the vascular type has many dilated vessels and occasionally granulation tissue and hemorrhage (Fig. 1-13); the hyaline type has fibrin-type material closely opposed to vascular spaces, while the fibrous type shows spindle cells in dense fibrous stroma (Fig. 1-16). The surface epithelium may become metaplastic, atrophic, keratotic, and hyperplastic. Inflammation is generally meager. Crystals can be seen in some polyps.

DIFFERENTIAL DIAGNOSIS

The differential diagnosis includes amyloidosis, myxoma, and rarely, neoplasms (granular cell tumor, spindle cell [sarcomatoid] squamous cell carcinoma [SCSCC]). The other histologic findings in these lesions allow for separation.

PROGNOSIS AND THERAPY

Excision of a polyp and treatment of the underlying cause of a nodule is generally sufficient therapy. Treatment of hypothyroidism can also be beneficial. Nodules may recur if the inciting factor is not identified and removed.

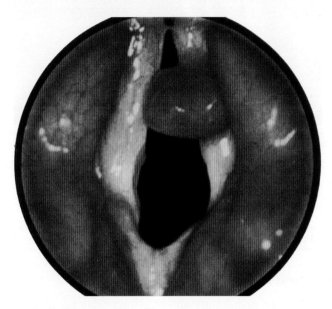

FIGURE 1-11

A polyp projects from the vocal cord on one side.

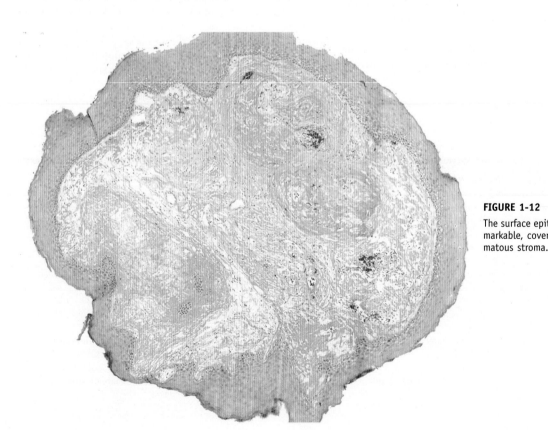

FIGURE 1-12

The surface epithelium of a polyp is unremarkable, covering the hypocellular, edematous stroma.

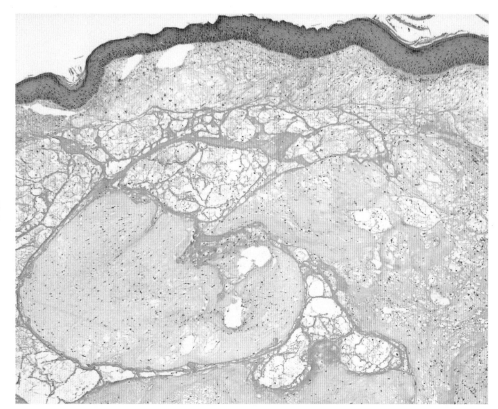

FIGURE 1-13

Large areas of degenerated material with edema and rich vascular investment in a polyp.

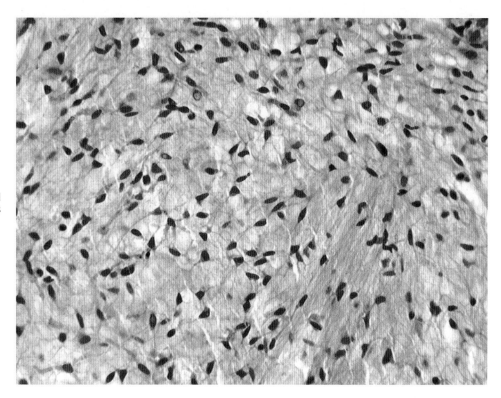

FIGURE 1-14

Laryngeal polyp. Basophilic myxoid material separates small stellate cells without cytologic atypia.

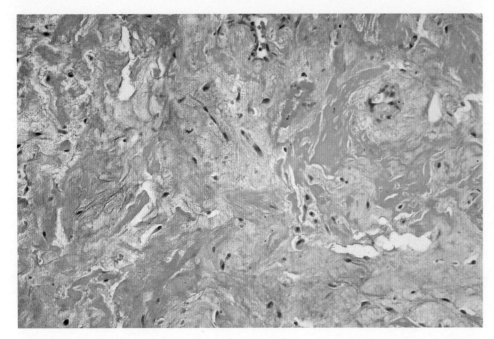

FIGURE 1-15
Degenerative changes can occur within polyps, such as the fibrinoid and myxoid change.

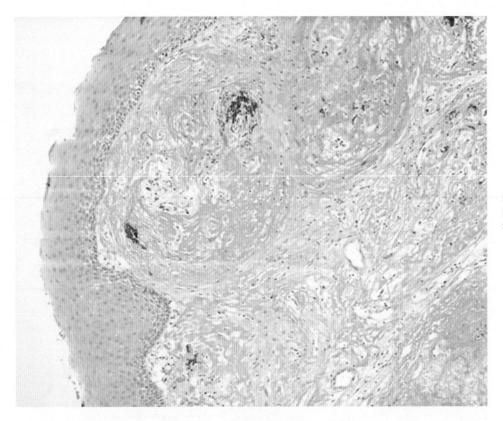

FIGURE 1-16
Hyaline change in a polyp which still shows edematous change.

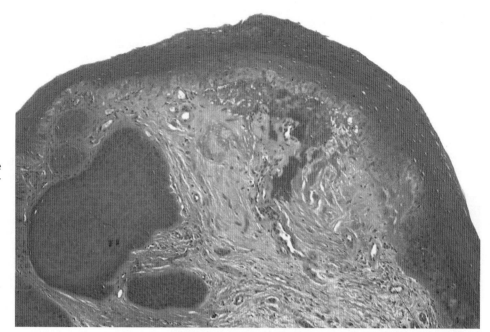

FIGURE 1-17

Laryngeal nodule. Fibrous connective tissue deposition beneath an unremarkable epithelium.

CONTACT ULCER

CLINICAL FEATURES

Also known as pyogenic granuloma, this benign condition generally occurs in adult men more frequently than women, with the patients presenting with hoarseness, sore throat, or pain. Patients often have chronic throat clearing or habitual coughing. Contact ulcer is associated with vocal abuse, intubation, and acid regurgitation. In the intubation setting, female patients are affected more commonly, especially in an emergent setting when an inappropriate size endotracheal tube has been selected. Gastric-laryngeal reflux or gastroesophageal reflux disease (GERD) is frequently missed as the patient is unaware of the underlying cause (hiatal hernia), although they may report heartburn and/or belching as a result of the acid reflux. Pepsin is thought to be the injurious agent and not the hydrochloric acid.

CONTACT ULCER DISEASE FACT SHEET	
Definition	Benign reactive response to an injury usually in the posterior larynx
Incidence and location	Frequent, especially in patients with GERD
	Posterior larynx is most common site
Gender, race, and age distribution	Male > Female (except in postintubation setting)
	Adults > children
Clinical features	Hoarseness, sore throat, and pain
	Chronic throat clearing and habitual coughing
	Vocal abuse/misuse
	Gastro-laryngeal reflux disease symptoms (heartburn, belching)
Prognosis and treatment	Excellent
	Resolve underlying cause, although surgery can be performed

CONTACT ULCER PATHOLOGIC FEATURES	
Gross findings	Ulcerated, polypoid nodular mass
	Posterior larynx
Microscopic findings	Surface ulceration with fibrinoid necrosis
	Exuberant granulation tissue
	Central areas may have hemosiderin laden macrophages
	Extensive inflammatory infiltrate and hyperplastic endothelial cells
	May have surface re-epithelialization with time
Pathologic differential diagnosis	Infectious agents
	Vascular lesions
	Epithelial neoplasms, specifically spindle cell (sarcomatoid) squamous cell carcinoma

PATHOLOGIC FEATURES

GROSS FINDINGS

Contact ulcer usually presents as an ulcerated, polypoid or nodular mass (Fig. 1-18), most frequently involving the posterior vocal cord. The lesion is red to tan-white in appearance, up to 3 cm in size, with frequent bilateral involvement of the cords, resulting in a "kissing ulcer" on the opposite side of the vocal cord lesion.

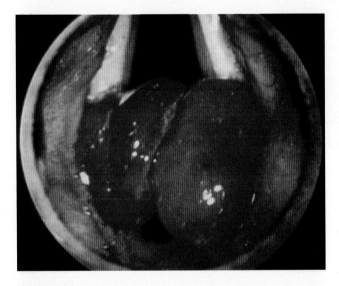

FIGURE 1-18
A laryngoscopic view of contact ulcer shows a polypoid, bilateral, beefy red mass involving the posterior vocal cords. A "kissing ulcer" is characteristic.

MICROSCOPIC FINDINGS

The surface is ulcerated, covered by fibrin and/or fibrinoid necrosis overlying an exuberant granulation tissue (Figs. 1-19, 1-20). The vessels in the granulation tissue are often arranged perpendicular to the surface, are lined by plump reactive endothelial cells, and are surrounded by acute and chronic inflammatory cells and histiocytes (Fig. 1-21). The vessels are haphazard in configuration, richly invested by lymphocytes, plasma cells, neutrophils and histiocytes (including giant-cell forms). Hemosiderin laden macrophages may be seen at the base of the polyp, especially in lesions of long clinical duration. Surface bacterial or fungal colonization is frequently identified. In the early stages, surface ulceration without granulation tissue may be identified. With the progression of time, the chronic phase of the disease may demonstrate an irregular hyperplastic epithelium resulting from the regenerative surface re-epithelialization, but a residuum of fibrinoid necrosis is often identified below the surface (Fig. 1-22). A prominent fibrosis may also be present in the stroma with progression of the disease.

DIFFERENTIAL DIAGNOSIS

The diagnosis of contact ulcer is usually a clinical pathologic correlation, as the histologic findings are often nonspecific. In light of this, the histologic differential diagnosis includes a variety of infectious agents, inflammatory conditions (Wegener's granulomatosis, inflammatory myofibroblastic tumor), vascular lesions (Kaposi's sarcoma, angiosarcoma) and epithelial

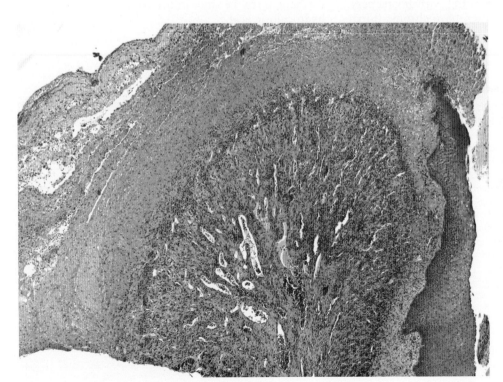

FIGURE 1-19
The polypoid nodule has most of the surface epithelium denuded and replaced by fibrinoid necrosis. The vessels are arranged perpendicular to the surface and are surrounded by a rich granulation-type tissue.

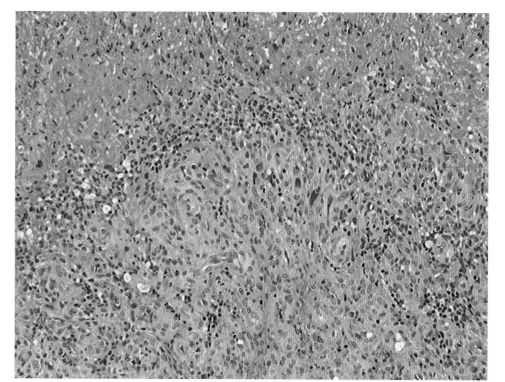

FIGURE 1-20

The fibrinoid necrosis replaces the surface epithelium and directly covers the granulation type tissue. Inflammatory elements are prominent.

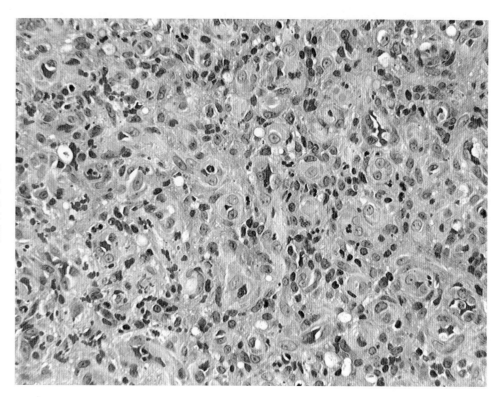

FIGURE 1-21

An exuberant granulation tissue with plump, reactive endothelial cells, acute and chronic inflammatory cells and histiocytes comprise the center of a contact ulcer. Mitotic figures within the endothelial cells are frequent as are extravasated erythrocytes.

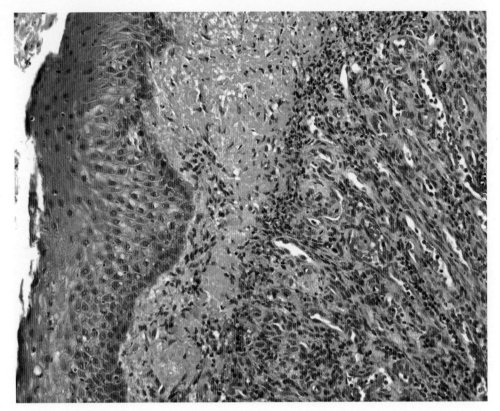

FIGURE 1-22
The surface epithelium has grown over the defect, but the fibrinoid necrosis and granulation tissue are still present to give a hint of the previous damage.

neoplasms (SCC, SCSCC). Special stains (GMS, PAS, Brown-Hopps [tissue Gram stain], Warthin-Starry) and culture should confirm an infectious agent. Wegener's granulomatosis has geographic bionecrosis combined with genuine vasculitis and helpful clinical findings (antineutrophil cytoplasmic antibodies titers). Kaposi's sarcoma and angiosarcoma are rare in the larynx, but show slit-like spaces with atypical cells, freely anastomosing vascular channels, spheroid hyaline globules (Kaposi's sarcoma), and atypical mitotic figures.

PROGNOSIS AND THERAPY

The ability to suggest the specific diagnosis with its causative factors is predicated on the correct morphologic interpretation. If the correct specific diagnosis of contact ulcer is made, appropriate identification and removal of the specific cause can eliminate the morbidity associated with surgery.

AMYLOIDOSIS

Amyloidosis encompasses a family of different types of benign accumulations of extracellular, fibrillar, insoluble protein deposits. Laryngeal amyloidosis is commonly

both localized and primary, and is the most common site of localized disease, although rare, accounting for <1% of benign laryngeal tumors. Multifocal disease is present in up to 15% of patients. There are a variety of classifications of amyloidosis, according to its distribution (localization), clinical type, and by the presence or

AMYLOIDOSIS DISEASE FACT SHEET	
Definition	Benign accumulation of extracellular, fibrillar insoluble protein deposits of amyloid
Incidence and location	<1% of all laryngeal neoplasms
	Usually in false vocal cord, but can be multifocal (15%)
Morbidity and mortality	Depends on primary or systemic disease and whether single or multifocal
	May be slowly progressive
Gender, race, and age distribution	Equal gender distribution
	Usually adults, but rarely children are affected
Clinical features	Hoarseness and voice changes
Prognosis and treatment	Good, although dependent on localized or systemic disease and whether primary or secondary
	Surgery is the treatment of choice
	Must exclude systemic disease with work-up

absence of underlying disease and its precursor protein (immunocytochemical nature) and patterns of extracellular deposition. Different sources of amyloidosis are recognized, with immunoglobulin light chains most common in the larynx.

CLINICAL FEATURES

Almost all patients experience hoarseness or voice changes, usually caused by mechanical factors, conditioned by the size and location of the amyloid. They usually present as adults, although children can rarely be affected, and there is no gender predilection.

PATHOLOGIC FEATURES

GROSS FINDINGS

Although there are conflicting data, the false vocal cord seems to be more frequently affected, showing a firm, "starch-like," waxy, translucent cut surface, measuring up to 4 cm in greatest dimension. Multifocal disease in the upper aerodigestive tract can be seen.

MICROSCOPIC FINDINGS

Amyloid consists histologically (irrespective of any associated findings) of a subepithelial, extracellular, acellular, hyaline-like, homogeneous, eosinophilic matrix material dispersed randomly throughout the stroma (Fig. 1-23), although revealing a predilection for vessels or mucoserous glands (Fig. 1-24). A sparse inflammatory infiltrate composed of lymphocytes and

plasma cells (Fig. 1-25) may be seen. Occasional histiocytes and a few giant cells may be either at the peripheral margin of or enclosed within the amyloid (Figs. 1-24, 1-26). Significant cytologic atypia of the lymphoplasmacytic infiltrate is not appreciated. The amyloidosis of the larynx is composed of a protein that is immunologically identical to the variable region of the light chain fragment of immunoglobulin.

AMYLOIDOSIS PATHOLOGIC FEATURES	
Gross findings	Firm, starch-like, waxy translucent cut surface Up to 4 cm
Microscopic findings	Subepithelial deposits
	Acellular, extracellular, eosinophilic, homogeneous matrix material
	Perivascular and periglandular predilection (compression atrophy may result)
	Lymphoplasmacytic infiltrate
	Foreign-body giant cell reaction can be seen
Special studies	Electron microscopy will show non-branching fibrils arranged in β-pleated sheets
	"Apple-green" birefringence with polarized light using a Congo-red stain (metachromatic with methyl violet)
	May show kappa or lambda light chain restriction and positive amyloid P immunoreactivity
Pathologic differential diagnosis	MALT lymphoma, vocal cord polyps, ligneous conjunctivitis, lipoid proteinosis
	Amyloid may be part of multiple myeloma, small cell carcinoma, and medullary thyroid carcinoma

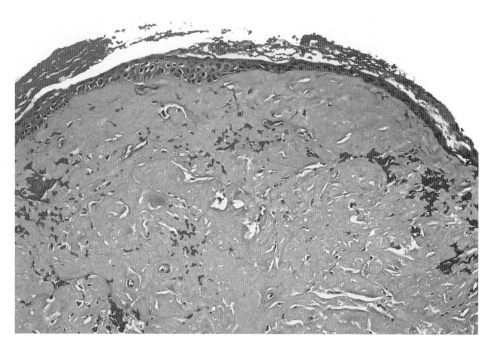

FIGURE 1-23

The acellular, eosinophilic, opaque amyloid deposition is noted below an intact surface epithelium without an obvious giant cell or inflammatory response.

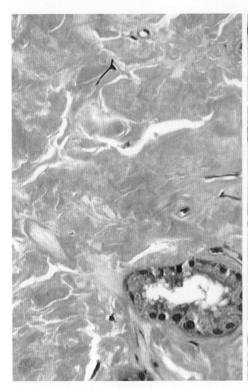
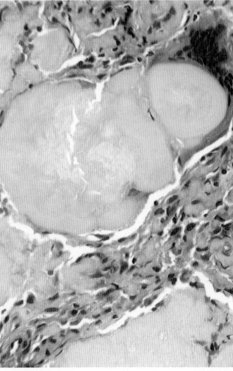

FIGURE 1-24
Left: periductal deposition with compression atrophy is characteristic for amyloid. *Right:* fragments of amorphous, acellular, eosinophilic amyloid material is found in the stroma, with a foreign body giant cell reaction.

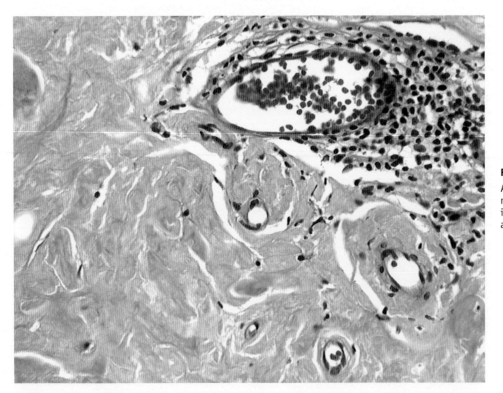

FIGURE 1-25
A sparse inflammatory infiltrate of mature lymphocytes and plasma cells is seen immediately around a vessel affected by amyloidosis.

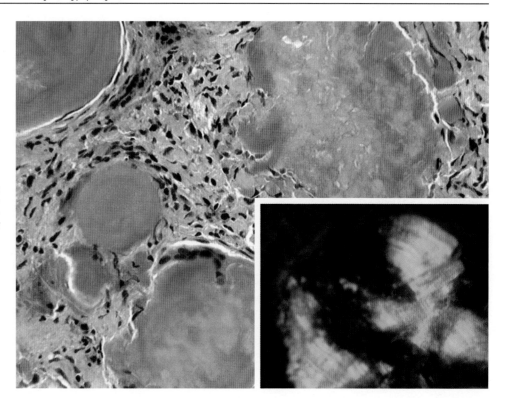

FIGURE 1-26
The foreign body giant cell reaction to amyloid. The inset shows Congo-red positive, "apple green" birefringence of amyloid when viewed under polarized light.

ANCILLARY STUDIES

ELECTRON MICROSCOPY

Electron microscopy reveals the characteristic interlacing meshwork of nonbranching fibrils as the protein arranges itself into ß-pleated sheets.

SPECIAL STAINS

Amyloid can be confirmed with histochemical techniques (Congo red, methyl violet [metachromatic pink-violet staining]), with apple-green birefringence under polarized light with Congo red (Fig. 1-26) proving to be the most reliable and easy-to-interpret technique.

IMMUNOHISTOCHEMICAL FEATURES

CD20 and CD3 highlight the admixture of B and T cells in the sparse lymphoplasmacytic infiltrate, respectively, although T cells tend to predominate, especially at the periphery of the amyloid deposits. Immunoreactivity with amyloid P and light chains (κ and λ) is more variable, although light chain restriction of the plasma cells can be seen.

DIFFERENTIAL DIAGNOSIS

The mucosal presentation of laryngeal amyloidosis, the recurrence and multifocal presentation in other mucosal sites, the monoclonal nature of the associated lymphoplasmacytic infiltrate in some cases, and a possible systemic plasma cell dyscrasias, all imply that at least a few laryngeal amyloid cases may be the result of an immunocyte dyscrasia or lymphoproliferative disorder with an origin from mucosa-associated lymphoid tissue (MALT). The differential diagnosis includes hyalinized vocal cord polyps (usually lacks an associated lymphoplasmacytic infiltrate), ligneous conjunctivitis, and lipoid proteinosis, all of which are negative for amyloid studies. It is important to note that amyloid may occur in association with multiple myeloma, small cell carcinoma, and medullary thyroid carcinoma. The determination of a serum calcitonin level can help to distinguish between a primary laryngeal small cell carcinoma tumor (serum elevation absent) versus a metastatic/invasive medullary thyroid carcinoma (serum elevation present).

PROGNOSIS AND THERAPY

There is a difference in the biologic behavior and clinical management between isolated laryngeal amyloidosis and other forms of amyloidosis. A clinical, radiographic, and laboratory investigation (including quantitative immunoglobulin assay, serological test for rheumatoid arthritis, urine and/or serum electrophoresis, Bence-Jones protein analysis) should be tailored to the individual patient to exclude multifocal or systemic disease. Prognosis for isolated laryngeal amyloidosis is excellent as the "tumors" are slow growing, although repeated surgeries (endoscopic) may be necessary for recurrent disease. There does not appear to be any prognostic significance of amyloid deposition in association with other tumors. In these cases, the prognosis is determined by the tumor morphology/type specifically.

INFLAMMATORY MYOFIBROBLASTIC TUMOR

CLINICAL FEATURES

This benign "reactive" lesion (similar to nodular fasciitis in other anatomic sites), presents as a change in

INFLAMMATORY MYOFIBROBLASTIC TUMOR DISEASE FACT SHEET	
Definition	Benign, reactive proliferation of myofibroblasts which form a tumor mass associated with inflammatory cells
Incidence and location	Rare
Gender, race, and age distribution	Male > Female Adult patients
Clinical features	May be associated with trauma, immunosuppression and/or HHV-8 Changes in phonation or dyspnea
Prognosis and treatment	Recurrence may develop if incompletely excised Surgery

phonation or dyspnea more commonly in adult men. There is no well-defined etiologic agent for this pseudoneoplastic "reactive" proliferation, but trauma, immunosuppression, and possibly human herpesvirus 8 have been suggested.

PATHOLOGIC FEATURES

GROSS FINDINGS

The lesion is usually a smooth polypoid or pedunculated mass involving the submucosal region of the true vocal cord, appearing firm or fleshy, tan to white, measuring up to 3 cm in greatest dimension. The lesions may demonstrate a myxomatous appearance, but do not have necrosis or hemorrhage.

MICROSCOPIC FINDINGS

The surface epithelium is usually intact and often hyperplastic, occasionally showing reactive epithelial atypia (Fig. 1-27). The proliferation respects the surface epithelium and surrounding mesenchymal tissues, although unencapsulated. The tumor is a loosely organized proliferation of spindle-shaped to stellate-appearing cells, in a myxoid or fibrous vascular background stroma, with variable inflammatory cells, occasionally demonstrating collagen deposition and calcifications (Figs. 1-28, 1-29). The inflammatory infiltrate is inconstant, varying from sparse to abundant, containing mature lymphocytes, histiocytes, plasma cells, neutrophils, and eosinophils, frequently in a rich vascular

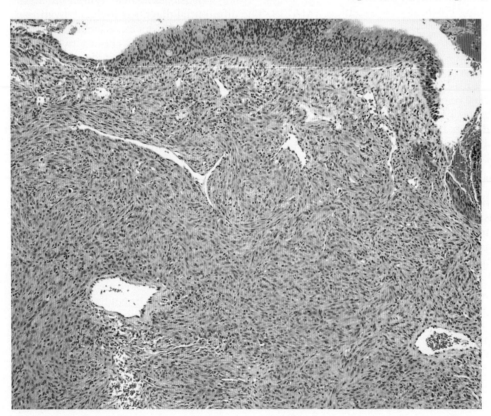

FIGURE 1-27

An intact respiratory type epithelium overlies a cellular spindle cell proliferation with an increased vascularity and inflammatory cells.

stroma. Russell bodies can be seen. The myofibroblasts have round to oval nuclei with dense chromatin surrounded by elongated cytoplasmic extensions ("tadpole cells") (Fig. 1-28). Atypia can be seen, but with a maintenance of a normal nuclear to cytoplasmic ratio. Mitotic figures, although infrequent, are not atypical.

INFLAMMATORY MYOFIBROBLASTIC TUMOR PATHOLOGIC FEATURES	
Gross findings	Smooth, polypoid or pedunculated mass
	Submucosal location
	Firm, fleshy, white-tan
	Up to 3 cm
Microscopic findings	Proliferation respects the epithelium
	Loosely organized proliferation
	Spindle-shaped to stellate cells ("tadpole")
	Myxoid-fibrous vascular background stroma
	Inflammatory cells
	Collagen deposition and calcifications are uncommon
Immunohistochemical features	Vimentin and actins are positive
	S-100 protein and keratins are non-reactive
	ALK overexpression and gene rearrangements
Pathologic differential diagnosis	Spindle cell (sarcomatoid) squamous cell carcinoma, inflammatory fibrosarcoma, peripheral nerve sheath tumors, and nonspecific inflammation

ANCILLARY STUDIES

The myofibroblasts react with vimentin, muscle-specific actin, and smooth muscle actin (Fig. 1-30). Cytoplasmic cytokeratin reactivity is rarely seen, but S-100 protein immunoreactivity is absent. Ultrastructural examination is not necessary, but demonstrates microfilaments arranged in parallel to the long axis along with intercalated dense bodies with rare junctional complexes. A few of these lesions in adults have been shown to have anaplastic lymphoma kinase (ALK) gene rearrangements and overexpression.

DIFFERENTIAL DIAGNOSIS

Spindle cell squamous cell carcinoma (SCSCC), inflammatory fibrosarcoma, nerve sheath tumors, and nonspecific inflammation should be included in the differential diagnosis. SCSCC has a surface or invasive component, with a greater degree of pleomorphism and atypical mitotic figures; when keratin is positive, it helps with the distinction. Inflammatory fibrosarcoma and leiomyosarcoma are exceedingly rare in the larynx, arise in the deep tissues of the larynx, and present with features of malignancy. A schwannoma usually has spindle cells, but nuclear palisading and S-100 protein immunoreactivity will help to distinguish between these two benign conditions. Nonspecific inflammation may be the harbinger of an infectious agent, and cultures or special stains should be performed to exclude this possibility.

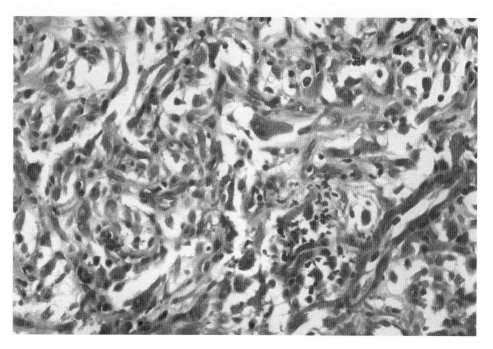

FIGURE 1-28
Hemorrhage, spindle cells, and inflammatory elements are haphazardly arranged. The myofibroblastic cells have a "tad-pole" like appearance.

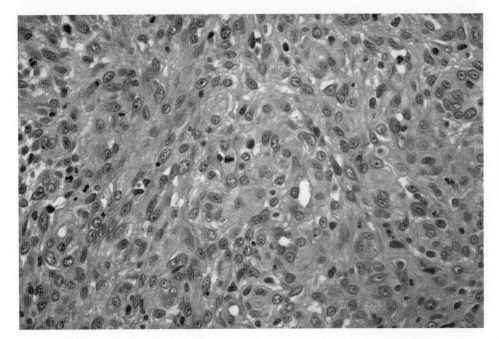

FIGURE 1-29

The myofibroblastic component has a tissue culture-like appearance. Mitotic figures are easily identified in this case, but are not atypical.

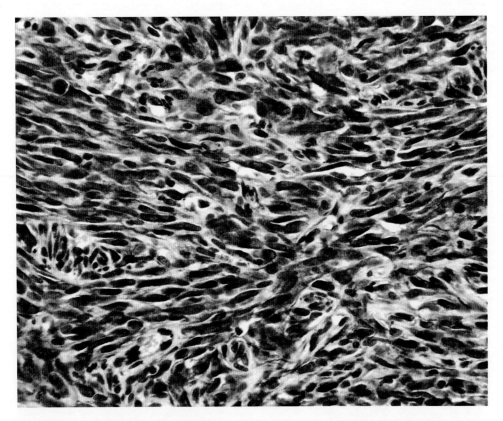

FIGURE 1-30

Inflammatory myofibroblastic tumor. The myofibroblasts are strongly and diffusely immunoreactive with actin.

PROGNOSIS AND THERAPY

The lesions may recur if incompletely excised, but regression has also been reported in patients managed by corticosteroid and nonsteroidal anti-inflammatory agents. No laryngeal lesion has directly caused the death of a patient.

REACTIVE EPITHELIAL CHANGES

There is a lack of uniformity and inconsistency of terminology used to describe reactive, hyperplastic, and "precancerous" epithelial lesions of the larynx, both clinically and histopathologically. This results in a lack of concordance with the term used and the biology of the lesion. Dozens of classification schemes have been proposed, but none has gained substantial support in either the clinical or pathology communities. No matter which system is used, it is imperative that the term used conveys to the clinician the potential biologic risk for the development of a malignant tumor.

CLINICAL FEATURES

The spectrum of laryngeal reactive epithelial lesions are usually in adults, men more frequently than women, and especially so after age 50 years. The incidence varies, but is correlated with the same "carcinogenic" factors which result in carcinoma, for the symptoms of reactive lesions are indistinguishable from those of carcinoma. Various factors may result in reactive or hyperplastic epithelial changes, including smoking and alcohol use/abuse, vocal abuse, chronic laryngitis, habitual throat clearing, industrial pollution, and/or occupational exposure to specific agents. Most of the lesions of the larynx present with symptoms of hoarseness, changes in phonation, and sore throat, often coupled with a nonproductive cough. Asymptomatic patients are occasionally identified. Leukoplakia, pachydermia, hyperplasia, pseudoepitheliomatous hyperplasia, metaplasia, keratosis, and contact ulcer are clinical and histologic terms that overlap with one another as well as with a number of distinctly different histologic lesions; i.e., leukoplakia clinically is a descriptive term designating a white patch or plaque, but histopathologically may describe keratosis, pseudoepitheliomatous hyperplasia, dysplasia, and SCC in situ. Therefore, these clinically macroscopic and microscopically morphologic diagnoses must be taken in context. Finally, there is a small, but well-accepted risk of certain "reactive" lesions representing preneoplastic processes, which left untreated may go on to carcinoma. Therefore, it is imperative to recognize these various epithelial processes and to place them in a teleologic arc of development when appropriate.

PATHOLOGIC FEATURES

GROSS FINDINGS

All of these epithelial reactions can be ulcerated, flat, polypoid, papillary, or verrucous in gross appearance, ranging from red (erythroplakic) to white (leukoplakic), involving a microscopic area or the entire larynx (pachyderma laryngis), mimicking neoplasia clinically. However, most of these reactive lesions occur along the true vocal cords, frequently bilateral, rarely involving the commissures. The lesions range from a circumscribed thickening of the mucosa to an ill-defined plaque, often exhibiting a rough surface. Unfortunately, no clinical appearance is consistently correlated to the underlying histology.

MICROSCOPIC FINDINGS

It is important to remember that the mucosal epithelia are different in the larynx, ranging from squamous epithelium on the epiglottis, transitional epithelium in the glottis, and respiratory-type epithelium in the supra- and infraglottic portions of the larynx. The areas of transition are normal, but in diseased states, the overall histology can vary considerably. (See Appendix A.)

The histologic findings may be focal or diffuse, with the overall degree or quantity influencing the diagnosis, since the characteristics become more "atypical" in aggregate. The degree of each of these changes takes on importance especially because of their known associa-

---

REACTIVE EPITHELIAL CHANGES
DISEASE FACT SHEET

Definition	Reactive, hyperplastic and precancerous epithelial changes, a subset of which have a biologic potential to develop into carcinoma
Incidence and location	Common and usually involve the vocal cords specifically
Morbidity and mortality	True reactive lesions have no potential mortality
Gender, race, and age distribution	Male > Female More common >50 yr
Clinical features	Smoking and alcohol use/abuse, vocal abuse, chronic laryngitis, habitual throat clearing, industrial pollution, and/or occupation exposure to specific agents Hoarseness, changes in phonation, sore throat and nonproductive cough
Prognosis and treatment	Excellent for reactive lesions Treat underlying etiology, although surgery is employed frequently (The precancerous lesions are discussed in dysplasia)

REACTIVE EPITHELIAL CHANGES PATHOLOGIC FEATURES			
Gross findings	Variable and include, ulcerated, flat, polypoid, papillary, verrucous, red, or white lesions Frequently bilateral and usually along the vocal cords		**Koilocytosis** has crenated nucleus, perinuclear halo, prominent, thick cell walls (usually in papilloma) **Keratosis** is an increased amount of keratin production
Microscopic findings	Aggregates of findings are necessary before a precancerous lesion is diagnosed **Hyperplasia** is an increase in cell number or cell layer **Verrucous hyperplasia** has hyperplastic epithelium with verrucous projections, hyperkeratosis, and sharp interface with stroma **Pseudoepitheliomatous hyperplasia** is exuberant, large, bulbous projections of epithelium contained by an intact basement membrane without cytologic atypia **Metaplasia** is transformation to a simpler epithelium		**Parakeratosis** has flat nuclei with the keratosis **Dyskeratosis** is abnormal keratinization, usually close to the basal zone **Radiation changes** incorporate nuclear enlargement but in cells with a low nuclear to cytoplasmic ratio, cytoplasmic vacuolization, cellular atrophy, and vascular proliferation **Necrotizing sialometaplasia** is a lobular arrangement of destroyed glands with metaplastic squamous epithelium growing through the mucoserous gland structures
		Pathologic differential diagnosis	Reactive and hyperplastic lesions, dysplasia, squamous cell carcinoma

tion with SCC. Critical judgment, including expert consultation or multiple biopsies taken sequentially over time, is essential to an accurate diagnosis. The presence alone of any one of these reactive epithelial changes is just a morphologic diagnosis and does not necessarily equate to a specific pathologic condition. The histologic appearance is variable, with architecture and histology used simultaneously to evaluate these lesions.

Reactive lesions include hyperplasia which is an absolute increase in the number of cells or cell layers (Fig. 1-31). This process may involve the surface or the deep, basal (Fig. 1-32) and parabasal cell layers. There is no cytologic atypia; *atypia* is used here in the context of inflammatory and regenerative changes particularly referring to cytologic features. This is not considered a precancerous lesion.

Verrucous hyperplasia and verrucous squamous cell carcinoma are very difficult to separate, and some have suggested that they vary only in stage and size, the lesions representing a developmental spectrum (Fig. 1-33). The distinction on histologic features alone, even when specialized studies have been performed

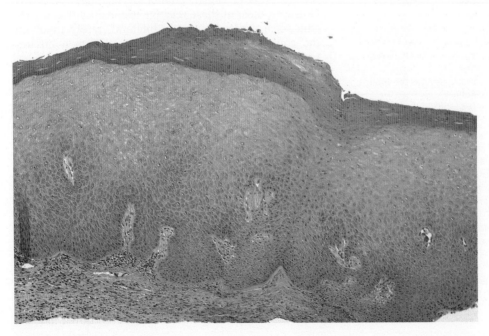

FIGURE 1-31

An increase in the number of layers of squamous epithelium is called hyperplasia, with the overlying increase in keratin termed keratosis.

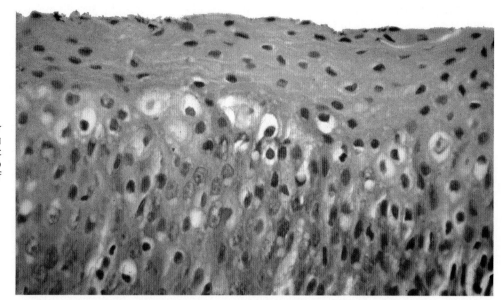

FIGURE 1-32

There is an increase of the number of cells in the basal zone, extending up to the middle one-third, where it comes to an abrupt stop. There is no cytologic atypia in this example of basal zone hyperplasia.

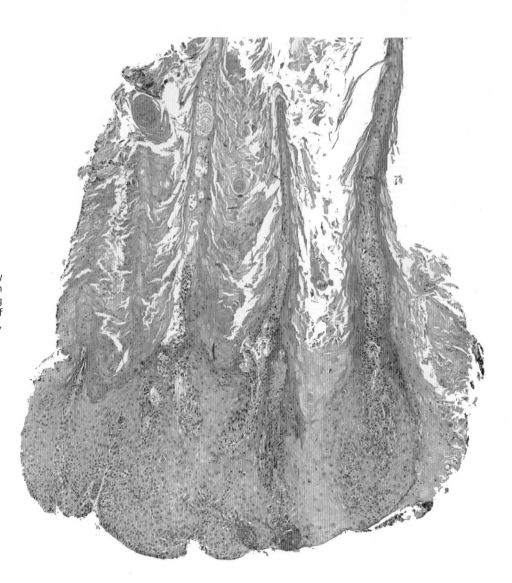

FIGURE 1-33

Verrucous hyperplasia with papillary fronds of squamous epithelium covered with keratin and lacking architectural and cytologic features of malignancy. The base is smooth, although an interface is lacking.

(including DNA analysis), is often not possible. However, true verrucous hyperplasia has a hyperplastic squamous epithelium with regularly spaced, verrucous projections with hyperkeratosis, and is sharply defined at the epithelial to stromal interface (Fig. 1-34). Parakeratotic crypting is not usually present. There is considerable overlap with verrucous carcinoma, which may require a larger biopsy coupled with excellent communication between the pathologist and surgeon.

Pseudoepitheliomatous hyperplasia (PEH) represents an exuberant reactive overgrowth of squamous epithelium without cytologic evidence of malignancy, often with large, bulbous projections into the underlying stroma, but always respecting the basement membrane (Fig. 1-35). This reactive condition is frequently confused with SCC. PEH is associated with fungal infections and granular cell tumor (Fig. 1-36).

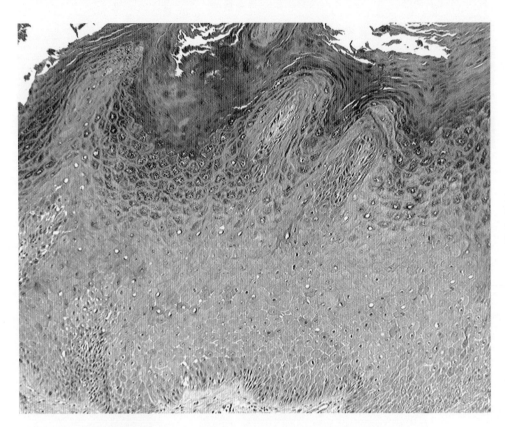

FIGURE 1-34

Verrucous hyperplasia is frequently associated with parakeratosis and shows an accentuated granulosa layer.

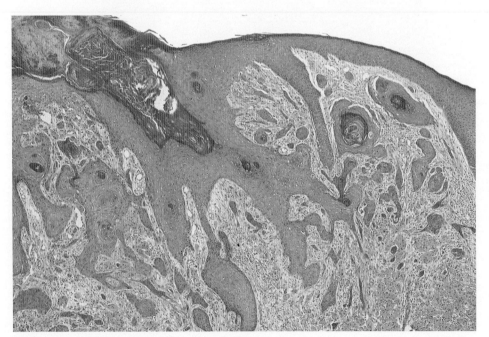

FIGURE 1-35

Pseudoepitheliomatous hyperplasia has a rounded type of growth into the underlying stroma, without nuclear atypia in the cells. Keratinization is frequent.

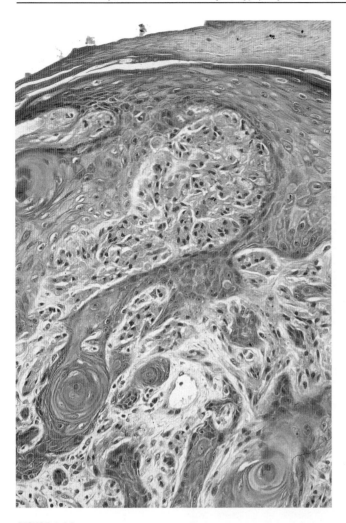

FIGURE 1-36
A granular cell tumor (small cells with granular, eosinophilic cytoplasm) is associated with pseudoepitheliomatous hyperplasia.

Metaplasia results when there is a change from a specialized respiratory epithelium to a more simple squamous epithelium and can occur anywhere within the larynx. Koilocytosis is defined by a centrally placed crenated nucleus surrounded by clear cytoplasm which forms a "halo," and prominent, thick cell walls/borders ("cookie cutter"). Koilocytosis is generally identified as part of papilloma (Fig. 1-37) or carcinoma, but is not identified in isolation, although glycogenation can sometimes cause diagnostic confusion.

Keratosis is separated from the other reactive and hyperplastic lesions because it may be part of all of them, and so is described in a little more depth. Keratosis is an abnormal production and accumulation of keratin at the surface of the laryngeal mucosa in which the nuclei are lost and the surface epithelial cells are completely replaced by keratin (Fig. 1-38). The keratin is often present in an exophytic pattern. Nuclear atypia or pleomorphism is not implied by "keratosis," although keratosis can have atypia (*atypia* is not synonymous with pleomorphism). When the nuclei remain with

incomplete keratinization, *parakeratosis* is the preferred term (Fig. 1-39). Keratosis is part of the complex response seen in the larynx and does not have any prognostic significance on its own. However, keratosis has been shown to have alterations in oncogenes and tumor suppressor genes (retinoblastoma protein, p53, p21, cyclin D1, Mcm-2, pTEN, tenascin, fibronectin), but not to the extent seen in dysplasia and carcinoma. This suggests there is an insufficient accumulation of the multiple genetic alterations which will result in the very early sequential transformation to carcinoma. There is an approximately 4% risk of subsequently identifying carcinoma in patients with an initial diagnosis of keratosis. Further, when keratinizing dysplasia is identified, there is a strong association with abnormalities of the DNA to a much greater extent seen in nonkeratinizing dysplasias, suggesting abnormal keratinization may be associated with a greater degree of DNA abnormalities.

Reactive epithelial changes can also be associated with radiation-induced changes. Nuclear enlargement (within epithelial or stromal cells which have a maintained nuclear to cytoplasmic ratio), multinucleation, cytoplasmic vacuolization, cellular atrophy, and vascular proliferation can be observed; but there are no readily identifiable changes of malignancy (recurrent or residual) (Fig. 1-40). The antecedent-inciting event (radiation) is generally known, and the difficulty generally arises in ruling out recurrent or residual disease rather than separation from a benign reactive epithelial response.

Necrotizing sialometaplasia (NS) is a benign, self-limited, reactive inflammatory process involving minor mucoserous or salivary glands. The histologic marker of this disease is the maintenance of the smooth contour and lobular architectural arrangement of the minor mucoserous glands after necrosis (Fig. 1-41). In an attempt at re-epithelialization, there is a squamous metaplasia of the residual glands and acini (Fig. 1-42). In the immediate area, remnants of uninvolved acini and ducts can be seen along with mucin-producing cells. There is frequently an associated acute and chronic inflammation in addition to mucus extravasation related to necrosis of the duct or acinar epithelium. The lobules of the mucoserous glands remain smooth in contour, now lined by a metaplastic squamous epithelium which is bland in overall appearance. However, as with any reparative or regenerative epithelium, enlarged nuclei, prominent nucleoli, apoptosis, and mitotic figures can be seen (Fig. 1-43). The difficulty distinguishing between NS and carcinomas is especially difficult when the biopsy is small. With deeper sections and sometimes a larger biopsy, the true nature of the lesion will become apparent.

ANCILLARY STUDIES

Immunohistochemical reactions for the subtypes of keratins have been proposed as a means for distinguishing between reactive epithelial changes and carcinoma

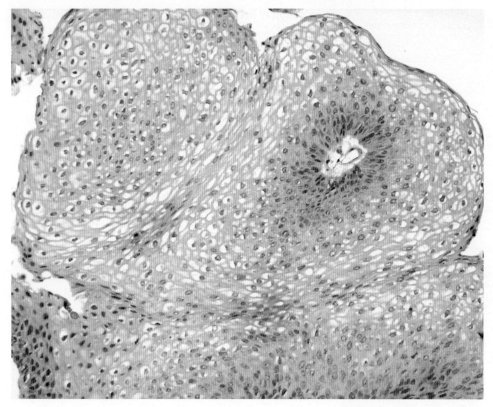

FIGURE 1-37
"Koilocytic" change (nuclear chromatin condensation, perinuclear halo and accentuation of the cell borders) seen in papillomas.

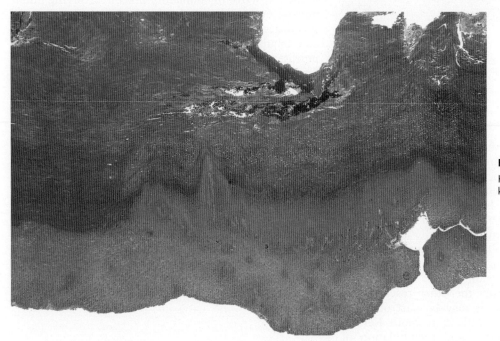

FIGURE 1-38
Keratosis is an accumulation of keratin at the surface.

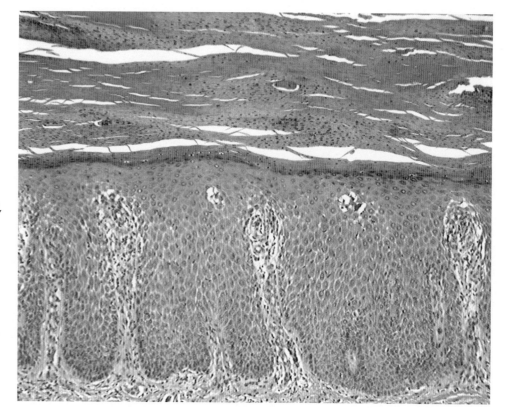

FIGURE 1-39

Keratin accumulation with nuclei, referred to as parakeratosis.

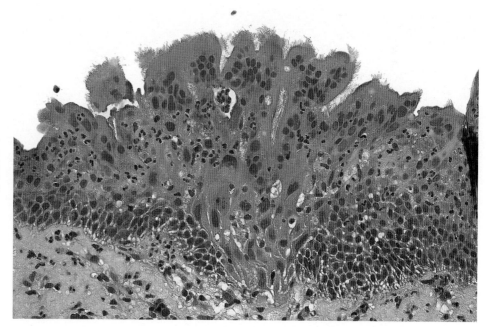

FIGURE 1-40

An area of papillary projection is comprised of remarkably enlarged cells with a low nuclear to cytoplasmic ratio and showing nuclear hyperchromasia and irregularity. Acute inflammation can be seen in this example of radiation injury.

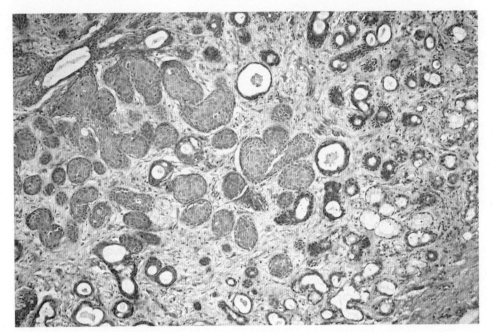

FIGURE 1-41

Necrotizing sialometaplasia is a lobular process, with areas of squamous metaplasia confined to the previous lobular architecture of a mucoserous gland. Uninvolved mucoserous glands can be identified at the periphery.

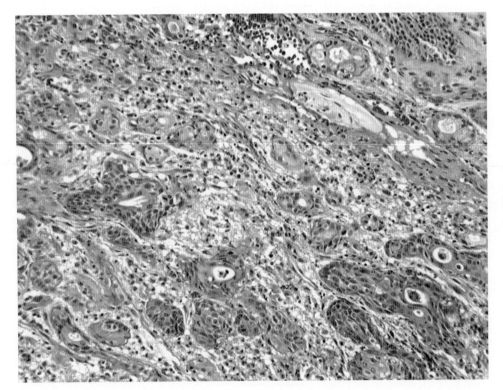

FIGURE 1-42

Extensive squamous metaplasia associated with acute inflammatory cells while mucus producing glands are seen at the periphery.

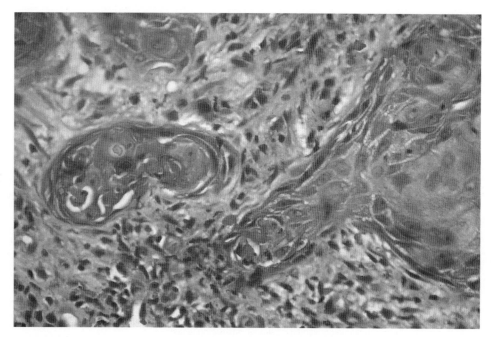

FIGURE 1-43

While well circumscribed and surrounded by an intact basement membrane, there is atypia in the epithelial cells. Inflammation is present in this example of necrotizing sialometaplasia examined at high power.

(CK13 is expressed in normal or reactive conditions, but is decreased or absent in dysplasia and carcinoma, respectively); but from a practical standpoint, these reactions are insufficiently reliable to be used in a clinical setting.

DIFFERENTIAL DIAGNOSIS

The differential diagnosis encompasses different lesions within the reactive and hyperplastic category as well as separation from dysplasia and carcinoma. It is well accepted that dysplasia (squamous intraepithelial lesion, squamous intraepithelial neoplasia) is a precancerous lesion, but the issue of how much *atypia* or *pleomorphism* makes a lesion dysplastic is not well established and poorly reproducible between practitioners. Since there is a sequential continuum, it is nearly impossible to rigidly place a lesion into reactive versus neoplastic, as no single combination of features consistently or accurately separates reactive from dysplastic. Therefore, degrees of atypia and subtle changes often portend of the impending carcinoma transformation but may at that time not represent a true "carcinoma." Dyskeratosis, a lack of maturity or irregular epithelial stratification toward the surface ("basal zone"-type cells identified above the basal zone), anisonucleosis (abnormal nuclear size), anisocytosis (abnormal cell size), pleomorphism (nuclear shape irregularities, chromatin distribution disturbance, nuclear hyperchromasia), changes in nuclear to cytoplasmic ratio, atypical mitotic figures, premature keratinization lower in the proliferating epithelium (toward the basal zone), and increased mitotic figures are markers of dysplasia and are not

seen in benign reactive conditions to any significant degree. It is imperative to repeat that there is a consecutive and cumulative alteration in the process of carcinogenesis.

PROGNOSIS AND THERAPY

True hyperplasia and reactive epithelial lesions are self-limiting and reversible, but when moderate to severe dysplasia exists, then the persistence and/or progression to carcinoma has a known risk. While diagnosis includes a biopsy, the underlying cause of the disorder should be sought and corrected. Due to the relative association with malignant tumors, clinicopathologic correlation is imperative in order to assure an excellent long-term prognosis. In hyperplasia no clinical follow-up is required, but clinical follow-up is necessary for patients with "dysplasia," as sampling inadequacies or progression of the lesion may result in inadequate clinical management.

SUGGESTED READING

Congenital and Developmental Abnormalities

1. Birzgalis AR, Farrington WT, O'Keefe L, et al.: Localized tracheopathia osteoplastica of the subglottis. J Laryngol Otol 1993;107:352–353.
2. Himalstein MR, Gallagher JC: Tracheobronchiomegaly. Ann Otol Rhinol Laryngol 1973;82:223–227.
3. Marchal G, Baert AL, van der HL: Calcification of larynx and trachea in infancy. Br J Radiol 1974;47:896–897.
4. Wenig BM, Devaney K, Wenig BL: Pseudoneoplastic lesions of the oropharynx and larynx simulating cancer. Pathol Annu 1995;30(Pt 1):143–187.

Infectious

1. Nash G, Foley FD: Herpetic infection of the middle and lower respiratory tract. Am J Clin Pathol 1970;54:857–863.
2. Yeh V, Hopp ML, Goldstein NS, et al.: Herpes simplex chronic laryngitis and vocal cord lesions in a patient with acquired immunodeficiency syndrome. Ann Otol Rhinol Laryngol 1994;103:726–731.

Vocal Cord Polyps and Nodules

1. Kambic V, Radsel Z, Zargi M, et al.: Vocal cord polyps: incidence, histology and pathogenesis. J Laryngol Otol 1981;95:609–618.
2. Kleinsasser O: Pathogenesis of vocal cord polyps. Ann Otol Rhinol Laryngol 1982;91:378–381.
3. Strong MS, Vaughan CW: Vocal cord nodules and polyps—the role of surgical treatment. Laryngoscope 1971;81:911–923.
4. Werner JA, Schunke M, Rudert, H, et al.: Description and clinical importance of the lymphatics of the vocal fold. Otolaryngol Head Neck Surg 1990;102:13–19.

Contact Ulcer

1. Fechner RE, Cooper PH, Mills SE: Pyogenic granuloma of the larynx and trachea. A causal and pathologic misnomer for granulation tissue. Arch Otolaryngol 1981;107:30–32.
2. Koufman JA: The otolaryngologic manifestations of gastroesophageal reflux disease (GERD): a clinical investigation of 225 patients using ambulatory 24-hour pH monitoring and an experimental investigation of the role of acid and pepsin in the development of laryngeal injury. Laryngoscope 1991;101:1–78.
3. McFerran DJ, Abdullah V, Gallimore AP, et al.: Vocal process granulomata. J Laryngol Otol 1994;108:216–220.
4. Ward PH, Zwitman D, Hanson D, et al.: Contact ulcers and granulomas of the larynx: new insights into their etiology as a basis for more rational treatment. Otolaryngol Head Neck Surg 1980;88:262–269.
5. Wenig BM, Heffner DK: Contact ulcers of the larynx. A reacquaintance with the pathology of an often underdiagnosed entity. Arch Pathol Lab Med 1990;114:825–828.

Amyloidosis

1. Barnes EL Jr, Zafar T: Laryngeal amyloidosis. Clinicopathologic study of seven cases. Ann Otol 1977;86:856–863.
2. Chen KTK: Amyloidosis presenting in the respiratory tract. Pathol Ann 1989;24:253–273.
3. Cohen SR: Ligneous conjunctivitis: an ophthalmic disease with potentially fatal tracheobronchial obstruction. Laryngeal and tracheobronchial features. Ann Otol 1990;90:509–518.
4. Lewis JE, Olsen KD, Kurtin PJ, et al.: Laryngeal amyloidosis: a clinicopathologic and immunohistochemical review. Otolaryngol Head Neck Surg 1992;106:372–377.
5. Michaels L, Hyams VJ: Amyloid in localised deposits and plasmacytomas of the respiratory tract. J Path 1978;128:29–38.
6. Thompson LD, Derringer GA, Wenig BM: Amyloidosis of the larynx: a clinicopathologic study of 11 cases. Mod Pathol 2000;13:528–535.

Inflammatory Myofibroblastic Tumor

1. Coffin CM, Watterson J, Priest JR, et al.: Extrapulmonary inflammatory myofibroblastic tumor (inflammatory pseudotumor). A clinicopathologic and immunohistochemical study of 84 cases. Am J Surg Pathol 1995;19:859–872.
2. Ereno C, Lopez JI, Grande J, et al.: Inflammatory myofibroblastic tumour of the larynx. J Laryngol Otol 2001;115:856–858.
3. Gomez-Roman JJ, Ocejo-Vinyals G, Sanchez-Velasco P, et al.: Presence of human herpesvirus-8 DNA sequences and overexpression of human IL-6 and cyclin D1 in inflammatory myofibroblastic tumor (inflammatory pseudotumor). Lab Invest 2000;80:1121–1126.
4. Pettinato G, Manivel JC, De Rosa N, et al.: Inflammatory myofibroblastic tumor (plasma cell granuloma). Clinicopathologic study of 20 cases with immunohistochemical and ultrastructural observations. Am J Clin Pathol 1990;94:538–546.
5. Wenig BM, Devaney K, Bisceglia M. Inflammatory myofibroblastic tumor of the larynx. A clinicopathologic study of eight cases simulating a malignant spindle cell neoplasm. Cancer 1995;76:2217–2229.
6. Wenig BM: Inflammatory myofibroblastic tumour. In: Barnes EL, Eveson JW, Reichart P, Sidransky D, eds. Pathology and Genetics of Head and Neck Tumours. Kleihues P, Sobin LH, series eds. World Health Organization Classification of Tumours. Lyon, France: IARC Press, 2005:153–154.

Cysts of the Larynx (Including Laryngocele)

1. Arens C, Glanz H, Kleinsasser O: Clinical and morphological aspects of laryngeal cysts. Eur Arch Otorhinolaryngol 1997;254:430–436.
2. Civantos FJ, Holinger LD: Laryngoceles and saccular cysts in infants and children. Arch Otolaryngol Head Neck Surg 1992;118:296–300.
3. DeSanto LW: Laryngocele, laryngeal mucocele, large saccules, and laryngeal saccular cysts: a developmental spectrum. Laryngoscope 1974;84:1291–1296.
4. Lundgren J, Olofsson J, Hellquist H: Oncocytic lesions of the larynx. Acta Otolaryngol 1982;94:335–344.
5. Matino Soler E, Martinez Vecina V, Leon Vintro X, et al.: [Laryngocele: clinical and therapeutic study of 60 cases]. Acta Otorrinolaringol Esp 1995;46:279–286.
6. Newman BH, Taxy JB, Laker HI: Laryngeal cysts in adults: a clinicopathologic study of 20 cases. Am J Clin Pathol 1984;81:715–720.
7. Thawley SE, Berlin BP, Berkowitz WP: Oncocytic hyperplasia of the larynx. J Laryngol Otol 1977;91:619–622.

Reactive Epithelial Changes

1. Blackwell KE, Fu YS, Calcaterra TC: Laryngeal dysplasia. A clinicopathologic study. Cancer 1995;75:457–463.
2. Calcaterra TC, Stern F, Ward PH: Dilemma of delayed radiation injury of the larynx. Ann Otol Rhinol Laryngol 1972;81:501–507.
3. Chatrath P, Scott IS, Morris LS, et al.: Aberrant expression of minichromosome maintenance protein-2 and Ki67 in laryngeal squamous epithelial lesions. Br J Cancer 2003;89:1048–1054.
4. Crissman JD: Laryngeal keratosis and subsequent carcinoma. Head Neck Surg 1979;1:386–391.
5. Crissman JD, Zarbo RJ: Quantitation of DNA ploidy in squamous intraepithelial neoplasia of the laryngeal glottis. Arch Otolaryngol Head Neck Surg 1991;117:182–188.
6. Cupic H, Kruslin B, Belicza M: Epithelial hyperplastic lesions of the larynx in biopsy specimens. Acta Otolaryngol Suppl 1997;527:103–104.
7. Gale N, Kambic V, Michaels L, et al.: The Ljubljana classification: a practical strategy for the diagnosis of laryngeal precancerous lesions. Adv Anat Pathol 2000;7:240–251.
8. Gale N, Pilch BZ, Sidransky D, Westra WH, Califano J: Epithelial precursor lesions. In: Barnes EL, Eveson JW, Reichart P, Sidransky D, eds. Pathology and Genetics of Head and Neck Tumours. Kleihues P, Sobin LH, series eds. World Health Organization Classification of Tumours. Lyon, France: IARC Press, 2005:140–143.
9. Gillis TM, Incze J, Strong MS, et al.: Natural history and management of keratosis, atypia, carcinoma-in situ, and microinvasive cancer of the larynx. Am J Surg 1983;146:512–516.
10. Hellquist H, Lundgren J, Olofsson J: Hyperplasia, keratosis, dysplasia and carcinoma in situ of the vocal cords—a follow-up study. Clin Otolaryngol 1982;7:11–27.
11. Ioachim E, Assimakopoulos D, Agnantis NJ, et al.: Altered patterns of retinoblastoma gene product expression in benign, premalignant and malignant epithelium of the larynx: an immunohistochemical study including correlation with p53, bcl-2 and proliferating indices. Anticancer Res 1999;19:541–545.
12. Koren R, Kristt D, Shvero J, et al.: The spectrum of laryngeal neoplasia: the pathologist's view. Pathol Res Pract 2002;198:709–715.
13. Vodovnik A, Gale N, Kambic V, et al.: Correlation of histomorphological criteria used in different classifications of epithelial hyperplastic lesions of the larynx. Acta Otolaryngol Suppl 1997;527:116–119.
14. Wu M, Putti TC, Bhuiya TA: Comparative study in the expression of p53, EGFR, TGF-alpha, and cyclin D1 in verrucous carcinoma, verrucous hyperplasia, and squamous cell carcinoma of head and neck region. Appl Immunohistochem Mol Morphol 2002;10:351–356.

2

Benign Neoplasms of the Larynx, Hypopharynx, and Trachea
Nina Gale

SQUAMOUS PAPILLOMA

CLINICAL FEATURES

Squamous papillomas (SPs) are the most common (84 % of cases) benign laryngeal tumors, caused by the human papillomavirus (HPV), specifically genotypes 6 and 11 and exceptionally by other HPV genotypes. Clinically, SP rarely occurs as a solitary lesion. Most frequently they arise, especially in children, as multiple and recurrent SPs, also known as recurrent respiratory papillomatosis (RRP). The most common sites of SPs

SQUAMOUS PAPILLOMA DISEASE FACT SHEET	
Definition	Benign epithelial tumor, exophytic, composed of branching fronds of squamous epithelium and fibrovascular cores, causally related to HPV infection usually genotypes 6 and 11
Incidence and location	Annual incidence 0.4–4.3/100,000-persons worldwide
	Predominantly larynx; extralaryngeal spread to surrounding aerodigestive areas (children in 30%, adults in 16%)
Morbidity and mortality	Overall mortality rate 4%–14%
Gender, race, and age distribution	Children: no gender predominance
	Adults: male predominance (M : F = 3 : 2)
	Bimodal age distribution; first incidence peak before age of 5 yr, second peak in ages 20–40 yr
Clinical features	Children:
	Symptoms include dysphonia, hoarseness and stridor; less frequently chronic cough, dyspnea, and respiratory distress
	Aggressive course of disease, multiple lesions, rapid recurrences, possible spread to tracheobronchial tree
	Adults:
	Symptom include dysphonia and hoarseness
	Less aggressive course of disease, frequently multiple lesions, less frequent recurrences, and extralaryngeal spread

Prognosis and treatment	Clinical course is unpredictable
	Presence of HPV in apparently normal mucosa presumed source of recurrences
	Disease in early childhood: increased risk of extralaryngeal spread and likelihood of mortality
	HPV genotypes 11 and 16 related to more aggressive disease, rapid recurrences and progression
	Malignant transformation: previously irradiated patients 14% of cases, nonirradiated patients 2% of cases
	Surgical removal(s) with CO_2 laser
	Adjuvant therapy such as interferon, indol-3-carbinol, and cidofovir may have potential benefit

occurrence within the larynx are the true and false vocal cords, Morgagni sinuses, and subglottic region. They may spread to the trachea, lungs, oral cavity, oropharynx, esophagus, and nasal cavity. The distribution of SPs follows a fairly predictive pattern at the juxtaposition of the squamous and respiratory epithelium. Artificially induced squamous metaplasia causes a new iatrogenic squamous–cilliary junction, which consequently provides a setting for further spread of the disease.

According to the characteristic bimodal age distribution, SPs have been traditionally divided into juvenile and adult groups. The first incidence peak appears before the age of 5 years, with no gender predominance. The course of disease in children, which is usually more aggressive than in adults, is characterized by multiple, recurrent and progressive disease requiring tracheotomy in 14 % of patients, risk of airway obstruction, and propensity to spread through the aerodigestive tract. The spread of disease to the tracheobronchial tree may be associated with tracheal stenosis, pneumatocoeles, and various kinds of infection. The relatively small diameter of airways in children is the most likely explanation for severe respiratory obstruction. The predominant presenting symptoms in children are dysphonia, hoarseness, and stridor and, less frequently, chronic cough, dyspnea, and life-threatening respiratory distress. The second incidence peak of SPs is between 20 to 40 years of ages with a slight male predominance (M : F = 3 : 2). The disease in adults is usually not dramatic, although frequent recurrences of multiple lesions with respiratory distress and other complications may also appear. Adults present mostly with dysphonia and hoarseness. It is generally believed that HPV transmission in children occurs in the perinatal period from infected mothers to newborns. The mode of adult infection remains unclear, but it could reflect viral reactivation present since birth or an acquired infection. Despite differences in the clinical courses, RRP is now considered a unified biological entity, caused by the same genotypes of HPV. In contrast to RRP, a solitary keratinizing SP (papillary keratosis) in adults is probably not related to HPV infection.

PATHOLOGIC FEATURES

GROSS FINDINGS

Grossly, SPs are exophytic, branching, pedunculated or broad-based lesions, pink or reddish with a finely lobular surface, occurring either in clusters or solitary, measuring up to 10 mm in diameter (Fig. 2-1).

MICROSCOPIC FINDINGS

Microscopically, SPs are characterized by exophytic, papillary, mucosal projections consisting of a mainly hyperplastic squamous epithelium overlying thin fibrovascular cores (Figs. 2-2, 2-3). One can identify secondary or tertiary branching of the papillae, which are covered by a thinner squamous epithelium. The development of papillary lesions is related to basal and parabasal cell proliferation and abnormal terminal differentiation of the squamous epithelium. Basal and parabasal cell hyperplasia, which is one of the most

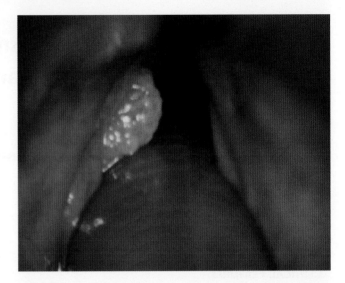

FIGURE 2-1
An endoscopic view of a cluster of papillomas located on the left vocal cord.

common epithelial abnormalities in SPs, shows a perpendicular orientation to the basement membrane. The increased number of basal and parabasal cells extend up to the midportion of the epithelium (Fig. 2-4). On the surface, there is only minimal or no cellular flattening. In other cases a thin parakeratotic layer may be seen. Mitotic figures are present mainly within the lower epithelial portion. Various amount of dyskeratotic cells are irregularly scattered throughout the epithelium. SPs may be infrequently lined with both squamous and respiratory epithelia and these lesions are believed to have an increased tendency to recur. In rare cases, SPs may show epithelial changes that are characterized as "atypical" or "dysplastic" and include abnormalities in the nuclear and cellular size and shape, hyperchromatism, increased nuclear-cytoplasmic ratio, and increased mitoses (Fig. 2-5). The only visible cytopathic effect of HPV infection, referred to as *koilocytosis,* is together with basal-parabasal cell hyperplasia regarded as the most decisive morphologic feature in SPs. Infected cells occur as a rule in the upper and superficial zone of the squamous epithelium where viral replication takes place. Irregularly scattered koilocytes show a characteristic morphology, with dark, wrinkled or enlarged, angulated, centrally located nuclei surrounded by a cleared area of cytoplasm (perinuclear halos) (Fig. 2-4). The surrounding rim of the cytoplasm is either seen at the periphery or is not visible at all.

ANCILLARY STUDIES

ULTRASTRUCTURAL FEATURES

Electron microscopy (EM) enables visualization of HPV particles in SPs, which appear in scattered form

SQUAMOUS PAPILLOMA PATHOLOGIC FEATURES	
Gross findings	Exophytic, warty, pedunculated or sessile growth, more frequently in clusters than single, fragile, pink to red with finely lobulated surface
Microscopic findings	Papillary, branching projections of squamous epithelium overlying fibrovascular cores
	Basal-parabasal cell hyperplasia
	Koilocytosis in superficial zone of squamous epithelium
	Rarely, a mild degree of cellular atypia
Immunohistochemical features	Detection of HPV infection
	In situ hybridization: the most reliable and useful method for routine detection of HPV in tissue specimens
Pathologic differential diagnosis	Adult papillary keratinizing papilloma, verrucous carcinoma, exophytic or papillary squamous cell carcinoma

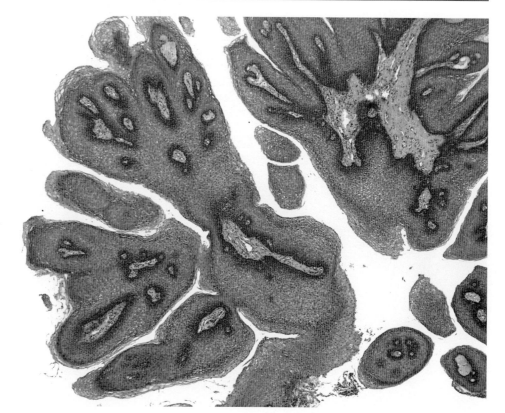

FIGURE 2-2

Branching of exophytic papillary projections consisting of squamous epithelium and thin fibrovascular cores.

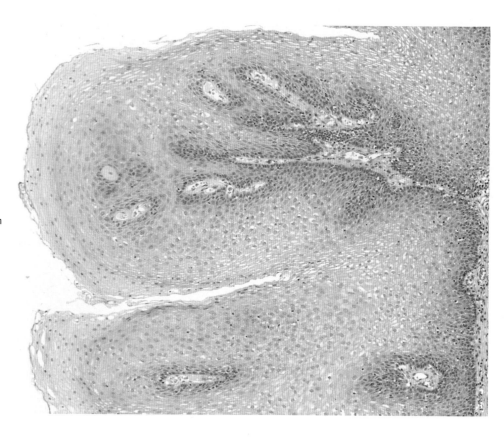

FIGURE 2-3

Papillary branches covered with hyperplastic squamous epithelium.

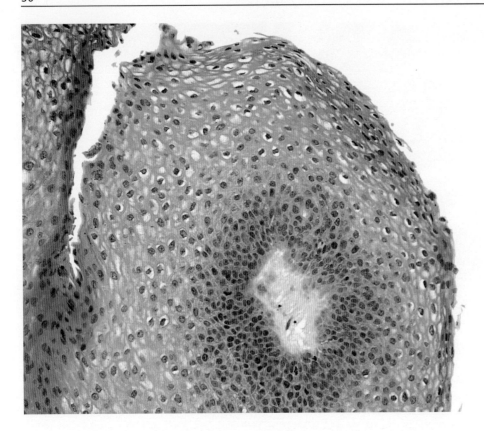

FIGURE 2-4
Covering epithelium of the papillary projections shows incipient basal-parabasal cell hyperplasia. Numerous koilocytes are seen in the upper part of the epithelium.

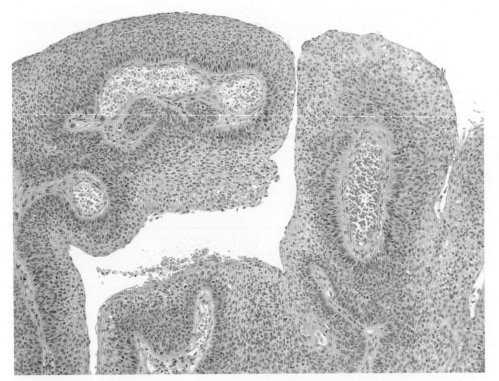

FIGURE 2-5
Pronounced epithelial abnormalities (atypical hyperplasia) are seen in the whole tissue specimen.

within the nuclei of the affected epithelial cells. However, due to its low sensitivity, EM has merely historical diagnostic value. Furthermore, even if HPV particles are detected, an identification of the specific HPV genotype present is not possible.

IMMUNOHISTOCHEMICAL FEATURES

Immunohistochemistry is the most consistent and reproducible traditional method for HPV detection. Inconsistencies in antigen detection may result from sampling error, variable expression of HPV capsid protein and destruction of antigens during tissue processing or lengthy storage.

MOLECULAR STUDIES

Molecular methods are at present considered as a key tool in the detection of HPV in SPs. They are be divided into two groups: those which enable the detection of viral DNA in tissue morphology content (e.g., in situ hybridization), and those in which tissue destruction is unavoidable for detection of HPV DNA (e.g., polymerase chain reaction).

In situ hybridization (ISH) routinely detects HPV in tissue specimens. HPV DNA specific ISH signals are found almost exclusively in the upper intermediate and superficial area of the squamous epithelium. The signals are usually confined to nuclei of koilocytes (Fig. 2-6). Improved protocols of ISH have recently proved very promising and also enable the detection of very low copy numbers and even genotyping of HPV.

Polymerase chain reaction is currently the most sensitive method for HPV detection. However, because of frequent contamination problems, it should be applied in diagnostic settings with great caution.

DIFFERENTIAL DIAGNOSIS

Distinguishing among various lesions with papillary structures and laryngeal SPs is a demanding task, especially if the biopsy specimen is small and superficial. An adult solitary keratinizing SP, in contrast to HPV-induced RRP, usually shows prominent surface keratinization with keratohyaline granules. There is no evidence of koilocytosis and the hyperplastic epithelium is frequently atypical. Verrucous carcinoma is covered by a prominent keratotic or parakeratotic layer, which is not a characteristic of SPs, and koilocytes are usually absent. Stromal fibrovascular projections are not present in verrucous carcinoma, which characteristically shows epithelial projections with central keratin pearls infiltrating underlying tissue in a pushing manner. Exophytic variant of squamous cell carcinoma is composed of broad-based projections of the neoplastic epithelium, but without fibrovascular cores, which are characteristically present in SPs. Papillary squamous carcinoma resembles the architectonic structures of SPs, but the covering epithelium is clearly neoplastic with the absence of maturation, loss of nuclear polarity, and possible evidence of invasive growth.

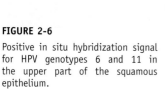

FIGURE 2-6

Positive in situ hybridization signal for HPV genotypes 6 and 11 in the upper part of the squamous epithelium.

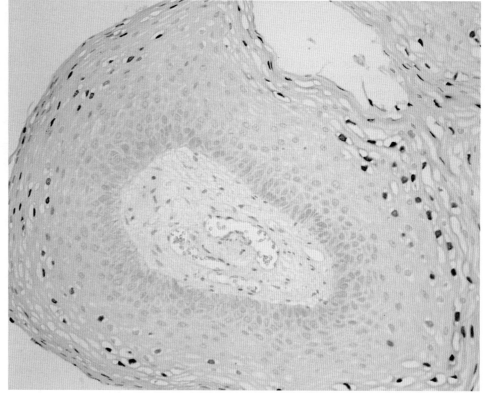

PROGNOSIS AND THERAPY

The clinical course of patients with SPs is unpredictable and includes periods of active disease and remissions. HPV present in apparently normal laryngeal mucosa seems to be a source of recurrences. Progression of disease in early childhood yields a greater risk of tracheotomy, eventual progression to the lower respiratory tract and likelihood of mortality. Malignant transformation, which is most frequently associated with HPV genotypes 11 and 16, occurs very rarely in adults and exceptionally in children. It mostly occurs in relation to additional predisposing factors such as previous radiation or heavy smoking. Malignant transformation in children is found preferentially in the tracheobronchial tree and has a very poor prognosis. In adults, it is more often in the larynx. The overall mortality rate of patients with SPs ranges from 4% to 14%, mostly related to asphyxia, pulmonary extension, and malignant transformation.

There is no single modality of therapy of laryngeal SPs that is effective in eradication of recurrent lesions. Children and adults usually require multiple surgical procedures to maintain a patent airway. A great variety of additional medical therapies have been used as a supplement to surgical treatment; however, no adjuvant therapy to date has cured SPs.

GRANULAR CELL TUMOR

CLINICAL FEATURES

Granular cell tumor (GCT) is a benign, slow-growing neoplasm of presumably Schwann cell origin. It typically appears between the fourth and fifth decades, and very rarely in children. Although GCT may occur at virtually any site, the head and neck region is the most common location, accounting for 30% to 50% of tumors. The tongue and subcutaneous tissue are most frequently affected, while laryngeal involvement comprises up to 10% of all cases. Rare cases have been also reported in the trachea. GCT occurs particularly in black patients with a female preponderance. Multiple synchronous or metachronous tumors have been reported. In the larynx, GCT most commonly appears in the posterior area of the vocal cords, half of the cases extended into the subglottic area as a smooth polypoid, sessile lesion, usually smaller than 2 cm in diameter (Fig. 2-7). Presenting symptoms of GCT in the upper aerodigestive tract consist of hoarseness, dysphagia, cough, and less frequently, stridor and hemoptysis. Patients with tracheal tumors may present with a long history of "intractable asthma." GCT may occasionally be asymptomatic.

GRANULAR CELL TUMOR DISEASE FACT SHEET	
Definition	Benign tumor of neural (Schwann cell) origin, composed of polygonal to spindle cells with abundant granular cytoplasm, filled with lysosomes
Incidence and location	Frequent tumor, with larynx accounting for about 10% of cases
	Predominantly affects skin and mucosal membranes of head and neck, especially tongue and larynx, rarely trachea
	Larynx: posterior area of vocal cords extending to subglottis
Gender, race, and age distribution	Female preponderance
	Predominantly in black patients (2/3 of cases)
	Peak 40–50 yr, rare in children
Clinical features	Hoarseness, stridor, airway obstruction
	Laryngoscopic appearance of a smooth, polypoid, sessile lesion, usually <2 cm in diameter
Prognosis and treatment	Excellent prognosis with low recurrence rate (2%–8%) after incomplete excision
	Conservative, complete surgical removal

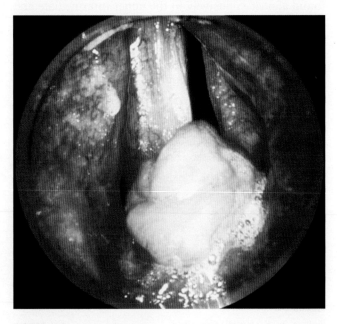

FIGURE 2-7

An endoscopic view of a posterior vocal cord, pale, polypoid mass, histologically confirmed to be a granular cell tumor.

RADIOLOGIC FEATURES

Imaging examination, including endoscopy and computed tomography (CT) are usually performed to determine the exact location, extension, and relation to surrounding structures. However, histopathological examination is required for the final diagnosis.

PATHOLOGIC FEATURES

GROSS FINDINGS

Gross pathology shows a rounded, firm, homogenous, usually nonulcerated lesion, with ill-defined margins, grayish-yellow on cut surface (Fig. 2-8).

MICROSCOPIC FINDINGS

Morphologically, the tumor consists of clusters and sheets of large rounded, polygonal or elongated cells with indistinct cellular borders giving a syncytial appearance (Fig. 2-9). Cells of GCT show either centrally or eccentrically located small, hyperchromatic to vesicular nuclei, enveloped by characteristically abundant, coarsely granular, and eosinophilic cytoplasm (Fig. 2-10). The granules are small, regular, periodic acid Schiff (PAS)-positive and diastase resistant; they may be also aggregated into larger fragments. There is usually no cytological pleomorphism, increased mitoses, or necrosis. If present, they may indicate more aggressive or even malignant potential of GCT.

Islands of tumor cells are separated by dense fibrovascular tissue. Abundant desmoplasia, which is often present in older lesions, may mask the presence of granular cells. GCT may grow around myelinated peripheral nerves or even infiltrate nerve fibers (Fig. 2-11). The periphery of GCT is not well delimited and clusters or

GRANULAR CELL TUMOR PATHOLOGIC FEATURES	
Gross findings	Rounded, firm, nonulcerated mass with ill-defined margins, grayish-yellow cut surface
Microscopic findings	Unencapsulated lesion
	Pseudoepitheliomatous hyperplasia of covering squamous epithelium
	Nested and trabecular growth pattern of rounded and polygonal cells giving a syncytial appearance
	Growth around myelinated peripheral nerves
	Cells contain abundant, coarsely granular cytoplasm, with small hyperchromatic to vesicular nuclei
	Aggressive or malignant potential: cytological atypia, pleomorphism, increased mitoses and necrosis
Ancillary studies	PAS-positive, diastase resistant cytoplasmic granules
	Positive for S-100 protein, vimentin, neuron-specific enolase, and myelin basic protein
	Negative for keratin and muscle markers
Pathologic differential diagnosis	Atypical and malignant variant of GCT, squamous cell carcinoma, adult-type rhabdomyoma, paraganglioma, reactive proliferation of histiocytes

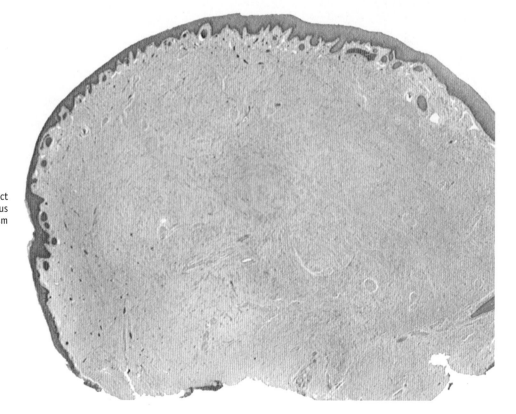

FIGURE 2-8

A polypoid mass with an intact slightly hyperplastic squamous mucosa. The polygonal cell neoplasm fills the stroma below the surface.

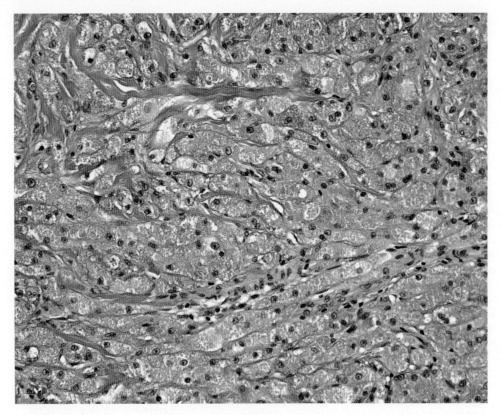

FIGURE 2-9

Tumor consists of rounded and polygonal cells with indistinct cellular borders and characteristically abundant, granular cytoplasm.

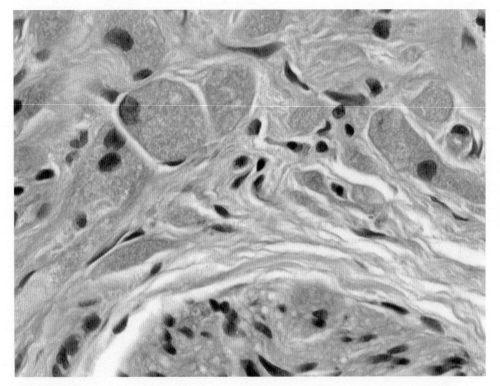

FIGURE 2-10

Nuclei are small, vesicular, and centrally or eccentrically located. Abundant granular cytoplasm is present. A nerve twig is noted at the bottom of the photograph.

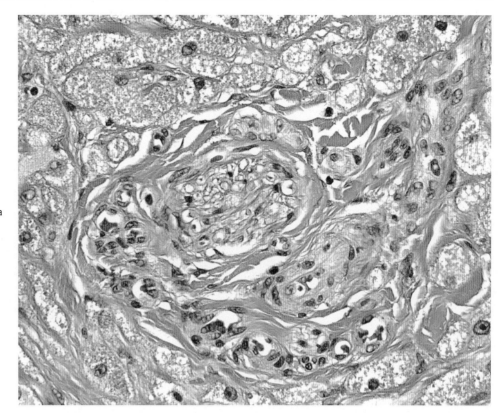

FIGURE 2-11
Growth of the granular cells around a peripheral nerve.

individual cells may infiltrate surrounding structures. If the tumor grows near the epithelial surface, secondary epithelial acanthosis, called pseudoepitheliomatous hyperplasia, may simulate invasive squamous cell carcinoma (Fig. 2-12). Pseudoepitheliomatous hyperplasia is seen in up to 60% of granular cell tumors of the larynx.

ANCILLARY STUDIES

ULTRASTRUCTURAL FEATURES

Ultrastructural examination shows a characteristic picture. Cells of GCT are often surrounded by a basal lamina. Abundant lysosomes are present in the cytoplasm in various stages of fragmentation and confer a granularity seen by light microscopy (Fig. 2-13). Lysosomes vary from discrete, dense, round bodies with a homogenous content to large structures with a lamellate appearance. Some of them, called angulated lysosomes, show a more angular than rounded profile and contain microtubules oriented parallel to the their long axis. Other organelles, such as mitochondria and cisternae of endoplasmic reticulum, are scarce.

IMMUNOHISTOCHEMICAL FEATURES

Immunohistochemically, GCTs express positivity for S-100 protein, vimentin, neurone-specific enolase, and

myelin basic proteins (Fig. 2-14). These findings are in accordance with the widely accepted theory of the Schwann cell origin, which is additionally supported by negative reaction for keratin and muscle markers. The positive reaction for CD68 supports the abundance of intracytoplasmic phagolysosomes rather than histiocytic lineage of the tumor.

DIFFERENTIAL DIAGNOSIS

GCT usually has a distinctive histological appearance and can be identified without further studies. Nevertheless, a rapid growth of the tumor with histologic evidence of pleomorphism and increased mitotic activity may suggest malignant behavior. The pseudoepitheliomatous hyperplasia associated with GCT can be misinterpreted as an invasive squamous cell carcinoma. However, the lack of epithelial atypia as well as increased mitotic activity may help to differentiate between these two entities. An adult-type rhabdomyoma differs from GCT in the appearance of large, granular, vacuolated cells with an abundance of glycogen and cross striations (highlighted with phosphotungstic acid-hematoxylin [PTAH] and immunohistochemical positivity for skeletal muscle markers). Paraganglioma typically shows an organoid growth pattern (i.e., Zellballen) of slightly basophilic granular cells and positive staining for neuroendocrine markers (chromogranin and synaptophysin).

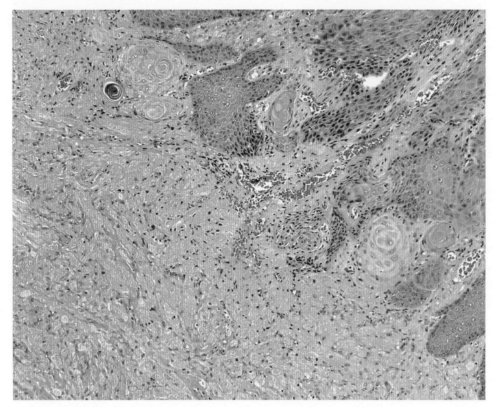

FIGURE 2-12

Pseudoepitheliomatous hyperplasia of the epithelium overlying a granular cell tumor may simulate invasive squamous cell carcinoma.

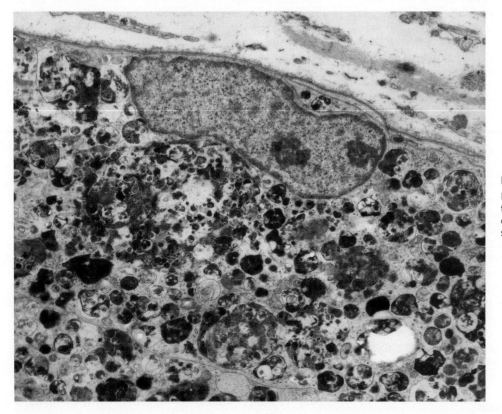

FIGURE 2-13

Electron microscopy reveals characteristic intracytoplasmic abundance of lysosomal structures in various stages of fragmentation.

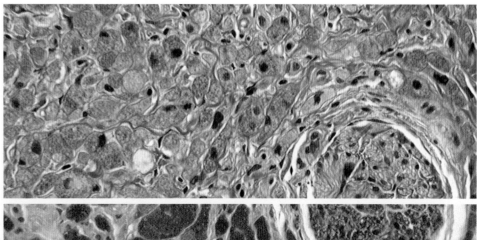
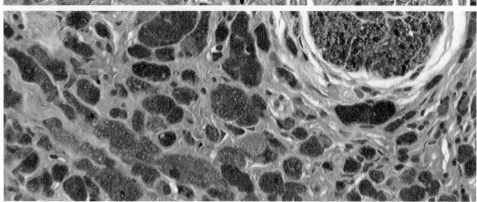

FIGURE 2-14
Upper: Granular cells are diffusely red with a Masson's trichrome while the fibrotic stroma is blue. *Lower:* The neoplastic cells are strongly and diffusely immunoreactive in the nuclei and cytoplasm for S-100 protein (perineural involvement is noted).

PROGNOSIS AND THERAPY

Complete excision of the tumor with an attempt to preserve normal structures is the treatment of choice. Larger tumors require a more extensive surgical procedure including laryngofissure or partial laryngectomy. The recurrence rate is low even if the surgical margins are positive.

ADULT RHABDOMYOMA

Rhabdomyomas are rare benign tumors of striated muscle differentiation. Topographically, they are divided in cardiac and extracardiac types. The latter is less common and additionally classified according to distinctive clinical and histological features into adult, fetal, and genital forms. Extracardiac rhabdomyomas (ERs) are developmentally linked to the head and neck region (90% of cases), since they arise from the unsegmented mesoderm of the third and fourth branchial arches and not from myotomes as do the rest of the skeletal muscles.

CLINICAL FEATURES

Most cases of adult rhabdomyomas (ARs) are found in adults from 16 to 82 years (mean, 52 yr). Only a few AR have been reported in children. Males are affected three to four times more commonly than females. The most frequent sites of AR are hypopharynx, supraglottic or glottic regions of the larynx, and floor of the mouth. Most ARs are solitary, but may be multinodular in the same anatomic location. The presenting symptoms differ among affected regions. The majority of patients with laryngeal tumors complain of hoarseness, progressive difficulties of breathing (airway obstruction) and swallowing, and of a slowly growing mass.

ADULT RHABDOMYOMA DISEASE FACT SHEET	
Definition	Benign tumor of skeletal muscle differentiation
Incidence and location	Very uncommon tumor
	Of extracardiac rhabdomyomas, 70% in head and neck region; most commonly in hypopharynx, larynx, floor of mouth
Gender, race, and age distribution	Male >> Female (3–4 : 1)
	Mean, 52 yr with wide age range (16–82 yr)
Clinical features	Common symptoms: dysphagia, hoarseness, dyspnea
	Slow-growing, well-demarcated mass without tenderness or pain
	Tumor size: 1.5–7.5 cm in diameter
Prognosis and treatment	Recurrences in up to 40% of cases after incomplete excision within 2–11 years after diagnosis
	No aggressive or malignant potential
	Complete surgical excision

PATHOLOGIC FEATURES

GROSS FINDINGS

Grossly, AR is usually a rounded, well-circumscribed, but not encapsulated submucosal lesion, grayish-red to brown. The lesion is a coarsely lobulated, polypoid, or pedunculated mass ranging up to 8 cm (mean, 3 cm). On the cut surface AR shows a finely granular, red-brown, soft, and lobulated appearance.

MICROSCOPIC FINDINGS

Histologically, ARs are composed of sheets, nests, and lobules of large, round to polygonal, closely packed cells, separated by thin fibrovascular stroma (Fig. 2-15). Their cytoplasm is abundant, eosinophilic, characteristically finely granular or vacuolated owing to the presence of glycogen removed during processing of the tissue (Fig. 2-16). An abundance of glycogen (PAS-positive, diastase sensitive) may lead to a spider-like appearance of cells with radially oriented strands of cytoplasm separating the vacuoles. Cytoplasmic cross-striation may be found in hematoxylin- and eosin-stained sections, as well as haphazardly arranged crystalline-like structures called jackstraw inclusions (Fig. 2-17). They are seen in a minority of cells. Both structures become intensely visible using PTAH staining (Fig. 2-17). The cells of AR contain one or more, peripherally or centrally located, small vesicular nuclei with prominent nucleoli. Mitotic figures are almost always absent.

ADULT RHABDOMYOMA PATHOLOGIC FEATURES	
Gross findings	Circumscribed, round or lobular lesion, with red-brown cut surface
Microscopic findings	Well-demarcated, unencapsulated lobules
	Closely packed, large polygonal cells
	Tumor cells have small, round nuclei, centrally or peripherally located with prominent nucleoli surrounded by abundant eosinophilic, granular, or vacuolated ("spider web") cytoplasm
	Cytoplasmic cross-striation and haphazardly arranged crystal-like structures
Ancillary studies	Cytoplasm is rich in glycogen (PAS-positive, diastase sensitive)
	Positivity for myoglobin, muscle-specific actin, desmin
	Focal positivity for α-smooth muscle actin, vimentin, S-100 protein, and Leu-7
	Negative for keratin, epithelial membrane antigen, glial fibrillary acid protein, and CD68
Pathologic differential diagnosis	Granular cell tumor, paraganglioma, oncocytoma, crystal-storing histiocytosis

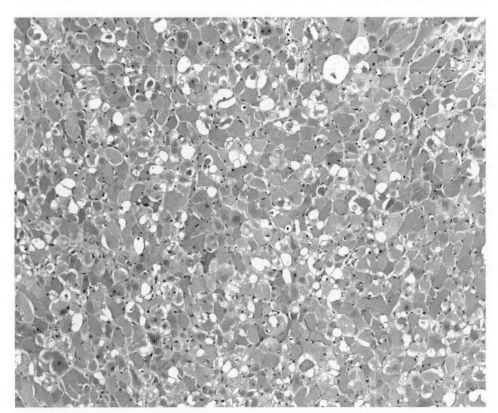

FIGURE 2-15

At low power, diffuse infiltration of polygonal cells with abundant, vacuolated cytoplasm and small nucleoli in this adult rhabdomyoma.

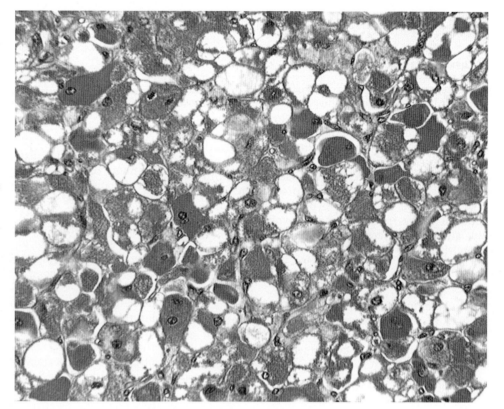

FIGURE 2-16

Characteristic polygonal cells of variable size, with eosinophilic, vacuolated, granular cytoplasm, and mainly peripherally located small hyperchromatic nuclei.

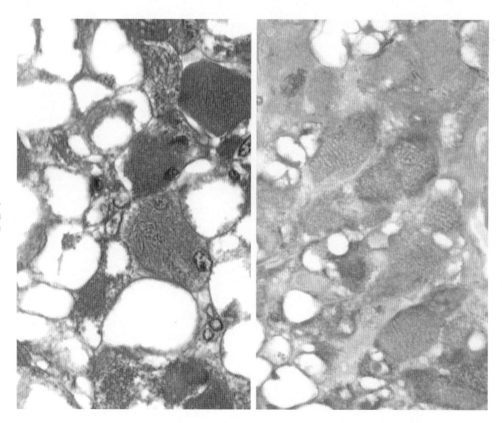

FIGURE 2-17

Crystalline-like structures and cross-striations in an adult rhabdomyoma (*left*) are highlighted by a PTAH stain (*right*).

ANCILLARY STUDIES

ULTRASTRUCTURAL FEATURES

Ultrastructurally, individual cells of AR are surrounded by a thin, continuous basal lamina. The most important diagnostic criterion refers to intracytoplasmic rudimentary myofibrils, found in virtually all cells. They are characterized by an alternation of thin (actin) and thick (myosin) myofilaments. Apparent condensation of myofibrils is readily identified as Z bands. Intracytoplasmic crystalline-like structures, seen by light microscopy, are considered hypertrophied Z bands. In addition to the intracytoplasmic myofilaments, a variable amount of glycogen and different number of mitochondria are always seen.

IMMUNOHISTOCHEMICAL FEATURES

The immunohistochemical profile confirms the skeletal muscle origin. The cells are usually positive for desmin, myoglobin, and muscle-specific actin. Focal and weak reactivity is also detected for smooth muscle actin, S-100, and Leu7. Additionally, AR characteristically lacks staining for cytokeratin, epithelial membrane antigen, and CD68.

OTHER ANCILLARY STUDIES

Intracytoplasmic cross-striation and crystalline-like structures are more evident if special stains such as PTAH and trichrome are applied (Fig. 2-17). Cytogenetic studies seem to support a neoplastic origin, rather than a hamartoma or hyperplasia (reciprocal translocation between chromosomes 15 and 17, and miscellaneous changes in the long arm of chromosome 10).

DIFFERENTIAL DIAGNOSIS

Differential diagnosis of AR includes benign and malignant tumors with distinctive abundant eosinophilic, granular, or vacuolated cytoplasm of tumor cells: GCT, paraganglioma, oncocytoma, and *crystal storing histiocytosis associated with lymphoplasmacytic neoplasm*. Particular similarity exists between AR and GCT. Both tumors exhibit a laryngeal predilection and consist of sheets and islands of large polygonal cells with abundant granular cytoplasm. The cells of GCT display indistinct cellular borders, lack cytoplasmic vacuolization, are S-100 protein positive, and show pseudoepitheliomatous hyperplasia. Paraganglioma is very rare in the larynx. It is composed of polyhedral cells organized in an organoid (Zellballen) pattern, which react with neuroendocrine markers (chromogranin and synaptophysin); while peripherally located sustentacular cells stain positively for S-100. Oncocytoma can be differentiated with histochemical (PAS-positive and diastase resistant) and electron microscopic studies confirming an abundance of intracytoplasmic abnormal mitochondria. Rhabdomyoma may also resemble a rare condition called *crystal-storing histiocytosis associated with lymphoplasmacytic neoplasm*, in which histiocytes containing sheaves of crystals are associated with a neoplastic lymphoplasmacytic infiltrate (Fig. 2-18).

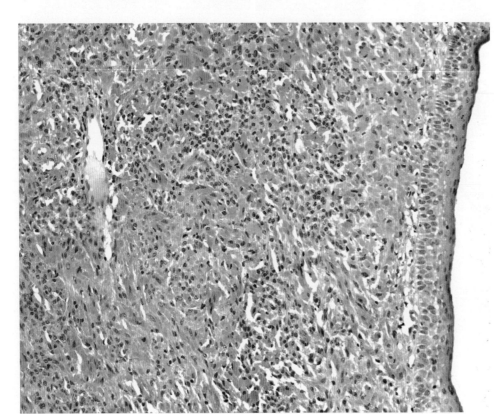

FIGURE 2-18
Crystal-storing histiocytosis associated with a lymphoplasmatic neoplasm may mimic a rhabdomyoma. The lesion is composed of crystal-storing histiocytes with abundant granular, eosinophilic cytoplasm, and small hyperchromatic nuclei, intermingled with lymphoplasmacytic infiltrate.

PROGNOSIS AND THERAPY

AR is a benign tumor that lacks aggressive behavior or malignant potential. The treatment of choice is complete surgical excision and endoscopic removal may often be suitable. Recurrences have been reported in up to 42 % of cases, months to years after incomplete excisions. One should be aware of possible multicentric AR occurring in either the same or a separate location.

CHONDROMA

CLINICAL FEATURES

Chondroma is a benign mesenchymal tumor, which occurs exceedingly rarely in the larynx and trachea. The most common localization is the posterior lamina of the cricoid cartilage. Other rare sites of origin in a decreasing order are thyroid, epiglottis, arytenoids, and tracheal cartilages. The lesion occurs more commonly in men than in women (2 : 1). Patients range from 24 to 79 years old (mean, 56 yr), slightly younger than chondrosarcomas. The tumor is typically a slowly growing endolaryngeal mass (Fig. 2-19). Clinical presentation depends on location and size. Subglottic lesions usually produce dyspnea, hoarseness, and stridor; while supraglottic lesions produce hoarseness, dyspnea, dysphagia, and odynophagia. Thyroid cartilage involvement may rarely produce a neck mass.

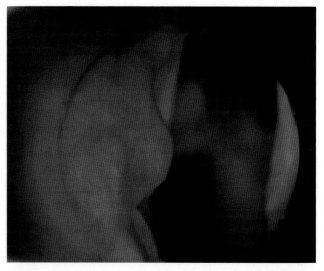

FIGURE 2-19
An endoscopic view of a chondroma shows a smooth endolaryngeal sessile mass in the left supraglottic region.

RADIOLOGIC FEATURES

Radiographic findings are very helpful in rendering a diagnosis. A plain anteroposterior radiograph usually shows a mucosal covered lesion arising from the laryngeal cartilage. CT, the superior diagnostic radiographic imaging, usually shows a hypodense, well circumscribed lesion with regular margins and minimal calcium deposits. The tumor-to-soft tissue relationship and extent of the lesion can be more sensitively delineated by MRI. However, radiological features cannot distinguish between chondroma and its malignant counterpart, chondrosarcoma.

PATHOLOGIC FEATURES

GROSS FINDINGS

Grossly, chondromas usually measure less than 2 cm in diameter and appear as firm, characteristically glassy, blue-white lesions on cut surface.

MICROSCOPIC FINDINGS

Light microscopic examination reveals a well-defined lobular pattern of the mature hyaline cartilage, confined by the perichondrium and identified below an intact squamous mucosa (Fig. 2-20). Chondroma typically shows a monotonous growth pattern with low cellularity with bland looking and evenly distributed individual chondrocytes within lacunae. The cells contain small, uniform, single, hyperchromatic nuclei, surrounded by clear to eosinophilic cytoplasm (Figs. 2-21, 2-22). Pleomorphism and mitoses are absent. Exceptionally, double-nucleated chondrocytes may be seen. Areas of

CHONDROMA DISEASE FACT SHEET	
Definition	Benign tumor of mature hyaline cartilage
Incidence and location	Extremely unusual in larynx and trachea
	Most common: cricoid and thyroid cartilages
Gender, race, and age distribution	Male > Female (M : F = 2 : 1)
	Peak in 6th decade (wide age distribution 24–79 yr)
Clinical features	Symptoms include hoarseness and dyspnea, rarely neck mass in extralaryngeal spread
	Slow growing endolaryngeal lesion, symptoms directly depend on location and size
	May be incidental finding
Prognosis and treatment	Excellent prognosis after conservative surgical excision
	Malignant alteration in 7% of cases
	Any recurrence of laryngeal cartilage tumor is considered chondrosarcoma

CHONDROMA
PATHOLOGIC FEATURES

Gross findings	Firm submucosal mass, less than 2 cm in size involving laryngeal cartilage
	Well-circumscribed, hard tumor, translucent, gray-blue cut surface
Microscopic findings	Lobular growth of benign, bland looking chondrocytes, resembling normal cartilage
	Monotonous appearance with low cellularity
	Single nucleus per lacuna
Pathologic differential diagnosis	Low-grade chondrosarcoma, chondrometaplasia on the vocal cord, tracheopathia osteoplastica, pleomorphic adenoma

calcifications, ossification and myxoid degeneration can be haphazardly distributed in the abundant basophilic stroma.

FINE NEEDLE ASPIRATION

A fine needle aspiration, if a specimen can be obtained from a laryngeal chondroma presenting as an external neck mass, may be of limited help. Normal looking cartilage or chondrocytes do not reliably argue for chondroma, and only examination of the whole lesion can differentiate between benign and malignant cartilaginous tumor.

DIFFERENTIAL DIAGNOSIS

The separation of chondroma from low-grade chondrosarcoma is difficult at best, and fraught with controversy in the medical literature. A small biopsy of a cartilaginous tumor resembling chondroma should be reported with caution. Meticulous examination of the whole specimen is required to avoid an incorrect diagnosis. Histologically, bone invasion/destruction, increased cellularity, loss of organization (nonlobular pattern), pleomorphism, multinucleation, increased mitotic activity, and necrosis are reliable features of chondrosarcoma. More remotely, chondrometaplasia, tracheopathia osteochondroplastica, and pleomorphic adenoma may be considered. Chondrometaplasia is characterized by an elastic-rich cartilage nodule, usually located on the vocal cord, with no relation to the laryngeal cartilages. Tracheopathia osteoplastica can be identified radiographically and laryngoscopically showing multiple submucosal nodules, usually attached to the cartilages. Pleomorphic adenoma can be easily differentiated by the presence of epithelial and myoepithelial components, which are incorporated in a myxochondroid stroma. This histologic pattern excludes the diagnosis of chondroma.

PROGNOSIS AND THERAPY

Surgical excision of the tumor with preservation of the larynx is the treatment of choice with an excellent

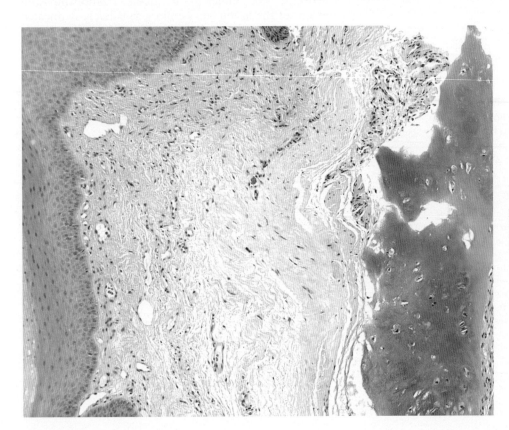

FIGURE 2-20

At low power, mature hyaline cartilage in laryngeal mucosa with characteristic low cellularity below an intact squamous mucosa.

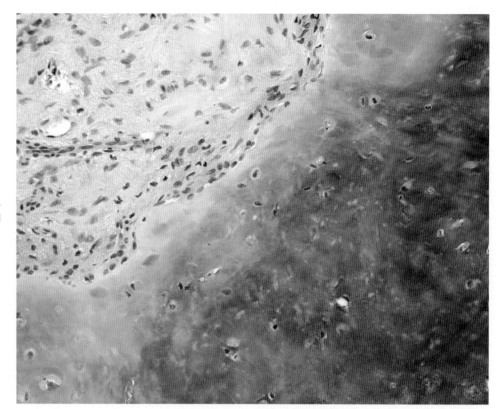

FIGURE 2-21

A well-defined border of the hypocellular neoplasm with the surrounding stroma.

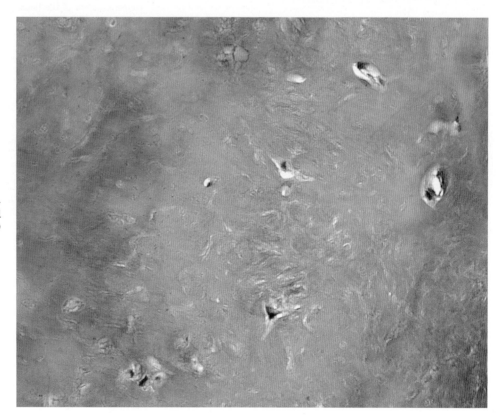

FIGURE 2-22

Bland-looking individual chondrocytes within lacunae with small hyperchromatic nuclei and clear to eosinophilic cytoplasm.

duration without recurrence. Any recurrence, however, should perhaps be considered as an originally under-diagnosed low-grade chondrosarcoma. The chondroma recurrence rate has been published to be 10%, with a mean time to recurrence of 9 years. Transformation to chondrosarcoma is seen in about 7% of cases. Furthermore, many chondrosarcomas (up to 60%) are superimposed on preexisting chondromas which have undergone ischemic change.

SUGGESTED READING

Squamous Papilloma

1. Derkay CS: Recurrent respiratory papillomatosis. Laryngoscope 2001;111;57–69.
2. Gale N, Poljak M, Kambič V, Ferluga D, Fischinger J: Laryngeal papillomatosis: molecular, histological and clinical evaluation. Virchows Arch 1994;425:291–295.
3. Gale N. Papilloma/papillomatosis. In: Barnes EL, Eveson JW, Reichart P, Sidransky D, eds. Pathology and Genetics of Head and Neck Tumours. Kleihues P, Sobin LH, series eds. World Health Organization Classification of Tumours. Lyon, France: IARC Press, 2005:144–145.
4. Kashima H, Mounts P, Leventhal B, Hruban RH: Sites of predilection in recurrent respiratory papillomatosis. Ann Otol Rhinol Laryngol 1993;102:580–583.
5. Lindeberg H: Laryngeal papillomas: histomorphometric evaluation of multiple and solitary lesions. Clin Otolaryngol 1991;16:257–260.
6. Poljak M, Seme K, Gale N: Detection of human papillomaviruses in tissue specimens. Adv Anat Pathol 1998;5:216–234.
7. Rihkanen H, Aaltonen LM, Syrjanen SM: Human papillomavirus in laryngeal papillomas and in adjacent normal epithelium. Clin Otolaryngol 1993;18:470–474.
8. Wiatrak BJ: Overview of recurrent respiratory papillomatosis. Curr Opin Otolaryngol Head Neck Surg 2003;11:433–441.

Granular Cell Tumor

1. Brandwein M, LeBenger J, Strauchen J, Biller H: Atypical granular cell tumor of the larynx: an unusually aggressive tumor clinically and microscopically. Head Neck 1990;12:154–159.
2. Curtis BV, Calcaterra TC, Coulson WF: Multiple granular cell tumor: a case report and review of the literature. Head Neck 1997;19:634–637.
3. Fine SW, Li M: Expression of calretinin and the alpha-subunit of inhibin in granular cell tumors. Am J Clin Pathol 2003;119:259–264.
4. Kamal SA, Othman EO: Granular cell tumor of the larynx. J Laryngol Otol 1998;112:83–85.
5. Lassaletta L, Alonso S, Ballestin C, Martinez-Tello FJ, Alvarez-Vincent JJ: Immunoreactivity in granular cell tumours of the larynx. Auris Nasus Larynx 1999;26:305–310.
6. Ordonez NG, Mackay B: Granular cell tumor: a review of pathology and histogenesis. Ultrastruct Pathol 1999;23:207–222.
7. Thompson LDR, Fanburg-Smith JC, Barnes L. Benign soft tissue tumours. In: Barnes EL, Eveson JW, Reichart P, Sidransky D, eds. Pathol-

ogy and Genetics of Head and Neck Tumours. Kleihues P, Sobin LH, series eds. World Health Organization Classification of Tumours. Lyon, France: IARC Press, 2005:152–155.
8. Victoria LV, Hoffman HT, Robinson RA: Granular cell tumor of the larynx. J Laryngol Otol 1998;112:373–376.

Adult Rhabdomyoma

1. Gibas Z, Miettinen M: Recurrent parapharyngeal rhabdomyoma. Evidence of neoplastic nature of the tumor from cytogenetic study. Am J Surg Pathol 1992;16:721–728.
2. Helliwell TR, Sissons MCJ, Stoney PJ, Ashworth MT: Immunohistochemistry and electron microscopy of head and neck rhabdomyoma. J Clin Pathol 1988;41:1058–1063.
3. Johansen ECJ, Illum P: Rhabdomyoma of the larynx: a review of the literature with a summery of previously described cases of rhabdomyoma of the larynx and a report of a new case. J Laryngol Otol 1995;109:147–153.
4. Kapadia SB, Enzinger FM, Heffner DK, Hyams VJ, Frizzera G: Crystal-storing histiocytosis associated with lymphoplasmacytic neoplasms. Report of three cases mimicking adult rhabdomyoma. Am J Surg Pathol 1993;17:461–467.
5. Kapadia SB, Meis JM, Frisman DM, Ellis GL, Heffner DK, Hyams VJ: Adult rhabdomyoma of the head and neck. A clinicopathologic and immunophenotypic study. Hum Pathol 1993;24:608–617.
6. LaBagnara J, Hitchcock E, Spitzer T: Rhabdomyoma of the true vocal cord. J Voice 1999;13:289–293.
7. Thompson LDR, Fanburg-Smith JC, Barnes L. Benign soft tissue tumours. In: Barnes EL, Eveson JW, Reichart P, Sidransky D, eds. Pathology and Genetics of Head and Neck Tumours. Kleihues P, Sobin LH, series eds. World Health Organization Classification of Tumours. Lyon, France: IARC Press, 2005:152–155.

Chondroma

1. Baatenburg de Jong RJ, van Lent S, Hogendoorn PC: Chondroma and chondrosarcoma of the larynx. Curr Opin Otolaryngol Head Neck Surg 2004;12:98105.
2. Casiraghi O, Martinez-Madrigal F, Pineda-Daboin K, Mamelle G, Resta L, Luna MA: Chondroid tumors of the larynx: a clinicopathologic study of 19 cases, including two dedifferentiated chondrosarcomas. Ann Diagn Pathol 2004;8:189–197.
3. Franco RA Jr, Singh B, Har-El G: Laryngeal chondroma. J Voice 2002;16:92–95.
4. Hyams VJ, Rabuzzi DD: Cartilaginous tumors of the larynx. Laryngoscope 1970;80:755–767.
5. Lewis JE, Barnes L, Tse LY, Hunt JL. Tumours of bone and cartilage. In: Barnes EL, Eveson JW, Reichart P, Sidransky D, eds. Pathology and Genetics of Head and Neck Tumours. Kleihues P, Sobin LH, series eds. World Health Organization Classification of Tumours. Lyon, France: IARC Press, 2005:156–159.
6. Saydem L, Koybasi S, Kutluay L: Laryngeal chondroma presenting as an external neck mass. Eur Arch Otorhinolaryngol 2003;260:239–241.
7. Thompson LDR, Gannon FH: Chondrosarcoma of the larynx. A clinicopathologic study of 111 cases with a review of the literature. Am J Surg Pathol 2002;26:836–851.

3

Malignant Neoplasms of the Larynx, Hypopharynx, and Trachea

Lester D. R. Thompson

PRECURSOR SQUAMOUS LESIONS

The definition of precursor lesions is difficult to quantify as they are lesions which have an increased likelihood of progressing to squamous cell carcinoma (SCC). A constellation of architectural and cytologic features comprise dysplasia or laryngeal intraepithelial neoplasia, but these features are not uniformly accepted or interpreted, thereby leading to difficulties in intra- and interobserver differences of interpretation. It is wise to use *atypia* in the context of reactive, inflammatory, or regenerative changes, while reserving *dysplasia* for the pre-malignant group of lesions. Whichever classification system is adopted, consistent application of the criteria will allow clinicians to correctly manage their patients.

CLINICAL FEATURES

Precursor lesions are mostly seen in the adult population (mean, 50 yr) and affect men more often than women, especially pronounced after the sixth decade. Strong association with tobacco smoking and alcohol abuse,

PRECURSOR LESIONS
DISEASE FACT SHEET

Definition	Squamous lesions with an increased risk/likelihood of progressing to squamous cell carcinoma
Incidence and location	Up to 10% of precursor lesions progress to carcinoma
	Supraglottic and glottic regions are most common
Gender, race, and age distribution	Male >> Female
	6th decade peak
Clinical features	Tobacco and alcohol abuse
	Hoarseness, throat irritation, sore throat, chronic cough
Prognosis and treatment	About 10% rate of malignant transformation
	Surgery and/or radiation, dependent on lesion

especially a combination of these two, is well known. The etiologic role of human papillomavirus (HPV) infection remains unsettled. Symptoms depend on the location and severity of the disease and are usually present for at least a few months before clinical attention. Hoarseness, throat irritation, sore throat, and/or chronic cough are frequently reported. Endoscopically, these lesions have a varied appearance: discrete to diffuse; leukoplakia to erythroplakia; a small, flat patch to a large, warty plaque. Leukoplakia, in contrast to erythroplakia, tends to be well demarcated. Although inconsistent, leukoplakia alone seems to have a lower risk of malignant transformation than pure erythroplakia.

PATHOLOGIC FEATURES

GROSS FINDINGS

There is no characteristic appearance of precursor lesions. They can be circumscribed or diffuse, smooth or irregular, flat or exophytic. The anterior true vocal cords are involved most commonly (usually not the commissure), although no region of the larynx is exempt. Bilateral disease is common (60%).

MICROSCOPIC FINDINGS

Dysplasia is an alteration of surface epithelium, which is more than hyperplasia but less than carcinoma. Needless to say, to identify the earliest forms of dysplasia and to arbitrarily separate and rigidly divide the dysplasias into different categories is fraught with tremendous intra- and interobserver variability and an overall lack of reproducibility.

Many architectural and cytologic features can be seen in dysplasia, although none in isolation is pathognomonic for dysplasia. In fact, many of these same features are more fully developed in carcinoma, and so a rigid segregation between lesions is nearly impossible. On a continuous spectrum, there is a quantitative increase of architectural and cytologic features for the diagnosis of dysplasia, with low-grade dysplasia usually limited to the lower one-third (Fig. 3-1) and severe dysplasia/carcinoma in situ (CIS) involving the full thickness (Fig. 3-2), with moderate dysplasia occupying the center (Fig. 3-3). In general, all of the various layers begin to resemble the basal layer cells as the lesion progresses from

PRECURSOR LESIONS PATHOLOGIC FEATURES	
Gross findings	Leukoplakia, erythroplakia, mixed (speckled), variegated
	Diffuse or discrete
	Flat patch or large warty plaque
	Anterior true vocal cord most often, with frequent bilateral disease (60%)
Microscopic findings	A continuum of architectural and cytologic features required, separated into low, moderate, and severe based on increasing thickness of the mucosa involved
	Increased cellularity, irregular maturation, lack of polarity, dyskeratosis, keratin pearl formation, parakeratosis, increased mitotic figures
	Increased nuclear to cytoplasmic ratio, increased nuclear size, anisocytosis, poikilocytosis, anisonucleolis, nuclear pleomorphism, nuclear hyperchromasia, nuclear chromatin condensation, increased nucleolar size and number, atypical mitotic figures
	No evidence of basement membrane invasion
Pathologic differential diagnosis	Hyperplasia, regeneration, repair, reactive and radiation changes, necrotizing sialometaplasia, papilloma, and squamous cell carcinoma

low-grade dysplasia toward carcinoma in situ. The cells are often monotonous, although all of the cells are monotonously atypical. Architectural features of dysplasia include increased cellularity, irregular maturation, lack of polarity, dyskeratosis (Fig. 3-4), keratin pearl formation within rete, parakeratosis, and increased number of mitotic figures, with mitotic figures above the basal zone (Fig. 3-5). Cytologic features of dysplasia include increased nuclear to cytoplasmic ratio, increased nuclear size, anisocytosis, poikilocytosis, anisonucleolis, nuclear pleomorphism, nuclear hyperchromasia (Fig. 3-6), nuclear chromatin condensation, and increased number and size of nucleoli. Atypical mitotic figures (misalignment of chromosomes, unbalanced distribution of chromosomes, and multipolar figures) are seen. While axiomatic, invasion of the basement is not present. However, an inflammatory infiltrate, occasionally intense, is common. How many features are necessary for the diagnosis? Here the art of pathology comes into play, with the clinical, gross, and histologic features interpreted collectively. Furthermore, invasive, synchronous SCC is frequently present.

Technical factors are important to accurate diagnosis. Multiple biopsies within the diseased area of sufficient size are necessary to assess the full extent of the lesion. Avoiding tangential sections is paramount, which usually precludes frozen section diagnoses. Additional deeper sections may be needed to fully demonstrate diagnostic features of dysplasia. Glandular/duct

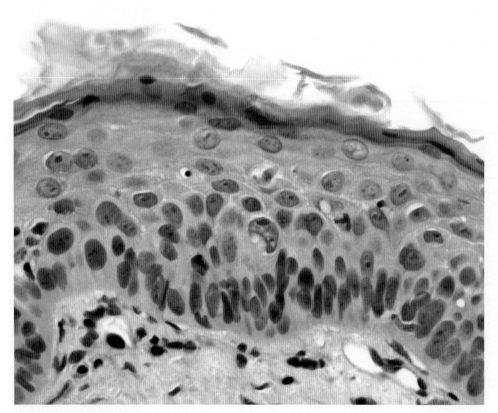

FIGURE 3-1

A mild dysplasia demonstrates focal disruption of the architecture and mild pleomorphism limited to the lower one-third of the mucosa. Parakeratosis is noted.

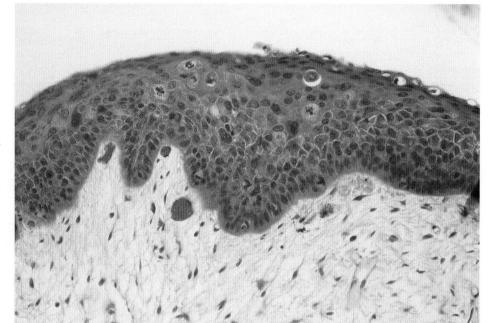

FIGURE 3-2

Severe dysplasia/carcinoma in situ. Full thickness replacement of the epithelium by markedly atypical cells, with numerous atypical mitotic figures, but without basement membrane penetration.

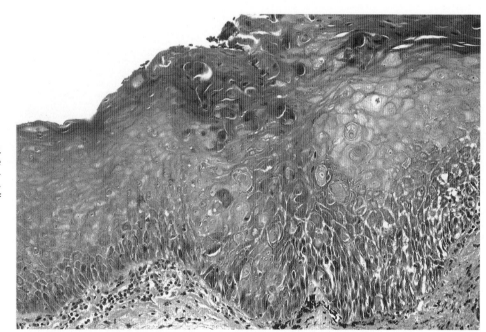

FIGURE 3-3

Moderate dysplasia has atypical features extending to the middle one-third of the epithelium. The thickened epithelium in the area of dysplasia sometimes makes determination of grade of dysplasia difficult.

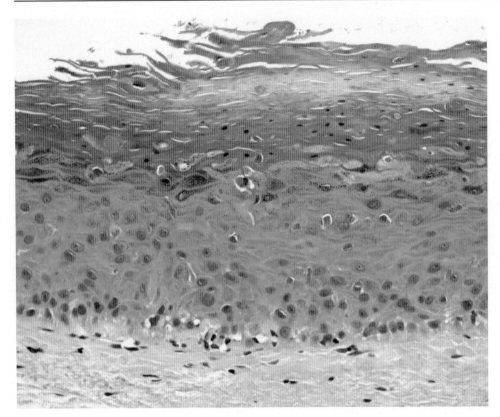

FIGURE 3-4
This atypical epithelium contains dyskeratosis, parakeratosis, keratosis, and loss of architecture, placing it in the mild dysplasia.

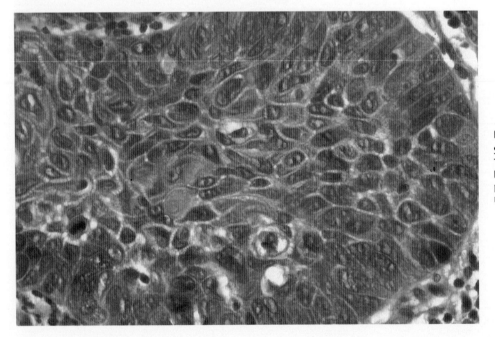

FIGURE 3-5
Severe dysplasia/carcinoma in situ. There is complete loss of maturation, loss of polarity, remarkable pleomorphism, mitotic figures, and atypical mitotic figures.

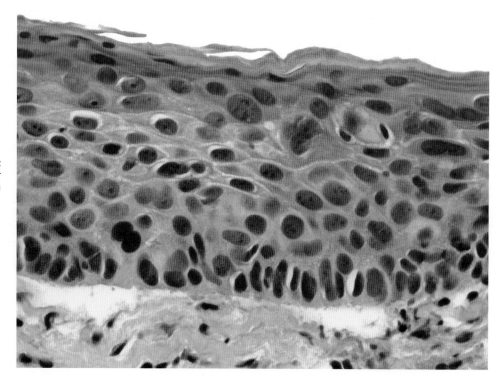

FIGURE 3-6

Increased nuclear to cytoplasmic ratio, nuclear pleomorphism, nuclear hyperchromasia, and binucleation in a dysplastic epithelium.

extension must not be interpreted as invasive disease. Various immunohistochemical and molecular studies have been proposed to separate hyperplasia, dysplasia, and carcinoma, but in practical application are currently too inconsistent and have too much overlap to be clinically meaningful.

DIFFERENTIAL DIAGNOSIS

Reactive, regenerative, reparative, or hyperplastic squamous proliferations (for example, in response to trauma, inflammation, irradiation, or ulceration) may manifest

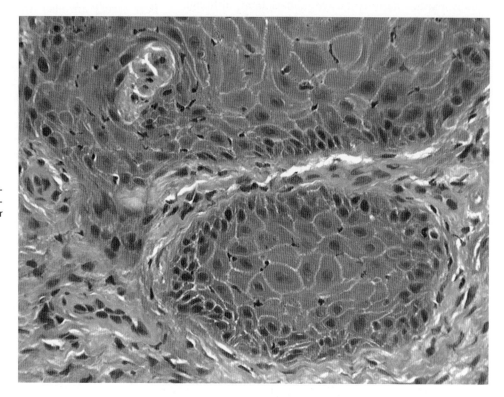

FIGURE 3-7

Reactive atypia with some irregularities to the periphery, but no cytologic atypia. This is not a precursor lesion.

architectural and cytologic atypia (Fig. 3-7). However, morphologic changes suggestive of the inciting event (e.g., ulceration, inflammation, hemorrhage, radiation-induced mesenchymal and/or endothelial nuclear enlargement, and hyperchromasia) may be present. Stratification and maturation is usually present and atypical mitotic figures are absent. The clinical history may also be helpful.

Transitional vocal cord epithelium is sometimes confused with dysplasia, but knowledge of the normal histology will help make this separation. Basal zone hyperplasia has a columnar arrangement to the basal cells which maintain a vertical polarity and hyperchromatic nuclei. There is an abrupt termination of the process at the upper edge of the prickle-layer with a very sharp zone of transition horizontally oriented (see benign reactive lesions, Fig. 1-32).

Inflammatory infiltrates caused by infectious agents should be excluded with special stains or cultures. Granular cell tumor can cause atypical epithelial changes, but the characteristic cells should confirm the diagnosis.

CONVENTIONAL SQUAMOUS CELL CARCINOMA DISEASE FACT SHEET	
Definition	A malignant neoplasm characterized by squamous cell differentiation
Incidence and location	About 1% of all cancers, but 90% of head and neck cancers
	Supraglottic and glottic regions are most common
Morbidity and mortality	Loss of phonation
	Up to 25% mortality (site and stage dependent)
Gender, race, and age distribution	Male >> Female
	6th–7th decades
Clinical features	Tobacco and alcohol abuse
	Hoarseness, dysphagia, dysphonia, changes in phonation
Prognosis and treatment	Site, size and stage specific, with approximately 90% 5-yr survival for T1 vs <50% for T4 lesions
	Surgery and radiation

PROGNOSIS AND THERAPY

Some precursor lesions are self-limiting and reversible, others persist and some progress to SCC. Lesions which arise in the anterior commissure nearly always convert to invasive SCC, while other topographic sites only convert about 15% of the time. Lesions classified as mild to moderate dysplasias have an approximately 10% rate of malignant transformation, implying the need for close clinical follow-up. Patients with carcinoma in situ usually require more extensive management, although clinically dictated.

SQUAMOUS CELL CARCINOMA

Squamous cell carcinoma is the most common malignancy of the head and neck and accounts for >95% of all laryngeal carcinomas. However, it still only accounts for about 1% of all carcinomas. There is a well-developed association with alcohol and tobacco use, with clinical stage and site playing an important role in patient management.

CLINICAL FEATURES

Men are affected much more frequently than women (about 85% of patients are men), although there is an increased incidence in women over recent years. All ages are affected, but patients usually present in the 6th–7th decades of life. The most important risk factors are, independently, tobacco (cigarette, cigar, pipe, smokeless) and alcohol use, while susceptibility (immunologic factors and age), environmental (including radiation), and occupational factors may also play a role. Smoking and alcohol abuse seem to have a multiplicative rather than additive effect in carcinoma development. Viruses (human papilloma virus, Epstein-Barr virus) are also linked to the developed of SCC, although association versus direct effect remains unresolved. Genetic predisposition to SCC is recognized, although comprises only a fraction of clinical SCC. All of these factors probably interact in a multistep process. Patients present with symptoms referable to the anatomic site of the primary, with hoarseness, dysphagia, dysphonia, difficulty swallowing, and changes in phonation.

Endoscopy is recommended to evaluate the extent of the disease, rule out other synchronous primaries (seen in up to 10% of patients), and to obtain a biopsy.

PATHOLOGIC FEATURES

GROSS FINDINGS

The anatomic sites—supraglottis, glottis, and sub-glottis—are embryologically distinct and separately compartmentalized, resulting in unique lymphatic drainage, and consequently have implications in the type of surgery and oncologic management. Glottic tumors for the most part are smaller (due to early clinical presentation), while supraglottic tumors are often

CONVENTIONAL SQUAMOUS CELL CARCINOMA PATHOLOGIC FEATURES	
Gross findings	Glottic, supraglottic, subglottic, transglottic
	Flat, well-defined, raised edge, polypoid, exophytic
	Surface ulceration is seen
Microscopic findings	In situ, superficially or deeply invasive
	Well, moderately, or poorly differentiated
	Keratinizing, nonkeratinizing
	Disorganized growth, lack of maturation, dyskeratosis, keratin pearl formation, intercellular bridges, increased nuclear to cytoplasmic ratio, nuclear chromatin distribution irregularities, prominent nucleoli, increased mitotic figures, atypical mitotic figures
	Inflammatory infiltrate and tumor desmoplasia
Pathologic differential diagnosis	Hyperplasia, radiation changes, necrotizing sialometaplasia, papilloma, variants of squamous cell carcinoma

clinically silent, resulting in a much larger tumor at the time of diagnosis. SCC can be ulcerative, flat, polypoid, verrucous or exophytic, ranging from minute mucosal thickened areas to large masses filling the luminal space (Fig. 3-8). Tumors can be erythematous to white to tan, frequently firm on palpation.

MICROSCOPIC FINDINGS

SCC is generally divided into three histologic categories: in situ (see Precursor Squamous Lesions), superficially invasive or deeply invasive carcinomas with additional modifiers based on histologic grade, including well (closely resembles normal squamous mucosa), moderately (distinct nuclear pleomorphism and less keratinization) or poorly differentiated (immature cells with little maturation or keratinization) along with the presence or absence of keratinization. "Conventional" SCC is composed of variable degrees of squamous differentiation, with the neoplastic cells invading through and disrupting the basement membrane (Fig. 3-9). The overlying surface may not be atypical, and yet invasion may develop from the base (Fig. 3-10). Broad infiltration or jagged, individual cell infiltration can be seen, the latter correlating with a worse prognosis. SCC shows disorganized growth, a loss of polarity, dyskeratosis, keratin pearls, intercellular bridges, an increased nuclear to cytoplasmic ratio, nuclear chromatin irregularities, prominent eosinophilic nucleoli, and mitotic figures (including atypical forms) (Fig. 3-11). Keratinizing type is not seen as frequently as the nonkeratinizing or poorly differentiated types (Fig. 3-12). Mitotic figures and necrosis tend to increase as the grade of the tumor becomes more poorly differentiated. A rich inflammatory infiltrate (usually of lymphocytes and plasma cells) is seen at the tumor to stroma junction,

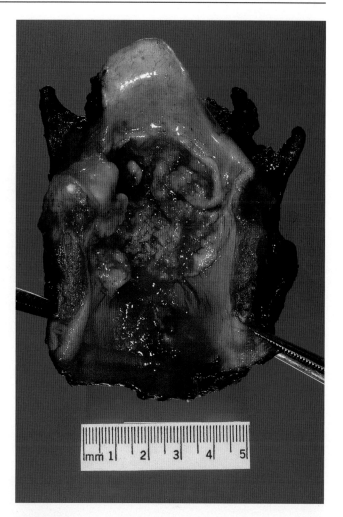

FIGURE 3-8

A laryngectomy specimen demonstrates a large, transglottic, exophytic squamous cell carcinoma. (Courtesy of Dr. J.A. Ohara.)

along with a dense, desmoplastic fibrous stroma (Fig. 3-13). Perineural invasion can be seen, with a positive correlation to metastatic potential. Special studies are rarely needed to document the epithelial nature of the tumor. Instead, tumor site, size, histology (poorly differentiated), degree of invasion, positive surgical margins of resection, lymph node metastases (especially when there is extranodal capsular extension), and multifocal disease, all correlate with a poorer prognosis. Separation of residual carcinoma from radiation changes in the postradiation sample may be difficult. While cellular enlargement is common, radiation usually does not change the nuclear to cytoplasmic ratio, but carcinoma does (Fig. 3-14).

DIFFERENTIAL DIAGNOSIS

The diagnosis of SCC is usually clear cut, although occasionally other lesions are included in the differential diagnosis, such as hyperplasia (with atypia),

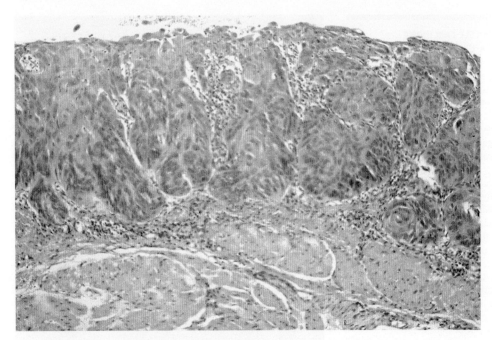

FIGURE 3-9

Squamous cell carcinoma with uneven, finger-like infiltration of the squamous cell carcinoma cells into the underlying stroma. Marked nuclear pleomorphism and cellular disarray is evident.

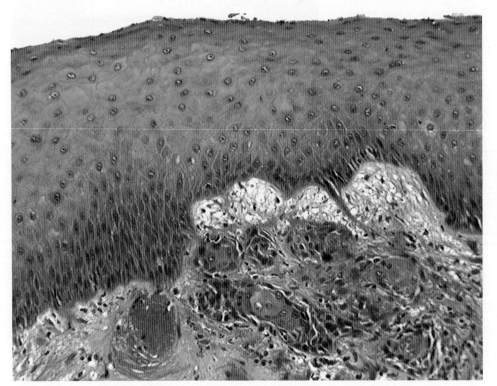

FIGURE 3-10

A well-differentiated squamous cell carcinoma is noted arising from an unremarkable surface epithelium, underscoring the necessity for a biopsy of adequate size and depth.

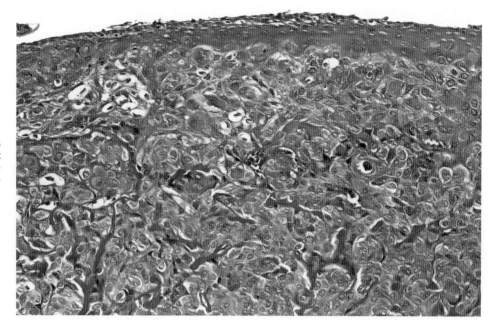

FIGURE 3-11

A moderately differentiated squamous cell carcinoma invading from an intact surface with loss of polarity, disorganization, increased nuclear to cytoplasmic ratio, and focal keratosis.

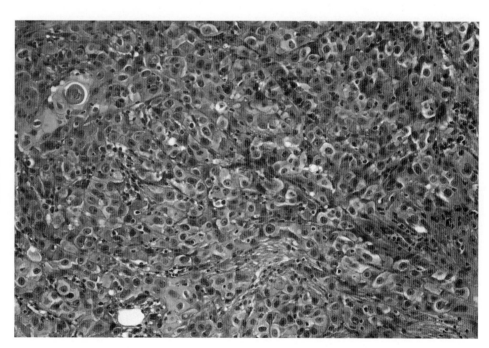

FIGURE 3-12

A poorly differentiated squamous cell carcinoma is arranged in a sheet-like distribution with only occasional cells (*upper left*) suggesting squamous differentiation.

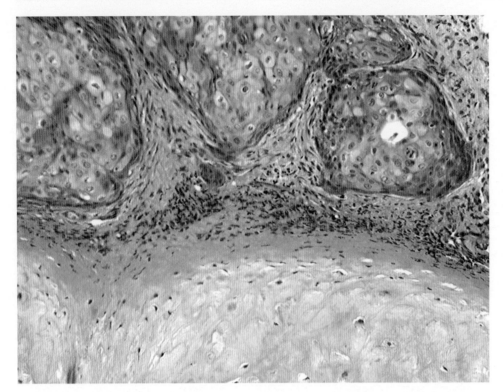

FIGURE 3-13

A moderately differentiated squamous cell carcinoma approaches but does not invade into the perichondrium of the laryngeal cartilage. Inflammation and fibrosis is noted.

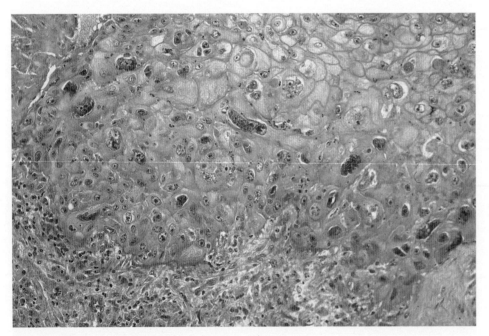

FIGURE 3-14

Radiation can induce changes in residual carcinoma, resulting in bizarre cells and nuclei, but the cells do not appear degenerated, nor do they have a low nuclear to cytoplasmic ratio. Nucleoli are frequently obvious in a squamous cell carcinoma after radiation therapy.

radiation, necrotizing sialometaplasia, and papilloma. Marked pseudoepitheliomatous hyperplasia (PEH) may be mistaken as SCC. However, the reactive nature of the proliferation, lack of "finger-like" invasion, and the association with infectious agents and granular cell tumor will help to make this distinction. Radiation changes affect epithelium, endothelial cells, and the stroma. Glands may become atrophic. There is often profound nuclear pleomorphism, but seen in cells with a very low nuclear to cytoplasmic ratio. Necrotizing sialometaplasia has a lobular architecture maintained, irrespective of the degree of cytologic atypia (Figs. 3-15, 3-16). A biopsy of sufficient size is necessary to secure this diagnosis. A papilloma does not have disorganized growth and unequivocal morphologic features of malignancy. SCC should be separated from the variants (discussed below), as there is often a difference in management and prognosis.

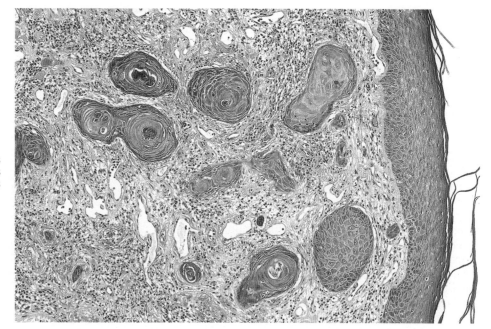

FIGURE 3-15

A hyperplastic squamous epithelium is identified over an area of squamous metaplasia of the mucoserous glands with necrotizing sialometaplasia.

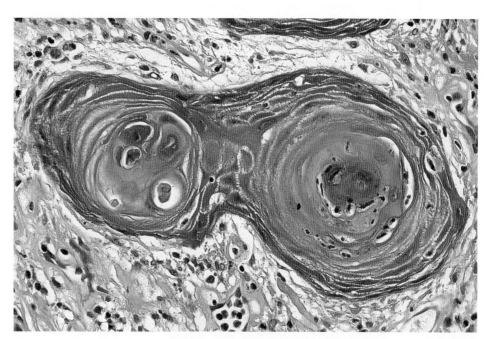

FIGURE 3-16

Keratin pearl formation, dyskeratosis, irregular polarity, and mitotic figures are contained with the basement membrane of this high-power view of squamous metaplasia.

PROGNOSIS AND THERAPY

The TNM tumor classification which incorporates site, size, and stage correlates closely with both disease-free and overall survival (see Appendix). Overall, 5-year survival rates approach 90% for T1 lesions, while <50% for T4 tumors. Laser excision, limited resection, and radiation therapy are variably employed to achieve the best potentially curative voice-sparing outcome. Occasionally, neoadjuvant chemotherapy and radiation therapy are used to maintain laryngeal function. However, if these modalities fail, delayed, salvaged

partial or total laryngectomy can still achieve a good patient outcome.

VARIANTS OF SQUAMOUS CELL CARCINOMA

Variants make up in aggregate up to 15% of all SCCs, and include among others: verrucous, exophytic or papillary, spindle cell (sarcomatoid) carcinoma, basaloid, and adenosquamous (Table 3-1). Rather than give an exhaustive review, only the unique features of each variant will be presented here.

VERRUCOUS SQUAMOUS CELL CARCINOMA (VSCC)

VSCC comprises about 3% of all SCC, is pathogenetically related to HPV, and has specific loss of heterozygosity patterns not identified in hyperplasia. The gross appearance is of a broad-based, warty, exophytic or fungating (Fig. 3-17) bulky, firm to hard, tan or white mass measuring up to 10 cm in greatest dimension.

VSCC is a highly differentiated type of SCC, composed of an exophytic, warty tumor with multiple filiform projections which are thickened and club-shaped, lined by well-differentiated squamous epithelium. The advancing margins of the tumor are usually broad or bulbous rete ridges with a pushing rather than an infiltrative appearance (Fig. 3-18), with a dense inflammatory response in the subjacent tissues. The epithelium is extraordinarily well differentiated without any of the normally associated malignant criteria identified in SCC. The cells are arranged in an orderly maturation towards the surface, with abundant surface keratosis (orthokeratosis; called "church-spire" keratosis; Fig. 3-19). Parakeratotic crypting is a common feature. Mitotic figures are not easy to identify, and when found are not atypical. Focal atypia/dysplasia must be limited to the basal zone if present (Fig. 3-20). Both a benign keratinizing hyperplasia (or verruca vulgaris) and a very well-differentiated SCC can share all of these features somewhere in the tumor, making separation of these lesions a most vexing problem. The relationship of the lesion to the stroma **must** be adequately assessed in a

VERRUCOUS SQUAMOUS CELL CARCINOMA VARIANT FACT SHEET	
Definition	Well-differentiated exophytic/verrucous growth with pushing border of infiltration in a cytologically bland, non-mitotic squamous epithelium
Prognosis and treatment	75% 5-yr survival
	Surgery
Gross findings	Broad-based, warty, exophytic, fungating mass
Microscopic findings	Broad border of pushing infiltration
	Multiple projections of well-differentiated squamous epithelium
	Maturation toward surface
	Abundant keratosis (ortho- and parakeratosis), parakeratotic crypting
	Limited mitotic figures if present at all
Pathologic differential diagnosis	Verrucous hyperplasia and conventional squamous cell carcinoma

sample of sufficient size which has been accurately oriented (not tangential) before rendering a definitive diagnosis.

The differential diagnosis rests between verrucous hyperplasia and conventional SCC. It is argued that the difference between verrucous hyperplasia and VSCC is only in stage and size, the lesions representing a developmental spectrum. The distinction on histologic features alone is often impossible. However, true verrucous hyperplasia does exist (hyperplastic squamous epithelium with regularly spaced, verrucous projections and hyperkeratosis, sharply defined at the epithelial to stromal interface; Fig. 3-21). VSCC can include an invasive component of "ordinary" SCC at the base or demonstrate atypical cytologic features; these tumors need to be managed as well-differentiated SCC.

Biologically, VSCC behaves as an "extremely well differentiated squamous cell carcinoma," with an approximately 75% 5-year survival depending on site and stage.

EXOPHYTIC AND PAPILLARY SQUAMOUS CELL CARCINOMA

Exophytic (ESCC) and papillary squamous cell carcinoma (PSCC) are uncommon but distinct variants of SCC, separable from VSCC (as outlined above). By definition, ESCC and PSCC are de novo malignancies without a pre- or co-existing benign lesion (i.e., squamous papilloma). The average size of exophytic and papillary tumors is between 1-1.5 cm. Most tumors present at a low tumor stage (T1 or T2), although multifocality is described. Macroscopically, ESCC and PSCC are polypoid, exophytic, bulky, papillary or fungiform tumors, soft to firm, arising from a broad base or from a narrow pedicle/stalk.

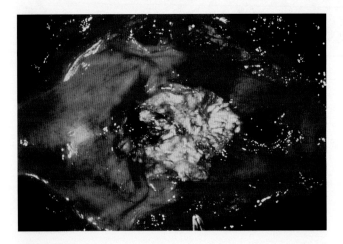

FIGURE 3-17

Multiple projections are seen in this macroscopic view of a large, transglottic verrucous squamous cell carcinoma.

FIGURE 3-18

A broad, pushing border of infiltration is noted immediately above the laryngeal cartilage. Extensive keratosis is noted along with an increased number of layers of squamous epithelium.

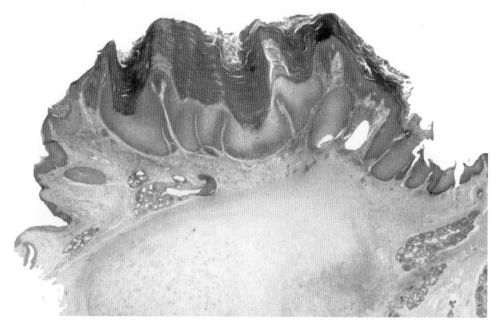

FIGURE 3-19

The size of the lesion is often a helpful indicator of the underlying diagnosis. Broad, pushing border of infiltration with extensive, "church-spire"-type keratosis, and parakeratotic crypting.

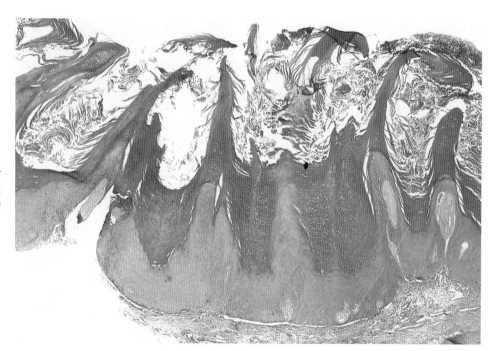

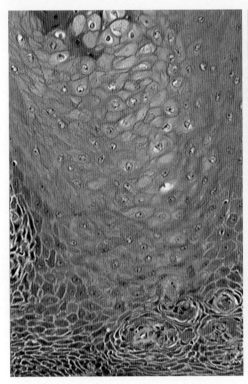
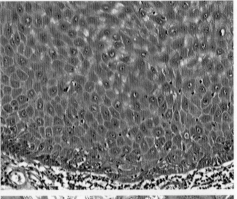
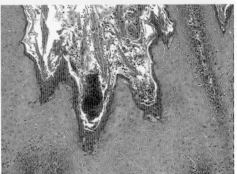

FIGURE 3-20

The proliferation in verrucous carcinoma is cytologically bland, shows maturation and appropriate polarity without mitotic figures (*left*); but demonstrates a broad, bulbous type infiltration into the stroma with associated inflammation (*right upper*). Keratosis is noted (*right lower*) along with parakeratosis and parakeratotic crypting.

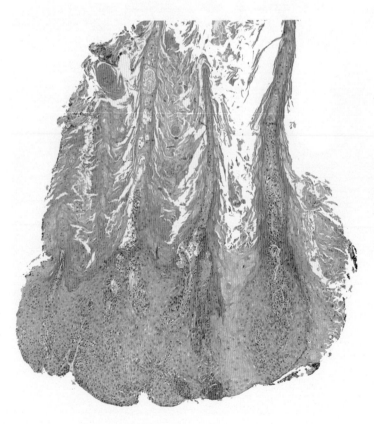

FIGURE 3-21

Verrucous hyperplasia with papillary fronds of squamous epithelium covered with keratin and lacking architectural and cytologic features of malignancy. The separation of verrucous hyperplasia from verrucous carcinoma is often difficult, demanding clinical correlation.

Table 3-1

Clinical and histologic features of squamous cell carcinoma variants

Feature	Variant				
	Verrucous	Papillary/Exophytic	Spindle cell (sarcomatoid)	Basaloid	Adenosquamous
Gender	M > F, except oral	M >> F	M >>> F	M >>> F	M slight > F
Location	Oral > Larynx	Larynx > Oral > Nasal	Larynx > Oral > Nasal	Base of tongue > supraglottic larynx	Tongue > Floor of mouth > nasal
Frequency (of all SCC)	~3%	~1%	~3%	<1%	<1%
Etiologic agent	HPV	? HPV	? Radiation	Unknown	Unknown
Macroscopic	Broad, based warty and fungating mass	Polypoid, exophytic, bulky, papillary, fungiform	Polypoid mass	Firm to hard with central necrosis	Indurated submucosal nodule
Size (cm)	Up to 10	1-1.5 (mean)	2 (mean)	Up to 6	1 (mean)
Microscopic	Pushing border of infiltration; abrupt transition with normal; large, blunt club-shaped rete pegs; no pleomorphism; no mitotic activity; abundant keratin, including parakeratotic crypting and "church-spire" keratosis	>70% exophytic or papillary architecture; "cauliflower-like" vs. "celery-like;" unequivocal cytomorphologic malignancy; surface keratinization; invasive, but difficulty to demonstrate; koilocytic atypia	Biphasic; SCC present, but ulcerated; blended/transition with atypical spindle cell population; hypercellular; variable patterns of spindle-cell growth; pleomorphism; opacified cytoplasm; increased mitotic figures	Biphasic; invasive; lobular; basaloid component most prominent; palisaded; high N:C ratio; abrupt squamous differentiation (metaplasia, dysplasia, CIS or invasive); increased mitotic figures; comedonecrosis; hyaline material	Biphasic; SCC and adenocarcinoma; undifferentiated component; separate or intermixed with areas of transition; infiltrative; increased mitotic figures; sparse inflammatory infiltrate
Special studies	HPV identified	None	~70% + with epithelial markers	Keratin, EMA, CK7 and 34βE12	Mucin positive
Differential diagnosis	Verrucous hyperplasia; SCC	In-situ SCC; Squamous papilloma; Reactive hyperplasia	Benign and malignant mesenchymal process; melanoma; synovial sarcoma	Adenoid cystic carcinoma; neuroendocrine carcinoma (small cell carcinoma)	BSCC; mucoepidermoid carcinoma; adenocarcinoma with squamous metaplasia
Treatment	Surgery; radiation is acceptable	Surgery ± radiation	Surgery with radiation	Surgery; radiation; chemotherapy	Surgery with neck dissection
Prognosis	75% 5-year survival	~70% 5-year survival	~70% 5-year survival	~40% 2-year survival	~55% 2-year survival
Pitfalls	Inadequate biopsy; tangential sectioning	Orientation; adequacy of specimen	No surface; mesenchymal markers; Needs "excisional" biopsy initially	Association with 2nd primary; High chance of nodal metastases	Separation on small biopsies from adenocarcinoma or SCC

EXOPHYTIC OR PAPILLARY SQUAMOUS CELL CARCINOMA VARIANT FACT SHEET	
Definition	Exophytic or papillary architecture in a squamous cell carcinoma
Prognosis and treatment	Recurrences in about 35%
	Better prognosis than conventional squamous cell carcinoma (site and stage dependent)
Gross findings	Mean of 1–1.5 cm
	Polypoid, exophytic, bulky, papillary or fungiform
Microscopic findings	>70% exophytic or papillary architecture
	Broad based, bulbous, rounded "cauliflower"-like growth
	Multiple, thin, delicate, filiform, finger-like projections
	Both types have malignant cytologic features
	Stromal invasion is difficult to identify
Pathologic differential diagnosis	Squamous papilloma, verrucous squamous cell carcinoma

By definition, the neoplastic squamous epithelial proliferation must demonstrate a dominant (>70%) exophytic or papillary architectural growth pattern with unequivocal cytomorphologic evidence of malignancy.

The exophytic pattern consists of a broad-based, bulbous to exophytic growth of the squamous epithelium (Fig. 3-22). The projections are rounded and "cauliflower-like" in growth pattern. Tangential sectioning yields a number of central fibrovascular cores, but the superficial aspect is lobular, not papillary. The papillary pattern consists of multiple, thin, delicate filiform, finger-like papillary projections (Fig. 3-23). The papillae contain a delicate fibrovascular core surrounded by the neoplastic epithelium (Fig. 3-24). Tangential sectioning yields a number of central fibrovascular cores, but appears more like a bunch of celery cut across the stalk. It is not uncommon to have extensive overlap between these patterns, and when that is the case, the ESCC should be the default. Both types have the features of SCC already described (Fig. 3-25). Invasion may be difficult to define, especially in superficial biopsies. However, the significant proliferation of this carcinomatous epithelium, often forming a large clinical lesion, is rather beyond the general concept of carcinoma in situ. When in doubt, the significantly proliferated appearance of the lesion should be heavily weighted in the direction of carcinoma. The cytomorphologic features of malignancy would exclude the diagnosis of a papilloma, as well as the consideration of a verrucous squamous cell carcinoma.

Approximately one-third of patients develop recurrence, frequently more than once. Patients with these variants seem to have a better prognosis when compared to site and stage-matched conventional SCC patients.

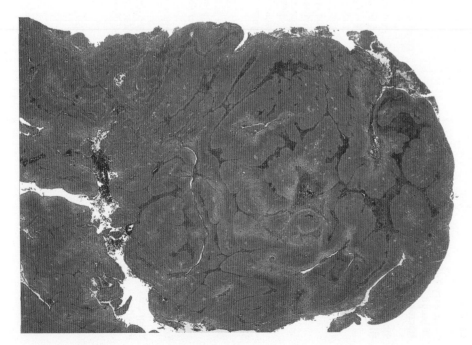

FIGURE 3-22

An exophytic squamous cell carcinoma has a rounded "cauliflower"-like projection to the projections.

FIGURE 3-23

A papillary squamous cell carcinoma demonstrates multiple papillary projections above the surface, but an invasive component is also noted. Keratinization is prominent.

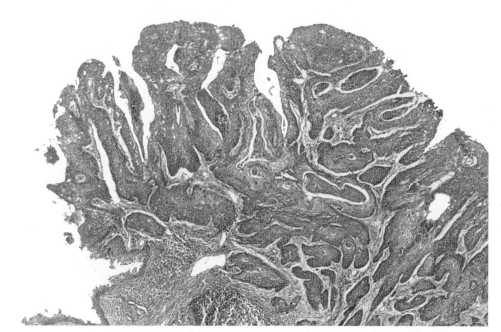

FIGURE 3-24

A papillary squamous cell carcinoma with individual, delicate, finger-like projections with fibrovascular cores.

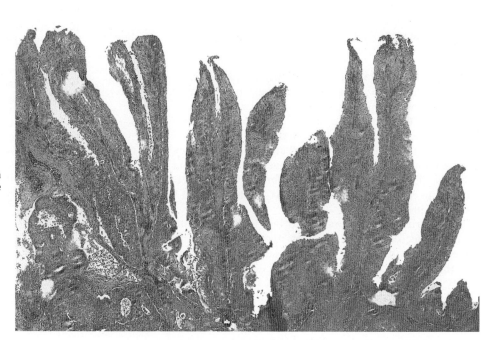

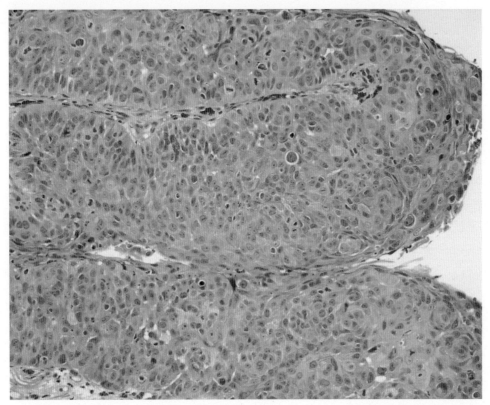

FIGURE 3-25
Papillary carcinoma. The papillary projections have thin fibrovascular cores and remarkably cytologically atypical epithelium lining the papillary projections. Dyskeratosis and jumbled architecture is prominent.

SPINDLE CELL (SARCOMATOID) SQUAMOUS CELL CARCINOMA (SCSCC)

SCSCC (Lane tumor) is recognized as a morphologically biphasic neoplasm containing an epithelioid and spindle-shaped neoplastic proliferation. It comprises up to 3% of SCC. There is a profound male to female ratio (11 : 1). Nearly all cases are described as *polypoid* masses with a mean size of about 2 cm (Fig. 3-26). They are frequently ulcerated with a covering of fibrinoid necrosis. They have a firm and fibrous cut surface. Similar to conventional SCC, most tumors are T1 lesions at presentation.

Considering the frequency of surface ulceration with fibrinoid necrosis (Fig. 3-27), it may be difficult to discern the transition between the surface epithelium and the spindle cell element. If meticulously and diligently sought, dysplasia, carcinoma in situ, or infiltrating SCC can be identified, although it is usually minor to inconspicuous with the sarcomatoid part dominating. Frank squamous differentiation can be found at the base of the polypoid lesion, the advancing margins, or within invaginations at the surface where the epithelium is not ulcerated or denuded. The carcinomatous and sarcomatoid components will abut directly against one another with areas of barely perceptible blending and continuity between them (Fig. 3-28). The sarcomatoid or fusiform fraction of the tumor can be arranged in a diverse array of appearances, including storiform, interlacing bundles or fascicles, and herringbone (Fig. 3-29). Generally hypercellular, hypocellular tumors with dense collagen deposition are also seen. Pleomorphism is often

SPINDLE CELL "SARCOMATOID" CARCINOMA VARIANT FACT SHEET	
Definition	Morphologically biphasic tumor with squamous cell and malignant spindle cell component with a mesenchymal appearance but an epithelial origin
Prognosis and treatment	80% 5-yr survival
	Surgery and radiation
Gross findings	Polypoid mass arising from true vocal cord
	Ulcerated surface and firm cut surface
Microscopic findings	Surface ulceration with fibrinoid necrosis
	Dysplasia, CIS, or infiltrating squamous cell carcinoma
	Blending of carcinoma with spindle cell population
	Storiform, interlacing fascicles, herringbone patterns
	Hypercellular, but hypocellular with collagen also
	Mitotic figures, but usually no necrosis
Immunohistochemical features	Keratin, epithelial membrane antigen, CK18 in epithelioid and spindle cell populations
Pathologic differential diagnosis	Inflammatory myofibroblastic tumor, synovial sarcoma

mild to moderate, without a severe degree of anaplasia. The tumor cells are plump fusiform cells, although they can be rounded and epithelioid. Opacified, dense, eosinophilic cytoplasm, gives a hint of squamous differentiation, but is difficult to quantify or qualify accu-

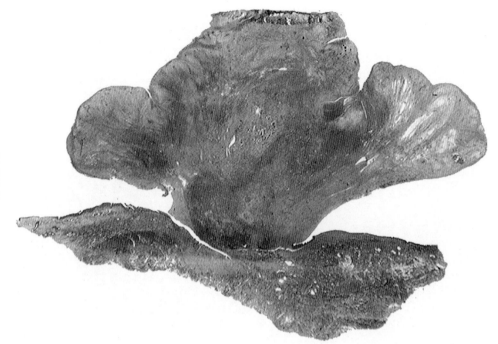

FIGURE 3-26

A macroscopic view of an SCSCC shows the polypoid projection attached to the underlying stroma by a narrow stalk. Surface ulceration has denuded most of the epithelium.

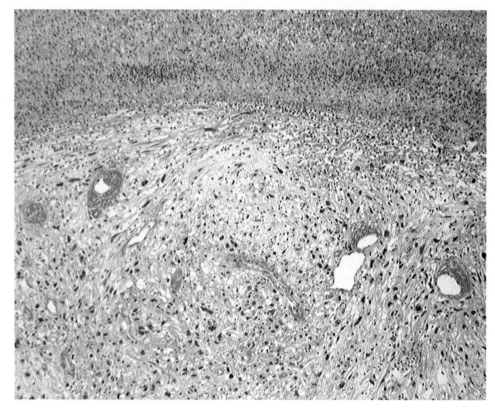

FIGURE 3-27

Complete loss of the surface epithelium with fibrinoid necrosis is characteristic for an SCSCC with markedly atypical, hyperchromatic nuclei identified within the spindle cells of the "stroma."

rately. Mitotic figures, including atypical forms, are easily counted in most tumors (Fig. 3-30). Rarely, metaplastic or frankly neoplastic cartilage or bone can be seen.

This is the one SCC variant in which immunohistochemistry may be of value. The individual spindle neoplastic cells react variably, although most sensitively and reliably with keratin (AE1/AE3), epithelial membrane antigen (EMA) (Fig. 3-31), and CK18, although only about 70% of cases will yield any epithelial immunoreactivity. Other mesenchymal markers can be identified focally, although this phenotypic plasticity or lineage infidelity supports the sarcomatoid transformation seen in SCSCC. Whereas a positive epithelial marker helps to

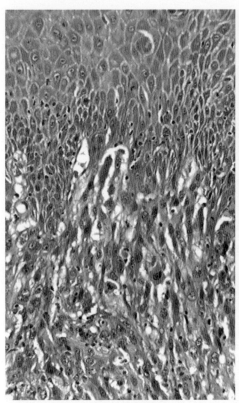 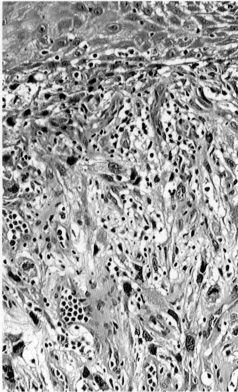

FIGURE 3-28
The surface epithelium blends imperceptibly with the spindled pattern of growth. Mitotic figures, pleomorphism, and inflammation are noted.

confirm the diagnosis of SCSCC, a nonreactive or negative result should not dissuade the pathologist from the diagnosis, especially in the right clinical setting.

The differential diagnosis includes any spindle cell lesion, but suffice it to say that authentic primary mucosal sarcomas or benign mesenchymal tumors of the larynx are exceptional. An inflammatory myofibroblastic pseudotumor has a tissue culture-like growth of spindle to stellate cells with inflammatory cells throughout. Synovial sarcoma (especially monophasic) may cause the most diagnostic difficulty, but the age at presentation (children), tumor location (usually hypopharynx and soft tissue rather than mucosal), and the presence of a specific chromosomal translocation t(X;18)(p11;q11) can aid in this distinction.

Surgery, usually followed by radiation therapy seems to yield the best long-term patient outcome, similar to conventional SCC, although site and stage specific. When metastatic disease develops, cervical lymph nodes and pulmonary involvement is most frequent. There is an overall 80% 5-year survival.

BASALOID SQUAMOUS CELL CARCINOMA (BSCC)

BSCC is a high-grade variant of SCC with a predilection for multifocal presentation, affects primarily men in the 7th decade with frequent cervical lymph node metastases at presentation. Macroscopically, these tumors are usually firm to hard with associated central necrosis, occurring as exophytic to nodular masses, measuring up to 6 cm in greatest dimension.

BASALOID SQUAMOUS CELL CARCINOMA VARIANT FACT SHEET	
Definition	High-grade squamous cell carcinoma variant with basaloid small cells arranged in a palisaded architecture, with focal areas of squamous differentiation
Clinical features	Multifocal, older men, high incidence of cervical lymph node metastases
Prognosis and treatment	40% survival
	Multimodality therapy (surgery, radiation, chemotherapy)
Gross findings	Firm tumors with central necrosis, up to 6 cm
Microscopic findings	Solid, lobular, *comedonecrosis*, cribriform, trabecular, glands, and cystic architecture
	Frequently ulcerated, easily identified lymphvascular invasion
	Basaloid cells with small closely opposed moderately pleomorphic cells with peripheral palisading
	Hyperchromatic nuclei with coarse nuclear chromatin
	Abrupt keratinization, squamous pearl formation, individual cell keratinization
	High mitotic index
	Prominent, eosinophilic, hyaline, "cylindrical" matrix material
Immunohistochemical features	Keratin, CAM5.2, epithelial membrane antigen, CK7, and 34ßE12
Pathologic differential diagnosis	Neuroendocrine carcinoma, adenoid cystic carcinoma, adenosquamous carcinoma, squamous cell carcinoma

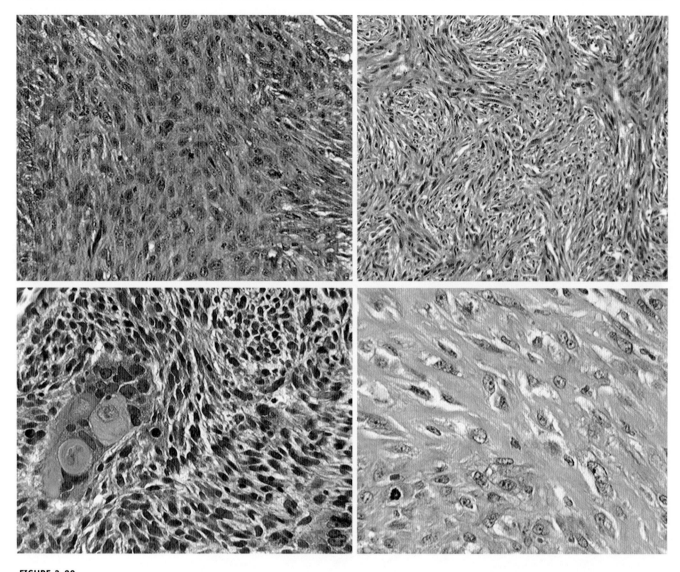

FIGURE 3-29

Variable patterns of growth, including solid-compact (*upper left*), fascicular and storiform (*upper right*), a focus of abrupt squamous differentiation (*lower left*), and a hypocellular atypical spindle cell population with mitotic figures (*lower right*).

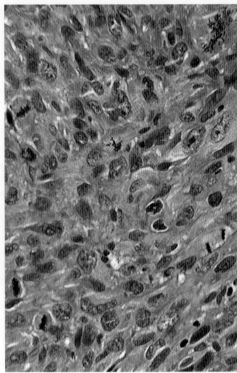

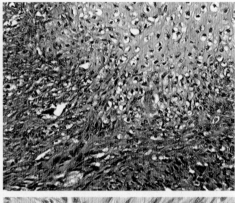

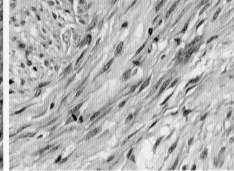

FIGURE 3-30

Left: SCSCC composed of haphazard atypical spindle cells with increased mitotic figures, including atypical forms. *Right upper:* Metaplastic cartilage has undergone malignant transformation into a chondrosarcoma within this SCSCC. *Right lower:* Deceptively bland spindle cells may be the dominant finding.

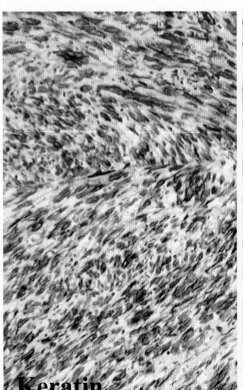

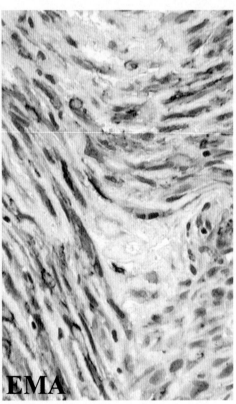

FIGURE 3-31

SCSCC. It is unusual to find such a strongly immunopositive keratin reaction (*left*), while the more focal epithelial membrane antigen stain is more characteristic of the quality of the reaction.

Many patterns are seen in this infiltrating tumor, including solid, lobular, comedonecrosis (Fig. 3-32), cribriform, cords, trabeculae, nests, and glands or cysts. Surface ulceration may belie the deeply invasive nature of the tumor, which has frequent lymphvascular invasion; neurotropism is less common. The basaloid component is the most diagnostic feature, incorporating small, closely opposed moderately pleomorphic cells with hyperchromatic nuclei and scant cytoplasm into a lobular configuration with peripheral palisading (Fig. 3-33). These basaloid regions are in intimate association with areas of squamous differentiation including abrupt keratinization in the form of squamous pearls (Fig. 3-34), individual cell keratinization, dysplasia, or SCC (in situ or invasive). Marked mitotic activity as well as comedonecrosis in the center of the neoplastic islands is common. The tumor cells are separated by a prominent dense pink hyaline material, often cylinder shaped, with small cystic spaces containing mucoid-type material. In metastatic disease, both basaloid and squamous cell components can be seen, although the basaloid features predominate.

A sample of sufficient depth to show the heterogeneous nature of the tumor will usually resolve the differential consideration of a neuroendocrine carcinoma, adenoid cystic carcinoma, adenosquamous carcinoma, and squamous cell carcinoma. A lack of neuroendocrine nuclear features and immunoreactivity eliminates neuroendocrine carcinoma from consideration. Adenoid cystic carcinoma does not have squamous differentiation, prominent pleomorphism, mitoses or necrosis. When the diagnosis of a basaloid squamous carcinoma is made, there is an increased possibility of a contemporaneous primary elsewhere. BSCC requires aggressive multimodality therapy, including radical surgery (including neck dissection), radiotherapy, and chemotherapy (especially for metastatic disease).

Despite aggressive therapy, the overall mortality rate is high (60 % die of disease).

ADENOSQUAMOUS CARCINOMA (ASC)

ASC is a high-grade variant of squamous cell carcinoma composed of an admixture of squamous cell carcinoma and adenocarcinoma. Most patients present with lymph node metastases (65 %). ASC occurs throughout the upper aerodigestive tract, often as an indurated submucosal nodule up to 5 cm in maximum dimension, although most are <1 cm.

ADENOSQUAMOUS CARCINOMA VARIANT FACT SHEET	
Definition	Composite of true adenocarcinoma and squamous cell carcinoma
Prognosis and treatment	Lymph node metastases in 65%
	Poor prognosis (55% 2-yr survival)
	Surgery
Gross findings	Indurated, submucosal nodule about 1 cm
Microscopic findings	Biphasic adenocarcinoma and squamous cell carcinoma
	Undifferentiated or transitional components between lesions
	Separate, intermixed, commingled, transitions
	Scant inflammatory infiltrate
Pathologic differential diagnosis	Basaloid squamous cell carcinoma, mucoepidermoid carcinoma, adenocarcinoma with squamous metaplasia

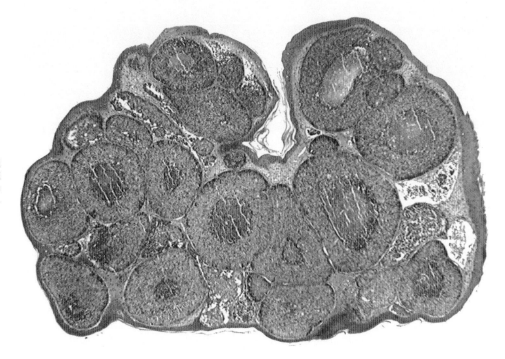

FIGURE 3-32

The neoplastic infiltrate is dominated by a lobular arrangement of basaloid cells with areas of comedonecrosis in this basaloid squamous cell carcinoma.

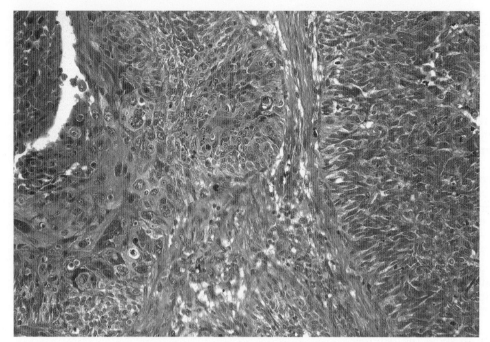

FIGURE 3-33
Frank squamous cell carcinoma is seen (*left*) with an area of necrosis, juxtaposed to the characteristic basaloid, small, peripherally palisaded nuclear architecture of a basaloid squamous cell carcinoma (*right*).

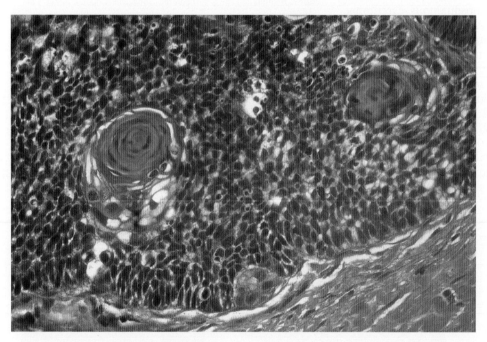

FIGURE 3-34
Abrupt keratinization intimately admixed with the basaloid cells which are smaller in size, have a high nuclear to cytoplasmic ratio and hyperchromatic nuclei in this basaloid squamous cell carcinoma.

By definition the tumor demonstrates biphasic components of adenocarcinoma and squamous cell carcinoma, with an undifferentiated cellular component in several tumors (Fig. 3-35). The SCC can be in situ or invasive ranging from well to poorly differentiated. Squamous differentiation is confirmed by pavemented growth with intercellular bridges, keratin pearl formation, dyskeratosis, or individual cell keratinization. The adenocarcinoma component can be tubular, alveolar, and glandular, although mucus-cell differentiation is not essential for the diagnosis. The cells in the adenocarci-noma can be basaloid and separation from basaloid squamous cell carcinoma can at times be arbitrary. The two carcinomas may be separate or intermixed, with areas of commingling and/or transition of the SCC to adenocarcinoma (Fig. 3-36). The "undifferentiated" areas between the two distinct carcinomas are often composed of clear cells. Both carcinomas may demonstrate frequent mitoses, necrosis, and infiltration into the surrounding tissue with affiliated perineural invasion. There is typically a sparse inflammatory cell infiltrate at the tumor-stromal interface.

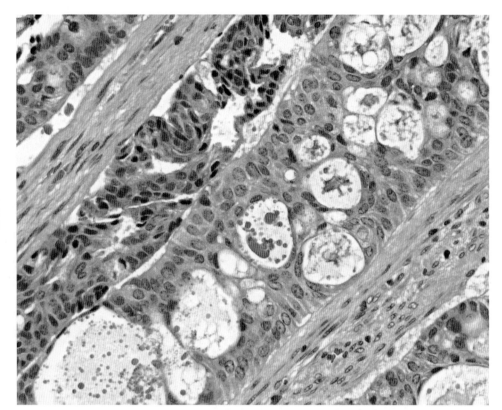

FIGURE 3-35

Adenosquamous carcinoma demonstrates blended adenocarcinoma and squamous cell carcinoma within a single tumor mass.

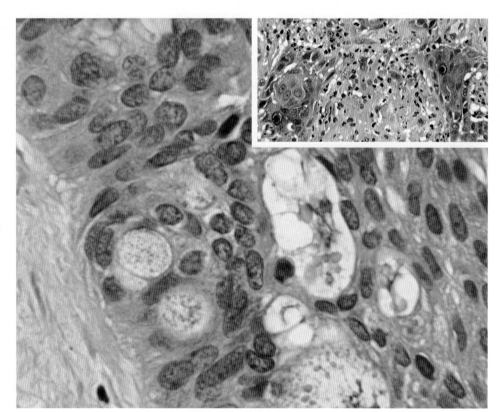

FIGURE 3-36

Adenosquamous carcinoma with small gland-like structures are seen blending with squamous epithelium that has intercellular bridges. The inset demonstrates a positive mucicarmine reaction.

In contrast to BSCC, ASC show a prominent squamous cell component, absence of basaloid cells with peripheral nuclear palisading, and the presence of glandular differentiation. Although separation of adenosquamous carcinoma from mucoepidermoid may be impossible in some cases, mucoepidermoid carcinoma demonstrates intermediate type cells, generally does not have true squamous cell differentiation, and does not have two distinctly separate carcinomas (adenocarcinoma and SCC). An adenocarcinoma with squamous metaplasia generally does not demonstrate the nuclear criteria of a malignant squamous cell component. A contemporaneous SCC and adenocarcinoma may affect the upper aerodigestive tract, but these lesions are usually temporally separated. Aggressive surgery with neck dissection yields an approximately 55% 2-year survival.

NEUROENDOCRINE CARCINOMA

The terminology for this family of neoplasms is fraught with a great deal of confusion and conflict. The terms carcinoid, atypical carcinoid, and small cell carcinoma, similar to pulmonary nomenclature has been suggested by the World Health Organization. Equivalent terminology includes well differentiated (carcinoid), moderately differentiated (atypical carcinoma), and poorly differentiated (small cell carcinoma) neuroendocrine carcinoma, respectively. Expression of hormones is often limited to immunohistochemistry, as it is most uncommon to have systemic manifestations or paraneoplastic syndromes.

CLINICAL FEATURES

Although there are slight differences among the various grades of neuroendocrine neoplasms, most patients are between 45–80 years of age with a peak in the 7th decade; the majority are men; and there is a strong tobacco association. As with all laryngeal tumors, dysphagia, hoarseness, sore throat, hemoptysis, and the feeling of a lump are the most common presenting symptoms. Atypical carcinoid represents the most common nonsquamous malignancy of the larynx. Patients will small cell carcinoma frequently have lymph node metastases (50%).

PATHOLOGIC FEATURES

GROSS FINDINGS

Neuroendocrine neoplasms occur most frequently in the supraglottic region, presenting as a submucosal mass in the aryepiglottic fold or arytenoid. The histogenesis is unsettled, but thought to be of epithelial origin. The

---

NEUROENDOCRINE CARCINOMA (CARCINOID, ATYPICAL CARCINOID, SMALL CELL CARCINOMA) DISEASE FACT SHEET

Definition	Malignant epithelial neoplasm with neuroendocrine differentiation
Incidence and location	Most common nonsquamous cell malignancy of the larynx
	Usually supraglottic
Morbidity and mortality	Variable based on histologic grade
	Metastatic disease is usual cause of death rather than recurrence
	Metastases are usually to lymph nodes, liver, lung, and bone
Gender, race, and age distribution	Male >> Female (3 : 1)
	Peak in 7th decade
Clinical features	Strong tobacco association
	Dysphagia, hoarseness, sore throat, hemoptysis, lump in throat
Prognosis and treatment	**Tumor type dependent:**
	Carcinoid: Good long-term prognosis; surgery alone
	Atypical carcinoid: 45% metastatic disease; 50% 5-yr survival; surgery and radiation
	Small cell carcinoma: Rapidly fatal; 16% 2-yr survival

NEUROENDOCRINE CARCINOMA (CARCINOID, ATYPICAL CARCINOID, SMALL CELL CARCINOMA) PATHOLOGIC FEATURES

Gross findings	Supraglottic
	Submucosal mass, with ulceration in higher grade tumors
	Polypoid, pedunculated
	Up to 4 cm in size
Microscopic findings	Carcinoid: Organoid and trabecular with monotonous cells with round nuclei and low N : C ratio and finely stippled chromatin
	Atypical carcinoid: Cords, solid and single-file infiltration, vascular invasion, vesicular to hyperchromatic nuclei with a higher N : C ratio, with nucleoli
	Small cell carcinoma: Sheets, ribbons and pseudorosettes, invasive growth, pleomorphism, high N : C ratio, nuclear molding, necrosis, mitoses, crush artifact
Immunohistochemical features	Keratin, epithelial membrane antigen, and carcinoembryonic antigen positive
	Chromogranin, synaptophysin, calcitonin, and other neuroendocrine markers and hormones are positive
Pathologic differential diagnosis	Poorly differentiated squamous cell carcinoma, medullary thyroid carcinoma, adenoid cystic carcinoma, melanoma, lymphoma, metastatic carcinoma

gross appearance ranges from polypoid, pedunculated to ulcerated, ranging in size up to 4 cm, but on average are 1.6 cm.

MICROSCOPIC FINDINGS

Neuroendocrine tumors are usually unencapsulated, although carcinoids and atypical carcinoids are circum-

scribed, covered by an uninvolved surface mucosa. The tumors present with a variety of different histologic patterns, including an organoid or trabecular growth in carcinoid tumors (Fig. 3-37); the addition of cords, solid, single-file, and cribriform patterns in atypical carcinoids (Fig. 3-38); and all of these patterns along with sheets, ribbons, pseudoglands, and rosette formations in small cell carcinoma. Atypical carcinoid and small cell

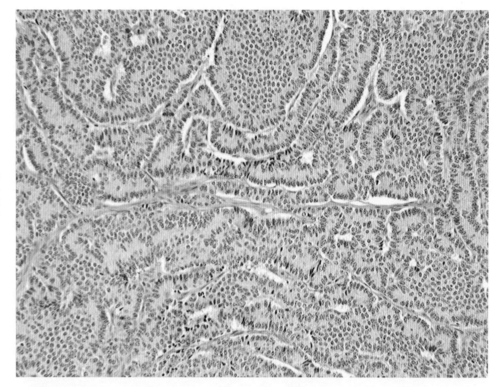

FIGURE 3-37
Well-differentiated cells arranged in ribbons and festoons in this carcinoid. The cells have pale cytoplasm surrounding round nuclei with granular, coarse nuclear chromatin.

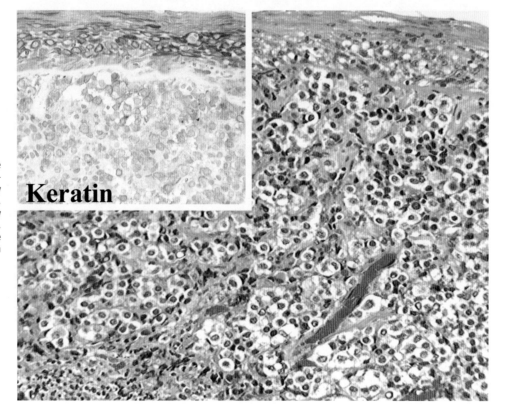

FIGURE 3-38
Atypical carcinoid. The surface epithelium is uninvolved by the neoplastic proliferation of moderately pleomorphic cells with coarse, hyperchromatic nuclei surrounded by ample, pale to basophilic cytoplasm. There is a rich vascularity. The neoplastic cells are strongly keratin immunoreactive (*inset*).

carcinoma may demonstrate surface ulceration. A fibrovascular stroma is generally absent in small cell carcinoma, although it is seen in carcinoids and atypical carcinoids. Lymphvascular, perineural, and soft tissue invasion is seen in the atypical carcinoids or small cell carcinomas. Amyloid and tumor cell spindling is occasionally noted. Concurrent squamous cell carcinoma may be present.

The cytologic appearance of the cells is determined by the subtype of neuroendocrine carcinoma. Glandular (with mucin production) or squamous differentiation can be seen in neuroendocrine neoplasms. The degree of cellular pleomorphism, mitotic activity and necrosis increases as the tumor becomes more poorly differentiated (small cell carcinoma). There is virtual absence of pleomorphism, necrosis, and mitoses in a carcinoid, while there is prominent pleomorphism, necrosis, and mitoses in a small cell carcinoma, with atypical carci-

noid exhibiting intermediate features (Fig. 3-39). Due to the fragility of the cells, crush artifact is frequently prominent in small cell carcinoma (Fig. 3-40).

Carcinoid tumors have small, monotonous cells with a low nuclear to cytoplasmic ratio, round vesicular nuclei with finely stippled chromatin (Fig. 3-37). Atypical carcinoid tumors have vesicular to more hyperchromatic nuclei within polygonal cells that have an increased nuclear to cytoplasmic ratio. The location of the nucleus is variable, surrounded by amphophilic to eosinophilic cytoplasm. Nucleoli are variable, from absent to prominent (Figs. 3-38, 3-39). Small cell carcinoma is comprised of cells with a high nuclear to cytoplasmic ratio, intensely hyperchromatic oval to spindled nuclei without nucleoli (Fig. 3-40). Mitotic figures, necrosis, and occasional multinucleated neoplastic giant cells are present. There is usually limited stroma, which may be mucoid. Laryngeal neuroendocrine

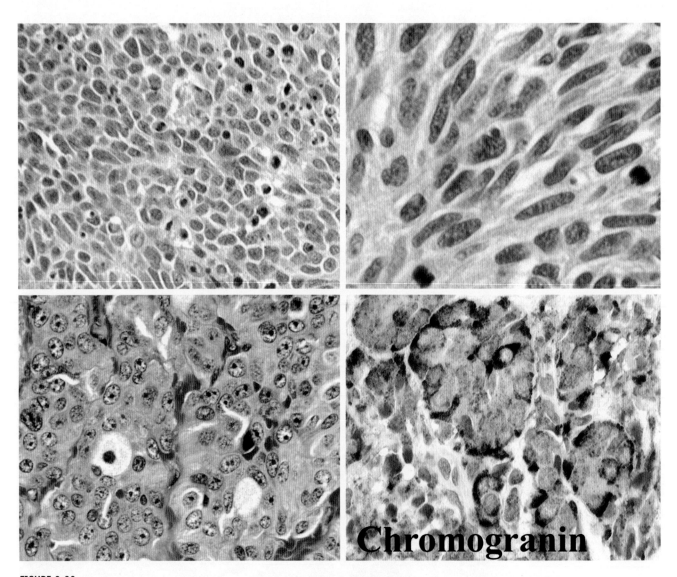

FIGURE 3-39

Atypical carcinoid. The cells of this neuroendocrine neoplasm can be arranged in solid sheets of cells with a high nuclear to cytoplasmic ratio (*upper left*), in fascicles of spindle cells with stippled nuclear chromatin (*upper right*), or in glandular profiles of cells with round nuclei, prominent nucleoli and "salt-and-pepper" chromatin distribution (*lower left*). The cytoplasm of the tumor cells shows a strong, granular chromogranin reaction (*lower right*).

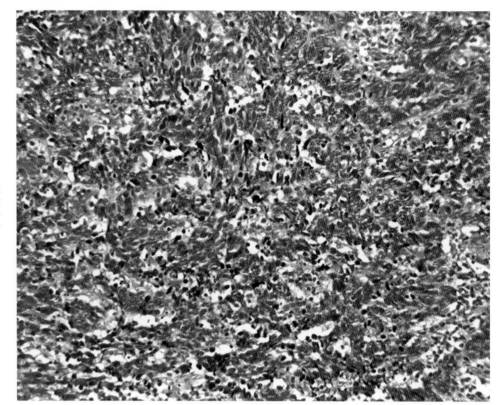

FIGURE 3-40

The "crush" artifact is characteristic for small cell carcinoma which has cells with high nuclear to cytoplasmic ratio and coarse nuclear chromatin distribution.

neoplasms are on a morphologically continuous spectrum, with an aggregate of features distinguishing between the tumors.

ANCILLARY STUDIES

ULTRASTRUCTURAL FEATURES

Electron microscopy will demonstrate membrane-bound, electron-dense neurosecretory granules, ranging from 50 to up 250 nm, decreasing in number as the tumor becomes less differentiated. Complex intercellular digitation and occasional intercellular junctions are present.

IMMUNOHISTOCHEMICAL FEATURES

All grades of tumor variably react with keratin (Fig. 3-38), epithelial membrane antigen (EMA), carcinoembryonic antigen, chromogranin (Fig. 3-39), synaptophysin, and calcitonin, while other neuroendocrine and hormone markers are variably reactive (neuron specific enolase, Leu7, neurofilament proteins). Almost all of these lesions are nonreactive for S-100 protein, glial fibrillary acid protein, and met-enkephalins.

DIFFERENTIAL DIAGNOSIS

The differential diagnosis is quite broad and includes squamous cell carcinoma, malignant melanoma, adenoid cystic carcinoma, lymphoma, metastatic carcinoma, and medullary thyroid carcinoma.

Part of the reason for making a definitive diagnosis regarding neuroendocrine tumors, is the differences in treatment protocols and patient outcome. A poorly differentiated SCC (which will be negative for neuroendocrine immunohistochemistry) will respond to radiation therapy, while atypical carcinoid is generally insensitive to this modality. A mucosal melanoma may have melanin pigment, more frequently involves the surface epithelium, will demonstrate greater pleomorphism and will have S-100 protein and HMB-45 reactivity in the tumor cells. It is imperative to exclude a metastatic tumor to the larynx, especially in small cell carcinoma, where a lung primary may have metastasized to the larynx and will usually be TTF-1 positive. Medullary carcinoma of the thyroid may metastasize to or directly invade into the larynx. The distinction between medullary carcinoma of the thyroid and neuroendocrine carcinoma of the larynx can be nearly impossible; amyloid and an increased serum calcitonin level is much more likely in a thyroid medullary carcinoma. Lymphomas, with crush artifact and a submucosal location, can be separated by lacking neuroendocrine differentiation (either immunohistochemically or ultrastructurally).

PROGNOSIS AND THERAPY

The reason for the distinction between of these tumor types relates to the differences in treatment and prognosis. Prognosis for carcinoid is excellent, while it gets progressively worse at the degree of differentiation decreases. Atypical carcinoid tumors frequently have metastases at presentation (45%), and are usually treated with surgery alone as they are rather insensitive to radiation or chemotherapy. Small cell carcinomas have metastasis at presentation in about 50% of patients, with a rapidly fatal clinical course. Death is usually due to metastatic disease, with the size of the tumor an important prognostic factor.

CHONDROSARCOMA

Only 2% to 5% of all chondrosarcomas arise in the head and neck, with laryngeal chondrosarcomas accounting for about 1% of all laryngeal malignancies. The proposed etiology for laryngeal chondrosarcomas is disordered ossification of the laryngeal cartilages, and specifically the cricoid cartilage (ossification usually develops in areas of muscle insertion and is attributed to the mechanical influence of the contracting muscles). The ossification is found in hyaline cartilages in older adult patients, the same age as the presentation of laryngeal chondrosarcoma. It has also been suggested that ischemic change in a chondroma subjected to mechanical trauma may be a precursor to malignant change. Interestingly, laryngeal chondromas develop on average about a decade earlier than chondrosarcomas, perhaps suggesting a developmental continuum.

CLINICAL FEATURES

Men are typically affected more frequently than women (4:1). Patients present in the mid 60s, although there is a wide age range (25–91 yr). As the airway is progressively narrowed or obstructed by the endolaryngeal growth, hoarseness, followed by dyspnea, dysphagia, difficulty breathing, and stridor results. Thyroid cartilage tumors are more likely to present as an anterior neck mass. Symptoms are frequently present for a long duration (mean, >2 yr), supporting the indolent tumor growth. Endoscopically, there is a subglottic swelling below an intact mucosa.

CHONDROSARCOMA DISEASE FACT SHEET	
Definition	Chondrosarcoma is a malignant tumor arising within the laryngeal cartilages and forming neoplastic cartilage
Incidence and location	Up to 1% of all laryngeal malignancies 75% of all laryngeal sarcomas Cricoid cartilage most commonly
Morbidity and mortality	Recurrences in up to 40% of patients Patients rarely die from tumor
Gender, race, and age distribution	Male >> Female (4:1) Mean, 60–65 yr
Clinical features	Hoarseness, dyspnea, dysphagia, stridor Thyroid cartilage lesions present as a neck mass Long duration of symptoms Subglottic submucosal swelling on endoscopy
Radiologic features	Fine, punctate, stippled to coarse calcifications Ill-defined, invasive, hypodense mass
Prognosis and treatment	>95% 10-yr survival Complete, but conservative, laryngeal-function preserving surgery

RADIOLOGIC FEATURES

Either plain films or computed tomography (CT) examinations will show fine, punctate stippled to coarse ("popcorn") calcification within a hypodense tumor mass (Fig. 3-41). After identifying the tumor as "cartilaginous," the remaining features are nonspecific, although most chondrosarcomas are centered in the

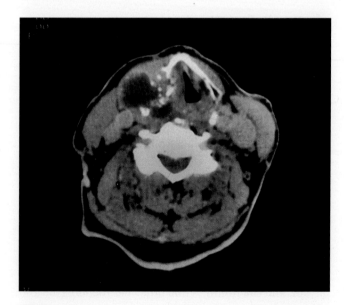

FIGURE 3-41

A computer tomography image of a chondrosarcoma destroying the posterior portion of the thyroid cartilage and demonstrating stippled to coarse ("popcorn") calcifications within the tumor.

cricoid cartilage, are frequently ill-defined, can be cystic, and illustrate an impulse for invasion, both endolaryngeal and extralaryngeal.

PATHOLOGIC FEATURES

GROSS FINDINGS

The cricoid cartilage (specifically the inner posterior lamina) is affected far more frequently (~75%) than other laryngeal cartilages, followed by the thyroid and arytenoid cartilages. The tumors range in size from 0.8–12 cm (mean, 3.5 cm). Tumors are hard, "crunchy" or "gritty," lobular, and glistening on cut surface, with a blue-gray, semitranslucent, myxoid-mucinous matrix material (Fig. 3-42). Dedifferentiated chondrosarcoma has fleshy areas.

MICROSCOPIC FINDINGS

Chondrosarcomas are recognized by their increased cellularity, nuclear atypia including bi- and multinucleation (Fig. 3-43), and propensity to invade and destroy surrounding structures. Most chondrosarcomas seem to involve only a single cartilage with very little tendency to infiltrate adjacent cartilages. When the native cartilage is included in the biopsy, the cartilage is frequently ossified, and will show neoplastic chondrocytes invading into the ossified regions (Fig. 3-44). The atypical, neoplastic chondrocytes are identified in a variable background of basophilic to metachromatic cartilaginous matrix material (Fig. 3-45). There is an overall loss of normal architecture and distribution of the chondrocytes ("cluster disarray"). The tumor cytomorphology varies from slightly cellular tumors composed of small, hyperchromatic nuclei surrounded by abundant cytoplasm to hypercellular neoplasms consisting of enlarged, bi- and multinucleated atypical cells with an increased nuclear to cytoplasmic ratio, nuclear chromatin distribution irregularities, and prominent nucleoli (Fig. 3-46). There is less stroma between the lacunar spaces as the grade of tumor increases. Mitotic figures, including atypical forms, are only infrequently noted and only in high-grade tumors. Tumor necrosis, usually focal and of limited geographic distribution, is usually restricted to higher grade tumors.

CHONDROSARCOMA PATHOLOGIC FEATURES	
Gross findings	Cricoid cartilage mass, posterior plate, midline mass
	Mean, 3.5 cm
	Hard, crunchy, lobular, glistening with myxoid-mucinous matrix
Microscopic findings	Bone invasion (ossification centers within cartilage)
	Increased cellularity
	Loss of normal architecture and distribution (cluster disarray)
	Nuclear atypia with bi- and multinucleation
	Increased nuclear to cytoplasmic ratio
	Basophilic to metachromatic cartilaginous matrix
	Mitotic figures and necrosis only in high grade tumors
Pathologic differential diagnosis	Chondroma and chondrometaplasia

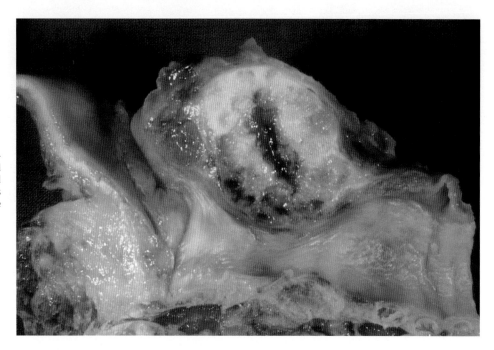

FIGURE 3-42
This macroscopic laryngectomy specimen shows a thin rim of bone invaded by the chondrosarcoma of the cricoid cartilage. A firm, lobular growth is noted, with central degenerative change.

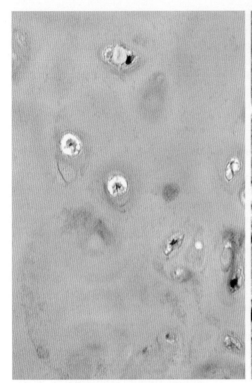
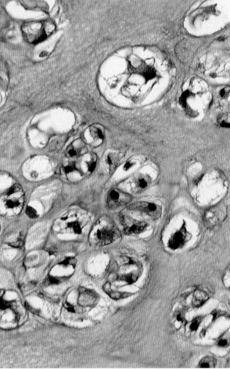

FIGURE 3-43

Left: Normal cartilage cellularity and lacunar size. *Right:* A chondrosarcoma has increased cellularity, pleomorphism and increased nuclear size.

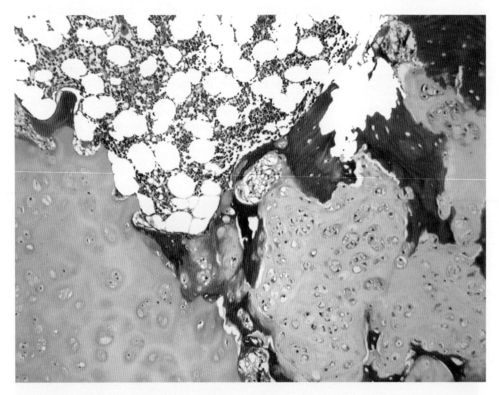

FIGURE 3-44

Hyaline cartilage with enchondral ossification is seen (*lower left*) immediately adjacent to the invasive component of a low-grade (grade I) chondrosarcoma (*lower right*). Normal bone marrow elements are noted in the upper portion of the field.

Chondrosarcomas are separated into grades based on increasing degrees of the aforementioned criteria. The vast majority (about 65%) are well differentiated (low-grade, grade I; Fig. 3-45), followed by moderately differentiated (intermediate-grade, grade II; 30%; Fig. 3-46), and poorly differentiated (high-grade, grade III; 5%; Fig. 3-46) neoplasms. In the larynx, the grade does not seem to affect the overall patient outcome. The vast majority of tumors are chondrocytic chondrosarcomas, but myxoid and dedifferentiated chondrosarcoma are described. Immunohistochemistry is unnecessary, although the tumor cells will be S-100 protein and vimentin immunoreactive.

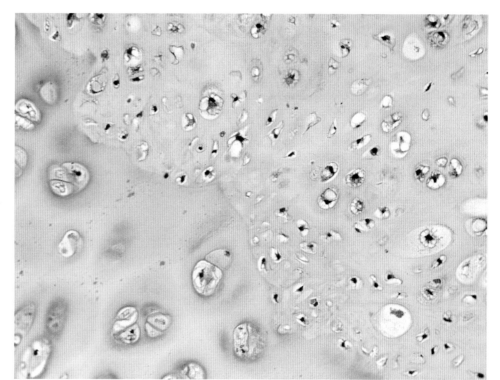

FIGURE 13-45

The lower left portion of the illustration demonstrates normal hyaline cartilage abutted by a grade I chondrosarcoma (*upper* and *right* side). Sampling is critical to accurate diagnosis of laryngeal cartilaginous neoplasms.

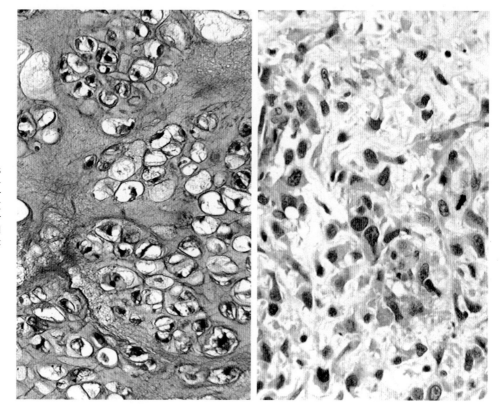

FIGURE 3-46

Left: A grade II chondrosarcoma has moderate cellularity with binucleation, nuclear atypia and nuclear hyperchromasia. *Right:* A grade III chondrosarcoma has marked nuclear pleomorphism, multinucleation and hyperchromatic nuclei. Mitotic figures are noted.

DIFFERENTIAL DIAGNOSIS

The differential diagnosis is limited in practical terms to chondroma and chondrometaplasia. In general, true laryngeal chondromas are considered exceedingly rare, and a number of authors consider all laryngeal chondromas to be erroneous descriptions of low-grade chondrosarcomas. Given the frequent association of chondroma with chondrosarcoma, it is quite possible that "biopsy" material does not sample the malignant component. Therefore, adequate tumor sampling (large biopsy) is critical to the accurate identification of tumor type and grade. While size alone is inaccurate in classification, tumors >3 cm are more likely to be chondrosarcomas. The microscopic separation of chondroma from chondrosarcoma can be a very difficult one, with chondromas containing slightly enlarged, albeit uniform nuclei with only slight architectural disorder. In practical terms, any recurrent cartilaginous tumor of the larynx should be considered a chondrosarcoma.

Chondrometaplasia of the larynx consists of elastic rich cartilage nodules usually located on the vocal cords, usually <1 cm, containing small, uniform chondrocytes without nuclear abnormalities. The margins of the lesions are indistinct with a peripheral zone of transition between the cartilage and the surrounding tissues. Multifocality can sometimes be confused for recurrence.

PROGNOSIS AND THERAPY

Laryngeal chondrosarcoma are considered low-grade neoplasms. Conservative, larynx function preserving surgery is the treatment of choice. When recurrences develop (in up to 40% of patients), wide excision can again be employed, depending on the extent of the tumor, until functional compromise and the inability to reconstruct an adequate airway dictates the necessity for total laryngectomy. The voice-preserving surgeries allow for an improved quality of life and for a longer morbidity-free survival which does not adversely impact the long-term patient survival.

Overall, there is a >95% survival with a mean follow-up of >10 years. Death from disease is very uncommon and is usually the result of uncontrolled local growth into vital structures of the neck. The presence of the myxoid subtype (>10% of the tumor volume) and age >60 years at initial presentation has been reported to portend a worse patient outcome. A higher grade tumor seems to suggest an increased chance of developing metastatic disease but not of dying from disease.

SYNOVIAL SARCOMA

Classifying soft tissue tumors of the larynx is often difficult for both surgeon and pathologist because of the potential similarities in appearance of epithelial tumors,

SYNOVIAL SARCOMA DISEASE FACT SHEET	
Definition	A high-grade mesenchymal spindle cell neoplasm with epithelial differentiation and a specific t(X;18) chromosomal translocation
Incidence and location	<1% of laryngeal neoplasms; about 5% of synovial sarcoma occur in the head and neck
	Hypopharynx
Morbidity and mortality	Variable, but generally <50% 5-yr survival
Gender, race, and age distribution	Young adults
	No gender bias
Clinical features	Progressive dysphagia, intermittent hoarseness, and airway compromise
Radiologic features	CT/MRI delineates tumor extent and site of origin
	Nonmucosal, heterogeneous septated mass with cysts and calcifications
Prognosis and treatment	Frequent recurrences (up to 80%)
	Multimodality therapy (wide surgical excision, radiation, chemotherapy)

metastatic lesions, and inflammatory processes. Up to 10% of synovial sarcomas (SS) arise in the head and neck, but primary SS of the larynx and hypopharynx is rare, while secondary involvement by direct extension from the neck is slightly more common.

CLINICAL FEATURES

Young adults (15–40 years) are usually affected although all ages can be affected, without a gender bias. Symptoms are nonspecific and include progressive dysphagia, intermittent hoarseness, deglutition difficulties, and gradual airway compromise. Radiographic studies (CT or MRI) are valuable in delineating tumor extent and site of origin, while a nonmucosal, heterogeneous, septated mass with cysts and calcifications may suggest the possibility of a synovial sarcoma.

PATHOLOGIC FEATURES

GROSS FINDINGS

The tumor mass is usually poorly circumscribed or partially encapsulated, with surface lobulation or bosselation in a submucosal location, most frequent in the retropharynx or hypopharynx and arytenoid, measuring up to 10 cm in size. The tumor may be exophytic or pedunculated, occasionally demonstrating surface ulceration. The cut surface is yellow, gray-white with a firm, gritty and friable, to soft, boggy and rubbery consistency, occasionally revealing areas of cystic, mucoid or hemorrhagic degeneration.

MICROSCOPIC FINDINGS

Arising from a pluripotential mesenchymal stem cell rather than mature synovial tissues, SS are high-grade neoplasms that express epithelial as well as supporting tissue features and are separated into monophasic and biphasic variants. In biphasic form, there is a mes-enchymal spindle component and a glandular epithelioid constituent, in variable proportions (Fig. 3-47). The monophasic variant will only have a spindle *or* epithelioid component. The spindle cells are arranged in orderly, densely packed, short interlacing fascicles of uniform plump cells. The cells contain oval to spindle, vesicular to hyperchromatic nuclei and scant cytoplasm with indistinct cellular boundaries. The epithelioid cells are cuboidal to columnar arranged in gland-like spaces, cords, and nests. There is abundant pale cytoplasm surrounding round to oval vesicular nuclei, with distinct cell membranes (Fig. 3-48). Mitotic activity is easily identified although not excessive. Mast cells and rarely calcifications may be seen in the spindle cell regions, more easily recognized in hypocellular foci or in areas of myxoid change or necrosis. A rich vascularity is often present. There is usually little collagen deposition.

SYNOVIAL SARCOMA PATHOLOGIC FEATURES	
Gross findings	Submucosal mass of considerable size
	Exophytic and pedunculated
	Yellow, gray-white, gritty, and occasionally cystic
Microscopic findings	Biphasic or monophasic variants
	Spindle cells arranged in densely cellular short interlacing fascicles of plump spindle cells
	Vesicular to hyperchromatic nuclei with indistinct cell borders
	Epithelioid cells are cuboidal or columnar arranged in gland-like spaces, cords or nests; distinct cell borders
	Mitotic figures are easily identified
	Mast cells common
	Calcifications may be seen
Immunohistochemical features	Epithelial and spindle cells will be keratin and epithelial membrane antigen reactive (although spindle cells may be focal and weak)
	Spindle cells are vimentin reactive
Molecular studies	t(X;18)(p11.2;q11.2) reciprocal chromosomal translocation
Pathologic differential diagnosis	SCSCC, mucosal malignant melanoma, malignant peripheral nerve sheath tumor

ANCILLARY STUDIES

ULTRASTRUCTURAL FEATURES

Electron microscopy will demonstrate glandular differentiation with microvilli, intercellular junctions, tonofilaments, and an intact basal lamina in the glandular portions, while the spindle cells demonstrate poorly formed rudimentary cellular junctions, non-branching cytoplasm, intermediate filaments and perhaps focal short cell processes surrounded by an external lamina.

IMMUNOHISTOCHEMICAL FEATURES

The epithelial and spindle cells will react with cytokeratin and EMA, while only the spindle cells will react with vimentin. Due to staining variability, both epithe-

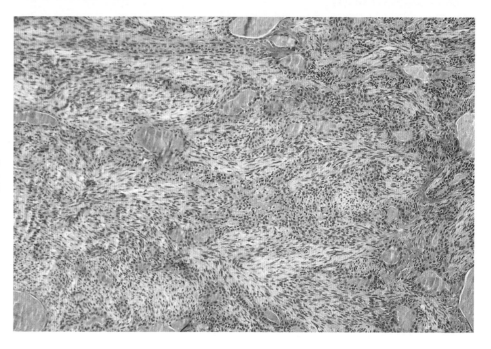

FIGURE 3-47

The intermingled of the glandular type epithelium with the spindle cell component is classic for a biphasic synovial sarcoma.

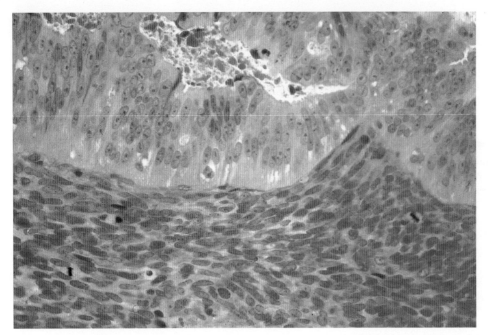

FIGURE 3-48
The epithelial component is well differentiated, arranged in a pseudostratified configuration. The spindle cell component is hypercellular with numerous mitotic figures and mild nuclear pleomorphism.

lial markers should be performed to help confirm the diagnosis, as the spindle cells may only show focal and weak epithelial reactivity.

HISTOCHEMICAL

Mucicarmine positive and diastase-resistant, periodic acid Schiff-positive *epithelial* mucin can be seen within the cytoplasm of the epithelial cells, within the glandular lumens and in intracellular areas, while hyaluronidase-sensitive alcian blue and colloidal iron *mesenchymal* mucin can be identified in the spindle cell and myxoid areas.

OTHER ANCILLARY STUDIES

By reverse transcriptase polymerase chain reaction or interphase fluorescence in situ hybridization, molecular studies reveal a characteristic reciprocal translocation t(X;18)(p11.2;q11.2) between chromosomes X and 18 which can confirm the diagnosis.

DIFFERENTIAL DIAGNOSIS

The biphasic tumor presents a unique differential diagnosis within the larynx specifically, and includes SCSCC, mucosal malignant melanoma, and rarely, malignant peripheral nerve sheath tumors (MPNST). An SCSCC will frequently demonstrate an in situ or invasive SCC in addition to the spindled component and will not have a glandular configuration. SCSCCs are infrequent in the hypopharynx. Molecular studies will cinch the diagnosis. Malignant melanoma will usually have a more epithelioid appearance with prominent

eosinophilic nucleoli, may have overlying surface mucosal (junctional) involvement, and will be reactive with S-100 protein and/or HMB45. MPNST may have a similar growth pattern, but will have nuclei with are more wrinkled and hyperchromatic and perhaps nuclear palisading. MPNST are usually S-100 positive and negative with epithelial markers, and EM will demonstrate the interdigitating processes indicating Schwann cell derivation. All of these tumor types (SS, malignant melanoma, MPNST) are extraordinarily rare in this location, with SCSCC much more likely.

PROGNOSIS AND THERAPY

The prognosis is variable and tends to be better than tumors arising in soft tissue. The inability to achieve adequate tumor-free surgical margins within the anatomic confines of the larynx and hypopharynx make recurrences more difficult to manage. SS are known to metastasize late, with limited survival after metastasis. Aggressive multimodality therapy with wide surgical excision, radiation and chemotherapy seems to achieve the best long-term patient outcome.

SUGGESTED READING

Precursor Lesions

1. Crissman JD, Zarbo RJ: Dysplasia, in situ carcinoma, and progression to invasive squamous cell carcinoma of the upper aerodigestive tract. Am J Surg Pathol 1989;13 (Suppl 1):5–16.
2. Devaney KO, Rinaldo A, Zeitels SM, Bradley PJ, Ferlito A: Laryngeal dysplasia and other epithelial changes on endoscopic biopsy: what does it all mean to the individual patient? ORL J Otorhinolaryngol Relat Spec 2004;66:1–4.

3. Gale N, Pilch BZ, Sidransky D, Westra WH, Califano J. Epithelial precursor lesions. In: Barnes EL, Eveson JW, Reichart P, Sidransky D, eds. Pathology and Genetics of Head and Neck Tumours. Kleihues P, Sobin LH, series eds. World Health Organization Classification of Tumours. Lyon, France: IARC Press, 2005:140–143.

4. Hellquist H, Lundgren J, Olofsson J: Hyperplasia, keratosis, dysplasia and carcinoma in situ of the vocal cords—a follow-up study. Clin Otolaryngol 1982;7:11–27.

5. Sanz-Ortega J, Valor C, Saez MC, Ortega L, Sierra E, Poch J, Hernandez S, Sanz-Esponera J: 3p21, 5q21, 9p21 and 17p13 allelic deletions accumulate in the dysplastic spectrum of laryngeal carcinogenesis and precede malignant transformation. Histol Histopathol 2003;18: 1053–1057.

6. Sengiz S, Pabuccuoglu U, Sarioglu S: Immunohistological comparison of the World Health Organization (WHO) and Ljubljana classifications on the grading of preneoplastic lesions of the larynx. Pathol Res Pract 2004;200:181–188.

Squamous Cell Carcinoma and Variants

1. Barnes L: Diseases of the larynx, hypopharynx, and esophagus. In: Barnes L. Surgical Pathology of the Head and Neck, 2nd ed. New York: Marcel Dekker, 2001:127–237.

2. Barnes L, Ferlito A, Altavilla G, MacMillan C, Rinaldo A, Doglioni C: Basaloid squamous cell carcinoma of the head and neck: clinicopathological features and differential diagnosis. Ann Otol Rhinol Laryngol 1996;105:75–82.

3. Batsakis JG, Hybels R, Crissman JD, Rice DH: The pathology of head and neck tumors: verrucous carcinoma, Part 15. Head Neck Surg 1982;5:29–38.

4. Cardesa A, Gale N, Nadal A, Zidar N. Squamous cell carcinoma. In: Barnes EL, Eveson JW, Reichart P, Sidransky D, eds. Pathology and Genetics of Head and Neck Tumours. Kleihues P, Sobin LH, series eds. World Health Organization Classification of Tumours. Lyon, France: IARC Press, 2005:118–121.

5. Cardesa A, Zidar N. Verrucous carcinoma. In: Barnes EL, Eveson JW, Reichart P, Sidransky D, eds. Pathology and Genetics of the Head and Neck Tumours. Kleihues P, Sobin LH, series eds. World Health Organization Classification of Tumours. Lyon, France: IARC Press, 2005:122–123.

6. Cardesa A, Zidar N, Ereño C. Basaloid squamous cell carcinoma. In: Barnes EL, Eveson JW, Reichart P, Sidransky D, eds. Pathology and Genetics of Head and Neck Tumours. Kleihues P, Sobin LH, series eds. World Health Organization Classification of Tumours. Lyon, France: IARC Press, 2005:124–125.

7. Cardesa A, Zidar N, Nadal A, Ereño C. Papillary squamous cell carcinoma. In: Barnes EL, Eveson JW, Reichart P, Sidransky D, eds. Pathology and Genetics of Head and Neck Tumours. Kleihues P, Sobin LH, series eds. World Health Organization Classification of Tumours. Lyon, France: IARC Press, 2005:126.

8. Cardesa A, Zidar N. Spindle cell carcinoma. In: Barnes EL, Eveson JW, Reichart P, Sidransky D, eds. Pathology and Genetics of Head and Neck Tumours. Kleihues P, Sobin LH, series eds. World Health Organization Classification of Tumours. Lyon, France: IARC Press, 2005:127–128.

9. Cardesa A, Zidar N, Alos L. Adenosquamous carcinoma. In: Barnes EL, Eveson JW, Reichart P, Sidransky D, eds. Pathology and Genetics of Head and Neck Tumours. Kleihues P, Sobin LH, series eds. World Health Organization Classification of Tumours. Lyon, France: IARC Press, 2005:130–131.

10. Crissman JD, Kessis T, Shah KV, et al.: Squamous papillary neoplasia of the adult upper aerodigestive tract. Hum Pathol 1988;19: 1387–1396.

11. Crissman JD, Zarbo RJ, Drozdowicz S, et al.: Carcinoma in situ and microinvasive squamous carcinoma of the laryngeal glottis. Arch Otolaryngol Head Neck Surg 1988;114:299–307.

12. Damiani JM, Damiani KK, Hauck K, Hyams VJ: Mucoepidermoid-adenosquamous carcinoma of the larynx and hypopharynx: a report of 21 cases and a review of the literature. Otolaryngol Head Neck Surg 1981;89:235–243.

13. Ferlito A, Recher G: Ackerman's tumor (verrucous carcinoma) of the larynx: a clinicopathologic study of 77 cases. Cancer 1980;46: 1617–1630.

14. Franceschi S, Talamini R, Barra S, et al.: Smoking and drinking in relation to cancers of the oral cavity, pharynx, larynx, and esophagus in northern Italy. Cancer Res 1990;50:6502–6507.

15. Gillison ML, Koch WM, Capone RB, et al.: Evidence for a causal association between human papillomavirus and a subset of head and neck cancers. J Natl Cancer Inst 2000;92:709–720.

16. Keelawat S, Liu CZ, Roehm PC, Barnes L: Adenosquamous carcinoma of the upper aerodigestive tract: a clinicopathologic study of 12 cases and review of the literature. Am J Otolaryngol 2002;23:160–168.

17. Koch BB, Trask DK, Hoffman HT, et al.: National survey of head and neck verrucous carcinoma: patterns of presentation, care, and outcome. Cancer 2001;92:110–120.

18. Lewis JE, Olsen KD, Sebo TJ: Spindle cell carcinoma of the larynx: review of 26 cases including DNA content and immunohistochemistry. Hum Pathol 1997;28:664–673.

19. Morice WG, Ferreiro JA: Distinction of basaloid squamous cell carcinoma from adenoid cystic and small cell undifferentiated carcinoma by immunohistochemistry. Hum Pathol 1998;29:609–612.

20. Nappi O, Wick MR: Sarcomatoid neoplasms of the respiratory tract. Semin Diagn Pathol 1993;10:137–147.

21. Suarez PA, Adler-Storthz K, Luna MA, et al.: Papillary squamous cell carcinomas of the upper aerodigestive tract: a clinicopathologic and molecular study. Head Neck 2000;22:360–368.

22. Thompson LD, Wenig BM, Heffner DK, Gnepp DR: Exophytic and papillary squamous cell carcinomas of the larynx: a clinicopathologic series of 104 cases. Otolaryngol Head Neck Surg 1999;120:718–724.

23. Thompson LD, Wieneke JA, Miettinen M, Heffner DK: Spindle cell (sarcomatoid) carcinomas of the larynx: a clinicopathologic study of 187 cases. Am J Surg Pathol 2002;26:153–170.

24. Vokes EE, Weichselbaum RR, Lippman SM, Hong WK: Head and neck cancer. N Engl J Med 1993;328:184–194.

25. Wu M, Putti TC, Bhuiya TA: Comparative study in the expression of p53, EGFR, TGF-alpha, and cyclin D1 in verrucous carcinoma, verrucous hyperplasia, and squamous cell carcinoma of head and neck region. Appl Immunohistochem Mol Morphol 2002;10:351–356.

Neuroendocrine Carcinoma

1. Barnes L. Neuroendocrine tumours. In: Barnes EL, Eveson JW, Reichart P, Sidransky D, eds. Pathology and Genetics of Head and Neck Tumours. Kleihues P, Sobin LH, series eds. World Health Organization Classification of Tumours. Lyon, France: IARC Press, 2005:135–139.

2. El-Naggar AK, Batsakis JG: Carcinoid tumor of the larynx. A critical review of the literature. ORL J Otorhinolaryngol Relat Spec 1991;53:188–193.

3. Ferlito A, Shaha AR, Rinaldo A: Neuroendocrine neoplasms of the larynx: diagnosis, treatment and prognosis. ORL J Otorhinolaryngol Relat Spec 2002;64:108–113.

4. Ferlito A, Barnes L, Rinaldo A, et al.: A review of neuroendocrine neoplasms of the larynx: update on diagnosis and treatment. J Laryngol Otol 1998;112:827–834.

5. Mills SE: Neuroectodermal neoplasms of the head and neck with emphasis on neuroendocrine carcinomas. Mod Pathol 2002;15:264–278.

6. Rinaldo A, Devaney KO, Ferlito A: Immunohistochemical studies in support of a diagnosis of small cell neuroendocrine carcinoma of the larynx. Acta Otolaryngol 2004;124:638–641.

7. Wenig BM, Gnepp DR: The spectrum of neuroendocrine carcinomas of the larynx. Sem Diag Pathol 1989;6:329–350.

8. Wenig BM, Hyams VJ, Heffner DK: Moderately differentiated neuroendocrine carcinoma of the larynx. A clinico-pathologic study of 54 cases. Cancer 1988;62:2658–2676.

Chondrosarcoma

1. Chiu LD, Rasgon BM: Laryngeal chondroma: a benign process with long-term clinical implications. Ear Nose Throat J 1996;75:540–549.

2. Garcia RE, Thompson LDR, Gannon FH: Dedifferentiated chondrosarcomas of the larynx: a report of two cases and review of the literature. Laryngoscope 2002;112:1015–1018.

3. Lewis JE, Olsen KD, Inwards CY: Cartilaginous tumors of the larynx: clinicopathological review of 47 cases. Ann Otol Rhinol Laryngol 1997;106:94–100.

4. Rinaldo A, Howard DJ, Ferlito A: Laryngeal chondrosarcoma: a 24-year experience at the Royal National Throat, Nose and Ear Hospital. Acta Otolaryngol 2000;120:680–688.

5. Thompson LDR, Gannon FH: Chondrosarcoma of the larynx: a clinico-pathologic study of 111 cases. Am J Surg Pathol 2002;26:836–851.

6. Tiwari R, Mahieu H, Snow G: Long-term results of organ preservation in chondrosarcoma of the cricoid. Eur Arch Otorhinolaryngol 1999;256: 271–276.

Synovial Sarcoma

1. Dei Tos AP, Dal Cin P, Sciot R, et al.: Synovial sarcoma of the larynx and hypopharynx. Ann Otol Rhinol Laryngol 1998;107:1080–1085.
2. Ferlito A, Caruso G: Endolaryngeal synovial sarcoma. An update on diagnosis and treatment. ORL J Otorhinolaryngol Relat Spec 1991;53: 116–119.
3. Hirsch RJ, Yousem DM, Loevner LA, et al.: Synovial sarcomas of the head and neck: MR findings. AJR Am J Roentgenol 1997;169: 1185–1188.
4. Roth JA, Enzinger FM, Tannenbaum M: Synovial sarcoma of the neck: a follow-up study of 24 cases. Cancer 1975;35:1243–1253.
5. Thompson LDR, Fanburg-Smith JC. Malignant soft tissue tumours. In: Barnes EL, Eveson JW, Reichart P, Sidransky D, eds. Pathology and Genetics of Head and Neck Tumours. Kleihues P, Sobin LH, series eds. World Health Organization Classification of Tumours. Lyon, France: IARC Press, 2005:147–149.

4

Non-Neoplastic Lesions of the Nasal Cavity, Paranasal Sinuses, and Nasopharynx

Margaret Brandwein-Gensler • Lester D. R. Thompson

SINONASAL POLYPS

CLINICAL FEATURES

Sinonasal polyps have a multitude of etiologies: allergy, vasomotor rhinitis, infectious rhinosinusitis, diabetes mellitus, cystic fibrosis, aspirin intolerance, and nickel exposure. However, they are most frequently the result of repeated bouts of sinusitis. They result by an influx of fluids into the Schneiderian mucosal lamina propria. Occasionally, antral (maxillary) polyps may expand and prolapse through sinus ostia, presenting intranasal, or

in the nasopharynx. These are referred to as antrochoanal polyps, and represent 4% to 6% of all sinonasal polyps. Angiomatous polyps are vascularized nasal choanal polyps that have been traumatized, often associated with fibrosis.

Between 10% and 20% of children with cystic fibrosis have nasal polyps. Generally, nasal polyps in children are uncommon, and 29% of such polyps in children are associated with cystic fibrosis. Nasal polyps may be also associated with aspirin intolerance and bronchial asthma (Sampter's triad). About 20% of patients with nasal polyps have asthma, and conversely about 30% of asthmatic patients have polyps. In general there is no specific age or gender findings, although children are uncommonly affected (unless they have cystic fibrosis). Patients will present with rhinorrhea, stuffiness, nasal discharge, headaches, sinusitis, and other nonspecific symptoms referable to the sinonasal tract.

RADIOLOGIC FEATURES

Sinonasal polyps may appear as solitary or multiple expansile masses within the nasal cavity and or paranasal sinuses. Mucous retention, or thickened mucosa within the affected sinus can be seen. If the ethmoid complex is involved, the ethmoid complex is widened but the delicate ethmoid septae are not destroyed. By distinction, a solid tumor (either benign or malignant) in this area will destroy the ethmoid septae. Angiomatous polyps are usually in the nasal fossae. On angiography, these polyps have only a few demonstrable feeding vessels as compared with the rich vascular supply of a nasopharyngeal angiofibroma.

PATHOLOGIC FEATURES

GROSS FINDINGS

Sinonasal polyps are usually smooth, glistening and translucent, gray pink in color. Antrochoanal polyps are firmer and not translucent.

SINONASAL POLYPS DISEASE FACT SHEET	
Definition	Multifactorial etiologies resulting in expansion of the lamina propria by fluids, protein, and fibrosis
Incidence and location	Uncommon sinonasal tract lesion
	Nasal cavity, paranasal sinuses (maxilla and ethmoids)
Morbidity and mortality	Bone destruction may lead to facial dysmorphia
Gender, race, and age distribution	Equal gender distribution
	Wide age distribution, but uncommon in children (raise the possibility of cystic fibrosis if in a child)
Clinical features	Rhinorrhea
	Nasal stuffiness, obstruction, and rarely anosmia
	Chronic headache
	Etiologies are legion, but include allergy, infection, diabetes, aspirin sensitivity, asthma, cystic fibrosis, nickel exposure
Prognosis and treatment	Prognosis is excellent, although management of underlying etiology is considered best treatment
	Conservative endoscopic removal and improved sinus ventilation

MICROSCOPIC FINDINGS

Typical sinonasal polyps contain a moderate degree of chronic inflammation within the lamina propria (Fig. 4-1). The mucoserous glands are present, and

SINONASAL POLYPS PATHOLOGIC FEATURES	
Gross findings	Smooth, glistening, gelatinous, translucent
	Antrochoanal polyp have a narrow stalk, firm, nontranslucent
Microscopic findings	Mucosa may be metaplastic, but is usually intact
	Edematous lamina propria with lymphoplasmacytic infiltrate, with occasional eosinophils (depends on etiology)
	Mucoserous glands may have goblet cell metaplasia
	May have "stromal atypia" in myofibroblastic cells
	Antrochoanal polyps are fibrotic with reduced or absent glands
	Pseudoangiomatous change, infarction, organization, and secondary infections may result
Pathologic differential diagnosis	Chronic sinusitis, Schneiderian papilloma (inverted type specifically), rhabdomyosarcoma, nasopharyngeal angiofibroma, allergic fungal sinusitis, lymphoma

may demonstrate goblet cell hyperplasia (Fig. 4-2). If the polyps are allergic in nature, then a prominent eosinophilic infiltrate is seen. Stalk torsion can result in dispersed, single, bizarre reactive fibroblasts within the lamina propria, so-called "stromal atypia" (Fig. 4-3). Antrochoanal polyps are fibrotic, and the underlying mucoserous glands are diminished or absent (Fig. 4-4). Pseudoangiomatous (lymphangiomatous) polyps contain proliferating thin-walled vessels in a loose, edematous to myxoid matrix (Fig. 4-5). Polyps of all types may undergo infarction, organization or secondary infection, sometimes giving rise to difficulties in diagnosis (Fig. 4-6). Polyps may co-exist with other sinonasal tract disorders, which should be carefully excluded.

DIFFERENTIAL DIAGNOSIS

Chronic sinusitis may give slightly edematous change in the stroma, but usually do not present as polypoid fragments of tissue. Schneiderian papillomas may be polypoid, but the proliferation of a transitional/respiratory epithelium and usually inverted growth separate these lesions from polyps. Rhabdomyosarcoma tends to be more cellular, with a layering or aggregation of atypical spindle cells. Muscle markers (myogenin, myo-D1, myoglobin, desmin) will also help to separate these lesions. Nasopharyngeal angiofibroma has variable sized vessels within the stroma, which also contains a collagen deposition and stellate stromal cells. There is also a difference in anatomic site. Polyps may become secondarily

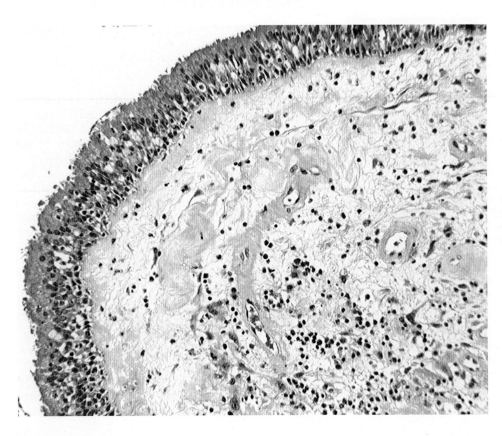

FIGURE 4-1

This polyp has an inflammatory infiltrate and a loose connective tissue stroma.

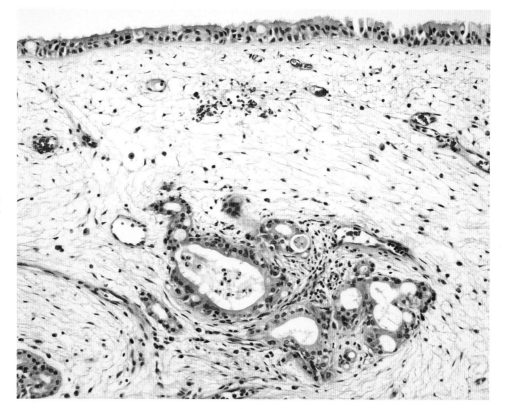

FIGURE 4-2

Seromucus glands are noted with chronic inflammation and an edematous stroma.

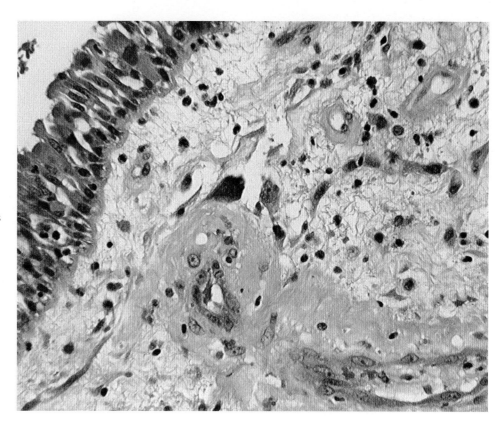

FIGURE 4-3

Atypical, single, myofibroblastic cells can be seen in polyps.

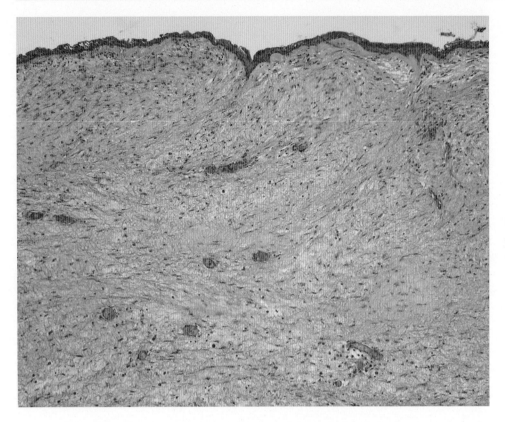

FIGURE 4-4
An antrochoanal polyp is heavily fibrotic and has decreased to absent mucoserous glands.

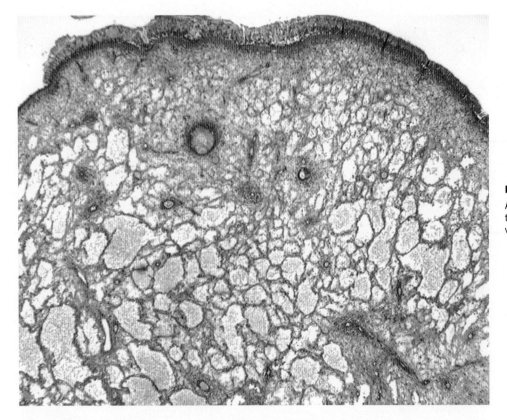

FIGURE 4-5
A pseudoangiomatous appearance in this polyp with multiple, dilated vascular channels.

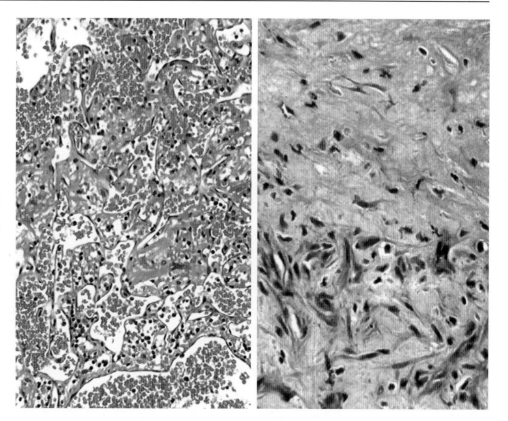

FIGURE 4-6

Left: An infarcted polyp undergoing organization with rich vascular ingrowth. *Right:* Fibrosis with reactive and atypia stroma myofibroblasts associated with a postinfarct.

infected, but if there is a heavy acute inflammatory infiltrate or allergic mucin, infectious agents must be excluded. Lymphomas within the sinonasal tract contain an atypical population of lymphoid cells and will show immunophenotypic restriction.

PROGNOSIS AND THERAPY

The prognosis is excellent, as these are benign reactive lesions. However, removal of the underlying etiologic agent, if known, results in significantly reduced morbidity. Polyps are usually amenable to conservative endoscopic removal and improved sinus ventilation.

NASAL GLIAL HETEROTOPIA

Nasal glial heterotopia (NGH) are congenital malformations of displaced normal, mature glial tissue (choristomas); continuity with the intracranial meningeal component has become obliterated. The term NGH is preferred to "glioma" which implies a tumor. By contrast, an encephalocele represents herniation of brain tissue and leptomeninges through a bony defect of the skull; continuity with the cranial cavity is maintained.

CLINICAL FEATURES

NGH most frequently presents during infancy, but occasionally may be identified in older children and adults. Most cases present as small, firm subcutaneous nodules at or near the bridge of the nose in children or infants.

NASAL GLIAL HETEROTOPIA DISEASE FACT SHEET	
Definition	Nasal glial heterotopia (NGH) are congenital malformations of displaced normal, mature glial tissue without an intracranial connection
Incidence and location	Uncommon lesions
	Location: extranasal (60%), intranasal (30%), mixed (10%)
Morbidity and mortality	If an encephalocele, meningitis and a CSF leak may develop
Gender, race, and age distribution	Equal gender distribution
	Most frequent during infancy, rare in adults
Clinical features	Mass, often over the glabella/nasal bridge
	Nasal obstruction
	Chronic sinusitis and nasal drainage
	Otitis media
Radiographic findings	Sharply demarcated mass without any identifiable intracranial connection
Prognosis and treatment	Excellent prognosis, although up to 30% may "recur" if incompletely excised

These are classified as extranasal NGH, and constitute the majority (60%) of NGH. Approximately 10% NGH are mixed, with subcutaneous and intranasal components. Lastly, approximately 30% NGH are intranasal, and manifest as polypoid lesions within the superior nasal cavity (Fig. 4-7). Patients present with nasal obstruction, along with nasal polyps, chronic sinusitis, nasal drainage, and chronic otitis media. It is important to obtain radiographic studies before biopsy to make certain continuity with the central nervous system is not present in order to avoid complications. The presence of meningitis and/or cerebrospinal fluid (CSF) rhinorrhea either before or after surgical manipulation may suggest encephalocele instead.

RADIOLOGIC FEATURES

NGH forms a sharply demarcated, expansile mass, either extranasally, or in the superior nasal cavity (Fig. 4-8). An intracerebral extension, seen as a tract, or cribriform plate defect, needs be ruled out. If an intracerebral communication, in particular a CSF communication is found, the lesion is better classified as an encephalocele. Even with high-resolution computed tomography scans and magnetic resonance imaging, the connection may be small and inapparent.

PATHOLOGIC FEATURES

GROSS FINDINGS

These tumors have a smooth, homogeneous, glistening cut surface, similar to brain tissue. They may be firm, due to a fibrous tissue component.

MICROSCOPIC FINDINGS

NGH resembles gliosis. The glial tissue is blended with fibrosis, often below an intact skin or surface mucosa (Fig. 4-9). It is composed of nests and masses of fibrillar neuroglial tissue with a prominent network of

NASAL GLIAL HETEROTOPIA PATHOLOGIC FEATURES	
Gross findings	Smooth, homogeneous, glistening cut surface
	Can be firm if there is extensive fibrosis
	Polyp if within the nasal cavity
Microscopic findings	NGH resemble gliosis
	Glial tissue blended with fibrosis below intact surface
	Astrocytic cells may show gemistocytic change
	Encephaloceles appear identical to normal brain tissue, but degeneration may result in loss of neurons
Ancillary studies	Trichrome highlights glial tissue red (fibrosis is blue)
	S-100 protein, GFAP react with glial tissue
Pathologic differential diagnosis	Encephalocele and fibrosed nasal polyp

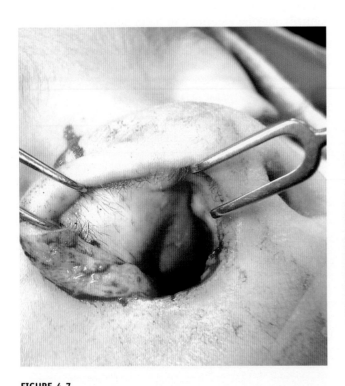

FIGURE 4-7
Nasal glial heterotopia can present as purely intranasal polyp.

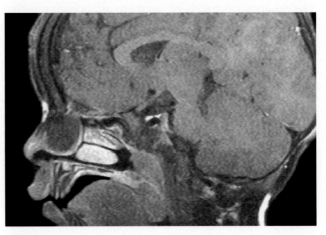

FIGURE 4-8
Sagittal T1-weighted, fat suppressed MRI of an anterior nasal fossa nasal glial heterotopia that comes up to the anterior skull base, but which has no intracranial component. There is no caudal distortion of the undersurface of the frontal lobe.

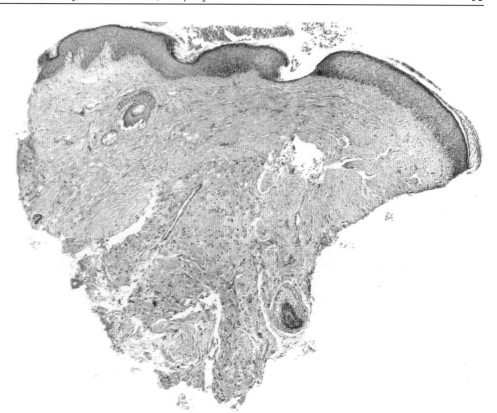

FIGURE 4-9

An intact skin overlies a proliferation of glial tissue and fibrosis. Note the intact adnexal structures.

glial fibers. Astrocytic cells may show gemistocytic changes (Fig. 4-10). Neuronal cells are rarely identified (10%). Choroid plexus, ependymal cells, and pigmented cells with retinal differentiation have rarely been reported. It is imperative to stress that the fibrosis may obscure the glial tissue (Fig. 4-11), often requiring special studies to separate the constituent parts. Encephaloceles appear identical to normal brain tissue,

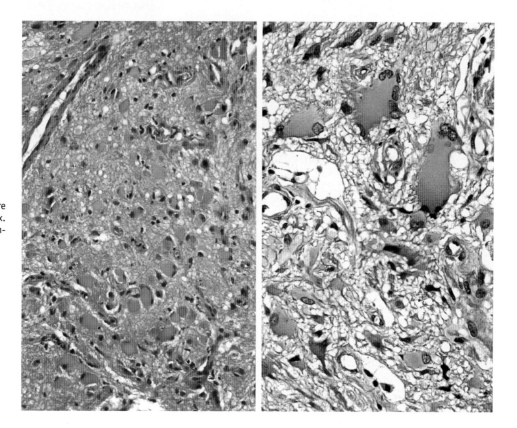

FIGURE 4-10

Left: Gemistocytic astrocytes are noted within a fibrillar neural matrix. *Right:* Ganglion-like cells with abundant neural matrix.

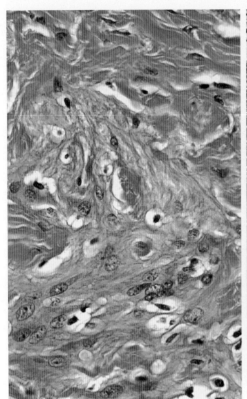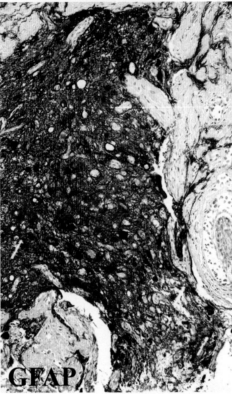

FIGURE 4-11
Left: Heavy fibrosis may sometimes obscure the more delicate glial tissues. *Right:* GFAP strongly and diffusely highlights the glial matrix.

but degeneration may result in loss of neurons. In such cases, distinction from NGH requires radiographic and clinical correlation.

ANCILLARY STUDIES

Trichrome will yield a separation of fibrous connective tissue from the glial tissue with glial tissue staining bright red and fibrosis staining blue. The glial tissues will reactive strongly and diffusely with glial fibrillary acidic protein (GFAP) (Fig. 4-11) and S-100 protein.

DIFFERENTIAL DIAGNOSIS

Separation of encephalocele and fibrosed nasal polyp are the most common considerations. The large astrocytic cells may be misinterpreted as histiocytes, but immunohistochemical expression of GFAP is diagnostic for glial cells. The diagnosis of a polyp can be made when no neural tissue is identified.

PROGNOSIS AND THERAPY

If there is adequate excision, the patients are cured, but recurrence may develop (up to 30%) if incompletely excised.

ALLERGIC FUNGAL SINUSITIS (EOSINOPHILIC FUNGAL RHINOSINUSITIS)

CLINICAL FEATURES

Fungi are much more common in chronic rhinosinusitis than previously appreciated, as almost everyone has commensal fungi in their nose. Allergic fungal sinusitis (AFS) is thought to be an allergic reaction initiated by ubiquitous fungal allergens, perpetuated and amplified by eosinophils. Patients usually have peripheral eosinophilia and elevated immunoglobulin (Ig)E to fungal antigens. The inflammation and secretions can cause an expansile mass, akin to mycetoma or mucocele (Fig. 4-12). In extreme cases, the mass effect can progress to cause facial dysmorphia and visual distur-

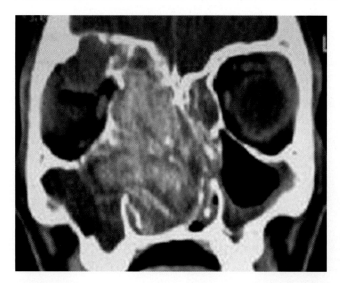

FIGURE 4-12
The radiographic image of a destructive expansile mass sometimes seen in allergic fungal sinusitis may mimic that of a neoplasm.

ALLERGIC FUNGAL SINUSITIS PATHOLOGIC FEATURES	
Gross findings	Secretions described as putty-like, peanut-butter-like, muddy
Microscopic findings	Alternating "tide-lines," waves, or ripples of mucin with degenerated debris, eosinophils, polymorphonuclear cells
	Charcot-Leyden crystals may be present (degenerated eosinophils)
	Fungal hyphae may be sparse, highlighted by silver stains
	Fungi cultured include *Aspergillus*, dermatiaceous fungi (bipolaris, curvularia, alternaria, exserohilum)
Pathologic differential diagnosis	Invasive fungal sinusitis, mycetoma, inflammatory polyps

ALLERGIC FUNGAL SINUSITIS DISEASE FACT SHEET	
Definition	An allergic response within the sinonasal tract to fungal allergens, amplified and perpetuated by eosinophils
Incidence and location	More common in warmer climates
Morbidity and mortality	Inflammatory mass may cause bone erosion, facial dysmorphia, and visual disturbances
Gender, race, and age distribution	Male = Female
	Most common in 3rd–7th decade
Clinical features	Allergic symptoms, nasal discharge and rhinorrhea
	Rare, facial dysmorphia and visual disturbances
	Peripheral eosinophilia with elevated anti-fungal IgE
Treatment and prognosis	Fungal desensitization helps to yield a good outcome
	Must obtain cultures to assist with desensitization
	Evacuation and aeration of affected sinus and/or intranasal steroids

bances. There is no gender or age predilection and symptoms of nasal discharge and rhinorrhea are often present for a long duration.

PATHOLOGIC FEATURES

GROSS FINDINGS

The secretions of AFS have been described as putty-like, peanut butter-like, muddy, and greasy. There is often an associated foul aroma.

MICROSCOPIC FINDINGS

The characteristic findings in AFS are alternating "tide-lines" or ripples of mucin with degenerating cellular debris, most commonly eosinophils (Fig. 4-13). The eosinophils often degenerate and degranulate (Fig. 4-14), occasionally forming Charcot-Leyden crystals, identified as long needle-shaped or bi-pyramidal crystals. Occasionally the mucin material may predominate, but the degenerated inflammatory cells can always be seen.

ANCILLARY STUDIES

A Gomori methenamine silver (GMS) stain reveals fungal hyphae (Fig. 4-15), but any fungal stain may be used. Organisms may be abundant to sparse, but do not usually show fruiting heads. Culture is necessary, with *Aspergillus* species most common, followed by dermatiaceous fungi (bipolaris, curvularia, alternaria, exserohilum), among others.

DIFFERENTIAL DIAGNOSIS

Invasive fungal infections, mycetoma, and sinonasal inflammatory polyps are included in the differential. Inflammatory polyps may have mucinous material, but do not have alternating mucin with inflammatory eosinophilic debris. Invasive fungal infections must have fungal organisms identified within the vessels or deep in the stroma of the respiratory epithelium (Fig. 4-16). A mycetoma is an aggregation of fungal elements, eliciting a limited response, but not invading the sinonasal tract tissues. Fruiting heads are more common in this form.

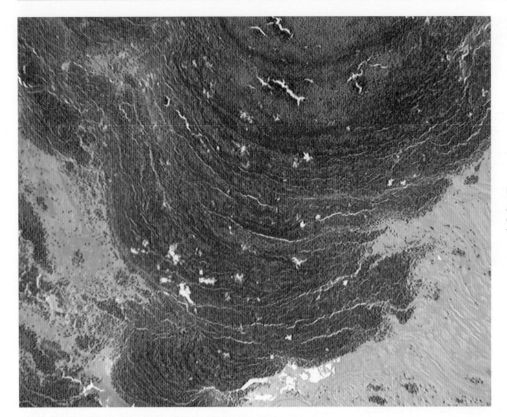

FIGURE 4-13
Alternating "tide-lines" or ripples of eosinophils and neutrophils characterize allergic fungal sinusitis.

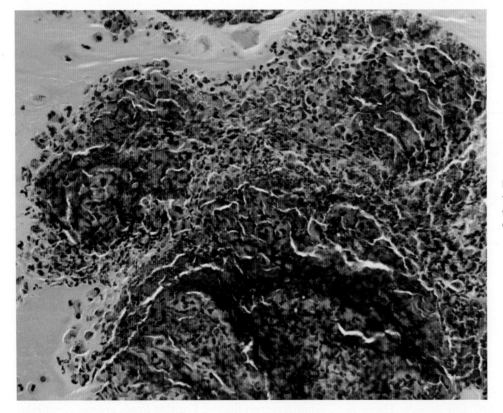

FIGURE 4-14
The background mucin is associated with abundant neutrophilic and eosinophilic debris.

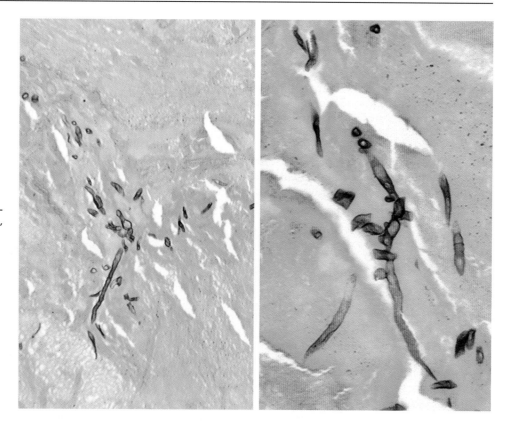

FIGURE 4-15

A silver impregnation stain highlights the fungal organisms (*left*), often *Aspergillus* species (*right*).

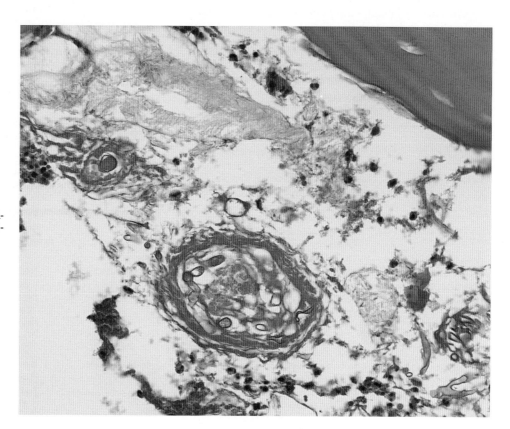

FIGURE 4-16

Bone is noted with a vessel infiltrated by mucor fungal hyphae, indicating invasive fungal sinusitis.

PROGNOSIS AND THERAPY

Identification of the exact fungal species on GMS stain is nearly impossible, and culture confirmation is necessary. Fungal identification is germane, as allergic desensitization is therapeutic after surgical evacuation and steroids. Steroid sprays may in fact lessen symptoms. If no fungal hyphae are found, but the patient has allergic symptoms, the preferred nomenclature is now eosinophilic fungal rhinosinusitis-like syndrome, although the management is often similar.

RHINOSCLEROMA

CLINICAL FEATURES

Rhinoscleroma is a chronic, progressive upper aerodigestive tract granulomatous infection caused by *Klebsiella rhinoscleromatis,* a gram-negative coccobacillus of low infectivity. The disease is considered endemic within Central America, Egypt, tropical Africa, India, Indonesia, and Eastern Europe, while rare in the United States. Whereas crowded conditions, poor hygiene, and poor nutrition appear necessary for transmission of the infectious agent, the actual pathogenesis of infection remains elusive. Females are affected slightly more commonly than males and the disease normally presents within the 2nd–3rd decades of life.

If untreated, the disease tends to progress through an arc of development in three stages: exudative, proliferative, and cicatrical. The "atropic catarrhal" or exudative stage is characterized by acute or chronic active infection with purulent rhinorrhea, mucosal congestion and erythema, with foul purulent discharge and crusting. The proliferative or "granulomatous" stage occurs months to years later, with multiple, small, firm, waxy, ulcerating inflammatory masses that distend and deform the mucosal surfaces, distorting the soft tissues and yielding a "rhinoceros-like" appearance. The final cicatrical "sclerotic" stage culminates in extensive scarring and possible stenosis.

PATHOLOGICAL FEATURES

GROSS FEATURES

In the granulomatous phase, rhinoscleroma causes friable inflammatory polypoid lesions. In the final stages, the involved tissues are densely scarred.

MICROSCOPIC FINDINGS

The histology varies with stage, with the disease most commonly biopsied and diagnosed in the proliferative phase. Microscopically, the connective tissue is highly vascular, characterized by a dense lymphoplasmacytic infiltrate and Russell bodies (Fig. 4-17). Most striking, however, are the groups, clusters or sheets of large (100–200 µm) vacuolated histiocytes (Fig. 4-18) containing the causative agent (called Mikülicz cells after the Polish surgeon Johann von Mikülicz). It is in this stage that the intracellular bacilli are easiest to find. The cicatrical stage displays nonspecific fibrosis.

ANCILLARY STUDIES

Although occasionally visible on standard H&E staining, the organisms are much more readily demonstrated

RHINOSCLEROMA DISEASE FACT SHEET	
Definition	A chronic, progressive, upper aerodigestive tract infection caused by *Klebsiella rhinoscleromatis*
Incidence and location	Endemic in Central America, tropical Africa, India, Indonesia, Egypt, Eastern Europe
	Crowded conditions, poor hygiene, poor nutrition seem necessary for transmission
Morbidity and mortality	May have facial deformity and stenosis
Gender, race, and age distribution	Female slightly > male
	Peak in 2nd–3rd decades
Clinical features	Three stages clinically: exudative, proliferative, cicatrical
	Purulent, foul rhinorrhea, mucosal congestion, and erythema
	Multiple small, firm, waxy ulcerated masses giving deformity
	Scarring and possible stenosis late in disease
Prognosis and treatment	Due to high relapse rate, continued clinical follow-up/therapy is necessary
	Surgery and prolonged antibiotic therapy

RHINOSCLEROMA PATHOLOGIC FEATURES	
Gross findings	Friable inflammatory polyps or dense fibrosis
Microscopic findings	Dense lymphoplasmacytic inflammation with Russell bodies
	Groups, clusters and sheets of large, vacuolated macrophages (Mikülicz cells), which contain the infective organisms
Ancillary studies	Warthin-Starry stain is most sensitive in detecting bacilli
	Immunohistochemistry against type III *Klebsiella* antigen
Pathologic differential diagnosis	Atypical mycobacterial infection, Lepromatous leprosy, syphilis

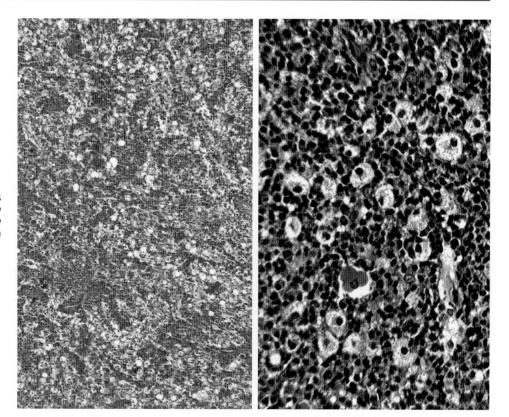

FIGURE 4-17

Left: Rhinoscleroma demonstrates abundant lymphocytes with foamy histiocytes. *Right:* A Russell body is noted within the histiocyte rich infiltrate.

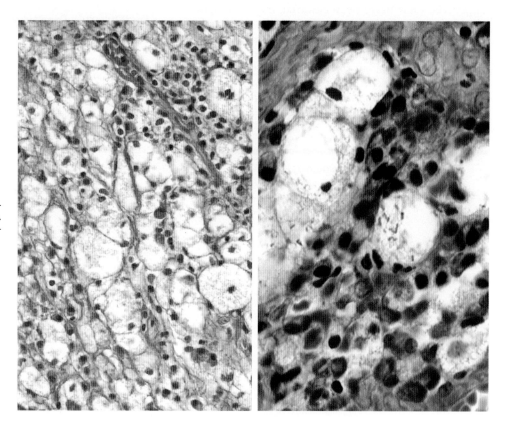

FIGURE 4-18

Left: The Mikülicz cells are in abundance in this granulomatous phase. *Right:* A Warthin-Starry stain highlights intracellular bacilli.

with the silver impregnation Warthin-Starry stain (Fig. 4-18). Immunohistochemistry against type III Klebsiella antigen are available, but are difficult to interpret. Other infectious agents, such as atypical mycobacterial infection, Lepromatous leprosy, and syphilis should be excluded, as necessary (Ziehl-Neelsen, Fite-Farraco stains).

PROGNOSIS AND THERAPY

Treatment for rhinoscleroma includes prolonged antibiotic therapy (doxycycline, ciprofloxacin, ceforanide, rifampicin, fluoroquinolone, streptomycin) followed by surgical debridement and correction of sclerotic defects. A high relapse rate is seen, however, and continued clinical follow-up is required.

RHINOSPORIDIOSIS

CLINICAL FEATURES

Rhinosporidium seeberi is the etiologic agent of a chronic and usually painless localized infection of the mucous membranes which occurs throughout the world, but has its highest incidence in India and Sri Lanka. *Rhinosporidium* has never been cultured, but is thought to be a blue-green algae, passed to humans from animals or possibly fomites. It is found in stagnant pools of water and dust. Infection is most common in the nasal cavity and the conjunctiva, but can also occur in the nasopharynx, larynx, tracheobronchial tree, esophagus, ear, and genital tract. Common symptoms include nasal obstruction, epistaxis, and rhinorrhea. Nasal and urethral infections have a male predominance; conjunctival infections have a female predominance.

PATHOLOGIC FEATURES

GROSS FEATURES

Grossly, the lesions are single or multiple polypoid, pedunculated, or sessile, friable red to pink masses. Due to the formation of a mass lesion, they may be mistaken clinically for a neoplasm.

MICROSCOPIC FEATURES

Intense acute and chronic inflammation is present, often induced by rupture of the large, round, thick-walled cysts (up to 300 μm sporangia). The overlying epithelium may be hyperplastic and may exhibit squamous metaplasia (Fig. 4-19). The thick cyst walls are birefringent, and stain with hematoxylin and eosin, Gomori methenamine silver, digested periodic acid-Schiff, and mucicarmine. The most mature and largest cysts are closest to the mucosal surface, but are not identified *within* the mucosa (Fig. 4-20). Hundreds to thousands of small (2–9 micron) endospores/algae are seen within mature cysts (Fig. 4-21). The spores are initially uni-nuclear, but upon maturation are multinucleated forming clusters of 12 to 16 "naked nuclei."

DIFFERENTIAL DIAGNOSIS

Schneiderian cylindrical cell papillomas have small cysts of mucin and nuclear debris *within* the epithelium and do not have a birefringent cyst wall. *Coccidioides immitis* may have a similar appearance, forming thick-walled spherules that contain endospores, but these spherules are 5–60 μm and are usually associated with a characteristic granulomatous reaction.

RHINOSPORIDIOSIS DISEASE FACT SHEET	
Definition	Infection by *Rhinosporidium seeberi*, a blue-green algae
Incidence and location	Highest incidence in India, Sri Lanka, Brazil, Argentina
	Associated with stagnant pools of water and dust
	Nasal cavity, conjunctiva, and genital tract
Morbidity and mortality	May cause destruction at local site
Gender, race, and age distribution	Male > Female (in the sinonasal tract)
	All ages may be affected
Clinical features	Nasal obstruction, epistaxis, and rhinorrhea
	Expansile, destructive polypoid process
Prognosis and treatment	As antibiotics are not effective, surgery is treatment of choice, but recurrence develops in 10% of patients

RHINOSPORIDIOSIS PATHOLOGIC FEATURES	
Gross findings	Single or multiple, polypoid, friable, red or pink masses
Microscopic findings	Overlying surface may be hyperplastic or metaplastic
	A dense lymphoplasmacytic response, especially if cysts rupture
	Subepithelial, large (300 μm) algae sporangial cysts with thick birefringent, walls
	Numerous small (2–9 μm) endospores within mature cysts
Pathologic differential diagnosis	Schneiderian papilloma, cylindrical cell type, *Coccidioides*

FIGURE 4-19

A metaplastic squamous mucosa covers a heavily inflamed submucosa. Multiple cysts with sporangia are noted, but all are below the mucosa.

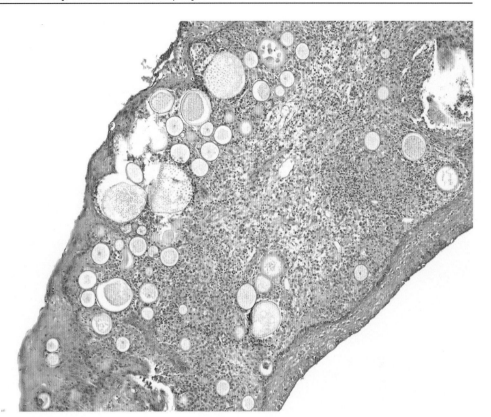

FIGURE 4-20

A rich inflammatory infiltrate surrounds the mature, trilaminar sporangia, these containing only rare spores.

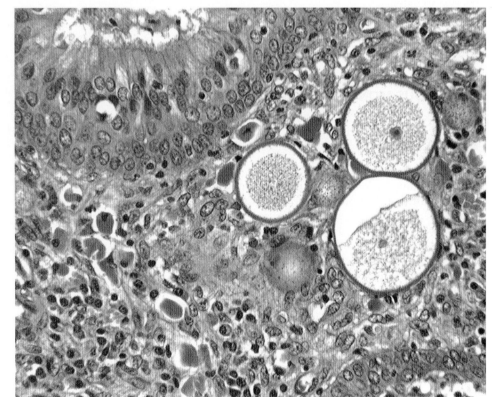

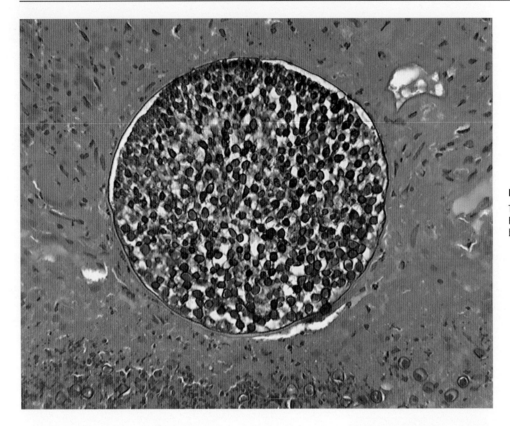

FIGURE 4-21
This cyst is filled with spores. Released spores are noted at the bottom.

PROGNOSIS AND TREATMENT

Treatment for *Rhinosporidium* is surgical, with up to a 10% recurrence rate. No antibiotics have proven effective to date.

INFECTIOUS MONONUCLEOSIS

CLINICAL FEATURES

Infectious mononucleosis (IM) is a benign, systemic, and self-limiting infectious lymphoproliferative disease, usually the acute clinical manifestation of primary Epstein-Barr virus (EBV) infection transmitted through oral secretions. EBV infection early in life is subclinical. However, primary infection is young adults (equal gender distribution) can lead to a worrisome clinical presentation, with a reported incidence of about 45 cases/100,000-population. Patients present with acute pharyngitis and tonsillitis, with symptomatology of fever, sore throat, headache, malaise, and cervical adenopathy after a nonspecific prodrome, 3–5 days long. Hepatosplenomegaly and hepatitis, with rare splenic rupture are possible complications. There is a leukocytosis, with atypical lymphocytosis. The pharyngitis and

INFECTIOUS MONONUCLEOSIS DISEASE FACT SHEET	
Definition	Infectious mononucleosis is benign, systemic and self-limiting infectious lymphoproliferative disease, usually the acute clinical manifestation of primary EBV infection
Incidence and location	Approximately 45/100,000-population Usually a disease of Western civilization
Morbidity and mortality	Upper airway obstruction, splenic rupture, encephalitis, myocarditis are serious complications
Gender, race, and age distribution	Equal gender distribution Usually Western societies Peak in young adults
Clinical features	Acute pharyngitis, tonsillitis Fever, sore throat, malaise, and headache Adenopathy of the anterior and posterior cervical chain Hepatosplenomegaly later in disease
Prognosis and treatment	Supportive care yields an excellent overall prognosis, although steroids are advocated for complications Complications include airway obstruction, thrombocytopenia, hemolytic anemia, CNS symptoms, pericarditis, myocarditis

tonsillitis may be ulcerative and exudative, and lead to peritonsillar abscess. In extreme cases, tonsillitis may cause upper airway obstruction. Multiple cranial nerve palsies may rarely occur, possibly secondary to brainstem encephalitis.

PATHOLOGIC FEATURES

GROSS FEATURES

The tonsils in infectious mononucleosis reveal a "dirty" gray membrane. Obstructive tonsillitis can result from massively hypertrophied tonsils. Associated enlarged lymph nodes may be found.

MICROSCOPIC FINDINGS

The histologic appearance of IM in tonsillectomy specimens may be startling in the extent of cytologic atypia. There is a marked lymphoid hyperplasia with enlarged and irregular germinal centers surrounded by a distinct mantle zone and with expansion of the interfollicular areas. There is no effacement of the tonsillar architecture. A full spectrum of inflammatory elements may be present, including mature lymphocytes, plasma cells, centrocytes, immunoblasts, Reed-Sternberg-like cells, histiocytes, eosinophils, and neutrophils (Fig. 4-22). Necrosis and mitotic figures may be present.

INFECTIOUS MONONUCLEOSIS PATHOLOGIC FEATURES	
Gross findings	Enlarged tonsils with gray membrane
Microscopic findings	Lymphoid hyperplasia with irregular germinal centers, but still have distinct mantle zone
	Expanded interfollicular zone with mature lymphocytes, plasma cells, centrocytes, immunoblasts, Reed-Sternberg–like cells, histiocytes, eosinophils, neutrophils
	Necrosis and mitotic figures are common
Immunohistochemical features	EBV-LMP or in situ hybridization for EBER
	Mixed B and T cell population without restriction
Pathologic differential diagnosis	Diffuse large B cell lymphoma, follicular lymphoma, Hodgkin lymphoma, carcinoma (rare in young patients)

ANCILLARY STUDIES

Obtaining a panel of B and T cell markers with kappa and lambda in addition to EBV-LMP or EBER is prudent in order to exclude a lymphoma (Fig. 4-23).

DIFFERENTIAL DIAGNOSIS

A hematologic malignancy, such as a diffuse large B cell lymphoma, follicular lymphoma, or Hodgkin lymphoma must be excluded through appropriate immunohistochemical studies. A carcinoma is also included in the differential, but given the young age at presentation and the known presence of the heterophile antibodies (positive "mono-spot" test), an accurate diagnosis is appropriately rendered.

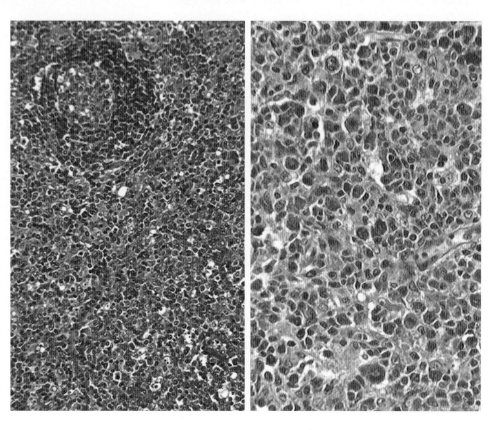

FIGURE 4-22

Left: A residual lymphoid follicle is surrounded by an increased interfollicular zone. *Right:* Remarkable cellular variability (pleomorphism) is seen within this EBV infection.

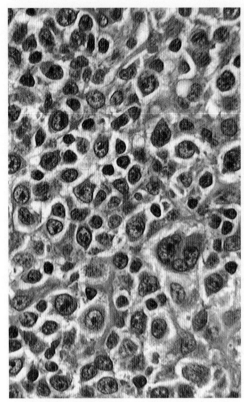
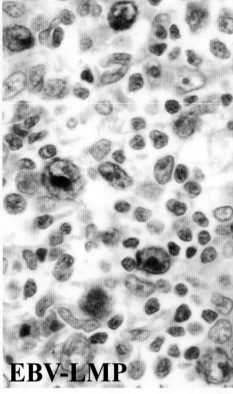

EBV-LMP

FIGURE 4-23

Left: A spectrum of reactive lymphoid cells, including a "Reed Sternberg" look-alike. *Right:* EBV latent membrane protein highlights the infected cells, often in a Golgi or paranuclear dot-like distribution.

PROGNOSIS AND TREATMENT

Treatment is largely supportive, because more than 95 % of cases resolve without specific therapy. Some advocate the use of corticosteroids, particularly in the setting of impending airway obstruction, thrombocytopenia, hemolytic anemia, CNS symptoms, pericarditis, or myocarditis. Antiviral therapy has not been shown to be of significant benefit.

HIV (TONSIL)

CLINICAL FEATURES

Primary HIV infection may be entirely asymptomatic, with seroconversion the only clue. More than half of patients infected with HIV may present with nonspecific symptoms such as fever, malaise, myalgias, diarrhea, pharyngitis, macular erythematous rash, lymphadenopathy, splenomegaly, and weight loss, findings similar to infectious mononucleosis. The acute illness occurs 3 to 6 weeks after primary exposure, and may last up to 2 weeks, though milder symptoms may persist for months. The tonsils have been shown to harbor HIV, although it is controversial as to whether

HIV (TONSIL) DISEASE FACT SHEET	
Definition	Tonsillar infection with human immunodeficiency virus
Incidence and location	HIV tonsillitis is rare
	Overall, approximately 40,000 new AIDS cases per year in US
	Much higher in Asia (1.2 million) and Africa (3.1 million) based on 2004 data
Morbidity and mortality	An ultimately fatal chronic disease
Gender, race, and age distribution	Male > Female (7 : 3), specifically in US
	In US, >50% of new infections are in blacks
	Peak in 3rd–5th decades
Clinical features	Often asymptomatic with seroconversion the only initial clue
	Nonspecific symptoms include fever, malaise, myalgias, weight loss, pharyngitis, mucosal ulcerations and discrete ulcers on palate, esophagus, and anogenital region
	Lymphadenopathy and splenomegaly
	Macular erythematous rash
Prognosis and treatment	A chronic disease which is considered fatal
	Drug cocktail (HART) slows progression

they may be the primary source of viral entry. The changing demographics of HIV make epidemiologic statements difficult, but there is an increased risk in homosexual men, IV drug users, and prostitutes, among others.

PATHOLOGY FEATURES

GROSS FEATURES

Tonsillectomy is usually performed for tonsillar enlargement, with the aim of excluding neoplasia. In some cases, HIV infection is unsuspected at the time of tonsillectomy.

MICROSCOPIC FEATURES

The findings of Waldeyer's ring tissue parallels those of the lymph nodes in HIV infected patients. Florid follicular hyperplasia, with or without follicular lysis, is seen in the early stage of HIV infection (Fig. 4-24). Multinucleated giant cells are randomly distributed throughout the lymphoid tissue, although there is an accentuation immediately below the lymphoepithelium (Fig. 4-25). In the burnt-out stage, the tonsils reveal effaced architecture, absent follicles, and an infiltrate of plasma cells, and immunoblasts.

ANCILLARY STUDIES

The presence of HIV can be confirmed by immunohistochemistry for p24 [which is specifically identified within the follicular dendritic cells (Fig. 4-25) and giant cells], and RNA in situ hybridization.

DIFFERENTIAL DIAGNOSIS

The giant cells of Warthin-Finkeldey may mimic those of HIV, but are usually centrally located within the tonsil, demonstrating a "grape-like" cluster. Other hematologic disorders, including lymphomas, may need to be excluded with pertinent immunohistochemistry studies.

PROGNOSIS AND TREATMENT

Prognosis for HIV infection has improved with current multimodality drug regimens, but there is no

HIV (TONSIL) PATHOLOGIC FEATURES	
Gross findings	Tonsils may be enlarged
Microscopic findings	Florid follicular hyperplasia with or without follicular lysis
	Multinucleated giant cells randomly distributed, although accentuated at the lymphoepithelium
	In late stage, effaced architecture, absent follicles, and a plasma cell infiltrate
Ancillary studies	p24 positive; may do in situ hybridization for HIV-RNA
Differential diagnosis	Warthin-Finkeldey giant cells, lymphoma

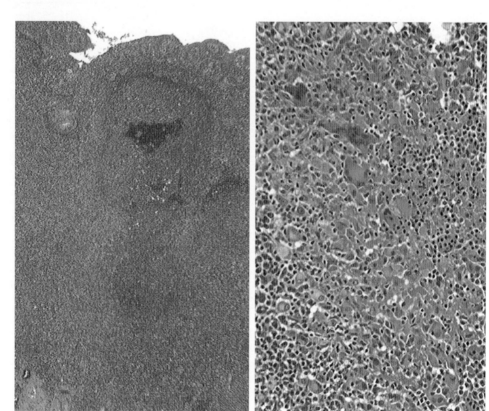

FIGURE 4-24

Left: Dissolution of the lymphoid tissue within a tonsil shows an expanded interfollicular zone. *Right:* Surface disruption and a hint of giant cell formation.

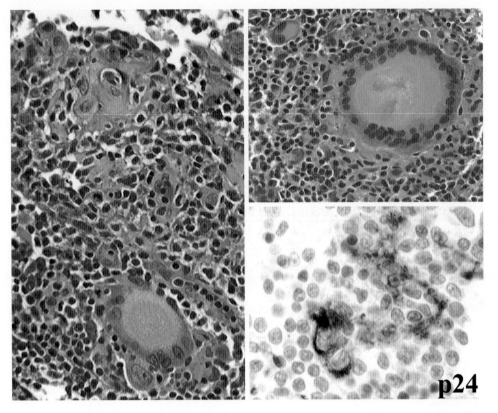

p24

FIGURE 4-25

Left: A giant cell with a wreath-like distribution is noted immediately below the surface epithelium. *Right upper:* A wreath-like giant cell. *Right lower:* p24 immunohistochemistry highlights the follicular dendritic cell population, while also being positive in giant cells.

specific or unique treatment required for tonsillar HIV changes.

WEGENER'S GRANULOMATOSIS

CLINICAL FEATURES

Wegener's granulomatosis (WG) has an unknown etiology, although an abnormal immune response seems to be at the heart of the disorder, along with possible environmental and genetic factors. Upper aerodigestive tract symptoms are presenting features in up to 90% of patients with WG. WG may be systemic with multiorgan involvement, or may be limited to a single organ system, such as the respiratory tract. The respiratory tract and renal systems are most frequently affected, the latter associated with a rapidly progressive glomerulonephritis. Pulmonary involvement can cause pulmonary infiltrates, pulmonary edema, or cavitary lesions. Skin lesions such as palpable purpura, vesicular bullous disease, or ulcers may also be manifest at presentation.

Patients of all ages can be affected and there does not seem to be a gender predilection. Patients complain of nasal pain and stuffiness, rhinitis, and hearing loss. The latter is due to eustachian tube involvement. Septal erosion and perforation may occur, and lead to saddle

WEGENER'S GRANULOMATOSIS DISEASE FACT SHEET	
Definition	Included in the small vessel vasculitides, WG is an abnormal immune response with possible environmental and genetic factors yielding a aerodigestive tract and kidney disease
Incidence and location	About 500 new cases per year in the US Kidney and lung most commonly affected, with sinonasal tract involvement in up to 90% of patients
Morbidity and mortality	Renal failure and pulmonary disease cause significant morbidity and possible mortality
Gender, race, and age distribution	Equal gender distribution Most patients are white Peak presentation, 41 yr
Clinical features	Nasal pain and stuffiness, rhinitis and hearing loss Septal erosion and perforation (saddle nose deformity) occur later in the disease Difficulty breathing as a result of subglottic stenosis
Prognosis and treatment	Prognosis depends on stage and extent of disease Relapses are common, often coinciding with a rising c-ANCA titer Immunosuppression (cyclophosphamide and steroids), with close monitoring of potential side effects

nose deformity, the latter more common in children. Laryngotracheal involvement may lead to subglottic stenosis, also more common in children.

RADIOLOGIC FEATURES

The imaging of the sinonasal tract varies from nonspecific mucosal changes to a localized soft tissue mass. Nasal cavity involvement usually precedes paranasal sinus involvement. The maxilla and ethmoids are the most frequently involved sinuses. Chest radiographs can reveal multifocal pulmonary opacities, infiltrates, or cavitation. Pulmonary effusions are common.

PATHOLOGIC FEATURES

GROSS FINDINGS

The sinonasal tract reveals chronic ulcerative disease, with fragments of necrotic-appearing tissue submitted.

MICROSCOPIC FINDINGS

While the microscopic findings encompass a number of features, the necrobiosis of the collagen ("collagenolytic necrosis") and mesenchymal tissues of the sinonasal tract is characteristic (Fig. 4-26). There is a finely to coarsely granular, basophilic, geographic-type

necrosis, a feature which is really quite unique in the head and neck. The basophilic debris results from karyorrhexis of the neutrophils and death of the endothelial cells and collagen (Fig. 4-27). Whereas the small vessel vasculitis is more easily identified in the lung and kidney, vasculitis in the sinonasal tract is often difficult to identify (Fig. 4-28). True granuloma are likewise challenging to demonstrate, and are often limited to just a few scattered giant cells (Fig. 4-29). Since the bionecrosis encompasses the soft tissues, smooth muscle-walled vessels will also be included in the areas of necrosis.

WEGENER'S GRANULOMATOSIS PATHOLOGIC FEATURES	
Gross findings	Chronic ulcerative disease with fragments of necrotic tissue
Microscopic findings	Geographic zones of bionecrosis (blue, granular debris)
	Vasculitis is often difficult to identify
	Granulomas not present, although giant cells may be seen
Immunofluorescence	Antineutrophil cytoplasmic antibodies in a cytoplasmic pattern against enzyme proteinase-3 (PR3)
Pathologic differential diagnosis	Granulomatous inflammation from infectious agents, microscopic polyangiitis, Churg-Strauss syndrome, extranodal NK/T cell lymphoma, nasal type, and cocaine use

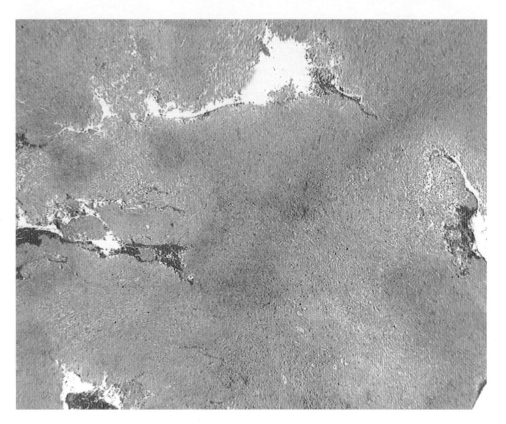

FIGURE 4-26
Sheets of blue, pink, granular bionecrotic material are characteristic for Wegener's granulomatosis.

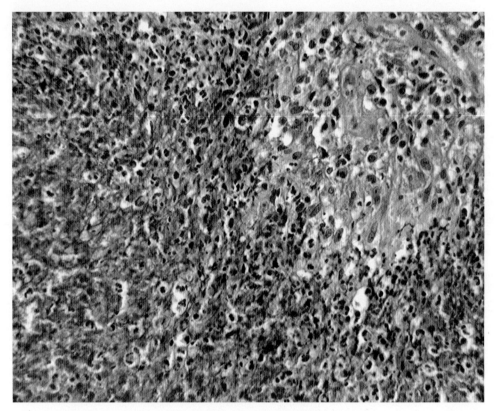

FIGURE 4-27

The blue, granular bionecrotic material associated with a small vessel being destroyed (*upper right*).

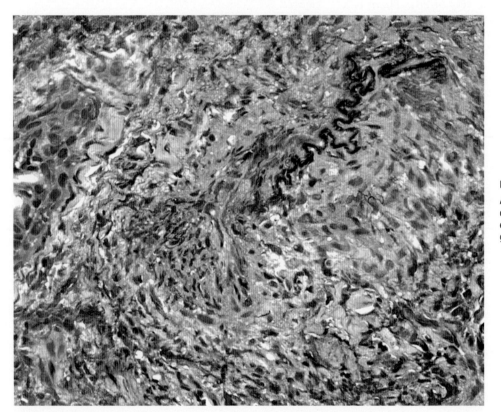

FIGURE 4-28

An elastic stain highlights the destruction of the vessel wall as an example of vasculitis in Wegener's granulomatosis.

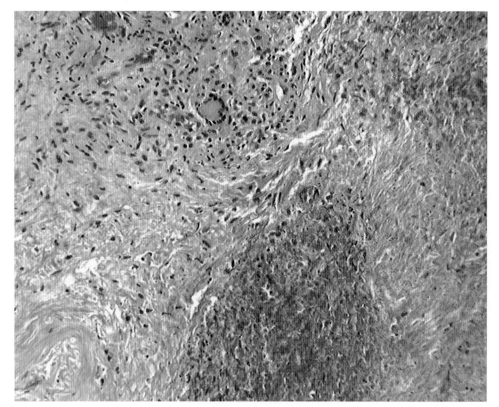

FIGURE 4-29
Rarely, giant cells may be present, but well-formed granulomas are absent. Note the vessel wall in lower left.

ANCILLARY STUDIES

Up to 85 % of patients with WG have elevated titers of antineutrophil cytoplasmic antibodies (ANCA) in a cytoplasmic pattern (c-ANCA), usually directed against enzyme proteinase-3 (PR3). However, 10 % to 15 % of patients with WG may be ANCA-negative. ANCA titers may persist after symptoms abate, but if there is a change or increase in titer, it suggests disease recrudescence. Some patients with WG have serum anti-endothelial antibodies that specifically recognize endothelia of the nasal cavity, lung, and kidney.

DIFFERENTIAL DIAGNOSIS

WG is often considered a diagnosis of exclusion, as a number of disorders may present with somewhat similar findings. Granulomatous inflammation from infectious agents, microscopic polyangiitis (MPA), Churg-Strauss syndrome, extranodal NK/T-cell lymphoma, nasal type, and cocaine are the most common considerations. Granulomatous inflammation from infections tends to have granulomas with increased numbers of giant cells. Special stains and cultures may help, although secondary infections may sometimes develop in WG patients. MPA is a related small vessel vasculitis that affects the lungs, kidneys, and skin. It is associated with ANCA against myeloperoxidase (MPO-ANCA). Churg-Strauss is usually a respiratory disease and has characteristic clinical findings. Lymphomas have cytologically atypical cells with vascular destruction, demonstrating specific immunohistochemical findings. Cocaine abuse may sometimes mimic the findings of WG. Using polarization may identify the talc used to cut cocaine, although many different agents are used to cut cocaine and talc is not always associated with cocaine use.

PROGNOSIS AND THERAPY

The patient outcome depends on limited or systemic disease, as well as the type of therapy. Therapy is directed at the disease severity, with disease relapses a common occurrence. Immunosuppression is the mainstay of treatment, with cyclophosphamide and glucocorticoids used in combination most often. Side effects of therapy need to be monitored.

RESPIRATORY EPITHELIAL ADENOMATOID HAMARTOMA

CLINICAL FEATURES

Respiratory epithelial adenomatoid hamartoma (READ) are benign overgrowths of minor mucoserous

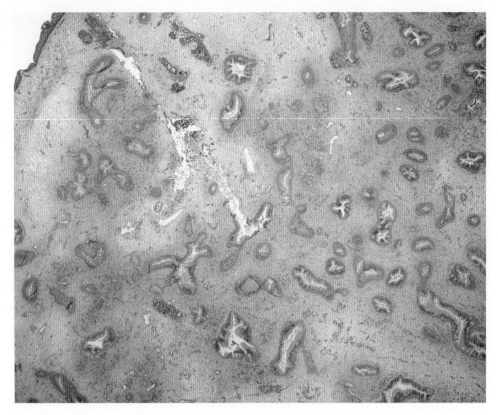

FIGURE 4-30
Multiple small glandular proliferations are noted in the stroma. The surface is noted at the upper left. There is no "stromal" reaction.

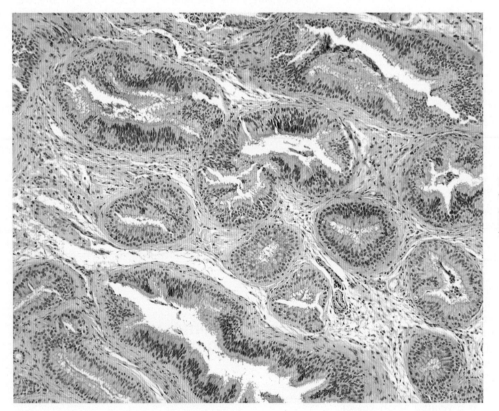

FIGURE 4-31
Well-circumscribed glandular profiles are surrounded by basement membrane material. There is a pseudostratified columnar epithelium.

RESPIRATORY EPITHELIAL ADENOMATOID HAMARTOMA (READ) DISEASE FACT SHEET	
Definition	A benign proliferation of mature sinonasal tissue presenting as a polypoid mass
Incidence and location	Rare
	READ usually in the nasal cavity
Gender, race, and age distribution	Male > Female
	Peak in 6th decade
Clinical features	Unilateral nasal obstruction
	Epistaxis
	Recurrent sinusitis
Prognosis and treatment	Cured with conservative but complete excision

RESPIRATORY EPITHELIAL ADENOMATOID HAMARTOMA (READ) PATHOLOGIC FEATURES	
Gross findings	Exophytic, polypoid, up to 6 cm masses
	Firm, tan-white to red-brown
Microscopic findings	Proliferation of mature respiratory glandular tissue with invagination from the surface epithelium
	Glands surrounded by thick basement membrane material
	Multilayered, columnar, respiratory epithelium with cilia
Pathologic differential diagnosis	Schneiderian papilloma, inverted type, intestinal-type adenocarcinoma, inflammatory polyps

glands of the sinonasal tract. These uncommon hamartomas are composed of small glandular epithelial islands in a mesenchymal background but lacking any components from other germ cell layers. These hamartomas usually present in men more commonly than women, with a peak in the 6th decade. Patients complain of unilateral nasal obstruction, epistaxis, and recurrent sinusitis.

RADIOLOGIC FEATURES

The radiograph reveals a unilateral nasal mass arising from the posterior nasal septum or the lateral nasal wall

in approximately 80% of cases. In the remaining cases, the mass may be in the nasopharynx or the paranasal sinuses.

PATHOLOGIC FEATURES

GROSS FINDINGS

READ are exophytic, polypoid, rubbery to firm, tan-white to red-brown lesions, measuring up to 6 cm in largest dimension.

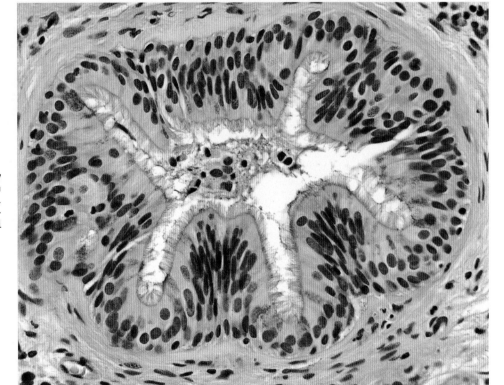

FIGURE 4-32
The epithelium is histologically benign with abundant cilia noted on the surface. There is stratification, expected for respiratory-type epithelium in this respiratory epithelial adenomatoid hamartoma.

MICROSCOPIC FINDINGS

These polyps are composed of prominent glandular proliferations lined with ciliated respiratory mucosa (Fig. 4-30). The glands are often in continuity with the surface, but are usually surrounded by a dense, pink basement membrane material which separates these invaginations from the fibrotic, edematous, and focally inflamed stroma (Fig. 4-31). The epithelium has multilayered, columnar, respiratory-type epithelium, with prominent cilia noted (Fig. 4-32). Occasionally cartilage or bone may also be present.

DIFFERENTIAL DIAGNOSIS

The differential diagnosis includes Schneiderian papilloma, inverted type (IP), intestinal-type adenocarcinoma (ITAC), and inflammatory polyps. The inverted islands of IP may retain luminal respiratory epithelium, but in general there is a thickened epithelium. Small mucus cysts filled with debris are present, but the epithelial groups are not usually surrounded by a thickened basement membrane. Well-differentiated ITAC is composed of back-to-back glands without a basal reserve layer or basement membrane material, and does not have ciliated respiratory epithelium. A lobular

architecture is maintained. Inflammatory polyps lack the "adenomatoid" appearance of epithelium within the stroma.

PROGNOSIS AND THERAPY

Conservative but complete excision is curative, with little chance of recurrence, if any.

RHINOPHYMA

CLINICAL FEATURES

Patients with rhinophyma suffer from progressive nasal distortion and enlargement. The nasal dome becomes progressively bulbous, bumpy, and telangiectatic (Fig. 4-33). These patients have a history of chronic roseacea. They also have a history of facial flushing after drinking hot liquids, alcohol, or eating spicy food. However, heavy alcoholic intake is present only in about half of those affected with rhinophyma. Men are affected more

FIGURE 4-33
A large, bulbous nose characteristic of rhinophyma.

RHINOPHYMA DISEASE FACT SHEET	
Definition	A hypertrophy of the sebaceous glands of the nasal dome in patients with long-standing acne roseacea
Incidence and location	Uncommon Nasal dome
Gender, race, and age distribution	Male > Female Older age
Clinical features	Enlarged, bumpy nasal dome with telangiectasia Chronic roseacea History of facial flushing with drinking hot liquids, alcohol, or eating spicy foods
Prognosis and treatment	Disease is often progressive and may be disfiguring Early stage managed with antibiotics, but dermabrasion, laser, and cryosurgery may be needed later

commonly than women, often in the later decades of life.

PATHOLOGIC FEATURES

Sebaceous hypertrophy and follicular plugging are present (Fig. 4-34). The fibrous variant of rhinophyma

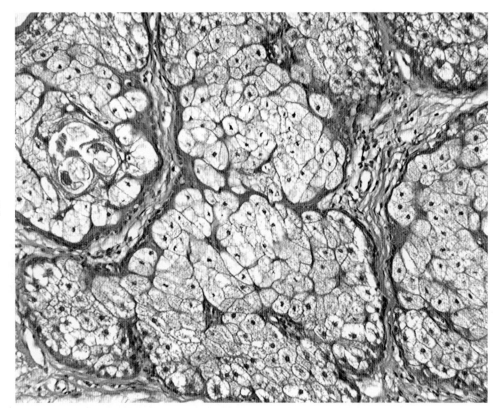

FIGURE 4-34
Increased sebaceous glands, often arranged in nests in this example of rhinophyma.

RHINOPHYMA PATHOLOGIC FEATURES	
Microscopic findings	Hyperplasia of sebaceous glands, follicular plugging, focal folliculitis, perifolliculitis, and telangiectasia No atypia or invasive growth
Pathologic differential diagnosis	Sebaceoma, sebaceous carcinoma

is characterized by diffuse dermal fibrosis, abundant mucin, obliterated pilosebaceous structures, and telangiectasia. Dilated follicles, focal folliculitis, and perifolliculitis may be seen.

DIFFERENTIAL DIAGNOSIS

Sebaceoma or sebaceous carcinoma are neoplasms, not arranged around hair follicles, and usually displaying significant cytologic atypia.

PROGNOSIS AND THERAPY

Early rhinophyma may be treated with antibiotics (topical metronidazole). More advanced cases may be treated surgically (dermabrasion, laser, cryosurgery).

SINUS HISTIOCYTOSIS WITH MASSIVE LYMPHADENOPATHY (ROSAI-DORFMAN DISEASE)

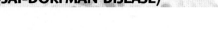

CLINICAL FEATURES

Rosai-Dorfman disease (sinus histiocytosis with massive lymphadenopathy, or SHML) is a rare, idiopathic, histiocytic proliferation usually seen in young black women (African and Caribbean origin). The massive lymphadenopathy most commonly involves the cervical lymph nodes. Nearly half of the affected patients have extranodal involvement, the majority of which (75%) occurs in sites in the head and neck, such as eyes, ocular adnexae, paranasal sinuses, and nasal cavity. Typically, patients present with nasal obstruction, proptosis, cranial nerve deficits and mass lesions, along with fever, and an elevated white count and erythrocyte sedimentation rate. Concurrent lymph node involvement may be seen.

RADIOLOGIC FEATURES

Paranasal sinus disease can appear as a bulky, homogenous mass, mimicking lymphoma.

SINUS HISTIOCYTOSIS WITH MASSIVE LYMPHADENOPATHY (ROSAI-DORFMAN) DISEASE FACT SHEET	
Definition	Rosai-Dorfman disease is a rare, idiopathic, histiocytic proliferation usually seen in young, black women
Incidence and location	Rare
	Majority have head and neck involvement, with about 50% demonstrating extranodal disease (ocular, paranasal sinuses)
Morbidity and mortality	Direct mass effect into the cranial cavity
Gender, race, and age distribution	Female > Male
	Predisposition in black patients
	Usually young
Clinical features	Nasal obstruction, proptosis, cranial nerve deficits, and mass lesion
	Cervical lymphadenopathy common
	Fever, elevated WBC, and erythrocyte sedimentation rate
Prognosis and treatment	Prognosis determined by extent and stage
	Spontaneous remission or death from complications both occur uncommonly
	Steroids conservatively manage localized disease, with surgery and/or radiation for more extensive disease

PATHOLOGIC FEATURES

GROSS FINDINGS

Sinonasal tract involvement results in polypoid masses, which may be fibrotic, with a gray to yellow cut surface.

MICROSCOPIC FINDINGS

There is a pronounced dilatation of the lymphoid sinuses, with an abundant lymphoplasmacytic infiltrate in the background (Fig. 4-35). Fibrosis may be seen in association with the dilated spaces. These sinuses are

SINUS HISTIOCYTOSIS WITH MASSIVE LYMPHADENOPATHY (ROSAI-DORFMAN) PATHOLOGIC FEATURES	
Gross findings	Polypoid masses in the sinonasal tract, which may be fibrotic
Microscopic findings	Marked dilation of the lymphoid sinuses
	Abundant lymphoplasmacytic infiltrate in the background
	Pale, histiocytic cells in the sinuses demonstrating lymphophagocytosis or *emperipolesis*
Immunohistochemical findings	S-100 protein, CD68, Leu M3, lysozyme positive
	Negative with CD1a
Pathologic differential diagnosis	Rhinoscleroma, lepromatous leprosy, histiocytic lymphomas

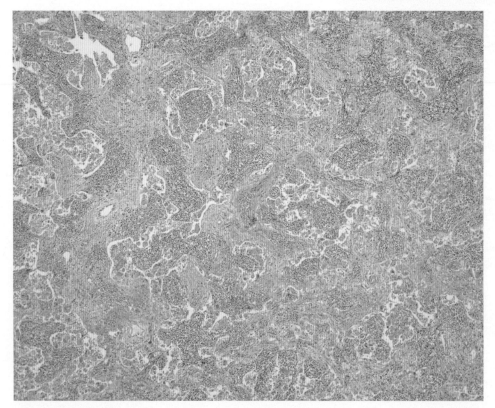

FIGURE 4-35

Lymphocytes are separated by lakes of histiocytes within expanded sinuses.

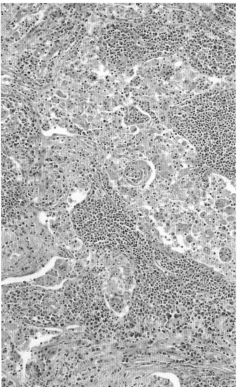 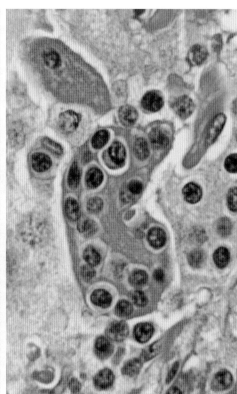

FIGURE 4-36

Left: Sinus histiocytosis composed of histiocytes with phagocytosis. *Right:* High power of a histiocyte with emperipolesis: numerous plasma cell and lymphocyte nuclei within the cytoplasm of the histiocyte.

filled with a plethora of pale, histiocytic cells that demonstrate the nearly pathognomonic lymphophago-cytosis or *emperipolesis* (Fig. 4-36). It is important to note that extranodal SHML tends to be more fibrotic with less emperipolesis than the nodal form. While axiomatic, special stains for organisms are negative.

ANCILLARY STUDIES

ULTRASTRUCTURAL FEATURES

The histiocytes contain fat vacuoles and lack Birbeck granules.

IMMUNOHISTOCHEMICAL FEATURES

The histiocytes are positive for S-100 protein and macrophage antigens such as CD68, Leu M3, lysozyme, alpha-1-chymotrypsin. However, they are negative for CD1a. These histiocytic cells are thought to be recently recruited blood monocytes.

DIFFERENTIAL DIAGNOSIS

The differential diagnosis includes other processes rich in histiocytes such as rhinoscleroma, lepromatous

leprosy, and rarely, histiocytic lymphomas. The histio-cytes of the infectious disease are smaller, not arranged within sinuses and lack S-100 protein reaction. B cell lymphomas may rarely exhibit emperipolesis, but will also be S-100 protein negative.

PROGNOSIS AND THERAPY

The prognosis is determined by the extent of the disor-der and "stage" of the disease. Patients may experience spontaneous remission, but occasionally patients may die of complications of the disorder (infectious and amyloid most commonly). Steroids may conservatively manage localized disease, but surgery (often extensive) and radiation may be necessary due to involvement of adjacent structures.

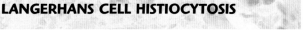

LANGERHANS CELL HISTIOCYTOSIS

CLINICAL FEATURES

Langerhans cell histiocytosis (LCH), formally Histio-cytosis X, represents a rare interrelated group of diseases including eosinophilic granuloma (EG),

LANGERHANS CELL HISTIOCYTOSIS (LCH) DISEASE FACT SHEET	
Definition	A interrelated group of disease which are manifestations of a unique histiocyte which contains Birbeck granules on electron microscopy
Incidence and location	Estimated prevalence in children is 1/200,000 per year
Morbidity and mortality	Morbidity can result from multifocal involvement of the skull
	Multiorgan involvement unresponsive to chemotherapy has a dismal prognosis
Gender, race, and age distribution	Equal gender distribution
	Usually young (<20 yr)
Clinical features	Head and neck involvement occurs in flat bones of the skull or jaws
	Present with otitis media and/or destructive temporal bone lesions (if the disease is localized)
Prognosis and treatment	Prognosis depends on stage and whether localized or systemic
	Disease progression is common if multiorgan involvement
	Surgery for localized disease has an excellent prognosis
	Combination chemotherapy if systemic disease

LANGERHANS CELL HISTIOCYTOSIS (LCH) PATHOLOGIC FEATURES	
Microscopic findings	Langerhans cells are enlarged cells with delicate, pale cytoplasm surrounding vesicular nuclei with indented, notched, lobated, folded, or grooved nuclei
	Increased eosinophils are often present, occasionally forming microscopic abscesses
Ultrastructural findings	Langerhans cells have folded, convoluted, and lobulated nuclei
	Cell membrane invaginations forming Birbeck or Langerhans granules: disk shaped, pentalaminar, giving a "tennis racquet" appearance
Immunohistochemical features	Broadly reactive with many histiocytic markers, a diagnosis is usually confirmed with S-100 protein, CD68, and CD1a
Pathologic differential diagnosis	Hodgkin lymphoma, extranodal NK/T cell lymphoma, Erdheim-Chester disease

Hand-Schüller-Christian syndrome, and Letterer-Siwe disease which are manifestations of a unique histiocyte which contains Birbeck granules on electron microscopy. The disease has an estimated prevalence of 1/200,000 children per year. The disease can be localized or systemic with multiorgan involvement. The head and neck is frequently involved in LCH, usually affecting the flat bones of the skull or the jaws, the ear, and the sinonasal tract. Patients range from a few months to the 6th decade, but a young age at initial presentation is most common (<20 yr). Patients have nonspecific findings including otitis media and destructive bone lesions.

RADIOLOGIC FEATURES

Radiographically osseous involvement by LCH produces sharply punched out radiolucencies. Extensive involvement of the alveolus causes the teeth to appear as if they are "floating in air."

PATHOLOGIC FEATURES

The Langerhans histiocytes are characterized by the presence of enlarged cells, containing delicate appearing pale or eosinophilic cytoplasm surrounding vesicular

nuclei with an indented, notched, lobated, folded, grooved, vesicular, or "coffee-bean"-shaped appearance, and one or two nucleoli (Figs. 4-37, 4-38). The cytoplasm is often finely vacuolated, occasionally showing phagocytized cellular debris. An increased number of eosinophils can be seen intermingled with the Langerhans cells, concentrated in collections around areas of necrosis.

ANCILLARY STUDIES

ULTRASTRUCTURAL FEATURES

Langerhans cells have folded, convoluted, and lobulated nuclei with cytoplasmic filipodial extensions, creating an uneven cell contour. The cell contains a variable number of invaginations of the cell membrane called Birbeck or Langerhans granules. The granules are disk shaped, but when cross-sectioned, appear rod-shaped. The granules are pentalaminar, showing cross-striations, often with the characteristic vesicular expansions imparting a "tennis racquet" appearance.

IMMUNOHISTOCHEMICAL FEATURES

The immunohistochemical antigenic profile of Langerhans cells is remarkably wide, but in practical terms S-100 protein, CD1a, and CD68 will yield a positive reaction with Langerhans cells. Occasionally, sialated Leu M1, peanut agglutinin, ATPase, or T-6 antigenic determinants, and HLA-DR CD74 may be used to confirm the diagnosis. The macrophage antigens generally demonstrate a concentration in the perinuclear space and Golgi region.

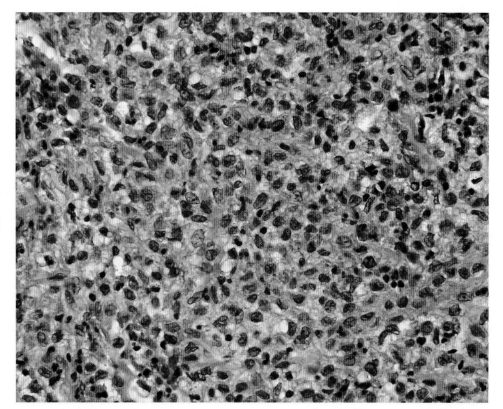

FIGURE 4-37
Langerhans cell histiocytosis demonstrates cleaved, "coffee bean"-shaped nuclei within a rich inflammatory background filled with eosinophils.

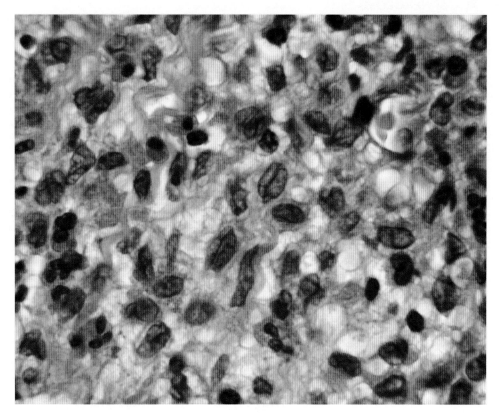

FIGURE 4-38
A cleave through the middle of the nucleus creates the characteristic lobulated "coffee-bean" appearance of Langerhans histiocytosis. Note the eosinophils in the background.

DIFFERENTIAL DIAGNOSIS

The differential in the head and neck is usually limited to Hodgkin lymphoma, extranodal NK/T cell lymphoma and perhaps Erdheim-Chester disease. Hodgkin lymphoma may have a pronounced eosinophilic infiltrate, but has Reed-Sternberg cells, with CD15 and CD30 but not CD1a immunoreactivity. NK/T cell lymphoma may have irregular and grooved nuclei, as well as eosinophils in the background, but will have angioinvasion, and a NK or T cell lineage. Erdheim-Chester disease is an idiopathic true histiocytic disorder, whose cells are S-100 protein positive, but negative for CD1a and lacks Birbeck granules.

PROGNOSIS AND THERAPY

LCH may be localized or systemic and a complex staging system is applied. However, localized disease, as is frequently the case in the head and neck, requires conservative surgery to achieve an excellent prognosis. If systemic disease is identified, combination chemotherapy is used.

MYOSPHERULOSIS

CLINICAL FEATURES

Myospherulosis is an iatrogenically introduced foreign body reaction resulting from the interaction of erythrocytes with petroleum, lanolin, or traumatized fat tissue. Patients who have had surgery with petroleum impreg-

nated packing used, will present with persistent sinusitis, facial pain, and swelling. These patients tend to have a significantly higher chance of developing adhesions and are likely to require additional therapy.

PATHOLOGIC FEATURES

Numerous small pseudocysts are seen with a "Swiss cheese" appearance. Heavy fibrosis surrounds the cysts (Fig. 4-39). These large (100 μm) cysts contain small collections with a nonrefractile thin membrane, containing brown, discolored, misshapen erythrocytes (Fig. 4-40). The erythrocytes will not stain with silver impregnation stains.

DIFFERENTIAL DIAGNOSIS

The differential diagnosis includes coccidiodomycosis and *Rhinosporidium.* The "capsule" of myospherulosis is approximately 1 micron thick, but is not as thick, double walled or birefringent, as are the capsules of *Coccidioidomyces* and *Rhinosporidium.*

PROGNOSIS AND THERAPY

Myospherulosis is amenable to conservative treatment, although patients who have this response to surgery are more likely to require revision surgery. Therefore, nasal packing with lipid-based ointments should be avoided in patients who have previously been diagnosed with myospherulosis.

MYOSPHERULOISIS
DISEASE FACT SHEET

Definition	Foreign body reaction to iatrogenic petroleum, lanolin, or traumatized fat tissue resulting in artifactually encysted erythrocytes
Incidence and location	Uncommon reaction
Morbidity and mortality	Patients who have myospherulosis tend to require multiple surgeries to manage adhesions
Clinical features	Persistent sinonasal symptoms after sinonasal procedure
Prognosis and treatment	Conservative therapy without future use of lipid-based packing

---

MYOSPHERULOISIS
PATHOLOGIC FEATURES

Microscopic findings	Numerous small pseudocysts in dense fibrosis
	Large (100 μm) cysts, with a nonrefractile thin membrane, containing brown, discolored, misshapen erythrocytes
Histochemical features	Hemoglobin stain confirms the spherules as erythrocytes
	Gomori methenamine silver and iron stains are negative
Pathologic differential diagnosis	*Coccidioidomyces, Rhinosporidium*

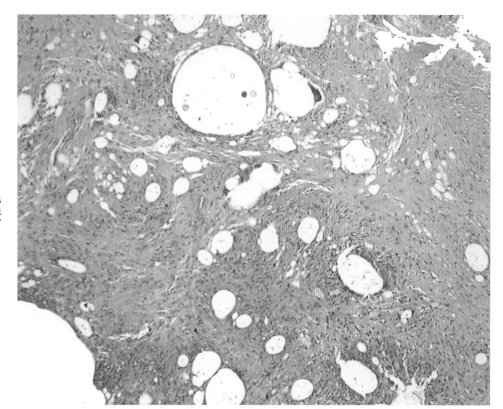

FIGURE 4-39

Heavy fibrosis and multiple vacuoles are noted with inflammation. Small aggregates of "eosinophilic globules" are seen in the spaces.

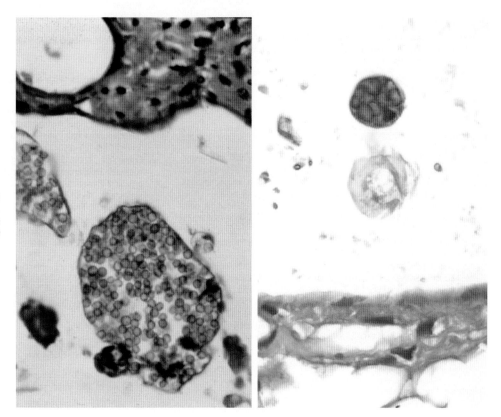

FIGURE 4-40

Left: The encysted erythrocytes in myospherulosis mimic fungal spores. *Right:* Small degenerated erythrocyte nuclei are housed in a ball within the lumen of this cyst.

SUGGESTED READING

Sinonasal Polyps

1. Gysin C, Alothman GA, Papsin BC: Sinonasal disease in cystic fibrosis: clinical characteristics, diagnosis, and management. Pediatr Pulmonol 2000;30(6):481–489.
2. Hellquist HB: Nasal polyps update. Histopathology. Allergy Asthma Proc 1996;17(5):237–242.
3. Nakayama M, Wenig BM, Heffner DK: Atypical stromal cells in inflammatory nasal polyps: immunohistochemical and ultrastructural analysis in defining histogenesis. Laryngoscope 1995;105:127–134.
4. Nishioka GJ, Cook PR: Paranasal sinus disease in patients with cystic fibrosis. Otolaryngol Clin North Am 1996;29(1):193–205.
5. Passali D, Bellussi L, Hassan HA, et al.: Consensus conference on nasal polyposis. Acta Otorhinolaryngol Ital 2004;24(2 Suppl 77):3–61.
6. Picado C: Aspirin intolerance and nasal polyposis. Curr Allergy Asthma Rep 2002;2(6):488–493.
7. Scadding GK: Comparison of medical and surgical treatment of nasal polyposis. Curr Allergy Asthma Rep 2002;2(6):494–499.
8. Zeifer B: Update on sinonasal imaging: anatomy and inflammatory disease. Neuroimaging Clin N Am 1998;8(3):607–630.
9. Zeitz HJ: Bronchial asthma, nasal polyps, and aspirin sensitivity: Samter's syndrome. Clin Chest Med 1988;9(4):567–576.

Nasal Glial Heterotopia

1. Cerda-Nicolas M, Fernandez de Sevilla CS, Lopez-Gines C, et al.: Nasal glioma or nasal glial heterotopia? Morphological, immunohistochemical and ultrastructural study of two cases. Clin Neuropathol 2002;21:66–71.
2. Mills SE, Gaffey MJ, Frierson HF: Neural, neuroendocrine, and neuroectodermal neoplasia. Tumors of the upper aerodigestive tract and ear, third series ed. Washington, DC: AFIP, 1997:119–200.
3. Patterson K, Kapur S, Chandra R: "Nasal gliomas" and related brain heterotopias: a pathologist's perspective. Ped Pathol 1986;5:353–362.
4. Penner CR, Thompson LDR: Nasal glial heterotopia: a clinicopathologic and immunophenotypic analysis of 10 cases with a review of the literature. Ann Diag Pathol 2003;7:354–359.
5. Wenig BM, Dulguerov P, Kapadia SB, Prasad ML, Fanburg-Smith JC, Thompson LDR. Neuroectodermal tumours. In: Barnes EL, Eveson JW, Reichart P, Sidransky D, eds. Pathology and Genetics of Head and Neck Tumours. Kleihues P, Sobin LH, series eds. World Health Organization Classification of Tumours. Lyon, France: IARC Press, 2005:65–75.

Infections

1. Corey JP, Delsupehe KG, Ferguson BJ: Allergic fungal sinusitis: allergic, infectious, or both? Otolaryngol Head Neck Surg 1995;113(1):110–119.
2. Kuhn FA, Swain R: Allergic fungal sinusitis: diagnosis and treatment. Current Opin Otolaryngol Head Neck Surg 2003;11: 1–5.
3. Lara JF, Gomez JD: Allergic mucin with and without fungus. A comparitive clinicopathologic analysis. Arch Pathol Lab Med 2001;125:1442–1447.
4. Ferguson BJ: Eosinophilic mucin rhinosinusitis. Laryngoscope 2000;110:799–813.
5. Makannaar JH, Chavan SS: Rhinosporidiosis: a clinicopathological study of 34 cases. Indian J Pathol Microbiol 2001;44:17–21.
6. Ahluwalia KB, Maheshwari N, Deka RC: Rhinosporidiosis: a study that resolves etiologic controversies. Am J Rhinol 1997;11:479–483.
7. Wenig BM, Thompson LDR, Franekl SS, et al.: Lymphoid changes of the nasopharyngeal and palatine tonsils that are indicative of human immunodeficiency virus infection: a clinicopathologic study of 12 cases. Am J Surg Pathol 1996;20:572–587.

Wegener's Granulomatosis

1. Frosch M, Foell D: Wegener granulomatosis in childhood and adolescence. Eur J Pediatr 2004;163:425–434.
2. Heffner DK: Wegener's granulomatosis is not a granulomatous disease. Ann Diagn Pathol 2002;6:329–333.

3. Holmen C, Christensson M, Petttersson E, et al.: Wegener's granulomatosis is associated with organ-specific antiendothelial cell antibodies. Kid International 2004;66:1049–1060.
4. Lamprecht P, Gross WL: Wegener's granulomatosis. Herz 2004;29:47–56.
5. Nishike S, Kato T, Nagai M, et al.: Management and follow-up of localized Wegener's granulomatosis: a review of five cases. Acta Otolaryngol 2004;124:1103–1108.
6. Rowshani AT, Schot LJ, Berge IJM: c-ANCA as a serological pitfall. Lancet 2004;363:782.
7. Seo P, Stone JH: The antineutrophil cytoplasmic antibody-associated vasculitides. Am J Med 2004;117:39–50.
8. Seyer BA, Grist W, Muller S: Aggressive destructive midfacial lesion from cocaine abuse. Oral Surg Oral Med Oral Pathol Oral Radiol Endod 2002;94:465–470.
9. Takwoingi YM, Dempster JH: Wegener's granulomatosis: an analysis of 33 patients seen over a 10-year period. Clin Otolaryngol 2003;28:187–194.
10. Yi ES, Colby TV: Wegener's granulomatosis. Semin Diagn Pathol 2001;18:34–46.

Respiratory Epithelial Adenomatoid Hamartoma (READ)

1. Wenig BM, Heffner DK: Respiratory epithelial adenomatoid hamartomas of the sinonasal tract and nasopharynx: a clinicopathologic study of 31 cases. Ann Otol Rhinol Laryngol 1995;104:639–645.
2. Wenig BM. Respiratory epithelial adenomatoid hamartoma. In: Barnes EL, Eveson JW, Reichart P, Sidransky D, eds. Pathology and Genetics of Head and Neck Tumours. Kleihues P, Sobin LH, series eds. World Health Organization Classification of Tumours. Lyon, France: IARC Press, 2005:33.

Rhinophyma

1. Curnier A, Choudhary S: Rhinophyma: dispelling the myths. Plast Reconstr Surg 2004;114:351–354.
2. Stucker FJ, Lian T, Sanders K: The ABCs of rhinophyma management. Am J Rhinol 2003;17:45–49.
3. Rohrich RJ, Griffin JR, Adams WP Jr: Rhinophyma: review and update. Plast Reconstr Surg 2002;110:860–869.

Sinus Histiocytosis With Massive Lymphadenopathy (Rosai-Dorfman Disease)

1. Carbone A, Passannante A, Gloghini A, Devaney KO, Rinaldo A, Ferlito A: Review of sinus histiocytosis with massive lymphadenopathy (Rosai-Dorfman disease) of head and neck. Ann Otol Rhinol Laryngol 1999;108:1095–1104.
2. Chan ACL, Chan JKC, Cheung MMC, Kapadia SB. Haematolymphoid tumours. In: Barnes EL, Eveson JW, Reichart P, Sidransky D, eds. Pathology and Genetics of Head and Neck Tumours. Kleihues P, Sobin LH, series eds. World Health Organization Classification of Tumours. Lyon, France: IARC Press, 2005:58–64.
3. Foucar E, Rosai J, Dorfman RF: Sinus histiocytosis with massive lymphadenopathy. An analysis of 14 deaths occurring in a patient registry. Cancer 1984;54:1834–1840.
4. Goodnight JW, Wang MB, Sercarz JA, Fu YS: Extranodal Rosai-Dorfman disease of the head and neck. Laryngoscope 1996;106:253–256.
5. Wenig BM, Abbondanzo SL, Childers EL, et al.: Extranodal sinus histiocytosis with massive lymphadenopathy (Rosai-Dorfman disease) of the head and neck. Hum Pathol 1993;24:483–492.

Langerhans Cell Histiocytosis

1. Davis SE, Rice DH: Langerhans' cell histiocytosis: current trends and the role of the head and neck surgeon. Ear Nose Throat J 2004;83:340–344.
2. Devaney KO, Putzi MJ, Ferlito A, Rinaldo A: Head and neck Langerhans cell histiocytosis. Ann Otol Rhinol Laryngol 1997;106:526–532.
3. Krishna H, Behari S, Pal L, et al.: Solitary Langerhans-cell histiocytosis of the clivus and sphenoid sinus with parasellar and petrous exten-

sions: case report and a review of literature. Surg Neurol 2004;62: 447–454.

Myospherulosis

1. Rosai J: The nature of myospherulosis of the upper respiratory tract. Am J Clin Pathol 1978;69:475–481.

2. Sindwani R, Cohen JT, Pilch BZ, Metson RB: Myospherulosis following sinus surgery: pathological curiosity or important clinical entity? Laryngoscope 2003;113:1123–1127.

3. Wheeler TM, Sessions RB, McGavran MH: Myospherulosis: a preventable iatrogenic nasal and paranasal entity. Arch Otolaryngol 1980;106:272–274.

5 Benign Neoplasms of the Nasal Cavity, Paranasal Sinuses, and Nasopharynx

Bayardo Perez-Ordoñez • Lester D. R. Thompson

SCHNEIDERIAN PAPILLOMAS

The mucosa of the nasal vestibule and the superior wall of the nasal cavity are lined by squamous and olfactory mucosa, respectively. The remaining nasal mucosa consists of ciliated columnar epithelium of ectodermal origin known as the Schneiderian membrane. Three benign neoplastic papillomatous proliferations arise from the Schneiderian membrane: exophytic, fungiform, or everted papillomas (EP), inverted or endophytic papillomas (IP), and columnar, cylindrical cell, or onco-cytic, papillomas (CCP). Although these entities share a number of features and are classified as "Schneiderian papillomas," there are sufficient clinical and microscopic differences to regard them as three distinctive clinicopathologic entities. The overall lack of mixed papillomas and their relation to human papilloma virus (HPV) are sufficiently different to lend further credence to this separation.

CLINICAL FEATURES

Sinonasal Schneiderian papillomas (SSP) are a rare disease with an estimated annual incidence of 0.6 per 100,000. Males are affected much more commonly than females (4:1), with most patients presenting in the latter years of life (range, 15–96 yr; mean, 56 yr). Clinical symptoms are nonspecific and include unilateral nasal obstruction, followed by epistaxis, rhinorrhea, facial pressure, and headaches. Often, patients report previous intranasal surgery before a diagnosis of SSP is firmly established. Physical examination usually demonstrates a unilateral polypoid mass in the nasal cavity. SSP show a remarkable anatomic distribution according to histologic type: EP arise almost exclusively on the

---

SCHNEIDERIAN PAPILLOMA: EXOPHYTIC TYPE
DISEASE FACT SHEET

Definition	A papilloma derived from the Schneiderian membrane composed of exophytic, papillary fronds with fibrovascular cores lined by multiple layers of well-differentiated stratified epithelial cells
Incidence and location	Uncommon (~6/1,000,000-population) Nasal septum
Morbidity and mortality	Morbidity associated with nasal obstruction and epistaxis No mortality
Gender, race, and age distribution	Male > Female (4:1) Adults (mean, 6th decade)
Clinical features	Unilateral nasal obstruction Epistaxis Rhinorrhea Headaches
Prognosis and treatment	Excellent long-term prognosis, although recurrences develop (up to 50%) Meticulous and complete surgical resection

---

SCHNEIDERIAN PAPILLOMA: ENDOPHYTIC TYPE
DISEASE FACT SHEET

Definition	A papilloma derived from the Schneiderian membrane with proliferation and invagination into the underlying stroma
Incidence and location	Uncommon (~6/1,000,000-population) Lateral nasal wall, middle meatus, and less often the paranasal sinuses (nasopharynx and middle ear are rare)
Morbidity and mortality	Intracranial invasion Malignant transformation in 10% of cases
Gender, race, and age distribution	Male > Female (4:1) Adults (mean, 6th decade) uncommon in children
Clinical features	Nasal obstruction Epistaxis Rhinorrhea Facial pressure Headaches
Prognosis and treatment	Excellent long-term prognosis (excluding cases with malignant transformation) Recurrences up to 60%, depending on type of surgery Malignant transformation in about 10% of cases Meticulous, complete surgical resection

SCHNEIDERIAN PAPILLOMA: CYLINDRICAL CELL TYPE DISEASE FACT SHEET	
Definition	A papilloma derived from the Schneiderian membrane displaying exophytic fronds and endophytic invaginations lined by multilayered columnar oncocytic cells
Incidence and location	Rare
	Lateral wall of nasal cavity
Morbidity and mortality	Nasal obstruction, bleeding
	Rare cases of malignant transformation
Gender, race, and age distribution	Equal gender distribution
	6th decade
Clinical features	Nasal obstruction
	Epistaxis
Prognosis and treatment	Excellent prognosis
	Rare examples of malignant transformation
	Meticulous and complete surgical resection

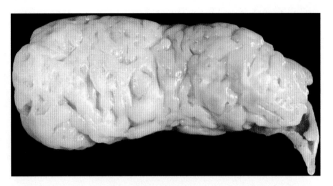

FIGURE 5-1

Surgical specimen of an inverted Schneiderian papilloma with a polypoid appearance. The cerebriform surface shows numerous clefts due to exuberant endophytic epithelial proliferation.

nasal septum; IP and CCP affect the lateral nasal wall, middle meatus, and less often the paranasal sinuses (maxillary, ethmoid, sphenoid, frontal sinuses). Less than 3% of cases are bilateral. Rarely, cases are seen as primary lesions in nasopharyngeal or middle ear mucosa.

RADIOLOGIC FEATURES

Plain x-rays, computed tomography (CT), and magnetic resonance imaging (MRI) routinely show a unilateral polypoid mass filling the nasal cavity. Displacement of the nasal septum and opacification of sinuses are also frequently seen. Pressure erosion of the bone is present in approximately 45% of cases. Intratumoral calcification is extremely rare.

SCHNEIDERIAN PAPILLOMA: EXOPHYTIC TYPE PATHOLOGIC FEATURES	
Gross findings	Grey-tan, cauliflower-like or verrucous papillary proliferation attached to mucosa by narrow stalk
Microscopic findings	Branching, exophytic proliferations with fibrovascular cores lined by well-differentiated stratified squamous epithelium
	Basal and parabasal cells, well-differentiated keratinized cells, granular cell layer, surface keratin
	Intraepithelial or luminal ciliated or goblet cells
	Stroma with seromucus glands
Pathologic differential diagnosis	Cutaneous squamous papilloma, inflammatory nasal polyp, papillary squamous cell carcinoma

SCHNEIDERIAN PAPILLOMA: ENDOPHYTIC TYPE PATHOLOGIC FEATURES	
Gross findings	Large, multinodular, firm polypoid lesions
	Deep clefts of inverted but intact mucosa
	Fragments of bone in surgical specimen
Microscopic findings	Markedly thick, inverted neoplastic proliferation replacing mucoserous glands and ducts (noninvasive)
	Transitional/squamoid epithelium with numerous intraepithelial microcysts containing macrophages, mucin, and cellular debris
	Distinct cell borders with glycogenation
	May have ciliated columnar cells or surface keratinization
	Foci of cytologic atypia
	Stroma ranging from edematous, myxomatous, to fibrous with an inflammatory infiltrate
	No seromucus glands in stroma
	Transformation to carcinoma (in situ or invasion) may occur (usually squamous cell carcinoma)
Immunohistochemical features	Co-expression of columnar and squamous epithelial keratins by the same cells
Pathologic differential diagnosis	Sinonasal polyp, READ, carcinoma

PATHOLOGIC FEATURES

GROSS FINDINGS

EP have been described as grey-tan cauliflower-like or mulberry-like verrucous papillary proliferations attached to underlying mucosa by a narrow stalk. IP usually are large, multinodular, firm polypoid lesions with deep clefts and intact mucosa (Fig. 5-1). Often, resections for IP included fragments of bone. Grossly, CCP are usually small and fragmented and consist of soft pink to tan papillary fragments of tissue.

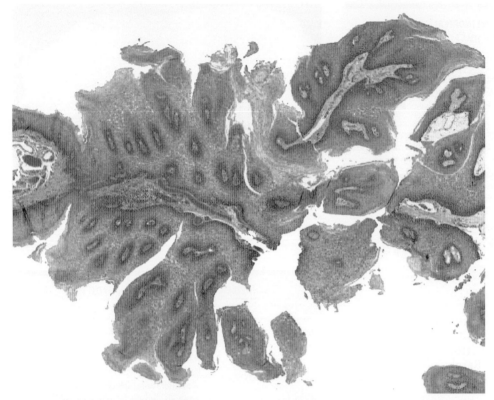

FIGURE 5-2

A basal-parabasal appearance to this exophytic Schneiderian papilloma is noted on the left, while a more well-differentiated keratinized epithelium with parakeratosis is noted on the right.

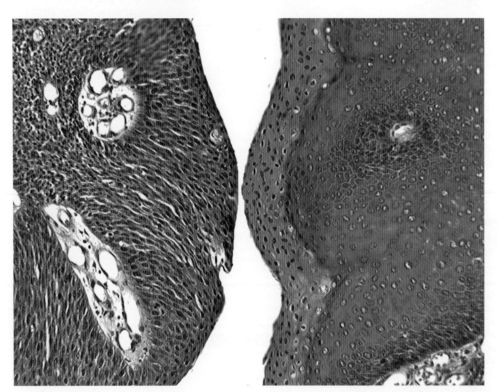

FIGURE 5-3

Exophytic Schneiderian papilloma of nasal septum lined by markedly thickened well-differentiated squamous epithelium.

MICROSCOPIC FINDINGS

Exophytic

EP consist of branching, exophytic proliferations composed of fibrovascular cores lined by well-differentiated stratified squamous epithelium (Fig. 5-2). The epithelium ranges from basal and parabasal cells (Fig. 5-

3) to well-differentiated keratinized cells with a granular cell layer and surface keratin with hyperkeratosis (Figs. 5-4, 5-5). There may be intraepithelial or luminal ciliated or goblet cells. The stroma usually contains variable numbers of seromucus glands. Mitotic figures and atypical cells are distinctly uncommon in EP. Malignant transformation is vanishingly rare.

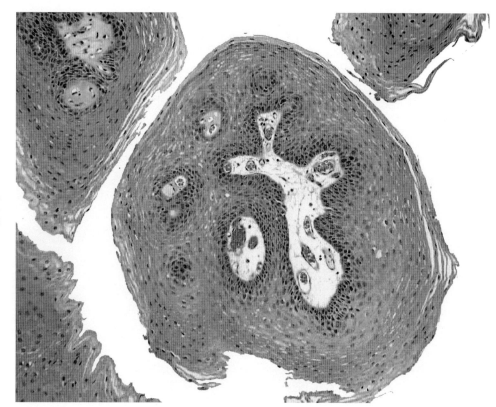

FIGURE 5-4

Exophytic Schneiderian papilloma with papillary "finger-like" projections with a fibrovascular core lined by squamous cells.

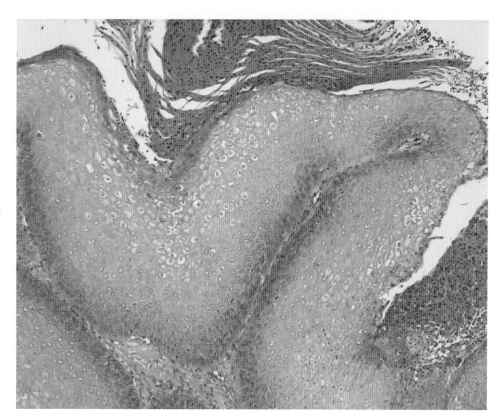

FIGURE 5-5

An exophytic Schneiderian papilloma with koilocytic atypia, hyperkeratosis, and parakeratosis.

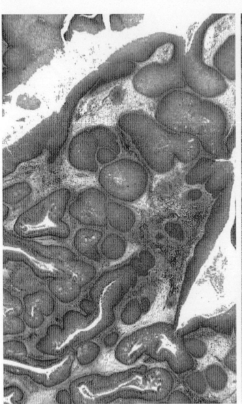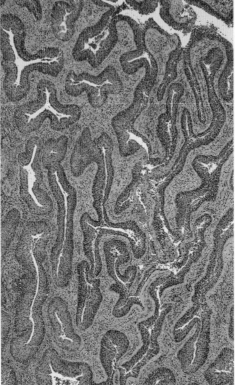

FIGURE 5-6
Inverted Schneiderian papillomas with nests of cells deep in the stroma.

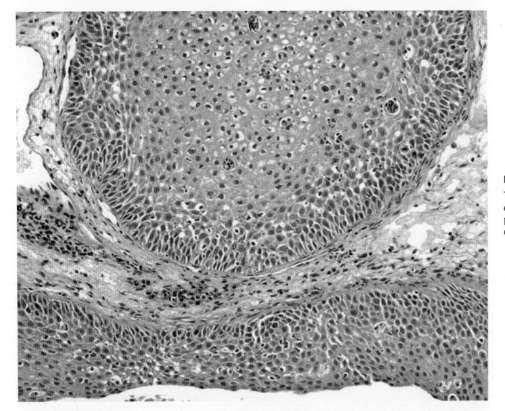

FIGURE 5-7
Typical nonkeratinizing squamous epithelium found in an inverted papilloma. Intraepithelial cysts with occasional macrophages are present.

Endophytic

IP consists of a markedly thick, inverted, or endophytic growth of nonkeratinizing transitional cells (Fig. 5-6). The inverted areas are surrounded by a well formed basement membrane and does not show "invasive" growth. The epithelium in IP undergoes squamous maturation with superficial cells adopting a flattened orientation (Fig. 5-7). Surface keratinization and a granular cell layer are uncommon (10%). Distinct cell borders and cleared cytoplasm (due to glycogen) are frequent findings. Cellular pleomorphism may be present, but is focal and not associated with dyskeratosis or increased mitotic activity. A characteristic feature is the presence of numerous intraepithelial microcysts containing macrophages, mucin, and cell debris (Fig. 5-8). These microcysts are more numerous close to the luminal surface. Mucous cells may be interspersed. Mitotic activity is variable, but usually limited to basal and parabasal cells. Occasionally, the luminal surface may be lined by ciliated columnar cells. The stroma ranges from edematous, myxomatous, to fibrous, usually showing a conspicuous absence of seromucus glands. An inflammatory infiltrate comprised of a variable mixture of neutrophils, eosinophils, small lymphocytes and plasma cells with occasional germinal centers is a consistent finding (Fig. 5-9).

Malignant transformation is seen in up to 10% of cases. The majority are conventional in situ and invasive squamous cell carcinomas (Fig. 5-10). When carcinoma is present, it is synchronous in 60%, while metachronous in 40%.

Cylindrical Cell

CCP are characterized by a proliferating multilayered columnar or oncocytic epithelium (Fig. 5-11). Most CCP have an exophytic branching papillary appearance with long delicate fibrous cores. The individual tumor cells show well-defined cell borders with eosinophilic or granular oncocytic cytoplasm. The nuclei are round, centrally located, and uniform. Small to medium nucleoli are readily seen. Occasional surface cells show well-defined cilia (Fig. 5-12). Numerous small intraepithelial mucous cysts are also typically seen in these tumors. Mitotic figures are uncommon in CCP. Unlike IP, seromucus glands are present in the submucosa of CCP. Malignant transformation of CCP is rare.

ANCILLARY STUDIES

ULTRASTRUCTURAL FEATURES

While unnecessary for diagnosis, electron microscopy shows that IP consist of stratified transitional-like cells with areas of basal and squamous cells characterized by cytoplasmic bundles of tonofilaments. Occasional goblet cells with mucin granules can be also identified. The tumor cells show long

SCHNEIDERIAN PAPILLOMA: CYLINDRICAL CELL TYPE PATHOLOGIC FEATURES	
Gross findings	Small fragments of soft, fleshy, pink, tan, papillary tissue
Microscopic findings	Both exophytic and endophytic patterns
	Multiple layers of columnar oncocytic epithelium
	Tumor cells have well defined borders with eosinophilic or granular oncocytic cytoplasm
	Round nuclei with small nucleoli
	Cilia may be present focally on the surface
	Intraepithelial cysts
	Rare malignant transformation
Immunohistochemical features	Mitochondrial histochemical stains (PTAH)–positive
	Cytochrome c oxidase positive
Pathologic differential diagnosis	Rhinosporidiosis and low-grade papillary sinonasal adenocarcinoma

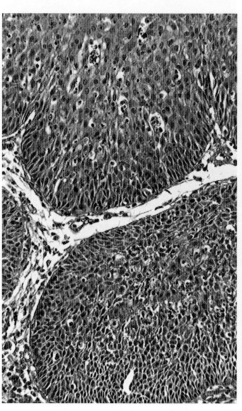
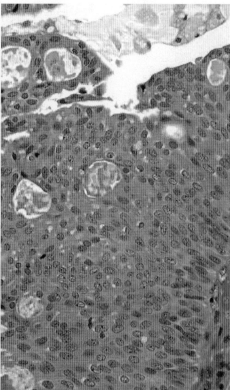

FIGURE 5-8

Squamoid proliferation with variable intraepithelial microcysts in an inverted type Schneiderian papilloma.

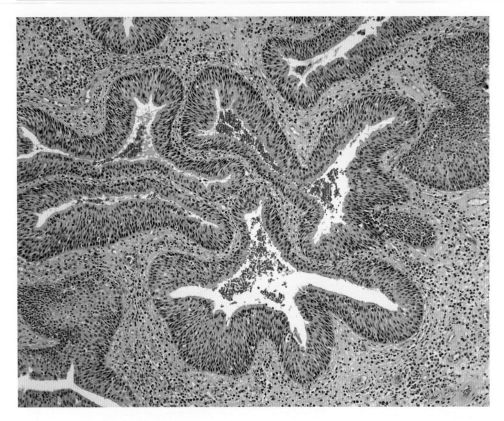

FIGURE 5-9
Inverted proliferation separated by a fibrous stroma with mixed inflammatory cells.

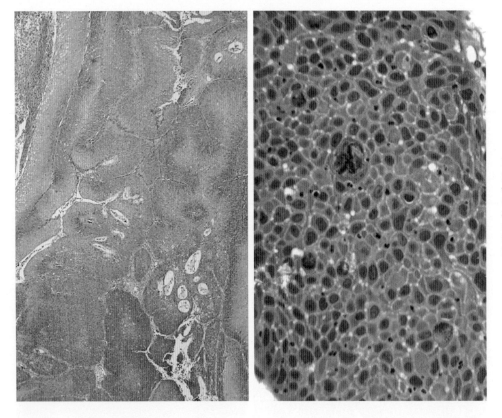

FIGURE 5-10
Malignant transformation of a inverted Schneiderian papilloma demonstrates an increased cellularity and lack of maturation (*left*), while nuclear pleomorphism and atypical mitotic figures are seen on high power (*right*).

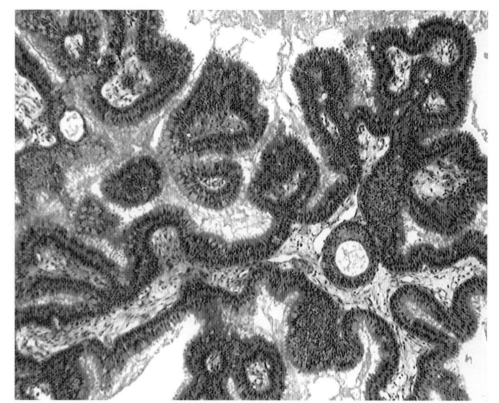

FIGURE 5-11

Multilayered oncocytic epithelium arranged in a focal "tram-track" architecture. Cilia are abundant at the surface of this complex papillary growth.

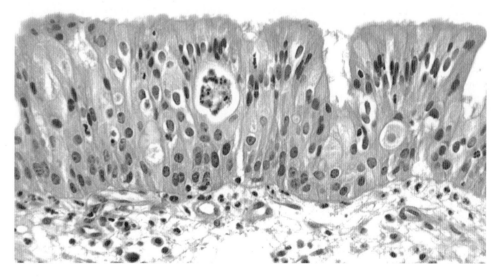

FIGURE 5-12

Cylindrical cell Schneiderian papilloma with stratified columnar respiratory epithelium with oncocytic cells and small neutrophilic abscesses.

microvilli-like processes joined by well-developed desmosomes. Cytoplasmic glycogen and lysosomes are prominent. The basement membrane is thin and discontinuous in many areas.

IMMUNOHISTOCHEMICAL FEATURES

Immunohistochemical studies are not necessary for the diagnosis or classification of SSP. Interestingly, the co-expression of keratins typical of columnar and squamous differentiation by the same cells appears to be characteristic of Schneiderian papillomas and is not seen in non-neoplastic mucosa. The cells of CCP are immunoreactive with cytochrome c oxidase as would be expected in an oncocytic cell.

MOLECULAR TECHNIQUES

In situ hybridization and polymerase chain reaction have convincingly demonstrated an etiologic role for HPV in SSP, although variation in technique and serotypes of HPV sought yield variable results. The low-risk HPV types 6 and 11 are by far the most common identified. The presence of HPV does not seem to increase the risk of malignant transformation.

DIFFERENTIAL DIAGNOSIS

The differential diagnosis depends on the histologic type of papilloma, and includes sinonasal polyps, cutaneous squamous papilloma, papillary squamous cell carcinoma, respiratory epithelial adenomatoid hamartoma (READ), low-grade papillary adenocarcinoma, and rhinosporidiosis. Sinonasal polyps have marked stromal edema and inflammation with a nonproliferative epithelium, lacking intraepithelial microcysts. Papillary squamous cell carcinomas are characterized by papillae with fibrovascular cores lined by clearly malignant squamous epithelium. It is important to bear in mind the possibility of a carcinoma arising in a Schneiderian papilloma. READ is a rare hamartoma with epithelium arranged in a glandular distribution. Low-grade papillary sinonasal adenocarcinoma has an infiltrative growth, with acinar, cystic, or trabecular growth. Rhinosporidiosis has characteristic sporangia and endospores within the stroma, below the epithelium rather than the microcysts within the epithelium of IP and CCP.

PROGNOSIS AND THERAPY

The long-term prognosis of SSP without in situ or invasive carcinoma is excellent. However, there is a considerable recurrence rate, often dependent on the extent of the tumor and initial surgical approach used. If inadequately removed, recurrences develop in up to 60% (more common for inverted than the other types), usually developing within 5 years of initial presentation.

Multiple recurrences are not uncommon. Given the anatomic confines, if neglected, significant morbidity may be experienced. There is no correlation between the number of recurrences and the development of carcinoma, if it occurs.

The treatment of choice is surgery, whether endoscopic, snare avulsion, or by a more radical excision (lateral rhinotomy and medial maxillectomy, Caldwell-Luc procedure, craniofacial resection or midfacial degloving). Meticulous removal is imperative if recurrences are to be averted.

LOBULAR CAPILLARY HEMANGIOMA (PYOGENIC GRANULOMA)

CLINICAL FEATURES

Lobular capillary hemangiomas (LCH) are a relatively common, benign vascular neoplasm representing about 25% of all nonepithelial sinonasal tract neoplasms. Although the term "pyogenic granuloma" preceded "lobular capillary hemangioma" as the diagnostic term for these lesions, it is a misnomer. LCH are not "purulent," "infectious," or "granulomatous." While the pathogenesis is unknown, local trauma and hormonal factors are suggested etiologic agents. About one-third of mucosal LCH arise in the nasal cavity. These lesions usually affect boys under the age of 15, females in their reproductive years, and less commonly older adults of either gender.

Patients typically present with intermittent, painless episodes of epistaxis. Large lesions may cause nasal obstruction. Rhinoscopy generally shows a well-defined, sessile or polypoid, red to purplish mass. Often, there is mucosal ulceration with a fibrinous exudate. Approximately 60% of cases arise from the anterior nasal

LOBULAR CAPILLARY HEMANGIOMA (PYOGENIC GRANULOMA) DISEASE FACT SHEET	
Definition	Benign vascular tumor with lobular architecture composed of variable size vessels with proliferating endothelial cells
Incidence and location	Common
	Anterior nasal septum (60%), nasal vestibule (20%), turbinates (20%)
Gender, race, and age distribution	Boys <15 yr
	Female in reproductive years
	Older adults no gender differences
Clinical features	Intermittent, painless epistaxis
	Nasal obstruction
Prognosis and treatment	Excellent prognosis with no significant recurrences
	Complete endoscopic resection with bleeding control

septum (Little's area), 20% involve the nasal vestibule, and 20% affect the turbinates.

PATHOLOGIC FEATURES

GROSS FINDINGS

LCH are polypoid (Fig. 5-13), nodular, or sessile masses with pink or gray-tan color. Frequently, the surgical specimen is ulcerated and partially covered with a yellow to white fibrinous exudate.

LOBULAR CAPILLARY HEMANGIOMA (PYOGENIC GRANULOMA) PATHOLOGIC FEATURES	
Gross findings	Sessile, polypoid, or nodular red to purplish mass
	Ulceration is common
Microscopic findings	Lobular architecture with mixture of thin and thick blood vessels
	Central vessel surrounded by cellular lobule of closely packed capillaries
	Plump endothelial cells with bland nuclear features and scanty to moderate eosinophilic cytoplasm
	Frequent mitotic figures
	Edematous to fibrotic stroma with mixed inflammatory infiltrate
	Ulcerated surface with fibrinous exudate simulating granulation tissue
Immunohistochemical features	Endothelial cells positive for CD31, CD34, factor VIII-RAg
	Actins positive in pericytes and smooth muscle cells
Pathologic differential diagnosis	Nasopharyngeal angiofibroma, glomangiopericytoma (sinonasal-type hemangiopericytoma), angiosarcoma

MICROSCOPIC FINDINGS

The term "lobular capillary hemangioma" properly describes the microscopic appearance of this benign vascular tumor. At low power, LCH exhibits a distinct lobular architecture with a mixture of thin and thick blood vessels comprising the center the lesion (Fig. 5-14). The lobules are quite cellular and composed of small, closely packed capillaries with slit-like or indistinct lumina (Fig. 5-15). The endothelial cells are plump with bland nuclear features and scanty to moderate eosinophilic cytoplasm (Fig. 5-16). Mitotic activity within the lobules is readily identified. The center and superficial portions of LCH show well-formed capillaries or large angulated vessels with branching lumina. These vessels may have thick walls resembling small arteries or venules. The stroma ranges from edematous to fibrotic. A variable inflammatory infiltrate composed of small lymphocytes, plasma cells, masts cells, and neutrophils is also present. The inflammatory infiltrate is most prominent in the surface of ulcerated tumors. Ulcerated tumors also exhibit a fibrinous exudate and areas indistinguishable from conventional granulation tissue.

ANCILLARY STUDIES

While unnecessary in the vast majority of cases, the endothelial cells are positive for vascular markers such as CD31, CD34, and factor VIII-RAg. Actin stains highlight pericytes and smooth muscle cells.

DIFFERENTIAL DIAGNOSIS

This benign tumor must be separated from nasopharyngeal angiofibroma (NPA), glomangiopericytoma

FIGURE 5-13

A lobular arrangement around large patulous vessels is seen in this lobular capillary hemangioma.

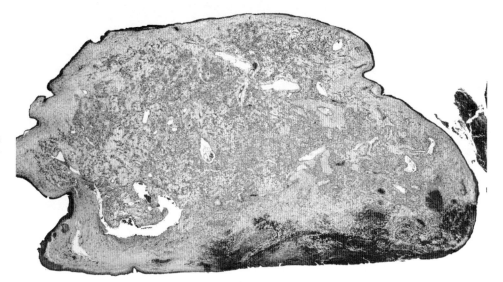

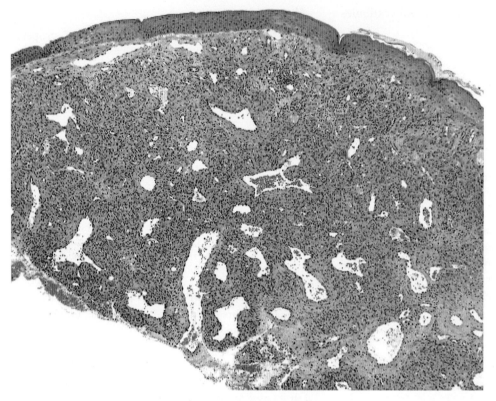

FIGURE 5-14
Lobular capillary hemangioma with lobular architecture demonstrating cellular lobules interspersed with larger dilated blood vessels.

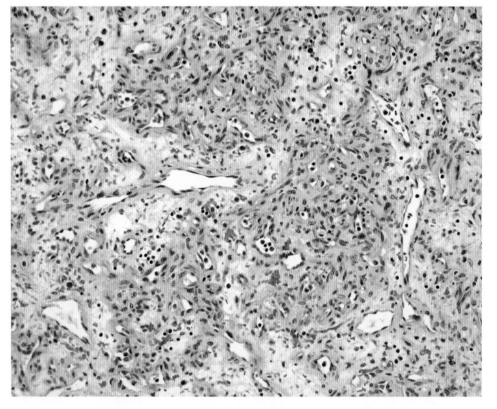

FIGURE 5-15
Central vessel surrounded by lobules of endothelial-lined capillaries.

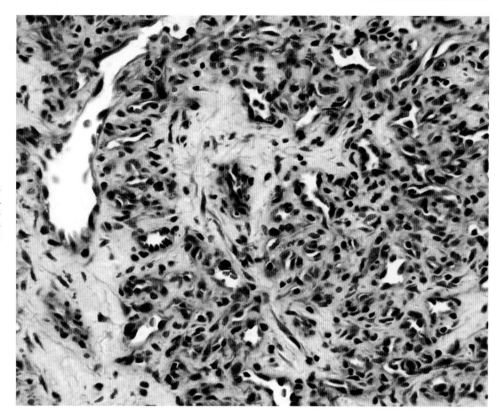

FIGURE 5-16
The lobule is quite cellular and is composed of prominent endothelial cells admixed with inconspicuous pericytes. The lobule contains and is surrounded by variably sized blood vessels.

(sinonasal-type hemangiopericytoma), and angiosarcoma. The lobular architecture is not seen in other vascular tumors. The vascular component of NPA is separated by thin to thick collagen fibers and spindle or stellate stromal cells. Glomangiopericytoma is a cellular tumor composed of fascicles of oval to spindle cells with a characteristic perivascular hyalinization and mast cells and eosinophils. Angiosarcoma is widely infiltrative, composed of atypical endothelial cells with increased mitotic figures.

PROGNOSIS AND THERAPY

LCH are benign tumors which do not recur after complete resection. Planning of the resection should include radiologic studies to investigate the extent of the tumor. Excision is best accomplished by wide endoscopic resection, utilizing YAG laser to control potential bleeding. The resection should include a rim of normal mucosa/submucosa.

GLOMANGIOPERICYTOMA (SINONASAL-TYPE HEMANGIOPERICYTOMA)

This tumor has been referred to by a number of names, including *hemangiopericytoma-like tumor, sinonasal-*

type hemangiopericytoma, and *glomangiopericytoma.* This is an uncommon sinonasal tract neoplasm demonstrating perivascular myoid phenotype, showing hybrid differentiation between glomus (myoid) and hemangiopericytoma (pericytic). Therefore, the preferred term is *glomangiopericytoma* (GPC). This lesion is distinctly different from soft tissue-type hemangiopericytoma.

CLINICAL FEATURES

GPC is a rare neoplasm (<0.5% of all sinonasal neoplasms), observed slightly more frequently in females than males. The age at presentation is variable and ranges from in utero to 86 years, with a mean in the 7th decade. Most patients complain of nasal obstruction, epistaxis, and less commonly nasal discharge, pain, and headaches. Physical examination usually reveals a unilateral, polypoid mass in the nasal cavity, with rare bilateral involvement. The paranasal sinuses are uncommonly affected.

RADIOLOGIC FEATURES

Radiologic studies are not distinctive. Plain x-rays and CT scans typically show sinus and nasal opacification by a polypoid nasal mass. Bone erosion and sclerosis is seen in a significant number of cases.

GLOMANGIOPERICYTOMA (SINONASAL-TYPE HEMANGIOPERICYTOMA) DISEASE FACT SHEET	
Definition	A sinonasal tumor demonstrating perivascular myoid phenotype
Incidence and location	Rare neoplasm (<0.5% of all sinonasal tract neoplasms)
	Lateral nasal cavity
	Paranasal sinuses uncommonly affected
Morbidity and mortality	Rare malignant tumors
Gender, race, and age distribution	Slight female predominance
	Mean, 7th decade (range, in utero to 86 yr)
Clinical features	Nasal obstruction
	Epistaxis
	Nasal discharge, pain, and headaches
Prognosis and treatment	Indolent neoplasm with excellent prognosis (>90% 5-yr survival)
	Recurrences in up to 30%
	Rare malignant neoplasms (2%)
	Complete surgical resection

PATHOLOGIC FEATURES

GROSS FINDINGS

The generally polypoid tumors range up to 8 cm (mean, ~3 cm). The tumors are beefy red to grayish pink, soft, edematous, fleshy to friable masses, often demonstrating hemorrhage.

MICROSCOPIC FINDINGS

GPC are a subepithelial well-delineated but unencapsulated cellular tumor, effacing or surrounding the normal structures (Fig. 5-17). It is comprised of closely packed cells, forming short fascicles and sometimes exhibiting a storiform, whorled, or palisaded pattern, interspersed with many vascular channels (Fig. 5-18). The latter are in the form of capillary-sized to large patulous spaces that may have a "staghorn" or "antler-like" configuration. A prominent peritheliomatous hyalinization is characteristic (Fig. 5-19). The neoplastic cells are uniform, elongated to oval, and possess vesicular to hyperchromatic, round to oval to spindle-shaped nuclei, and lightly eosinophilic cytoplasm (Fig. 5-20). The cells are often syncytial in appearance. Mild nuclear pleomorphism and occasional mitotic figures may be present, but necrosis is not found. Extravasated erythrocytes, mast cells, and eosinophils are nearly ubiquitously present (Fig. 5-21). Occasionally, tumor giant cells, fibrosis or myxoid degeneration may be seen. Moderate to severe nuclear atypia and a mitotic rate of >4/10 HPF have been associated with an increased risk of developing recurrent disease or dying with disease.

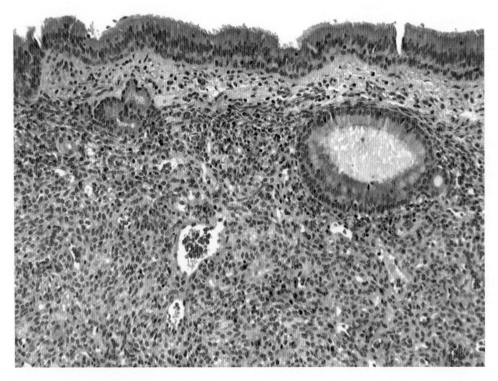

FIGURE 5-17

Characteristic diffuse growth within the submucosa with effacement of the normal components of the submucosa and preservation of minor salivary glands. The overlying respiratory epithelium remains intact.

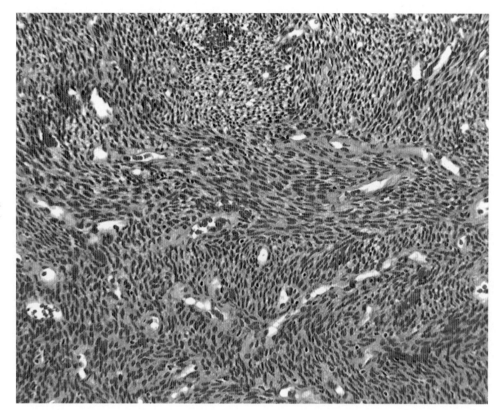

FIGURE 5-18
Closely packed cells in short fascicles with vague storiforming. Many vessels are present.

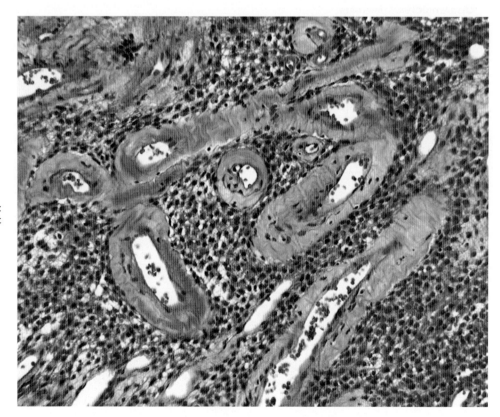

FIGURE 5-19
A characteristic histomorphologic feature is the presence of prominent perivascular hyalinization.

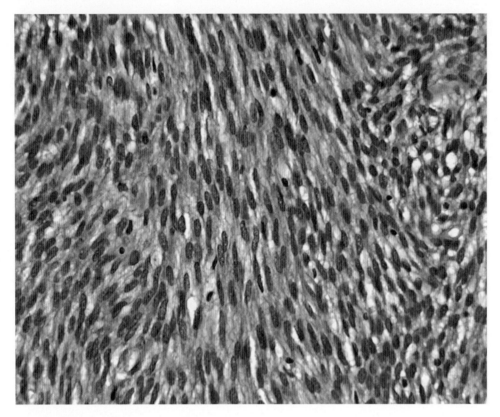

FIGURE 5-20
A syncytial arrangement of stream-ing, short spindled cells. The nuclei are oval. Vascular spaces are not prominent in this field.

ANCILLARY STUDIES

ULTRASTRUCTURAL FEATURES

Electron microscopy studies have shown that GPC are composed of spindle and stellate cells surrounding non-neoplastic vessels and endothelial cells. The tumor cells contain bundles of microfilaments with dense bodies and subplasmalemmal plaques consistent with true pericytic differentiation. Micropinocytotic vesicles are demonstrable in some tumors.

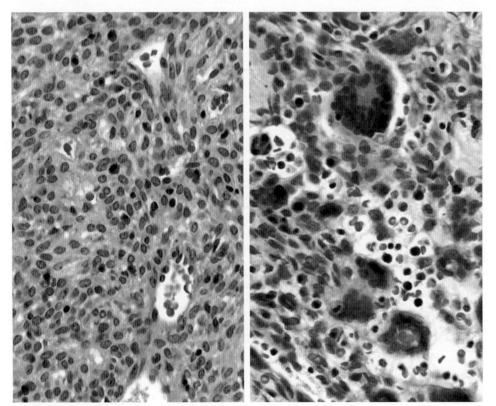

FIGURE 5-21
Left: Eosinophils and mast cells are common in GPC. *Right:* Occasionally tumor giant cells can be seen.

GLOMANGIOPERICYTOMA (SINONASAL-TYPE HEMANGIOPERICYTOMA) PATHOLOGIC FEATURES

Gross findings	Polypoid masses Mean, 3 cm Solid, beefy, fleshy masses with areas of hemorrhage		Mast cells and eosinophils Moderate to severe nuclear atypia and a mitotic rate of >4/10 HPF associated with an increased risk of developing recurrent disease or dying with disease
Microscopic findings	Subepithelial unencapsulated cellular tumor Closely packed cells, short fascicles, and storiform-whorled pattern Vascular channels (staghorn) demonstrating prominent peritheliomatous hyalinization Uniform, syncytial arrangement of oval to elongated cells Round to spindled nuclei	Immunohistochemical features	Positive for vimentin, smooth muscle actin, muscle-specific actin, factor XIII Negative bcl-2, keratins, CD31, factor VIII-RAg, desmin, CD117
		Pathologic differential diagnosis	Hemangioma, solitary fibrous tumor, glomus tumor, leiomyoma, monophasic synovial sarcoma, fibrosarcoma, and malignant peripheral nerve sheath tumor

IMMUNOHISTOCHEMICAL FEATURES

The tumor cells are diffusely positive for vimentin, smooth muscle actin, muscle-specific actin, and factor XIII (Fig. 5-22). Occasional focal staining for CD34 is noted. The cells are negative with bcl-2, keratins, CD31, factor VIII-RAg, desmin, CD99, and CD117.

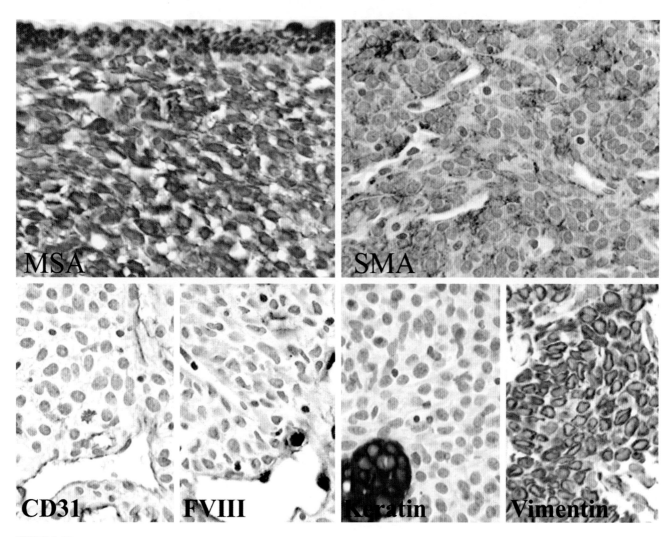

FIGURE 5-22

Positive immunostaining for actins and vimentin, while there is no reaction of the tumor cells with CD31, factor VIII-RAg, or keratin.

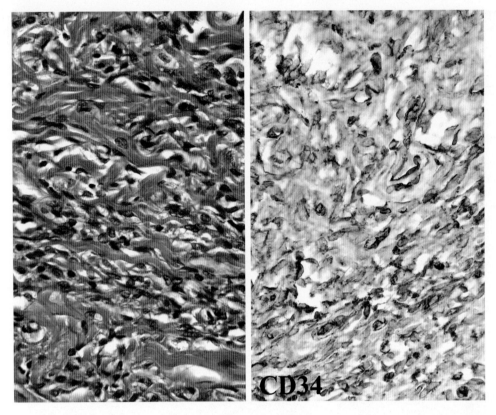

FIGURE 5-23

Left: A solitary fibrous tumor has haphazard cellular arrangement with heavy fibrosis. *Right:* CD34 strongly highlights the lesional cells.

DIFFERENTIAL DIAGNOSIS

The differential diagnosis of GPC includes a variety of benign and malignant spindle cell tumors, but usually can be limited to hemangioma, solitary fibrous tumor, glomus tumor, leiomyoma, monophasic synovial sarcoma, fibrosarcoma, and malignant peripheral nerve sheath tumor. Hemangiomas are lobular, frequently exhibit surface ulceration and do not grow in a fascicular architecture. Solitary fibrous tumor (SFT) is often hypocellular, has thick stromal collagen, and are diffusely positive for CD34 and bcl-2 (Fig. 5-23). Glomus tumors are comprised of round, epithelioid cells forming cellular nests with organoid appearance and are exceptionally rare in the sinonasal tract. Leiomyomas of the sinonasal tract show a perivascular distribution with larger spindle cells. They are desmin positive in addition to the actins. All the sarcomas usually have significant pleomorphism, mitotic activity, and necrosis.

PROGNOSIS AND THERAPY

GPC are indolent, with an overall excellent survival rate (>90% 5-yr survival) achieved with complete surgical

excision. Recurrence, which develops in up to 30% of cases, usually occur within one year, but may occur many years after the initial surgery. Aggressive-behaving GPC (malignant GPC) are uncommon (2%), and usually exhibit the following features: large size (>5 cm), bone invasion, severe nuclear pleomorphism, increased mitotic activity (>4/10 HPF), atypical mitotic figures, necrosis, and proliferation index >10%.

NASOPHARYNGEAL ANGIOFIBROMA

The term "juvenile" angiofibroma is a misnomer since angiofibromas do not arise exclusively in the young. Nasopharyngeal angiofibromas (NPA) are benign, highly cellular and richly vascularized mesenchymal neoplasms that arise in the roof of the nose nasopharynx in males. It is rare, accounting for <1% of all nasopharyngeal tumors, arising in the fibrovascular stroma of the posterolateral wall of the roof of the nose. Localization studies have determined that the point of origin for most NPA is the region where the sphenoidal process of the palatine bone meets the horizontal ala of the vomer and pterygoid process. This junction forms the superior margin of the sphenopalatine foramen and the posterior margin of the middle turbinate.

CLINICAL FEATURES

NPA affects almost exclusively boys and adolescent to young men, with a mean age of 15 years. NPA are uncommon tumors with an estimated incidence of 1 in 150,000 males, with fair-skinned and red-haired males more commonly affected. If a female is affected, testicular feminization has to be excluded by chromosome analysis. There is an association with familial adenomatous polyposis. The most common symptoms of NPA are nasal obstruction, spontaneous epistaxis, and nasal drainage. Other patients may present with facial deformities, proptosis, rhinolalia, deafness, sinusitis, otitis, and a bulging palate resulting from extension of the tumor into soft tissues of the face and orbit. Endoscopic examination usually shows a mass involving the posterior nasal wall. Various staging systems have been proposed, with size and location determining the outcome (Chart 1).

RADIOLOGIC FEATURES

On plain x-rays, NPA are characterized by a soft tissue mass causing bowing of the posterior wall of the maxillary sinus and distortion and posterior displacement of the pterygoid plates (Holman-Miller sign). Bony margins may be eroded, but are obvious. CT and MRI show the extent of the tumor as well as possible surgical approach (Fig. 5-24). Angiography identifies the feeding vessel(s) and allows for presurgical embolization. The dense tumor blush is characteristic (Fig. 5-24). Due precautions are suggested before taking biopsies from these tumors because of the risk of life-threatening bleeding.

PATHOLOGIC FEATURES

GROSS FINDINGS

Most NPA are round or nodular, nonencapsulated masses with a sessile or pedunculated base. The tumors may be large, although the mean size is 4 cm. The surface of the tumors is largely covered by intact mucosa

---

Chart 5-1

System for staging juvenile nasopharyngeal angiofibroma

Stage	Description
Stage I	Tumor limited to the nasopharynx with no bone destruction
Stage II	Tumor invading the nasal cavity, maxillary, ethmoid, and sphenoid sinuses with no bone destruction
Stage III	Tumor invading the pterygo-palatine fossa, infra-temporal fossa, orbit and parasellar region
Stage IV	Tumor with massive invasion of the cranial cavity, cavernous sinus, optic chiasm, or pituitary fossa

---

**NASOPHARYNGEAL ANGIOFIBROMA
DISEASE FACT SHEET**

Definition	A benign, highly cellular, and richly vascularized mesenchymal neoplasm that arises in the nasopharynx in males		Sinusitis, rhinolalia, otitis, tinnitus, deafness
Incidence and location	Uncommon, incidence of 1/150,000 males <1% of nasopharyngeal tumors Posterior nasal wall, roof of nose and nasopharynx	Radiographic features	Soft tissue density with bowing of the posterior maxillary sinus Bony margins may be eroded Angiography identifies feeder vessels and permits presurgical embolization
Morbidity and mortality	Intracranial extension in some patients Mortality up to 9% related to hemorrhage and intracranial extension	Prognosis and treatment	Benign but locally aggressive neoplasm Recurrences in about 20%, most commonly intracranially, and usually within first 2 yr
Gender, race, and age distribution	Males (exclusively) Peak age, 15 yr (range, 6–29 yr)		Mortality up to 9% related to hemorrhage or intracranial extension
Clinical features	Nasal obstruction, spontaneous epistaxis, nasal drainage Facial deformities, proptosis, and a bulging palate		Complete surgical resection with preoperative embolization or hormonal therapy Radiotherapy for unresectable intracranial tumors

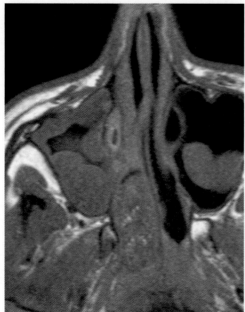

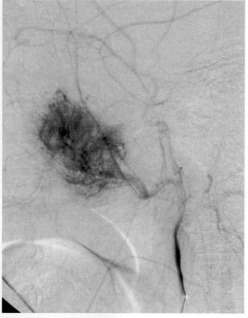

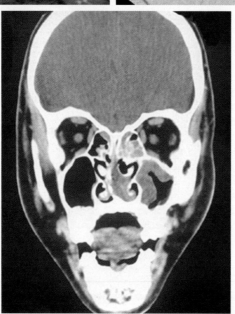

FIGURE 5-24

Left upper: A computed tomography scan shows a large mass within the nasopharynx, nasal cavity, and maxillary sinus. The posterior wall of the maxillary sinus is bowed. *Right upper:* A dense blush showing the rich vascularity of the angiofibroma and the feeder vessel. *Lower:* CT demonstrating a mass in the nasal cavity, filling the maxillary and ethmoid sinus.

NASOPHARYNGEAL ANGIOFIBROMA PATHOLOGIC FEATURES	
Gross findings	Round or nodular, nonencapsulated masses with sessile or pedunculated base
	Intact mucosa with focal areas of ulceration and superficial hemorrhage
	Cut surface showing dilated vascular channels which give the tumors a spongy appearance or solid, fibrotic tumors
	Mean size, 4 cm
Microscopic findings	Combination of abnormal vascular network, a connective tissue stroma, and stromal cells
	Vascular network with variable sized vessels, from thin-walled, slit-like to large irregular vessels
	Muscle layer is absent, focal, pad-like, or circumferential
	Endothelium is attenuated, but can be plump
	Spindle, stellate, angular stromal cells in collagenized background
	Inflammatory cells usually absent
	Increased fibrosis with treatment; embolic material may be seen
Immunohistochemical features	Vessel walls positive with vimentin and
	Endothelial cells positive for CD34, CD31, androgen receptors, factor VIII-RAg
	Stromal cells positive for vimentin, β-catenin, androgen receptors
Pathologic differential diagnosis	Lobular capillary hemangioma, sinonasal polyps, peripheral nerve sheath tumor, solitary fibrous tumor, desmoid tumor (desmoid-type fibromatosis)

with focal areas of ulceration and superficial hemorrhage. The cut surface is variable and shows dilated vascular channels, which give the tumors a spongy appearance. In less vascular areas, the tumors appear solid and fibrotic (Fig. 5-25).

MICROSCOPIC FINDINGS

The microscopic appearance of NPA resides in the dynamic combination of three elements: an abnormal

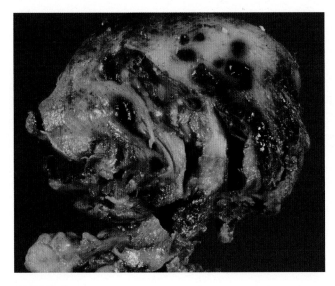

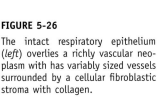

FIGURE 5-25
Nasopharyngeal angiofibroma with smooth surface. The cut surface shows a solid mass with large hemorrhagic areas corresponding to feeding vessels.

vascular network, a connective tissue stroma, and stromal cells (Fig. 5-26). The vascular network consists of mostly thin-walled, slit-like ("staghorn") or dilated vessels, with calibers ranging from capillary to large, patulous vessels (Fig. 5-27). The muscular layer can be absent, focal and pad-like, or circumferential. The vascular spaces and lining endothelium appear to be resting directly on the connective tissue stroma (Fig. 5-28). The endothelial cells may be plump but are usually attenuated. The fibrous connective tissue stroma consists of plump spindle, angular, or stellate-shaped cells, and a varying amount of fine and coarse collagen fibers (Fig. 5-29). Focally, the stroma may be acellular with a hyalinized appearance, or show myxoid changes (especially in embolized specimens). The nuclei of the stromal cells are generally cytologically bland (Fig. 5-30), but they may be multinucleated or show some degree of pleomorphism in the more cellular areas. The chromatin is finely and evenly dispersed. Large stromal cells with abundant cytoplasm resembling ganglion cells can be identified. Mitotic activity and nuclear atypia are not features of typical NPA. Mast cells may be seen, but other inflammatory elements are usually absent (except if there is surface ulceration). Long-standing lesions show increased fibrosis and diminished vasculature. Treatment with hormones results in increased collagenization of the stroma with fewer, but thicker walled vessels. In specimens excised after embolization treatment, the tumour often shows areas of infarction, and emboli can be seen in some blood vessels (Fig. 5-31). Sarcomatous transformation is an exceedingly uncommon event, usually following radiation therapy.

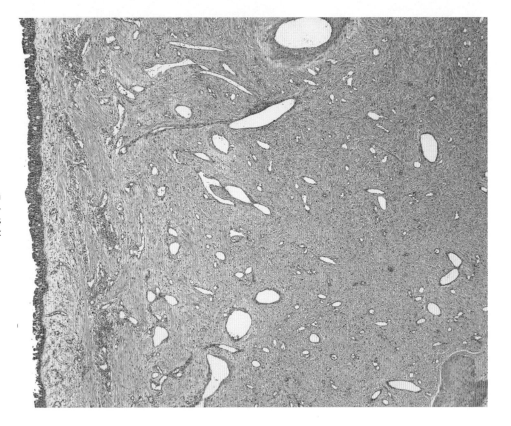

FIGURE 5-26
The intact respiratory epithelium (*left*) overlies a richly vascular neoplasm with has variably sized vessels surrounded by a cellular fibroblastic stroma with collagen.

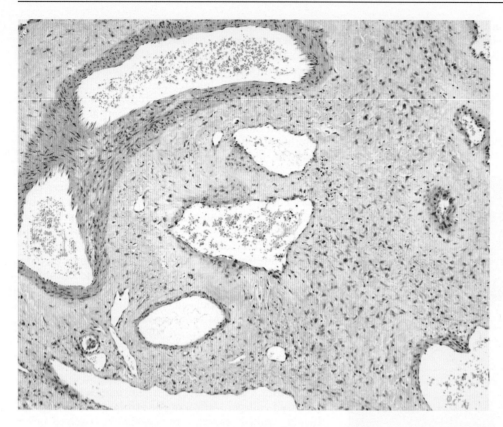

FIGURE 5-27
Smooth muscle walled vessels, patulous vessels, and capillaries are all surrounded by the characteristic collagenized stroma.

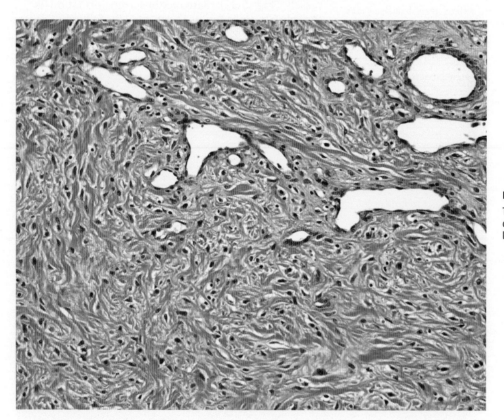

FIGURE 5-28
Thin-walled vessels surrounded by dense, "keloid-like" collagen. Stellate fibroblasts are noted.

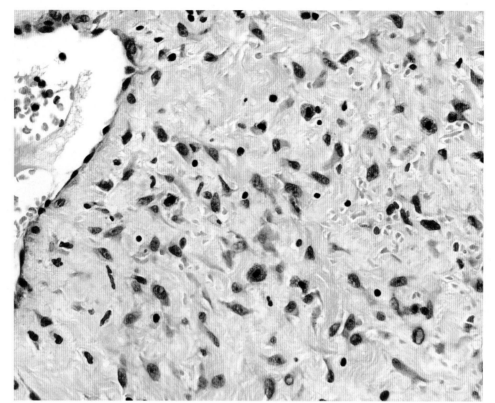

FIGURE 5-29

A large thin-walled vessel is associated with fibrous connective tissue, inflammatory cells, and stellate fibroblasts.

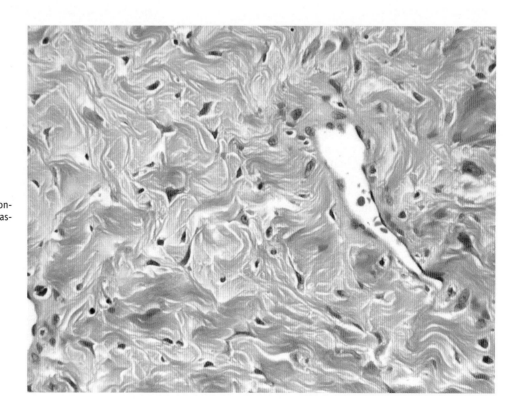

FIGURE 5-30

Heavily collagenized stroma demonstrates only a few stellate fibroblastic cells with a single vessel.

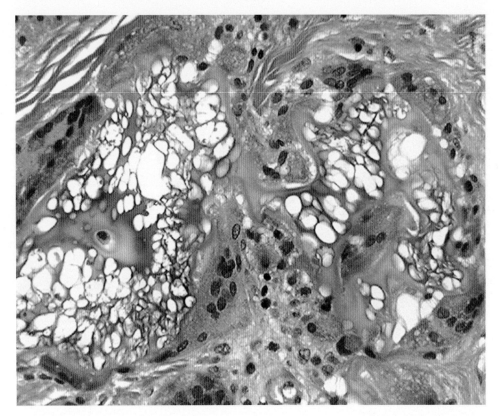

FIGURE 5-31
Embolic material surrounded by mult-inucleated giant cells in this NPA.

ANCILLARY STUDIES

ULTRASTRUCTURAL FEATURES

Ultrastructurally, the stromal cells contain lobulated nuclei, intranuclear inclusions, variable amounts of rough endoplasmic reticulum and thin filaments, hemidesmosomes, focal basal lamina, and prominent pinocytotic vesicles, suggesting a hybrid mesenchymal cell (myofibroblast). The presence of intranuclear dense bodies in stromal fibroblasts is an uncommon, but characteristic feature. These nuclear bodies resemble large perichromatin granules. The stromal fibroblasts are surrounded by abundant mature collagen fibers.

IMMUNOHISTOCHEMICAL FEATURES

The vessel wall cells are immunoreactive with vimentin and smooth muscle actin (SMA), whereas the stromal cells are immunoreactive with vimentin only, except in areas of increased fibrosis, where focal SMA may be identified. Desmin may be focally immunoreactive in larger vessels at the periphery of the tumor. Factor VIII R-Ag, CD34, and CD31 highlight the endothelium, but not the stromal cells. Stromal and endothelial cells are usually reactive with androgen receptors (75 %), while progesterone receptors are occasionally reactive. Other markers, including nuclear staining for ß-catenin, CD117, platelet-derived growth factor B, basic fibroblast growth factor, insulin-like growth factor type II, and nerve growth factor are also reactive.

DIFFERENTIAL DIAGNOSIS

The main differential diagnoses of NPA include LCH, sinonasal polyps, peripheral nerve sheath tumors, SFT, and desmoid tumor. LCH have a lobular architecture and lack the stromal cells and collagen of angiofibroma. Polyps with stromal atypia have inflammatory cells and lack the vascular pattern. Peripheral nerve sheath tumors have a fascicular architecture and are S-100 protein positive. SFT show increased cellularity, do not have the vascular pattern, and strongly express CD34. A desmoid tumor or desmoid-type fibromatosis has long sweeping fascicles and infiltrative borders without the prominent vascularity of NPA.

PROGNOSIS AND THERAPY

This benign tumour is characterized by local aggressive growth, with recurrences in about 20 % of patients (>50 % in older series), most commonly intracranially, and usually within the first 2 years after diagnosis. Mortality has ranged up to 9 % due to hemorrhage and intracranial extension, but this figure has dropped with improved radiographic and surgical techniques. Patients may be managed with selective angiographic embolization or hormonal therapy prior to definitive surgical resection (usually via a lateral rhinotomy). Radiation therapy has been successfully implemented to manage large, intracranial, or recurrent tumors, but surgery is still the therapy of choice. The rare case of malignant transformation represents postradiation sarcoma.

MYXOMA

Myxomas are an intraosseous neoplasm characterized by stellate and spindle-shaped cells embedded in an abundant myxoid or mucoid extracellular matrix. When a relatively greater amount of collagen is evident, the term myxofibroma may be used. Tumors arise within bone or soft tissue. The prevailing opinion is that myxomas arise from altered fibroblasts or myofibroblasts that produce an excess of mucopolysaccharides and are usually incapable of producing mature collagen. This, however, is not an "all or none" phenomenon, as some cells may retain the capacity to form collagen.

CLINICAL FEATURES

Myxomas of bone are rare and develop almost exclusively in the jaws, affecting the mandible more often than the maxilla, more often in the posterior portions.

The strong predilection for the jaws suggests an odontogenic origin, further supported by the association with impacted or missing teeth. The true incidence of myxomas is difficult to estimate; however, the incidence has been calculated as being 0.07 per million. Most tumors affect young adults in the 2nd–5th decades (mean, 30 yr). Myxoma has shown a slight female predominance. Most patients are asymptomatic, but if symptomatic, they report pain, headache, orbital protuberance, nasal stuffiness or obstruction, or facial asymmetry. Loosening and displacement of teeth occurs if the tumor affects tooth-bearing areas. Gnathic and sinonasal tract tumors are not a feature of Carney's complex, although soft tissue myxomas are associated with fibrous dysplasia and/or Albright's syndrome.

RADIOLOGIC FEATURES

In conventional radiographs and CT scans, myxomas are homogeneous, unilocular or multilocular radiolucent tumors with expansion or invasion of cortical bone (Fig. 5-32). Tumors with interlaced bone trabeculae often show a "soap-bubble" or "honeycomb" appearance. Tooth displacement and tooth resorption is frequently seen in large lesions.

PATHOLOGIC FEATURES

GROSS FINDINGS

Macroscopically, myxomas are described as unencapsulated but well-circumscribed, lobular or multinodular tumors with tan, grey to white color. They have a glistening mucoid, gelatinous, translucent to firm consis-

MYXOMA DISEASE FACT SHEET	
Definition	Benign mesenchymal neoplasm composed of stellate and spindle cells surrounded by loose myxoid or mucoid extracellular stroma
Incidence and location	Rare tumor; incidence of .07 per million
	Mandible and maxilla (posterior), rarely sinonasal
Morbidity and mortality	Mortality associated with intracardiac myxoma only
Gender, race, and age distribution	Females slightly more common than males (1:1.2)
	Mean age, 30 yr (2nd–4th decades)
Clinical features	Most jaw lesions are asymptomatic
	May be associated with pain, headache, nasal stuffiness, and facial asymmetry
	Loosening or displacement of teeth
	Bone lesions are not associated with syndromes
Radiographic features	Well-circumscribed, unilocular radiolucency, or a multilocular destructive lesion
	Soap-bubble or honeycomb appearance
	Teeth may be displaced
Prognosis and treatment	Good prognosis, although insidious local invasion may make recurrences a problem
	Recurrences in about 25%, most within 5 yr
	Rarely death if there is cranial base extension
	Complete surgical resection with margin of normal tissue

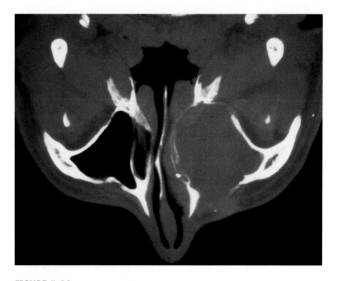

FIGURE 5-32

Radiolucent, homogeneous mass with expansion of cortical bone typical of myxoma.

MYXOMA
PATHOLOGIC FEATURES

Gross findings	Unencapsulated but well circumscribed
	Lobular or multinodular tumors
	Tan, grey to white
	Glistening mucoid, gelatinous, translucent to firm consistency
	Invasion or destruction of cortical bone may be present
	Lobular or multinodular tumors
Microscopic findings	Hypocellular tumors composed of stellate and spindle cells with delicate cytoplasmic processes and no atypia
	Large amounts of myxoid or mucoid stroma with scant vessels
	Scanty collagen usually; may be increased (fibromyxoma)
	Occasionally foci of inactive odontogenic epithelium
Ultrastructural features	Fibroblasts or myofibroblasts with rudimentary cell junctions
	Well-developed rough endoplasmic reticulum
	Cytoplasmic intermediate filaments and microfilaments
	Extracellular amorphous material with collagen fibers
Immunohistochemical features	Vimentin, laminin, and actin positive; rarely desmin positive
	Negative for keratins, S-100 protein, GFAP, CD34
Pathologic differential diagnosis	Dental papilla, mucocele, nasal polyp with myxoid change, neurothekeoma, benign peripheral nerve sheath tumor, low-grade myxofibrosarcoma, myxoid chondrosarcoma

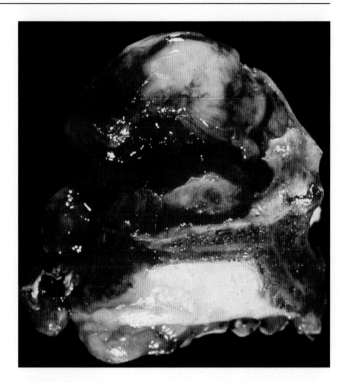

FIGURE 5-33
Partial maxillectomy for myxoma specimen demonstrating a glistening, gelatinous mass in the maxilla.

ANCILLARY STUDIES

ULTRASTRUCTURAL FEATURES

The tumor cells in myxoma show ultrastructural features of fibroblasts and myofibroblasts with spindle or stellate cells with slender cytoplasmic cell process occasionally joined by rudimentary cell junctions. Many cells display a well-developed rough endoplasmic reticulum, Golgi apparatus, and mitochondria. Bundles of cytoplasmic intermediate filaments (vimentin) and microfilaments (actin) are often seen. The microfilaments can be abundant along the cell membrane. The extracellular material consists of amorphous substance of low-electron density with thin bundles of collagen fibers.

IMMUNOHISTOCHEMICAL FEATURES

Myxomas are typically positive for vimentin and laminin, with variable actin and desmin reactions. The cells are negative with keratins, S-100 protein, glial fibrillary acidic protein, and vascular markers.

DIFFERENTIAL DIAGNOSIS

The differential diagnosis includes any tumor with myxoid change, only a few of which are suggested here. A dental papilla, the embryonic precursor of the dental

tency (Fig. 5-33). Invasion or destruction of cortical bone may also be identified (Fig. 5-34). Small cysts and bands of fibrosis may be seen on cut surface.

MICROSCOPIC FINDINGS

Myxomas are paucicellular neoplasms composed of randomly distributed stellate to spindle cells with poorly defined long, delicate cytoplasmic processes. The tumor cells show no cytologic or nuclear atypia (Fig. 5-35). The nuclei are small and hyperchromatic and mitotic figures are rare or inconspicuous. These cells lie in a hypovascular intercellular matrix, rich in mucopolysaccharides (hyaluronic acid and chondroitin sulfate) and appearing myxoid or mucoid. This stroma contains delicate reticulin fibers. Characteristically, myxomas contain little collagen; however, some tumor may show variable areas with increased vascularity or condensed collagen, the latter referred to as "fibromyxoma" (Fig. 5-36). Occasional tumors contain inactive odontogenic epithelium resembling rests of Malassez.

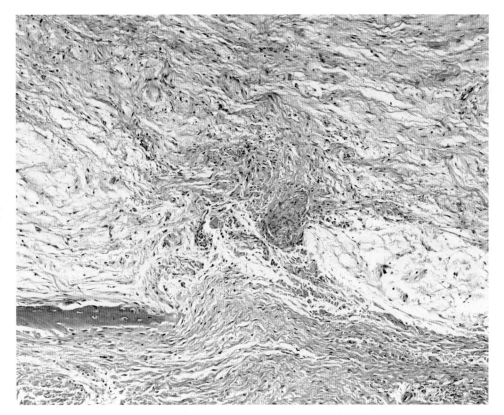

FIGURE 5-34

This collagenized myxoma shows focal invasion and destruction of cortical bone.

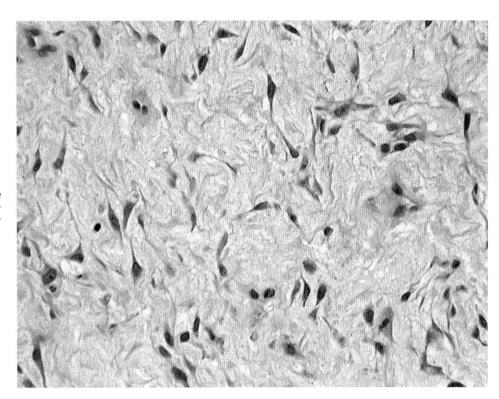

FIGURE 5-35

Myxoma composed of slender spindle and stellate cells with delicate cytoplasmic processes and small hyperchromatic nuclei.

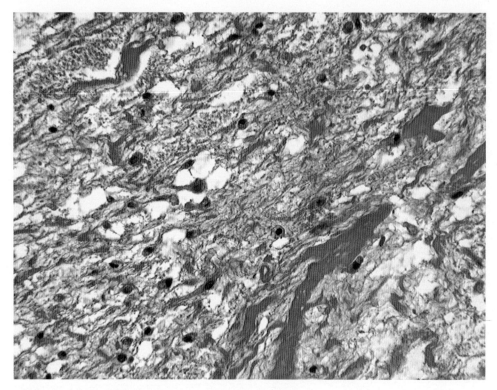

FIGURE 5-36
A fibromyxoma has a myxoid background with scant spindle cells and delicate to heavy collagen deposition.

pulp, is an incidental finding, is always circumscribed, usually small, and often has odontoblasts with dentinoid material. A mucocele lacks fibroblasts/myofibroblasts. A nasal polyp with myxoid change has inflammatory cells and usually a polypoid appearance. Neurothekeoma and benign peripheral nerve sheath tumors are more cellular than most myxomas and are S-100 protein positive. Low-grade myxofibrosarcoma and myxoid chondrosarcomas have cytologically atypical cells, have a distinct nodular or lobular architecture and chondrosarcomas will be S-100 protein positive.

PROGNOSIS AND THERAPY

Myxomas are benign neoplasms with no metastatic potential. However, untreated tumors can reach large sizes, and may invade adjacent bone and soft tissues. Recurrences develop in about 25 % of patients, usually within 5 years of therapy. Rarely death may result from cranial base extension. The treatment of choice is conservative but complete resection with a rim of normal tissue surrounding the tumor, a difficult achievement in the sinonasal tract especially.

ECTOPIC PITUITARY ADENOMA

A benign pituitary gland neoplasm occurring separately from and without involvement of the sella turcica (i.e., with normal anterior pituitary gland) is referred to as ectopic pituitary adenoma. Involvement of the

sinonasal tract by pituitary adenomas is encountered more commonly as direct extension of an intrasellar neoplasm, while only rarely as an ectopic neoplasm. It has been estimated that secondary extension into the sinonasal tract is seen in approximately 2 % of intrasellar pituitary adenomas. The sphenoid bone and sinus are the most frequent locations for ectopic lesions, although rarely the nasal cavity, nasopharynx, and petrous temporal bone may be affected. Embryologic remnants along the migration path of the Rathke's pouch are presumed to be the source of pituitary adenomas.

CLINICAL FEATURES

Similarly to sellar adenomas, sinonasal pituitary adenomas are more common in females than males (2 : 1), with a mean age at presentation of 49 years (range, 16–65 yr). Patients usually have nonspecific complaints such as nasal obstruction, chronic sinusitis, bloody nasal discharge or epistaxis, headaches, and diplopia or other visual field defects. Approximately 50 % of patients affected will have clinical evidence of hormonal hyperactivity, including Cushing disease, acromegaly, hyperparathyroidism, hyperthyroidism, amenorrhea, and hirsutism. In endocrinologically silent tumors, the diagnosis is often unsuspected before surgery.

RADIOLOGIC FEATURES

CT and MRI studies of ectopic pituitary adenomas define the extent and location of the tumor, character-

ECTOPIC PITUITARY ADENOMA DISEASE FACT SHEET	
Definition	A benign pituitary neoplasm occurring separately from, and without involvement of the sella turcica (a normal anterior pituitary gland)
Incidence and location	Rare
	Sphenoid sinus most common location followed by nasal cavity
Morbidity and mortality	Morbidity associated with hormonal manifestations and local invasion
Gender, race, and age distribution	Females > Males (2 : 1)
	Mean age, 49 yr (range, 16–65 yr)
Clinical features	Nasal obstruction
	Chronic sinusitis
	Bloody nasal discharge or epistaxis
	Headaches
	Visual field defects (diplopia)
	About 50% have hormone hyperactivity
Radiographic features	CT and MR define extent and location of tumor
	Sellar may be involved by upward extension, although usually normal
Prognosis and treatment	Excellent prognosis with control of endocrine abnormalities after complete surgical resection
	Recurrence may develop in large tumors
	Malignant transformation exceptionally rare
	Surgery is curative, but only if completely removed
	Drugs (dopamine-agonists, somatostatin analog) and radiation may be used postoperatively for control

ECTOPIC PITUITARY ADENOMA PATHOLOGIC FEATURES	
Microscopic findings	Submucosal location of unencapsulated tumor
	Tumors arranged in solid, organoid, and trabecular patterns separated by delicate fibrovascular septa
	Monotonous population of round, or polygonal epithelial cells with eosinophilic cytoplasm
	Round or oval nuclei with "salt-and-pepper" chromatin and inconspicuous or small nucleoli
	Nuclear pleomorphism, mitoses and necrosis are rare
Ultrastructural features	Intracytoplasmic neurosecretory granules, type dependent on the tumor hormone production
Immunohistochemical features	Strong keratin, chromogranin, synaptophysin, NSE reactivity
	May stain for the hormone peptides, including ACTH, prolactin, TSH, GH, FSH, and LH
Pathologic differential diagnosis	Olfactory neuroblastoma, ES/PNET, carcinoma, neuroendocrine carcinoma, lymphoma, melanoma

ized by the presence of an irregular sphenoidal or nasal mass with bone destruction in the presence of a normal pituitary gland. Upward invasion with sellar involvement may be seen in large ectopic adenomas (Fig. 5-37). Tumor size does not seem to correlate with symptom severity.

PATHOLOGIC FEATURES

The surface epithelium is usually intact and uninvolved, subtended by the unencapsulated neoplasms (Fig. 5-38). Delicate fibrovascular septa separate the tumor into solid, organoid, and trabecular patterns. The neoplasms are histologically identical to their intrasellar counterparts. Most neoplasms are composed of a monotonous population of round to oval epithelial cells with eosinophilic cytoplasm, usually characterized as chromophobe adenomas. The nuclei are round or oval and contain clumped chromatin with inconspicuous or small nucleoli (Fig. 5-39). Focal pleomorphism can be seen, as with all endocrine-type neoplasms. Mitotic activity and necrosis are not seen.

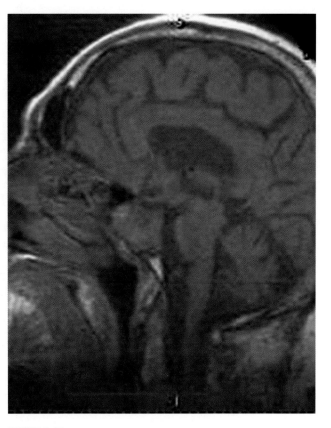

FIGURE 5-37

Large prolactinoma of sphenoidal sinus with secondary invasion of sella.

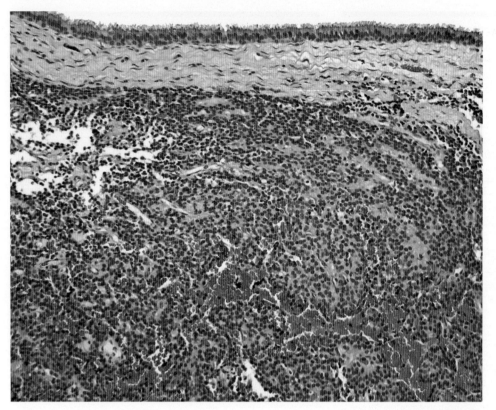

FIGURE 5-38

Ectopic pituitary adenoma of the sphenoid sinus underlying respiratory-ciliated mucosa. The tumor consists of lobules of monotonous epithelial cells with eosinophilic cytoplasm. Note the thin delicate fibrovascular septa separating the tumor lobules.

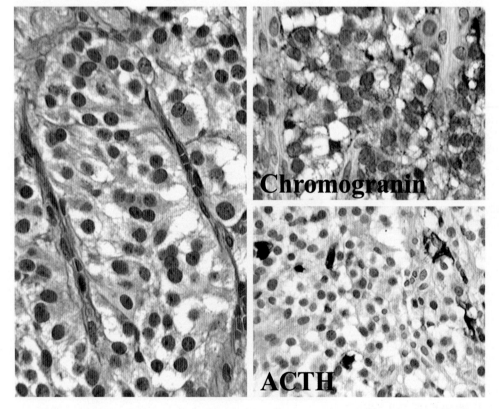

FIGURE 5-39

Left: Delicate, salt-and-pepper nuclear chromatin distribution. *Right upper:* Chromogranin immunoreactivity. *Right lower:* This tumor was ACTH immunoreactive.

ANCILLARY STUDIES

ULTRASTRUCTURAL FEATURES

The identification of intracellular neurosecretory granules confirms the neuroendocrine nature of the process, with variable size and shape of the granules specifically associated with hormone production.

IMMUNOHISTOCHEMICAL FEATURES

The tumor cells have strong and diffuse reactions with keratin, chromogranin, synaptophysin and neuron specific enolase. Specific hormones may be produced by the tumor, and should be sought to confirm the diagnosis. These include adrenocorticotropin (ACTH), prolactin, growth hormone, thyroid-stimulating hormone (ß-TSH), pituitary-specific transcription factor (Pit-1), ß-subunit and α-subunit of glycoprotein hormones, soluble fibrin (SF-1), follicle-stimulating hormone, and luteinizing hormone. The most common immunohistochemically expressed hormones have been ACTH and prolactin.

DIFFERENTIAL DIAGNOSIS

Keen attention to the morphologic and immunophenotypic features is necessary if the diagnosis is to be correct. Anatomic location is a key tip-off to the diagnosis. The differential diagnosis includes olfactory neuroblastoma, low-grade neuroendocrine carcinoma (carcinoid tumor), lymphoma, ES/PNET (Ewing sarcoma/primitive neuroectodermal tumor), and carcinoma/NOS (not otherwise specified). Neuroendocrine features alone will not separate these first two lesions, but olfactory neuroblastoma has a neurofibrillary background, rosette formation, and usually negative keratin expression. The separation with carcinomas can be extremely difficult, often resting with the identification of specific pituitary hormones or electron microscopy. ES/PNET is most uncommon in this location and usually has scant cytoplasm with CD99 immunoreactivity. Lymphoma usually has a dispersed architecture and CD45RB immunoreactivity.

PROGNOSIS AND THERAPY

While histologically benign, there is a potential for significant morbidity related to their local mass effects (invasion into bone and cranial cavity) and hormonal manifestations. Recurrences develop, especially if the tumors are large and incompletely excised. Malignant transformation is exceptionally are. Most tumors are amenable to surgery, with follow-up drugs or radiation therapy if necessary to control hormone symptoms.

SUGGESTED READING

Schneiderian Papillomas

1. Barnes L, Tse LLY, Hunt JL. Schneiderian papillomas. In: Barnes EL, Eveson JW, Reichart P, Sidransky D, eds. Pathology and Genetics of Head and Neck Tumours. Kleihues P, Sobin LH, series eds. World Health Organization Classification of Tumours. Lyon, France: IARC Press, 2005:28–32.
2. Barnes L, Bedetti C: Oncocytic Schneiderian papilloma: a reappraisal of cylindrical cell papilloma of the sinonasal tract. Hum Pathol 1984;15:344–351.
3. Buchwald C, Franzmann MB, Tos M: Sinonasal papillomas: a report of 82 cases in Copenhagen County, including a longitudinal epidemiological and clinical study. Laryngoscope 1995;105:72–79.
4. Buchwald C, Lindeberg H, Pedersen BL, Franzmann MB: Human papilloma virus and p53 expression in carcinomas associated with sinonasal papillomas: a Danish Epidemiological study 1980–1998. Laryngoscope 2001;111:1104–1110.
5. Califano J, Koch W, Sidransky D, Westra WH: Inverted sinonasal papilloma: a molecular genetic appraisal of its putative status as a precursor to squamous cell carcinoma. Am J Pathol 2000;156:333–337.
6. Hyams VJ: Papillomas of the nasal cavity and paranasal sinuses. A clinicopathological study of 315 cases. Ann Otol Rhinol Laryngol 1971;80:192–206.
7. Kapadia SB, Barnes L, Pelzman K, Mirani N, Heffner DK, Bedetti C: Carcinoma ex oncocytic Schneiderian (cylindrical cell) papilloma. Am J Otolaryngol 1993;14:332–338.
8. Kaufman MR, Brandwein MS, Lawson W: Sinonasal papillomas: clinicopathologic review of 40 patients with inverted and oncocytic Schneiderian papillomas. Laryngoscope 2002;112:1372–1377.
9. Kraft M, Simmen D, Casas R, Pfaltz M: Significance of human papillomavirus in sinonasal papillomas. J Laryngol Otol 2001;115: 709–714.
10. Lawson W, Kaufman MR, Biller HF: Treatment outcomes in the management of inverted papilloma: an analysis of 160 cases. Laryngoscope 2003;113:1548–1556.
11. Michaels L, Young M: Histogenesis of papillomas of the nose and paranasal sinuses. Arch Pathol Lab Med 1995;119:821–826.
12. Phillips PP, Gustafson RO, Facer GW: The clinical behavior of inverting papilloma of the nose and paranasal sinuses: report of 112 cases and review of the literature. Laryngoscope 1990;100:463–469.
13. Schwerer MJ, Kraft K, Baczako K, Maier H: Coexpression of cytokeratins typical for columnar and squamous differentiation in sinonasal inverted papillomas. Am J Clin Pathol 2001;115:747–754.
14. Syrjanen KJ: HPV infections in benign and malignant sinonasal lesions. J Clin Pathol 2003;56:174–181.
15. Vrabec DP: The inverted Schneiderian papilloma: a 25-year study. Laryngoscope 1994;104:582–605.
16. Ward BE, Fechner RE, Mills SE: Carcinoma arising in oncocytic Schneiderian papilloma. Am J Surg Pathol 1990;14:364–369.

Lobular Capillary Hemangioma (Pyogenic Granuloma)

1. Fu YS, Perzin KH: Non-epithelial tumors of the nasal cavity, paranasal sinuses, and nasopharynx: a clinicopathologic study. I. General features and vascular tumors. Cancer 1974;33:1275–1288.
2. Heffner DK: Problems in pediatric otorhinolaryngic pathology. II. Vascular tumors and lesions of the sinonasal tract and nasopharynx. Int J Pediatr Otorhinolaryngol 1983;5:125–138.
3. Iwata N, Hattori K, Nakagawa T, Tsujimura T: Hemangioma of the nasal cavity: a clinicopathologic study. Auris Nasus Larynx 2002;29: 335–339.
4. Miller FR, D'Agostino MA, Schlack K: Lobular capillary hemangioma of the nasal cavity. Otolaryngol Head Neck Surg 1999;120:783–784.
5. Mills SE, Cooper PH, Fechner RE: Lobular capillary hemangioma: the underlying lesion of pyogenic granuloma. A study of 73 cases from the oral and nasal mucous membranes. Am J Surg Pathol 1980;4: 470–479.
6. Ozcan C, Apa DD, Gorur K: Pediatric lobular capillary hemangioma of the nasal cavity. Eur Arch Otorhinolaryngol 2004;261:449–451.
7. Thompson LDR, Fanburg-Smith JC. Benign soft tissue tumours. In: Barnes EL, Eveson JW, Reichart P, Sidransky D, eds. Pathology and Genetics of Head and Neck Tumours. Kleihues P, Sobin LH, series eds. World Health Organization Classification of Tumours. Lyon, France: IARC Press, 2005:46–50.

Glomangiopericytoma (Hemangiopericytoma)

1. Compagno J: Hemangiopericytoma-like tumors of the nasal cavity: a comparison with hemangiopericytoma of soft tissues. Laryngoscope 1978;88:460–469.
2. Compagno J, Hyams VJ: Hemangiopericytoma-like intranasal tumors. A clinicopathologic study of 23 cases. Am J Clin Pathol 1976;66:672–683.
3. Eichhorn JH, Dickersin GR, Bhan AK, Goodman ML: Sinonasal hemangiopericytoma. A reassessment with electron microscopy, immunohistochemistry, and long-term follow-up. Am J Surg Pathol 1990;14:856–866.
4. El-Naggar AK, Batsakis JG, Garcia GM, Luna ML, Goepfert H: Sinonasal hemangiopericytomas. A clinicopathologic and DNA content study. Arch Otolaryngol Head Neck Surg 1992;118:134–137.
5. Li XQ, Hisaoka M, Morio T, Hashimoto H: Intranasal pericytic tumors (glomus tumor and sinonasal hemangiopericytoma-like tumor): report of two cases with review of the literature. Pathol Int 2003;53:303–308.
6. Thompson LD, Miettinen M, Wenig BM: Sinonasal-type hemangiopericytoma: a clinicopathologic and immunophenotypic analysis of 104 cases showing perivascular myoid differentiation. Am J Surg Pathol 2003;27:737–749.
7. Thompson LDR, Fanburg-Smith JC, Wenig BM. Borderline and low malignant potential tumours of soft tissues. In: Barnes EL, Eveson JW, Reichart P, Sidransky D, eds. Pathology and Genetics of Head and Neck Tumours. Kleihues P, Sobin LH, series eds. World Health Organization Classification of Tumours. Lyon, France: IARC Press, 2005:43–45.
8. Tse LLY, Chan JKC: Sinonasal haemangiopericytoma-like tumor: a sinonasal glomus tumor or haemangiopericytoma. Histopathology 2002;40:510–517.

Nasopharyngeal Angiofibroma

1. Abraham SC, Montgomery EA, Giardiello FM, Wu TT: Frequent beta-catenin mutations in juvenile nasopharyngeal angiofibromas. Am J Pathol 2001;158:1073–1078.
2. Beham A, Beham-Schmid C, Regauer S, et al.: Nasopharyngeal angiofibroma: true neoplasm or vascular malformation? Adv Anat Pathol 2000;7:36–46.
3. Beham A, Fletcher CD, Kainz J, et al.: Nasopharyngeal angiofibroma: an immunohistochemical study of 32 cases. Virchows Arch A Pathol Anat Histopathol 1993;423:281–285.
4. Beham A, Regauer S, Beham-Schmid C, et al.: Expression of CD34-antigen in nasopharyngeal angiofibromas. Int J Pediatr Otorhinolaryngol 1998;44:245–250.
5. Giardiello FM, Hamilton SR, Krush AJ, et al.: Nasopharyngeal angiofibroma in patients with familial adenomatous polyposis. Gastroenterology 1993;105:1550–1552.
6. Hwang HC, Mills SE, Patterson K, Gown AM: Expression of androgen receptors in nasopharyngeal angiofibroma: an immunohistochemical study of 24 cases. Mod Pathol 1998;11:1122–1126.
7. Neel HB, Whicker JH, Devine KD, Weiland LH: Juvenile angiofibroma. Review of 120 cases. Am J Surg 1973;126:547–556.
8. Thompson LDR, Fanburg-Smith JC. Nasopharyngeal angiofibroma. In: Barnes EL, Eveson JW, Reichart P, Sidransky D, eds. Pathology and Genetics of Head and Neck Tumours. Kleihues P, Sobin LH, series eds. World Health Organization Classification of Tumours. Lyon, France: IARC Press, 2005:102–103.

Myxoma

1. Andrews T, Kountakis SE, Maillard AA: Myxomas of the head and neck. Am J Otolaryngol 2000;21:184–189.
2. Barker BF: Odontogenic myxoma. Semin Diag Pathol 1999;16:297–301.
3. Fu Y-S, Perzin KH: Non-epithelial tumors of the nasal cavity, paranasal sinuses and nasopharynx: a clinico-pathologic study. Cancer 1977;39:195–203.
4. Gregor RT, Loftus-Coll B: Myxoma of the paranasal sinuses. J Laryngol Otol 1994;108:679–681.
5. Kawai T, Murakami S, Nishiyama H, et al.: Diagnostic imaging for a case of maxillary myxoma with a review of the magnetic resonance images of myxoid lesions. Oral Surg Oral Med Oral Pathol Oral Radiol Endod 1997;84:449–454.
6. Buchner A, Odell EW. Odontogenic myxoma/myxofibroma. In: Barnes EL, Eveson JW, Reichart P, Sidransky D, eds. Pathology and Genetics of Head and Neck Tumours. Kleihues P, Sobin LH, series eds. World Health Organization Classification of Tumours. Lyon, France: IARC Press, 2005:315–316.
7. Sato H, Gyo K, Tomidokoro Y, Honda N: Myxoma of the sphenoid sinus. Otolaryngol Head Neck Surg 2004;130:370–380.
8. Simon ENM, Merkx MAW, Vuhahula E, et al.: Odontogenic myxoma: a clinicopathological study of 33 cases. Int J Oral Maxillofac Surg 2004;33:333–337.
9. Thompson LDR, Fanburg-Smith JC. Benign soft tissue tumours. In: Barnes EL, Eveson JW, Reichart P, Sidransky D, eds. Pathology and Genetics of Head and Neck Tumours. Kleihues P, Sobin LH, series eds. World Health Organization Classification of Tumours. Lyon, France: IARC Press, 2005:46–50.

Pituitary Adenoma

1. Asa SL: Pituitary adenomas. In: Atlas of Tumor Pathology. Tumors of the pituitary gland. Washington, DC: Armed Forces Institute of Pathology; 1998:47–147.
2. Coire CI, Horvath E, Kovacs K, et al.: Cushing's syndrome from an ectopic pituitary adenoma with peliosis: a histological, immunohistochemical, and ultrastructural study and review of the literature. Endocr Pathol 1997;8:65–74.
3. Hosaka N, Kitajiri S, Hiraumi H, et al.: Ectopic pituitary adenoma with malignant transformation. Am J Surg Pathol 2002;26:1078–1082.
4. Langford L, Batsakis JG: Pituitary gland involvement of the sinonasal tract. Ann Otol Rhinol Laryngol 1995;104:167–169.
5. Lloyd RV, Chandler WF, Kovacs K, Ryan N: Ectopic pituitary adenomas with normal anterior pituitary glands. Am J Surg Pathol 1986;10:546–552.
6. Luk SC, Chan JKC, Chow SM, Leung S: Pituitary adenoma presenting as sinonasal tumor: pitfalls in diagnosis. Hum Pathol 1996;27:605–609.
7. Luna MA, Cardesa A, Barnes L, et al.: Benign epithelial tumours. In: Barnes EL, Eveson JW, Reichart P, Sidransky D, eds. Pathology and Genetics of Head and Neck Tumours. Kleihues P, Sobin LH, series eds. World Health Organization Classification of Tumours. Lyon, France: IARC Press, 2005:99–101.
8. Matsushita H, Matsuya S, Endo Y, et al.: A prolactin producing tumor originated in the sphenoid sinus. Acta Pathol Jpn 1984;34:103–109.
9. Pasquini E, Faustini-Fustini M, Sciarretta V, et al.: Ectopic TSH-secreting pituitary adenoma of the vomerosphenoidal junction. Eur J Endocrinol 2003;148:253–257.

Malignant Neoplasms of the Nasal Cavity, Paranasal Sinuses, and Nasopharynx

Lester D. R. Thompson

Malignant sinonasal tract tumors comprise <1% of all neoplasms and about 3% of those of the upper aerodigestive tract. Squamous cell carcinoma (SCC) and adenocarcinoma are strongly associated with environmental factors, including tobacco, alcohol, and occupational exposures, such as heavy metal particles (nickel, chromium), and workers in the leather, textile, furniture, and wood industries.

Sinonasal tract malignancies most commonly affect maxillary sinus (~60%), followed by nasal cavity (~22%), ethmoid sinus (~15%), and frontal and sphenoid sinuses (<3%). Sinonasal tract tumors are diverse with the majority being squamous cell carcinoma and its variants (55%), followed by nonepithelial neoplasms (20%), glandular tumors (15%), undifferentiated carcinoma (7%), and miscellaneous tumors (3%).

Carcinoma of the nasopharynx differs in many aspects from that of the nasal cavity and paranasal sinuses and will be discussed separately.

The clinical presentations, radiologic features, and pattern of tumor spread for SCC, adenocarcinoma and most of the other malignant neoplasms of the sinonasal tract are similar. These features will be discussed in detail under the section on SCC and not repeated elsewhere. Gross appearance of the sinonasal tract and nasopharyngeal malignancies has limited value in aiding diagnosis, because the initial diagnosis depends on tissue obtained by endoscopes or polypectomy. The treatment of choice for most sinonasal tract malignancies, with the exception of nasopharyngeal carcinoma, malignant lymphoma, and rhabdomyosarcoma, is surgical resection with clear margins. Treatment for SCC will be used as a model.

SQUAMOUS CELL CARCINOMA

CLINICAL FEATURES

SCC has a male predilection (2 : 1), with a peak incidence in the 6th–7th decades. The location in order of frequency is maxillary sinus, nasal cavity, ethmoid sinus, frontal sinus, and sphenoid sinus. Early diagno-sis is difficult because symptoms and signs are nonspecific and closely resemble those of chronic sinusitis, allergic reaction, and nasal polyposis. Initial symptoms are related to the effects of the mass causing unilateral nasal obstruction. Secondary infection is common, giving rise to a mucoid or purulent discharge. Epistaxis develops when the mucosa is ulcerated or tumor extends into the sinus wall. Tumors involving the ethmoid, maxillary, or frontal sinuses may cause proptosis, restriction of eye movements, diplopia, or loss of vision. Epiphora results from lacrimal sac or duct obstruction by the tumor. Compression of the nerve at the primary site or perineural space invasion can compromise the functions of cranial nerves. A mass or discolored lesion may be visualized endoscopically and biopsied.

Late manifestations include facial swelling and cheek paresthesia resulting from anterior maxillary extension into the soft tissue and infraorbital nerve involvement, respectively. Inferior extension into the oral cavity forms a visible mass in the palate or alveolar ridge. Posterior extension can cause trismus from pterygoid muscle invasion. Ear symptoms suggest possible involvement of nasopharynx, eustachian tube, and pterygoid plates. Upward extension into the skull base may lead to cranial nerve involvement and dura invasion. In the initial workup, it is rare to find cervical lymph node metastasis.

RADIOLOGIC FEATURES

Computed tomography (CT) and magnetic resonance imaging (MRI) have largely replaced conventional radiographs in imaging sinonasal tract disease. CT and MRI complement each other, helping to separate inflammatory disorders and benign and malignant neoplasms and to provide pretreatment information, including location, size, extent, local invasion, and regional and distant metastasis. Of particular interest, is tumor extension into the pterygopalatine and infratemporal fossae, and tumor relationship to the blood vessels (especially internal carotid artery and cavernous sinus), nerves, and cranial cavity. CT highlights bony structures, with bony destruction and soft tissue invasion usually indicative of an aggressive lesion. MRI is supe-

SQUAMOUS CELL CARCINOMA
DISEASE FACT SHEET

Definition	Malignant neoplasm of squamous epithelial cells
Incidence and location	Most common malignant neoplasm of sinonasal tract; about 60%–70% of sinonasal tract carcinomas
	Paranasal sinuses: maxillary sinus > ethmoid sinus
	Nasal cavity: lateral nasal wall and nasal septum
Morbidity and mortality	Mortality is 30%–40% at 5 yr
Gender, race, and age distribution	Male > Female (2 : 1)
	6th–7th decades
Clinical features	Nasal obstruction, nasal discharge, epistaxis, pain
	Orbital and eye symptoms and signs
	Cranial nerve involvement
	Mass in the nasal cavity
Radiographic findings	CT and MRI complement each other
	MRI separates inflammatory from neoplastic and shows relationship to soft tissue
	CT is best for highlighting bony destruction and yielding extent, location, and size of tumor
Prognosis and treatment	**Nasal cavity:**
	Prognosis: if confined, 80% 5-yr survival
	Surgery, with postoperative radiotherapy (T3, T4)
	Paranasal sinuses:
	Prognosis less favorable than nasal cavity, with common recurrences, extending into cranial vault
	Cervical lymph node metastasis in about 15%
	Radical en bloc resection, if possible, with postoperative radiotherapy and/or chemotherapy (pre- or postoperatively)

PATHOLOGIC FEATURES

GROSS FINDINGS

Nasal tumors are usually exophytic and prone to become friable, necrotic, and ulcerated with increasing tumor size. Sinus tumors may be well circumscribed, filling the sinus cavity in an expansile fashion with erosion of the bone wall, while others are more destructive, necrotic, and hemorrhagic.

MICROSCOPIC FINDINGS

Most authors use a three-grade system based on (a) extent of keratinization, (b) mitotic activity, and (c) nuclear features. This grading method correlates to some extent with the tumor behavior. In general, SCC of the nasal cavity is well differentiated and keratinizing, whereas sinus counterparts are nonkeratinizing and moderately or poorly differentiated.

SCC is classified by cell type into keratinizing and nonkeratinizing. In keratinizing squamous cell carcinomas, the tumor cells exhibit keratinization, intercellular bridges, and squamous "pearls" (Fig. 6-1). Tumor cells usually have enlarged, hyperchromatic nuclei, with a variable degree of nuclear anaplasia. Mitotic figures are usually easy to find. Stromal invasion by irregular nests and cords of cells in a desmoplastic stroma, which is often associated with chronic inflammatory response (Fig. 6-2) is noted. However, in superficial biopsies, the only sign of stromal invasion may be in the form of single cells becoming isolated from the base of rete pegs or the tip of tongue-like protrusions.

Nonkeratinizing type of SCC form solid nests of variable sizes, frequently with relatively smooth borders. Individual tumor cells reveal uniform large, round, or

rior to CT in its ability to delineate sinus tumors from inflammatory disease and it can better delineate tumor from the adjacent soft tissues. Using MRI, inflamed mucosa, polyps, and non-inspissated secretions, with a high water content, have high signal intensity on T2-weighted images. In contrast, cellular paranasal neoplasms have lesser amounts of water and demonstrate intermediate signal intensities on T2-weighted images. Perineural spread is best demonstrated by a gadolinium contrasted MRI and T1-weighted images with fat suppression. CT helps detect cervical lymph node metastasis, especially when there are multiple, clustered lymph nodes exceeding 1.5 cm. The status of cervical lymph node is best determined by positron emission tomography (PET) using ^{18}fluorodeoxyglucose (^{18}FDG-PET) to detect tissue with increased metabolism, i.e., nodal metastasis.

SQUAMOUS CELL CARCINOMA
PATHOLOGIC FEATURES

Gross findings	Exophytic, friable mass
	Local soft tissue infiltration and bony destruction
Microscopic findings	**Nasal cavity:**
	Well-differentiated, keratinizing
	Squamous pearls, intercellular bridges, hyperchromatic nuclei
	Paranasal sinus:
	Moderately to poorly differentiated, nonkeratinizing
	Spindle cell, papillary, endophytic, verrucous types recognized
Immunohistochemical features	Positive with CK5/6, CK8, CK13
	Negative with CK10
Pathologic differential diagnosis	Pseudoepitheliomatous hyperplasia, sinonasal tract papilloma with dysplasia/carcinoma in situ

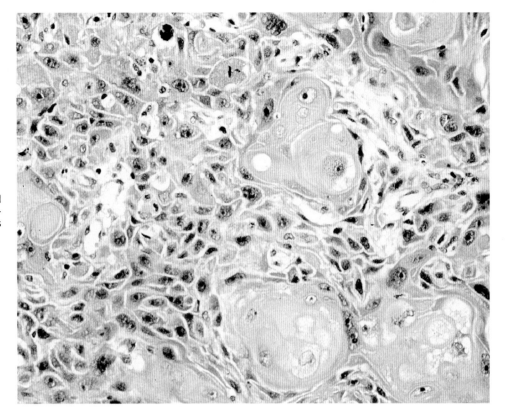

FIGURE 6-1

Tumor cells form irregular nests and sheets with keratinizing pearl formation in this keratinizing squamous cell carcinoma.

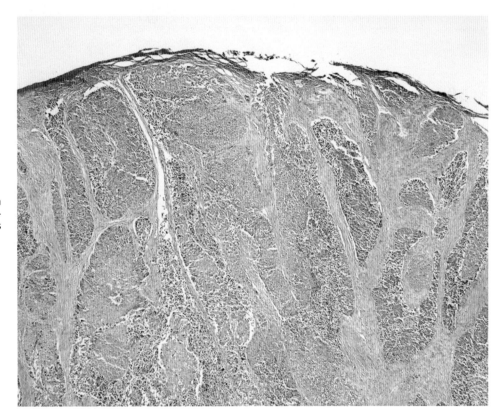

FIGURE 6-2

Tumor cells form solid sheets with infiltrative borders and stromal fibrosis in this nonkeratinizing squamous cell carcinoma.

oval nuclei with prominent nucleoli (Fig. 6-3). The cytoplasm varies from pale acidophilic to amphophilic to vacuolated. The cells may have distinct borders. Occasionally, individual cell keratinization may be identified (Fig. 6-4). Spindled tumor cells may be seen, and when

predominant, they are diagnosed as spindle cell squamous cell carcinoma. Papillary and endophytic patterns can be seen. The papillary type has a dysplastic epithelium lining thin fibrovascular cores (Fig. 6-5). The inverted type is often poorly differentiated, referred to

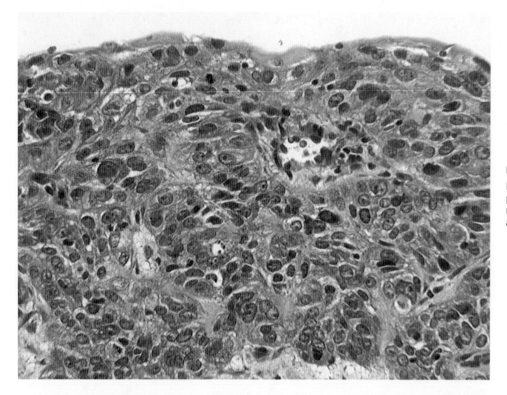

FIGURE 6-3

Poorly differentiated squamous cells present with irregular hyperchromatic nuclei, small nucleoli, and a moderate amount of cytoplasm.

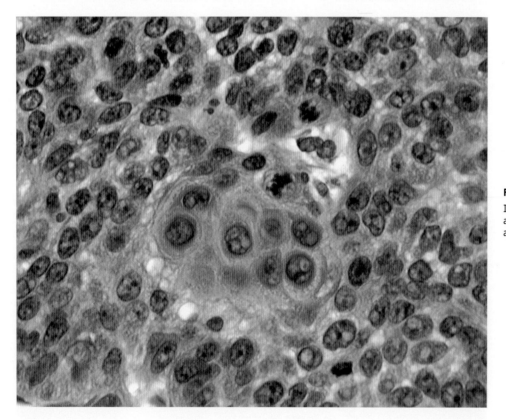

FIGURE 6-4

Isolated focus of individual cell keratinization in this otherwise nonkeratinizing squamous cell carcinoma.

as "transitional cell carcinoma" or "Schneiderian carcinoma." The tumor cells are arranged in broad sheets, which have smooth borders and are surrounded by basement membrane-like material (Fig. 6-6). In superficial or small biopsies evidence of stromal invasion is usually absent. In these cases, correlation with radiologic evidence of local destruction confirms the invasive nature of the malignancy. Similarly, biopsies of verrucous squamous carcinoma and papillary squamous carcinoma are prone to be under-diagnosed without

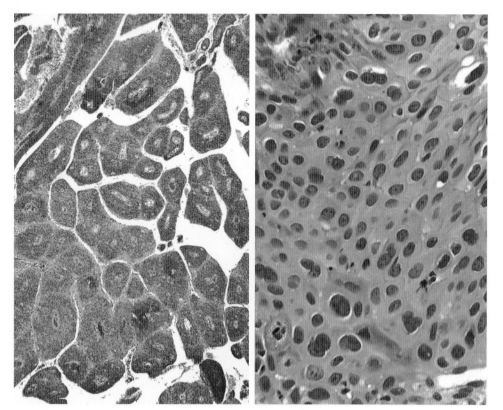

FIGURE 6-5

Left: Papillary pattern of a sinonasal squamous cell carcinoma. *Right:* Obvious cytologic atypia and loss of polarity is seen within the epithelium lining the papillary projections.

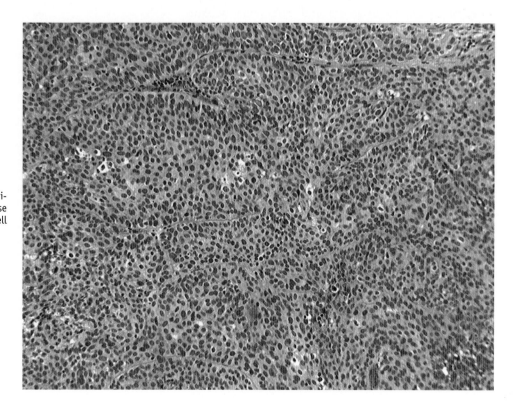

FIGURE 6-6

Sheets of smooth bordered "transitional" type epithelium comprise this nonkeratinizing squamous cell carcinoma.

including the base of the lesion. Variants of SCC, such as verrucous carcinoma and basaloid type are rare in the sinonasal tract.

ANCILLARY STUDIES

The diagnosis of SCC seldom requires immunohistochemistry, but the cells are CK5/6, CK8, and CK13 positive, while CK10 negative.

DIFFERENTIAL DIAGNOSIS

Pseudoepitheliomatous hyperplasia in the sinonasal tract region is most commonly associated with mucosal ulcer with or without prior medical interventions, and may be associated with rhinoscleroma, fungal infection, and neoplastic disease. The latter includes granular cell tumor, malignant lymphoma, and fibrohistiocytic tumors. The elongated and thickened rete pegs extend into the underlying connective tissue and have smooth, sharp, and sometimes pointed borders. There is no desmoplastic stroma. The cells resemble each other and have uniform nuclei without nuclear atypia and rare mitotic figures. Schneiderian and squamous papillomas may occasionally have malignant transformation, with areas of squamous dysplasia and carcinoma in situ. When broad sheets of cytologically malignant squamous cells are seen in biopsies, the diagnosis of SCC should be considered, even though stromal invasion is not demonstrable. Clinical and radiologic findings should by requested to aid decision making.

PROGNOSIS AND THERAPY

If SCC is confined to the nasal cavity, the 5- and 10-year survival rates are in the range of 80%. Involvement of the paranasal sinuses adversely affects the prognosis. Most treatment failures are related to locally advanced disease and tumor recurrence in areas inaccessible to surgical resection, such as skull base, dura, and brain. Cervical lymph node metastasis develops in up to 20% of patients, with rare distant metastases.

Treatment depends on the tumor location and extent. T1 and T2 nasal tumors are treated by surgical resection, while T3 and T4 tumors receive postoperative radiotherapy. Various surgical approaches are employed, with lateral rhinotomy or a mid-face degloving for septal tumors, medial maxillectomy or an en bloc ethmoidectomy for superior and lateral nasal cavity carcinomas. Paranasal sinus tumors are managed by radical en bloc surgical resection (including craniofacial combinations) followed by radiotherapy. Chemotherapy may be used as a neoadjuvant or postoperatively.

SINONASAL ADENOCARCINOMA

Malignant glandular neoplasms of sinonasal tract can originate from the respiratory epithelium or the underlying mucoserous glands, with the majority arising from the mucoserous glands (60%). The respiratory epithelial derived tumors tend to develop high in the nasal cavity and ethmoid sinus, while salivary gland neoplasms develop more frequently in the lower nasal cavity and maxillary sinus.

SINONASAL TRACT ADENOCARCINOMA DISEASE FACT SHEET	
Definition	Salivary-type adenocarcinoma arising from mucoserous glands
	Nonsalivary gland-type adenocarcinoma arising from respiratory mucosa
Incidence and location	Second most common carcinoma of sinonasal tract
	15% of sinonasal tract carcinomas
	Paranasal sinuses > nasal cavity
Morbidity and mortality	Salivary gland-type adenocarcinomas have 40%–60% mortality
	Nonsalivary gland-type adenocarcinomas have about 60% mortality, but grade dependent
Gender, race, and age distribution	**Salivary gland-type adenocarcinoma:**
	Equal gender distribution
	3rd–8th decades
	Nonsalivary gland-type adenocarcinoma:
	Male >>> Female (specifically with industrial exposure)
	6th–7th decades (low grade: 6th decade; high grade: 7th decade)
Clinical features	Unilateral nasal obstruction
	Epistaxis
	Purulent or clear rhinorrhea
	Pain or visual disturbances if large
	Intestinal-type has very strong association with wood workers and leather workers (500x increase incidence)
Radiographic findings	CT and MRI define extent of the tumor and identify invasion
Prognosis and treatment	**Salivary gland-type adenocarcinoma:**
	Prognosis depends on stage of tumor type (50% 10-yr survival for adenoid cystic)
	Recurrences common (60%)
	Complete surgical resection with optional radiation
	Nonsalivary gland-type adenocarcinoma (intestinal type):
	80% 5-year survival for papillary ITAC, but 40% 5-yr survival for poorly differentiated
	Complete surgical resection with radiation

CLINICAL FEATURES

SALIVARY GLAND-TYPE ADENOCARCINOMA

The genders are equally affected with a wide age range, although most are older patients (mean, 55 yr). The majority develop in the maxillary sinus (about 60%) or combination of sinuses and nasal cavity. Symptoms are nonspecific, and include obstructive symptoms, epistaxis, and pain. Palatal swelling may be seen.

NONSALIVARY GLAND-TYPE ADENOCARCINOMA

These are divided into two major categories: intestinal-type adenocarcinomas and nonintestinal-type adenocarcinoma. The intestinal type has a strong male predominance (about 90%), and tends to affect older aged males (mean, 60 yr). There is a well-known occupational exposure, specifically in wood workers and leather workers. While the carcinogenic substance is unknown, it is felt to be particulate in nature, as spouses of these workers also have an increased risk. Prolonged occupational exposure is necessary, and is frequently decades. These tumors tend to occur in the ethmoid sinus and nasal cavity, specifically the lower and middle turbinate in the latter (Fig. 6-7). Unilateral

obstruction, rhinorrhea, and epistaxis are the most common symptoms.

The nonintestinal-type adenocarcinomas are separated into low- and high-grade adenocarcinoma. Tumors tend to develop in men slightly more commonly, with a wide age range, although low-grade tumors tend to occur in patients about a decade younger than those of high grade (54 yr vs. 63 yr, respectively). The ethmoid and maxillary sinus tend to be affected more commonly than other sites.

PATHOLOGIC FEATURES

GROSS FINDINGS

Salivary gland-type adenocarcinoma tend to be large, firm, solid masses, extensively infiltrative at the time of diagnosis. Intestinal-type adenocarcinoma tend to be fungating, with an ulcerated friable surface. Cut surface reveals gray, translucent, mucoid parenchyma.

MICROSCOPIC FINDINGS

Salivary Gland–Type Adenocarcinoma

Adenoid cystic carcinoma (ACC) is the most common salivary-type adenocarcinoma to occur in the sinonasal tract. Other salivary gland tumors, such as mucoepidermoid carcinoma, acinic cell carcinoma, and low-grade papillary adenocarcinoma, rarely involve this region. ACC is invasive with perineural and bone invasion

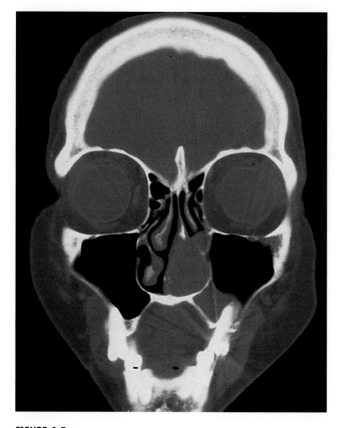

FIGURE 6-7
An adenocarcinoma of the nasal cavity has eroded the bone, with involvement of the maxillary sinus in this CT image.

SINONASAL TRACT ADENOCARCINOMA PATHOLOGIC FEATURES	
Gross findings	**Salivary gland-type adenocarcinoma:** Submucosal mass
	Nonsalivary gland-type adenocarcinoma: Fungating, ulcerated mass
Microscopic findings	**Salivary gland-type adenocarcinoma:** Adenoid cystic carcinoma most common, with cribriform and cystic pattern, small basaloid cells with hyperchromatic nuclei
	Nonsalivary gland-type adenocarcinoma: Intestinal and nonintestinal types
	Papillary, colonic, solid, and mucinous as major categories
	Usually tall, nonciliated, columnar cells
	Frequently have background of necrosis and inflammation
Immunohistochemical features	Intestinal-type are CK7, CK20, and CEA positive
	Sialosyl-Tn antigen, c-erbB-2 expression, and H-ras point mutation may have prognostic value
Pathologic differential diagnosis	Schneiderian papilloma, metastatic colon carcinoma, high-grade carcinoma, lymphoma, olfactory neuroblastoma

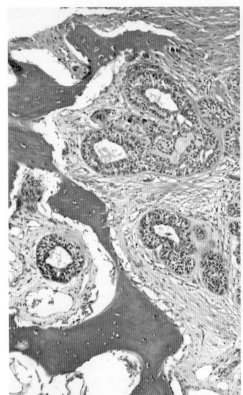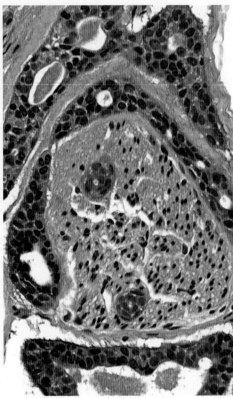

FIGURE 6-8
Adenoid cystic carcinoma with bone and perineural invasion.

(Fig. 6-8), composed of small basaloid cells with hyperchromatic nuclei and scant cytoplasm arranged in tubules, cribriform glands, and solid sheets. Reduplicated basement membrane material and mucinous or hyaline material within the cysts are common (Fig. 6-9). Predominantly solid ACC can be distinguished from undifferentiated small cell carcinomas and basaloid squamous cell carcinoma by its low mitotic activity and the presence of myoepithelial cell differentiation by immunohistochemistry.

Nonsalivary Gland-Type Adenocarcinoma

This is a heterogeneous group of tumors that is divided into intestinal and nonintestinal types, with the intestinal type further separated into papillary, colonic, solid, and mucinous types.

Intestinal-Type Adenocarcinoma. Intestinal-type of adenocarcinoma is made up of absorptive cells and goblet cells forming glands, nests, and abundant mucin. The degree of differentiation varies. Some are extremely well differentiated, having the appearance of a colonic tubular and villous adenomas, with nuclear stratification and mild nuclear atypia (Fig. 6-10). Some tumors contain small intestinal type cells, such as Paneth cells and enterochromaffin cells (Fig. 6-11). Occurring at the base of glands are a few layers of smooth muscle cells simulating muscularis mucosae. Other tumors resemble moderately differentiated colonic adenocarcinoma with confluent glands (Fig. 6-12), nuclear pleomorphism, prominent nucleoli, and increased mitotic activity. Some tumor cells produce abundant mucinous material (Fig. 6-13). Necrosis is common. Papillary and solid patterns are also recognized (Fig. 6-14). In biopsies, the presence of mucous pools and necrotic debris in the stroma should raise the suspicion of the possibility of malignancy. In all cases, the patient should be examined for evidence of intestinal tumor before the neoplasm is accepted as a primary lesion of the upper respiratory tract.

Nonintestinal-Type Adenocarcinoma. The nonintestinal-type adenocarcinomas are also divided into low grade and high grade, based on architecture, nuclear features, and mitotic activity. Low-grade adenocarcinoma has uniform cells arranged in compact acini, back to back, confluent glands, cystic spaces, and papillae. They maintain tall columnar to cuboidal configuration and arrange in a single layer without nuclear stratification (Fig. 6-15). The cytoplasm is abundant, but variable in appearance, eosinophilic (Fig. 6-16), basophilic, granular, or mucinous. The nuclear atypia is mild to moderate. Nucleoli may be prominent. The mitotic activity is generally low. High-grade adenocarcinomas are often solid, demonstrating nuclear pleomorphism, prominent nucleoli, and high mitotic activity. Some contain abundant signet-ring cells (Fig. 6-17). Special stains are helpful to identify mucus secretion.

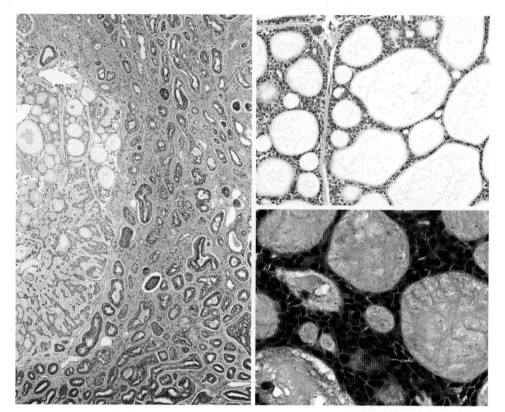

FIGURE 6-9

Left: Tumor cells form predominantly tubules with abundant hyalinized stroma. Some cribriforming is present. *Right:* Small cells with hyperchromatic, angular nuclei surround blue mucinous or pale material.

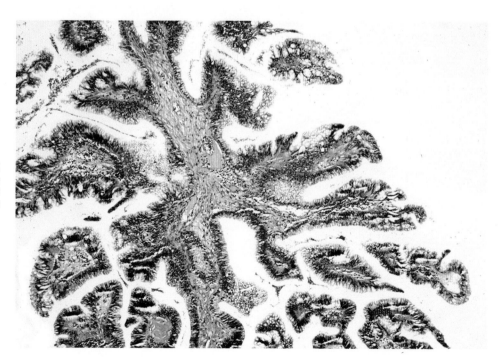

FIGURE 6-10

This intestinal type, well-differentiated adenocarcinoma of ethmoid sinus resembles villous adenoma of colon with multiple papillary projections and smooth borders at the base.

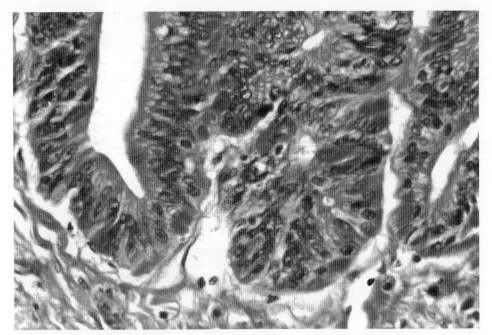

FIGURE 6-11
Tumor cells demonstrate nuclear stratification, mild nuclear atypia and Paneth cells with abundant granular eosinophilic cytoplasm in an ITAC. (Courtesy of Yao S. Fu, MD, Senior Pathologist, Providence St. Joseph Medical Center, Burbank, CA.)

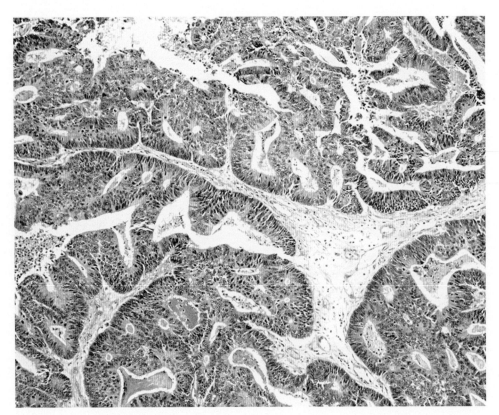

FIGURE 6-12
A moderately differentiated adenocarcinoma consists of cribriform glands with central comedonecrosis.

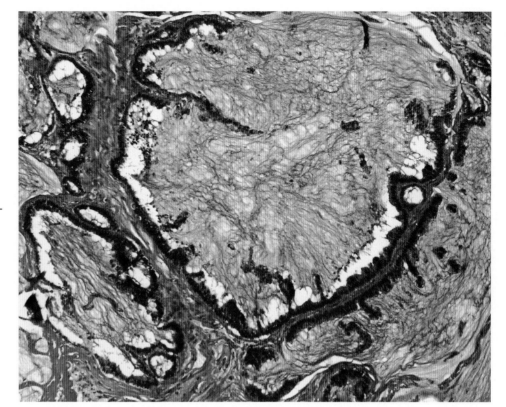

FIGURE 6-13

Neoplastic glands producing abundant mucin.

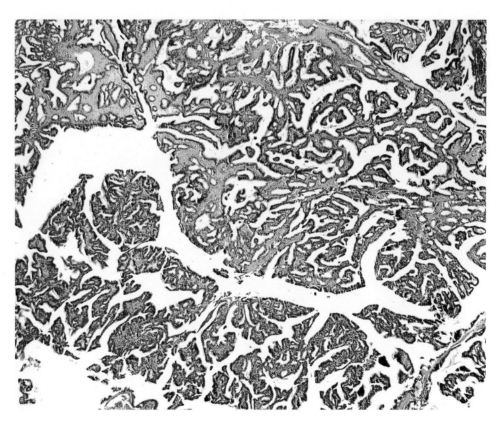

FIGURE 6-14

A papillary pattern of growth predominates in this ITAC, papillary type.

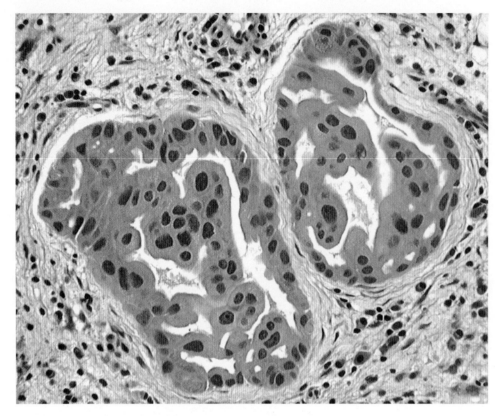

FIGURE 6-15
This nonintestinal-type low-grade adenocarcinoma shows complex glands with nuclear atypia, but no stratification.

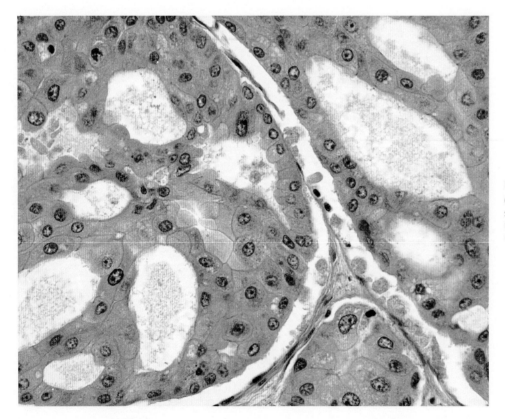

FIGURE 6-16
Columnar to cuboidal cells without stratification or marked nuclear pleomorphism. A mitotic figure is seen (*upper left*).

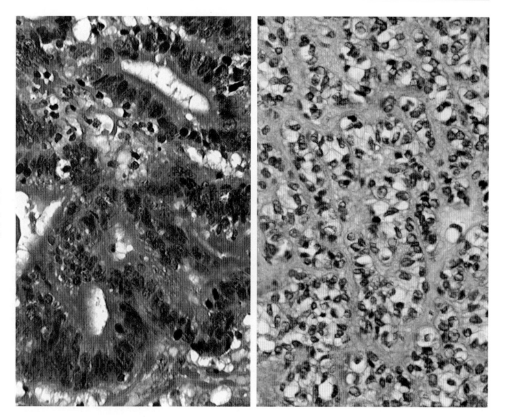

FIGURE 6-17
Left: A high-grade adenocarcinoma with hyperchromatic nuclei and increased mitotic figures. *Right:* A clear-cell to signet-ring morphology can be seen in adenocarcinomas of the sinonasal tract.

ANCILLARY STUDIES

Most adenocarcinomas do not require immunohistochemical stains. ACC is keratin, CK7, S-100 protein, calponin, and p63 positive. Intestinal-type adenocarcinomas show keratin, CMA, B72.3, CK7, CK20, and CDX-2 immunoreactivity. Immunohistochemical stains for sialosyl-Tn antigen and c-erbB-2 oncoprotein may provide prognostic information. K- or H-ras point mutations tend to be associated with a poor prognosis.

DIFFERENTIAL DIAGNOSIS

Adenoid cystic carcinoma must be separated from high-grade carcinomas, lymphoma, and olfactory neuroblastoma. Schneiderian papilloma (oncocytic variant specifically) with their complex back to back, confluent glands and papillary architecture may be over-diagnosed as low-grade adenocarcinoma, but the cells are cytologically benign.

PROGNOSIS AND THERAPY

The overall 10-year survival rate for ACC is 40% to 60%. Aggressive local therapy is warranted even in patients with distant metastases, since a significant number of patients will live for many years with their disease. Recurrences are common (up to 60%). The treatment of choice for adenoid cystic carcinoma is surgical resection with clear margins often accompanied by postoperative radiotherapy to improve local control, especially in cases with positive or close margins. The propensity for perineural spread makes obtaining clear margins difficult.

Among patients with nonsalivary gland-type adenocarcinoma, histologic grade affects outcome. Well-differentiated tumors with predominantly papillary and tubular structures have better prognosis (80% 5-yr survival) than those poorly differentiated counterparts (40% 5-yr survival). Patients with industrial exposure have a better outcome than the sporadic cases, but perhaps because they are detected earlier due to regular surveillance. Recurrences develop in about 50% of patients with distant metastasis in about 15%. Overall survival is about 40%, with death in about 3 years. Treatment is radical surgical resection with postoperative radiotherapy.

SINONASAL UNDIFFERENTIATED CARCINOMA

This is a rare and highly aggressive undifferentiated carcinoma, showing pleomorphism and necrosis, but separated from olfactory neuroblastoma. The taxonomy is not well developed or accepted.

SINONASAL UNDIFFERENTIATED CARCINOMA DISEASE FACT SHEET	
Definition	High-grade aggressive undifferentiated carcinomas with locally extensive disease
Incidence and location	Rare
	Nasal cavity, maxillary sinus, ethmoid sinus, often in combination
Morbidity and mortality	Mortality of 80% in 5 yr
Gender, race, and age distribution	Male > Female (2–3 : 1)
	Wide age range (20–76 yr), mean 6th decade
Clinical features	Nasal obstruction
	Epistaxis
	Proptosis, periorbital swelling, and facial pain
	Destructive lesion
	May have cranial nerve involvement
Prognosis and treatment	Median survival is about 18 mo, with 20% 5-yr survival
	About 30% have cervical lymph node metastasis
	Radical resection, multimodality chemotherapy, and radiation

CLINICAL FEATURES

This type of undifferentiated carcinoma is a distinct clinicopathologic entity. The majority of patients present with locally advanced disease with frequent bony, cranial or orbital involvement at diagnosis. The median age is in the 6th decade with a male predominance (2–3:1). Previous radiation may be an etiologic factor. Patients have nonspecific symptoms, indistinguishable from other sinonasal tract tumors. The nasal cavity, maxillary sinus and ethmoid sinus are usually involved, frequently showing spread into directly contiguous sites.

PATHOLOGIC FEATURES

GROSS FINDINGS

Tumors are usually large (>4 cm) with bone invasion and poorly defined margins.

MICROSCOPIC FEATURES

The cells are arranged in nest, lobules and sheets without any squamous or glandular differentiation. The cells have a high nuclear to cytoplasmic ratio with medium to large nuclei surrounded by scant cytoplasm (Figs. 6-18, 6-19). Nucleoli are usually prominent and single. Necrosis, including comedonecrosis is common. Mitotic figures are increased. Lymph-vascular invasion is a common finding.

SINONASAL UNDIFFERENTIATED CARCINOMA PATHOLOGIC FEATURES	
Gross findings	Large fungating mass (>4 cm) with bone destruction/invasion
Microscopic findings	Nests, lobules and sheets of undifferentiated cells (no squamous or glandular differentiation)
	High nuclear to cytoplasmic ratio with medium to large nuclei
	Single, prominent nucleoli
	High mitotic activity
	Tumor necrosis is common
Immunohistochemical features	Usually pan-keratin, CK7, CK8, CK19 positive
	Occasionally EMA, NSE, and p53 positive
	Rarely has S-100 protein, CD99 (MIC2), chromogranin, and synaptophysin reaction
Pathologic differential diagnosis	Olfactory neuroblastoma, neuroendocrine carcinoma, lymphoma, malignant melanoma, rhabdomyosarcoma, ES/PNET

ANCILLARY STUDIES

The majority of tumors react with keratins (simple keratins especially, CK7, CK8, and CK19) (Fig. 6-20). Epithelial membrane antigen (EMA), neuron-specific enolase (NSE), and p53 may be positive. Chromogranin and synaptophysin are rarely positive. Epstein-Barr virus–encoded RNA (EBER) in situ hybridization is negative.

DIFFERENTIAL DIAGNOSIS

Separation of sinonasal undifferentiated carcinoma from olfactory neuroblastoma and neuroendocrine carcinoma remains controversial. Olfactory neuroblastoma have a specific anatomic site of involvement, lobular architecture, and neural features. Neuroendocrine carcinomas may overlap with sinonasal undifferentiated carcinoma, a separation which at present does not have clinical implications. Immunohistochemical stains are valuable to diagnose lymphoma, melanoma, rhabdomyosarcoma, and Ewing sarcoma/primitive neuroectodermal tumor (see Chart 6-1).

PROGNOSIS AND THERAPY

Prognosis is usually poor, with median survival of <18 months. Overall survival is about 20% at 5 years. There is frequent recurrence with metastasis to lymph nodes and distant sites. A combination of radical surgery,

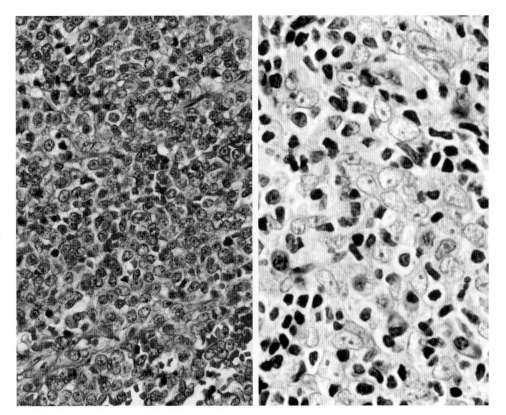

FIGURE 6-18

Left: A sheet of malignant small tumor cells reveal nuclear molding, resulting from high-nuclear cytoplasmic ratios. *Right:* Vesicular open nuclear chromatin with prominent nucleoli.

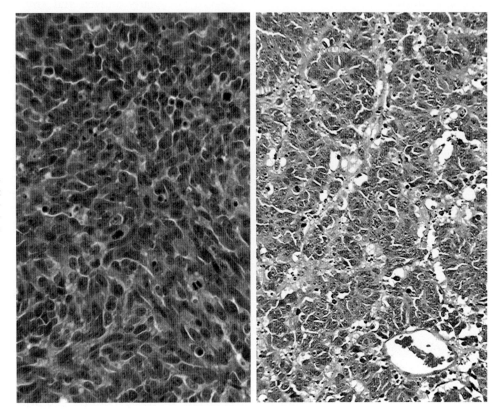

FIGURE 6-19

Left: The tumor cells have medium-sized round to oval hyperchromatic nuclei, a moderate amount of cytoplasm and increased nuclear cytoplasmic ratios. *Right:* Vascular stroma may separate the nodules of tumor. Mitotic figures are increased.

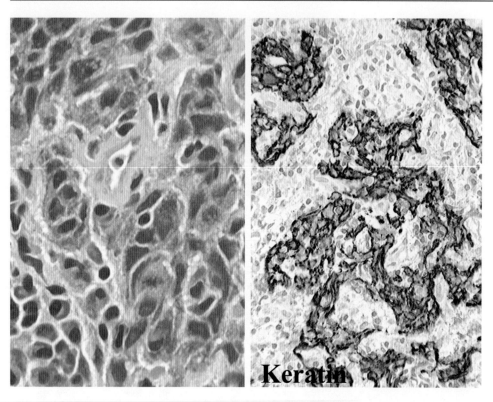

Keratin

FIGURE 6-20
Left: Irregular, polygonal to spindle-shaped cells can be seen in sinonasal undifferentiated carcinoma. *Right:* Tumor cells are positive for keratin.

chemotherapy, and radiotherapy provides the best chance of survival.

NASOPHARYNGEAL CARCINOMA

The nomenclature for carcinomas of the nasopharynx has undergone several iterations, but at present adeno-carcinomas and salivary gland-type carcinomas are excluded from this category. Nasopharyngeal carcinoma (NPC) encompasses nonkeratinizing carcinoma, keratinizing squamous cell carcinoma, and basaloid squamous cell carcinoma. In the past, synonyms included lymphoepithelial carcinoma, Schmincke-type carcinoma, Regaud lymphoepithelioma, undifferentiated carcinoma, and anaplastic carcinoma. These terms have been abandoned in favor of the current nomenclature.

CLINICAL FEATURES

NPC is epidemic in southern parts of China and Southeast Asian countries (Thailand, Philippines, Vietnam), but it is still an uncommon tumor, accounting for <0.5% of all carcinomas. The high-risk populations experience a decreased risk in subsequent generations in new places to which they migrate. There is a strong etiologic association with Epstein-Barr virus (EBV) (especially early antigen and viral capsid antigen), diets high in volatile nitrosamines (salted fish, fermented foods), and other environmental factors (smoking, formaldehyde, chemical fumes). Men are affected more commonly than women (3:1), with a wide age range at initial presentation (7–77 yr), with a peak incidence in the 5th decade of life. Due to the anatomic location, NPC may remain clinically silent. The most common initial presentation is metastasis in the cervical lymph node (up to 70%). This is followed by nasal symptoms, such as nasal obstruction, discharge, postnasal drip, and epistaxis. Middle ear complaints, such as tinnitus, ear ache, discharge, and hearing loss secondary to eustachian tube obstruction, are common. With disease progression, cranial nerve involvement becomes apparent, especially cranial nerves III, V, VI, IX, and X.

DIAGNOSTIC TECHNIQUES

RADIOLOGIC FEATURES

Both CT and MRI are equally sensitive in the study of the roof and lateral wall of nasopharynx. However, MRI provides a better separation of tumor from benign tissue. Both CT and MRI are used in assessing the local extent of the tumor for treatment planning. Status of cervical lymph nodes is best assessed by positron emission tomography (PET), which is also used in the detection of residual tumor after treatment.

NASOPHARYNGEAL CARCINOMA
DISEASE FACT SHEET

Definition	A malignant neoplasm arising from the nasopharynx mucosa which shows evidence of squamous differentiation
Incidence and location	Incidence varies by location and population (highest in Asians)
	<0.5% of all carcinomas
	Nasopharynx
Morbidity and mortality	5-yr survival improved up to 80% in low-stage patients; usually 55%–60% 5-yr survival
Gender, race, and age distribution	Male > Female (3 : 1)
	Peak, 40–60 yr
Clinical features	Neck mass, nasal obstruction, epistaxis, hearing loss, tinnitus, cranial nerve involvement
	Endoscopy may show mass, fullness, or no lesion
	Migration of population from high-risk to low-risk areas does not change carcinoma risk, but subsequent generations have a reduced risk
	Strong association with EBV and high levels of volatile nitrosamines in foods
Radiographic findings	MRI is study of choice, showing extent of tumor, especially bony invasion
	PET is best for lymph node evaluation
Prognosis and treatment	Overall, 55%–60% 5-yr survival (stage dependent)
	Recurrences common, most during first 3 yr post-diagnosis
	Radiotherapy is cornerstone of management, although best for nonkeratinizing type
	Chemotherapy used for advanced disease

NASOPHARYNGEAL CARCINOMA
PATHOLOGIC FEATURES

Gross findings	Superior or lateral wall mass, especially fossa of Rosenmüller
	Cervical metastases common finding
Microscopic findings	**Nonkeratinizing carcinoma:**
	Most common type with possible surface involvement
	Solid sheets, islands, and nests with intimate lymphoid infiltrates
	Syncytial, large cells with indistinct borders, vesicular nuclei with prominent, eosinophilic nucleoli, and scant cytoplasm
	Prominent mitotic figures; necrosis
	Keratinizing squamous cell carcinoma:
	Invasive carcinoma with obvious squamous differentiation and keratinization
	Distinct tumor borders, intercellular bridges
	Frequent surface involvement
	Basaloid squamous cell carcinoma:
	Identical to BSCC in other head and neck sites (rare)
Immunohistochemical features	Positive with pan-keratin, CK5/6 34βE12, EBER in situ hybridization
Pathologic differential diagnosis	Lymphoma, Hodgkin lymphoma, rhabdomyosarcoma, metaplasia/reactive atypia (epithelial or lymphoid), sarcomas

LABORATORY STUDIES

In nonkeratinizing carcinoma about 90 % of patients will have EBV titers, including immunoglobulin IgG or IgA against early antigens or IgA against viral capsid antigens. EBER-1 (EBV encoded early RNA) or EBNA-1 can be detected in the serum or plasma of patients by quantitative polymerase chain reaction (PCR), one of the most sensitive tests for NPC.

PATHOLOGIC FEATURES

GROSS FINDINGS

Nasopharyngeal carcinoma arises most frequently in the superior wall or vault, followed by the pharyngeal recess in the lateral wall. By nasopharyngoscopy, tumors appear as a bulging (elevated, full), infiltrative, exophytic and lobulated, or ulcerative mass. In some cases, there is no visible lesion, the tumor identified by random blind biopsies of the nasopharynx only.

MICROSCOPIC FINDINGS

The World Health Organization (WHO) histologic typing system for NPC includes nonkeratinizing carcinoma, keratinizing squamous cell carcinoma, and basaloid squamous cell carcinoma.

Nonkeratinizing Carcinoma

The tumor is arranged in irregular islands, solid sheets, trabeculae, and single neoplastic cells. The neoplastic cells are intimately intermingled with lymphocytes and plasma cells. The cells are syncytial-appearing, large tumor cells lacking cell borders. The nuclei are usually vesicular with large, central, prominent nucleoli (Figs. 6-21, 6-22). Sometimes a greater degree of "differentiation" is appreciated with cellular pavementing and stratification. Necrosis and mitotic figures are usually easy to find. A desmoplastic stroma is uncommon. At times the lymphoid population may separate the tumor islands into individual cells, bring the previous term "lymphoepithelial carcinoma" to mind. Eosinophils and amyloid deposits may be seen. Tumor cells may uncommonly be spindled (Fig. 6-23). In metastatic deposits, the lymphoid mixture is similar to the primary, although a desmoplastic stroma and epithelioid granulomas may obscure the metastatic foci.

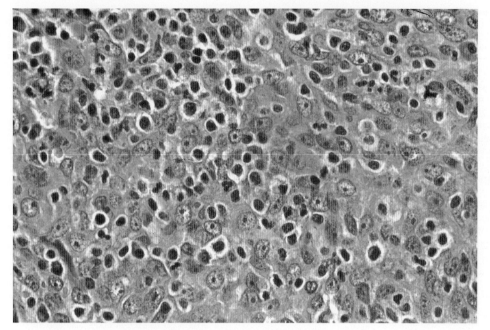

FIGURE 6-21

Loosely cohesive tumor cells are intermingled with small lymphocytes in this nonkeratinizing carcinoma. The tumor cells have large round to oval nuclei, prominent nucleoli, and ill-defined cell borders. (Courtesy of Yao S. Fu, MD, Senior Pathologist, Providence St. Joseph Medical Center, Burbank, CA.)

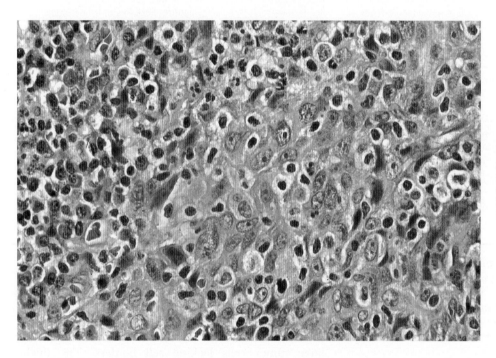

FIGURE 6-22

Nests of epithelium are noted, surrounded by lymphocytes and plasma cells. (Courtesy of Yao S. Fu, MD, Senior Pathologist, Providence St. Joseph Medical Center, Burbank, CA.)

Keratinizing Squamous Cell Carcinoma

The tumor cells have demonstrable intercellular bridges and keratin pearl formation, opaque, glassy, eosinophilic cytoplasm and well-defined cell borders (Fig. 6-24). The cells grow in compact nests rather than syncytial loose cohesive aggregates. Surface epithelium is frequently affected, representing carcinoma in situ. The tumors can be graded as well, moderately and poorly differentiated (Fig. 6-25). There is a desmoplastic stroma with inflammatory cells. This tumor tends to be a locally aggressive neoplasm, metastasizing less commonly than the nonkeratinizing type.

Basaloid Squamous Cell Carcinoma

Morphologically identical to tumors in other head and neck sites, but vanishingly rare in this location.

ANCILLARY STUDIES

NPC as a group show strong and diffuse reactions with pan-keratin, often highlighting wisps of cytoplasm in a reticular pattern as they surround lymphocytes

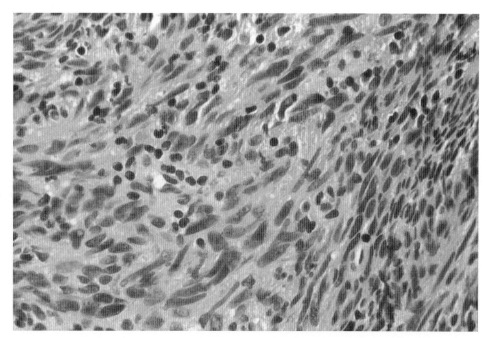

FIGURE 6-23

Spindle cell variant of nonkeratinizing carcinoma of the nasopharynx. (Courtesy of Yao S. Fu, MD, Senior Pathologist, Providence St. Joseph Medical Center, Burbank, CA.)

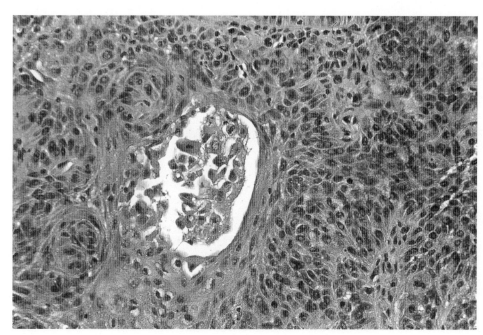

FIGURE 6-24

Keratinizing squamous cell carcinoma reveals individual cell keratinization, concentric whorls, and desquamated parakeratotic cells in the center. (Courtesy of Yao S. Fu, MD, Senior Pathologist, Providence St. Joseph Medical Center, Burbank, CA.)

(Fig. 6-26). High-molecular weight keratins (CK5/6, 34ßE12) are positive, while CK7 and CK20 are negative. EBV is found in nearly 100% of tumors, but the technique and antigen sought influence the positivity rate: EBV latent membrane protein-1 (LMP1) is weak, patchy, and only positive in about 30% of cases. The easiest and most reliable way to identify EBV is using the in situ hybridization technique for EBER, which will show strong nuclear labeling in nearly all tumor cells. The lymphoid cells react with a compartmentalized mixture of B and T cells, supporting a reactive population.

DIFFERENTIAL DIAGNOSIS

The histologic diagnosis of NPC can be difficult and challenging, because of small biopsy size and crush artifacts. The most common differential diagnosis includes large cell lymphoma, Hodgkin lymphoma, metaplastic or reactive epithelial atypia, and spindle cell sarcomas. Immunohistochemical stains are essential for reaching a definitive diagnosis as management is different for each tumor type.

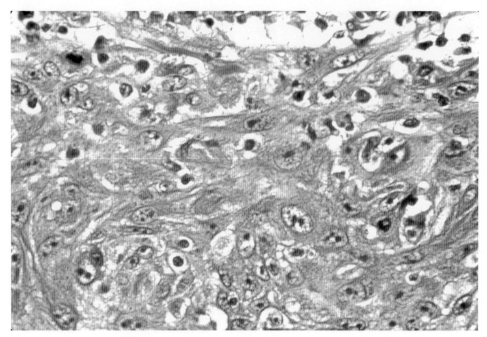

FIGURE 6-25
This keratinizing squamous cell carcinoma is moderately differentiated with cellular pavementing, large round to oval hyperchromatic nuclei, abundant eosinophilic cytoplasm, and well-defined cell borders with bridges. (Courtesy of Yao S. Fu, MD, Senior Pathologist, Providence St. Joseph Medical Center, Burbank, CA.)

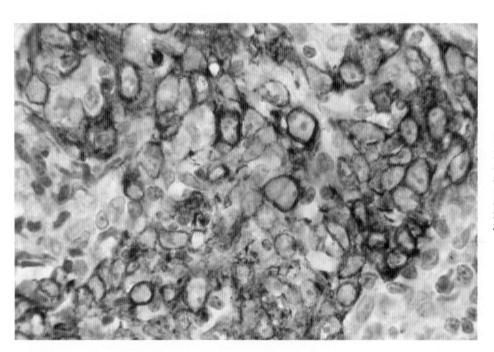

FIGURE 6-26
Immunohistochemical stain for pankeratin reveals keratin positive tumors and background keratin negative lymphocytes to confirm the diagnosis of carcinoma. (Courtesy of Yao S. Fu, MD, Senior Pathologist, Providence St. Joseph Medical Center, Burbank, CA.)

PROGNOSIS AND THERAPY

Overall, there is a relatively good prognosis of 55% to 60% at 5 years for nonkeratinizing type, but this is stage dependent, with stage I showing 98% 5-year survival and stage IV decreasing to 70%. Prognosis is influenced by tumor stage at presentation, tumor type, young age, female gender, and tumor aneuploidy. Recurrences are common. Keratinizing carcinomas have <20% 5-year survival, probably reflecting radioresistance. Radiation is the cornerstone of therapy, with specific shielded ports employed. When there is advanced disease, chemotherapy may be added (pre-, concurrent, or postradiation).

Post-therapy biopsies are sometimes difficult to interpret, especially if taken with 3 months of the initiation of therapy. Radiation will induce changes in the surrounding mucosa as well as affecting the tumor cells. Maintenance of the nuclear to cytoplasmic ratio favors reactive changes. In situ EBER reaction would favor residual/recurrent tumor. In some cases, monitoring the serologic EBV DNA titer may suggest disease relapse, although it is usually a late finding.

MALIGNANT MELANOMA

CLINICAL FEATURES

Malignant melanoma of the sinonasal tract is rare, accounting for <1% of all melanomas, and <5% of all sinonasal tract neoplasms. There is an equal gender distribution, with patients affected from the 5th to 8th decades of life. There appears to be an increased incidence in Japanese patients. In the sinonasal tract, the most frequently involved site is the anterior septum, followed by maxillary antrum. Clinically, the majority of patients have symptoms of nasal obstruction, epistaxis, nasal discharge, polyps, and pain.

PATHOLOGIC FEATURES

GROSS FINDINGS

Nasal melanomas at the time of diagnosis have usually reached a few centimeters in size, have a polypoid appearance, and vary in color from white to gray, brown, or black (Fig. 6-27).

MICROSCOPIC FINDINGS

Sinonasal tract malignant melanomas have a protean histology. A helpful, albeit uncommon diagnostic feature is the presence of junctional activity and epidermal migration (Fig. 6-28). Most sinonasal tract melanomas grow in sheets, nests, fascicles, and/or interlacing bundles (Fig. 6-29). A peritheliomatous distribution is unique (Fig. 6-30). Large polygonal epithelioid to plasmacytoid or rhabdoid cells have vesicular nuclei, prominent nucleoli, and intranuclear cytoplasmic inclusions (Fig. 6-31). Some tumor cells have small hyperchromatic nuclei and scant cytoplasm resembling anaplastic small cell carcinoma. Melanin-containing tumor cells may be found (Fig. 6-32). Mitotic figures are common and inflammation may also be seen adjacent to the tumor. Tumor depth of invasion and/or thickness is not meaningful in the sinonasal tract.

MALIGNANT MELANOMA DISEASE FACT SHEET	
Definition	Malignant neoplasm of melanocytic cells
Incidence and location	<1% of all melanomas
	<5% of all sinonasal tract neoplasms
	Anterior nasal septum > maxillary sinus
Morbidity and mortality	Mortality of 50%–80% at 5 yr
Gender, race, and age distribution	Equal gender distribution
	Increased incidence in Japanese patients
	Usually 5th–8th decades
Clinical features	Nasal obstruction
	Epistaxis or nasal discharge
	Polyp
	Pain uncommon
Prognosis and treatment	Generally poor prognosis (17%–47% 5-yr survival)
	Recurrences common
	Poor prognosis with advanced age, tumors >3 cm, mixed anatomic sites, vascular invasion
	Radical surgery with palliative radiation

MALIGNANT MELANOMA PATHOLOGIC FEATURES	
Gross findings	Grey, brown, or black bulky mass with friable or gelatinous appearance
Microscopic findings	Junctional activity and epidermal migration confirm primary
	Epithelioid, small, spindle, and pleomorphic cell types
	Peritheliomatous growth is unique, often associated with necrotic tumors
	Usually large cells with high nuclear to cytoplasmic ratio, prominent nucleoli, intranuclear cytoplasmic inclusions
	Pigment may be present
	Mitotic figures are easily identified
Ultrastructural features	Premelanosomes and melanosomes present in the cytoplasm, without cell junctions
Immunohistochemical features	S-100 protein, melan A, HMB45, vimentin positive
	Keratin and muscle markers are negative
Pathologic differential diagnosis	Undifferentiated carcinoma, lymphoma (anaplastic), angiosarcoma, sarcomas (rhabdomyosarcoma, leiomyosarcoma, fibrosarcoma), metastasis to sinonasal tract

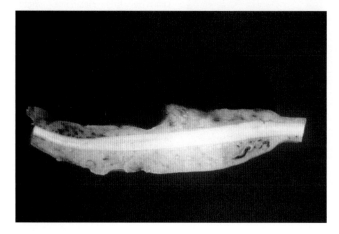

FIGURE 6-27
A black polypoid mass on the nasal septal cartilage was histologically a melanoma.

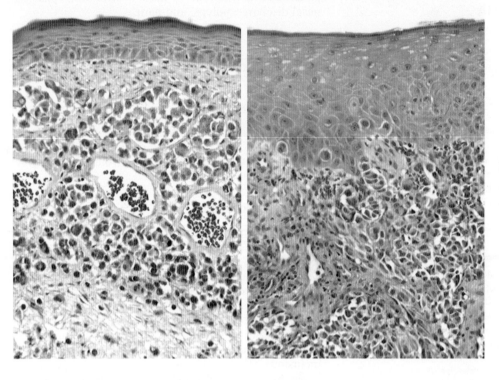

FIGURE 6-28

Left: A zone of separation between the neoplastic cells and the surface. *Right:* Pagetoid spread and involvement of the base shows a junctional component in this melanoma.

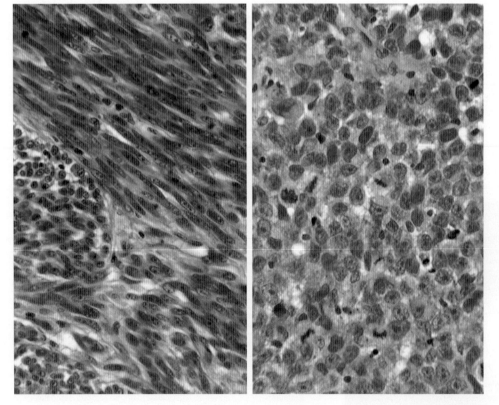

FIGURE 6-29

Left: Tight fascicles of spindle cells comprise this melanoma. *Right:* An epithelioid to undifferentiated solid sheet of cells comprises this melanoma.

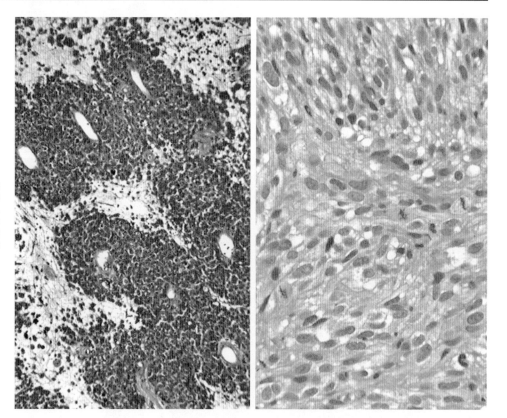

FIGURE 6-30

Left: A peritheliomatous arrangement of the neoplastic cells is quite unique to melanoma of the sinonasal tract. *Right:* A storiform pattern with atypical spindled cells simulates a leiomyosarcoma. Mitotic figures are increased.

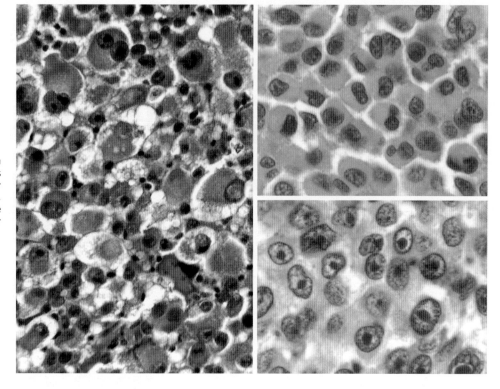

FIGURE 6-31

Left: Plasmacytoid architecture with intranuclear cytoplasmic inclusions comprise this melanoma. *Right upper:* Rhabdoid cells with abundant, opaque eosinophilic cytoplasm are seen in this melanoma. *Right lower:* Prominent, eosinophilic nucleoli.

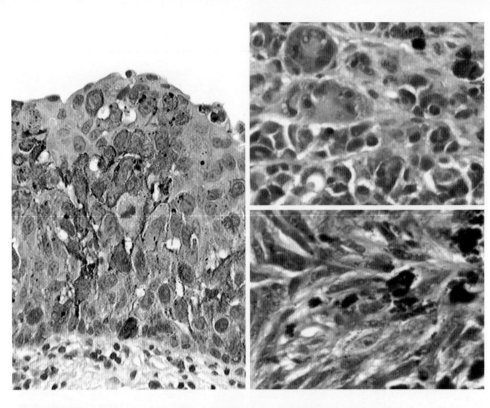

FIGURE 6-32
Pigment can be seen, identified in an in situ melanoma (*left*), in an epithelioid type (*right upper*), and in a spindle cell type (*right lower*).

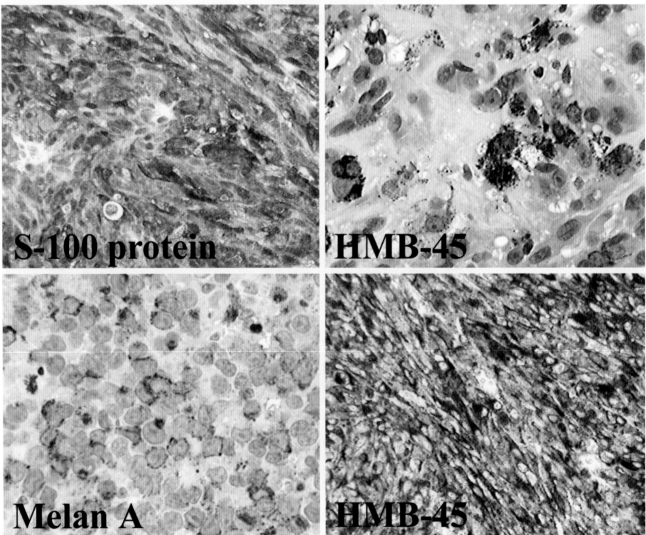

S-100 protein

HMB-45

Melan A

HMB-45

FIGURE 6-33
The neoplastic cells are reactive with S-100 protein (*left upper*), melan A (*right upper*), and HMB45 (*lower*) to a variable degree, ranging from strong, diffuse, and heavy reactions to light, granular, and sparse reactivity.

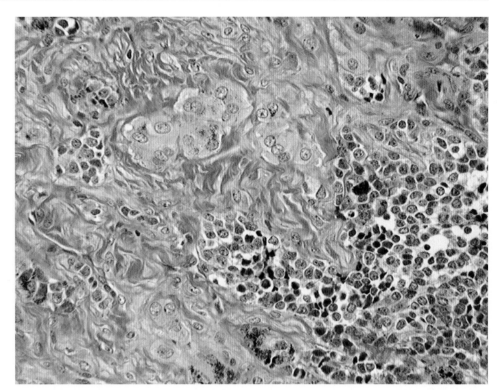

FIGURE 6-34
A melanocytic neuroectodermal tumor of infancy has a dual population of large, pigmented cells with small, primitive cells. A dense fibrous stroma separates the biphasic populations. There is little pleomorphism and mitotic activity is scarce. The young age at presentation helps with clinical separation from melanoma.

ANCILLARY STUDIES

ULTRASTRUCTURAL FEATURES

The presence of premelanosomes and melanosomes confirms melanocytic origin.

IMMUNOHISTOCHEMICAL FEATURES

The neoplastic cells are immunoreactive with S-100 protein, HMB45, melan A, microphthalmia transcription factor, tyrosinase, and vimentin (Fig. 6-33).

DIFFERENTIAL DIAGNOSIS

The wide morphologic diversity includes many malignant neoplasms such as undifferentiated carcinoma, lymphoma, melanotic neuroectodermal tumor of infancy (Fig. 6-34), rhabdomyosarcoma, leiomyosarcoma, fibrosarcoma, angiosarcoma and rare, metastatic melanoma to the sinonasal tract (Chart 6-1). Pertinent immunohistochemical studies allows for appropriate separation. Metastatic melanoma to the SNT, if it devleops, is usually a late event, and part of systemic disease.

PROGNOSIS AND THERAPY

The overall prognosis for sinonasal tract melanoma is poor, with a 5-year survival ranging from 17% to 47%.

Recurrences are common, with a poor prognosis associated with advanced stage, tumor >3 cm, mixed anatomic sites of involvement and vascular invasion. Wide local excision is the treatment of choice, with radiation providing only palliation.

OLFACTORY NEUROBLASTOMA

Olfactory neuroblastomas (esthesioneuroblastoma) are malignant neuroectodermal neoplasms thought to arise from the specialized sensory neuroepithelial (neuroectodermal) olfactory cells normally found in the upper part of the nasal cavity, including the superior nasal concha, the upper part of septum, the roof of nose, and the cribriform plate of the ethmoid sinus.

CLINICAL FEATURES

Olfactory neuroblastomas (ONB) account for approximately 5% of sinonasal tract malignancies. There is an equal gender distribution and may occur at any age, with a bimodal age distribution peak at 11–20 years and 51–60 years. These slow growing tumors most commonly cause unilateral nasal obstruction, epistaxis, and a mass high in the nasal cavity and ethmoid region.

Chart 6-1

Differential diagnostic comparison of sinonasal tract "small round cell malignant neoplasms"

Feature	Squamous cell carcinoma	Sinonasal undifferentiated carcinoma	Malignant melanoma	Olfactory neuroblastoma	Extranodal NK/T cell lymphoma, nasal	Rhabdomyosarcoma	Ewing sarcoma/PNET
Mean age	55–65 yr	55–60 yr	40–70 yr	40–45 yr	50–60 yr	<20 yr	<30 yr
Site	Nasal cavity and/or sinuses	Multiple sites usually	Anterior nasal septum > maxillary sinus	Roof of nasal cavity	Nasal cavity > paranasal sinuses > nasopharynx	Nasopharynx > sinonasal tract	Maxillary sinus > nasal cavity
Radiographic studies	Little destruction/ spread	Marked destruction/ spread	Central destructive mass	"Dumbbell-shaped" cribriform plate mass	Early changes non-specific; midline destruction later	Size, extent of tumor	Mass lesion, with bone erosion
Prognosis	60% 5-year (stage and tumor type dependent)	<20% 5-year survival	17%–47% 5-year survival	60%–80% 5-year survival	30%–50% 5-year survival (stage dependent)	44%–69% (age, stage, subtype dependent)	60%–70% 5-year (stage, size, FLI1)
Cranial nerve involvement	Uncommon	Common	Uncommon	Sometimes	Sometimes	Uncommon	Sometimes
Pattern	Syncytial	Sheets and nests	Protean	Lobular	Diffuse	Sheets, alveolar	Sheets, nests
Cytology	Squamous differentiation, keratinization, opaque cytoplasm	Medium cells, inconspicuous nucleoli	Large, polygonal, epithelioid, rhabdoid, plasmacytoid, spindle; pigment	Salt and pepper chromatin, small nucleoli (grade dependent)	Polymorphous, small to large, folded, cleaved and grooved nuclei	Round, strap, spindled, rhabdomyoblasts, primitive	Medium, round cells, vacuolated cytoplasm, fine chromatin
Anaplasia	Present	Common	Common	Occasionally and focally	Common	Common	Minimal
Mitotic figures	Present	High	High	Variable	High	Variable	Common
Necrosis	Limited	Prominent	Limited	Occasionally	Prominent (60%)	Limited	Frequent
Vascular invasion	Rare	Prominent	Rare	Occasionally	Prominent (60%)	Rare	Rare

Chart 6-1

Differential diagnostic comparison of sinonasal tract "small round cell malignant neoplasms"—Cont'd

Feature	Squamous cell carcinoma	Sinonasal undifferentiated carcinoma	Malignant melanoma	Olfactory neuroblastoma	Extranodal NK/T cell lymphoma, nasal	Rhabdomyosarcoma	Ewing sarcoma/PNET
Neurofibrillary stroma	Absent	Absent	Absent	Common	Absent	Absent	Absent
Pseudorosettes	Absent	Absent	Rare	Common	Absent	Absent	Present
Keratin	Positive	>90%	Negative	Focal, weak	Negative	Negative	Rare
CK 5/6	Present	Negative	Negative	Negative	Negative	Negative	n/a
EMA	Present	50%	Rare	Negative	Negative	Negative	n/a
NSE	Negative	50%	Negative	>90%	Negative	Negative	Positive
S-100 protein	Negative	<15%	Positive	+ (sustentacular)	Negative	Negative	Rare
Chromogranin/ Synaptophysin	Negative	<15%	Negative	>90% (can be weak)	Negative	Negative	Positive
HMB45	Negative	Negative	Positive	Negative	Negative	Negative	Negative
CD45RB	Negative	Negative	Negative	Negative	Positive[a]	Negative	Negative
CD56	Negative	Negative	Negative	Positive	Positive	Negative	Rare
CD99	Negative	<10%	Negative	Negative	Negative	Rare	>99%
Vimentin	Negative	Negative	Positive	Negative	Positive	Positive	Positive
Desmin	Negative	Negative	Negative	Negative	Negative	Positive[b]	Negative
In situ EBER	Absent	Absent	Absent	Absent	Nearly 100%	Negative	Negative
Electron microscopy	Epithelial junctions	Junctions, rare neurosecretory granules	Premelanosomes, melanosomes	Neurite-like processes, neurofilaments, neurosecretory granules	n/a	Thick and thin filaments, sarcomeres, Z-bands, glycogen	Glycogen; primitive cells

[a]Lymphoma is positive with CD3e, CD2, CD56, perforin, TIA1, granzyme B.
[b]Rhabdomyosarcoma is positive with desmin, actin, myoglobin, fast myosin, myo-D1 and myogenin.

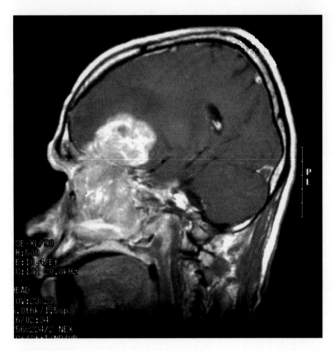

FIGURE 6-35

A T1-weighted gadolinium constrast MRI image shows a dumbbell-shaped mass extending through the cribriform plate and filling the nasal vault and the intracranial cavity.

OLFACTORY NEUROBLASTOMA DISEASE FACT SHEET	
Definition	Malignant neuroectodermal neoplasm arising from olfactory epithelium
Incidence and location	Approximately 5% of sinonasal tract malignancies
	About 0.4/1,000,000-population
	Encompasses cribriform plate
Morbidity and mortality	Stage-dependent mortality, overall about 60% 5-yr survival
Gender, race, and age distribution	Equal gender distribution
	Bimodal distribution: peak at 11–20 and 51–60 yr, respectively
Clinical features	Unilateral nasal obstruction and epistaxis most common
	Anosmia, headaches, pain, and ocular disturbances
	Often slow growing
Radiographic features	Dumbbell-shaped mass on either side of the cribriform plate
	MRI shows intense signal on T2-weighted images, with striking enhancement on T1-weighted gadolinium contrast images
	CT shows bone erosion (cribriform plate, lamina papyracea, fovea ethmoidalis)
	Calcifications may be seen
Prognosis and treatment	Prognosis is stage and grade dependent, with 75%–90% 5-yr survival (stage A) to 45% (stage C); 80% low grade vs 40% high grade
	Approximately 30% recurrence rate, usually within 2 yr
	Metastasis develops in lymph nodes or lungs and bone (about 20%)
	Meticulous surgical eradiation (combined craniofacial approach) achieves best outcome with postoperative radiotherapy
	Chemotherapy and bone marrow transplant shows promise

RADIOGRAPHIC FEATURES

The classic presentation is with a "dumbbell-shaped" mass encompassing the cribriform plate in the nasal vault (Fig. 6-35). MRI pre- and postcontrast images, which show striking enhancement on T1-weighted gadolinium contrast images. T2-weighted images also show an intense signal but contrast independent. Calcifications may be identified, generally on CT studies.

PATHOLOGIC FEATURES

GROSS FINDINGS

The excised tumors vary from a small polypoid nodule to large masses involving the ethmoids and nasal cavity bilaterally with extension into the adjacent paranasal sinuses. The cut surface appears gray-tan to pink-red and hypervascular.

MICROSCOPIC FINDINGS

The histologic appearance of olfactory neuroblastomas varies by degree of differentiation, although a semblance of lobular architecture seems to be maintained throughout (Fig. 6-36). The tumor cells are

identified below an intact mucosa, often immediately subtending the olfactory epithelium. Low-grade tumors contain cellular nests surrounded by fine fibrovascular septa in an organoid fashion. These relatively uniform cells, which are slightly larger than lymphocytes, lie in a finely fibrillar stroma. The cells have small, round to oval nuclei with uniformly distributed fine or coarse nuclear chromatin (Fig. 6-37). Homer Wright pseudorosettes are characterized by rings of neoplastic cells with finely fibrillar or granular material in the center (Fig. 6-38). True Flexner-Wintersteiner rosettes form duct-like spaces lined by nonciliated columnar cells with basally placed nuclei, but are only rarely identified (Fig. 6-39).

As the olfactory neuroblastomas become higher grade (less differentiated), pseudorosettes and fibrillar stroma are less common. The nuclei become more pleomorphic, chromatin is more coarse, mitotic figures increase, and tumor necrosis is present (Figs. 6-40, 6-41, 6-42).

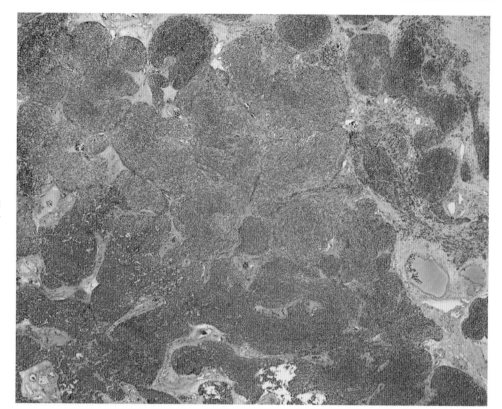

FIGURE 6-36

Well-formed lobules of closely packed cells separated by a highly vascularized stroma.

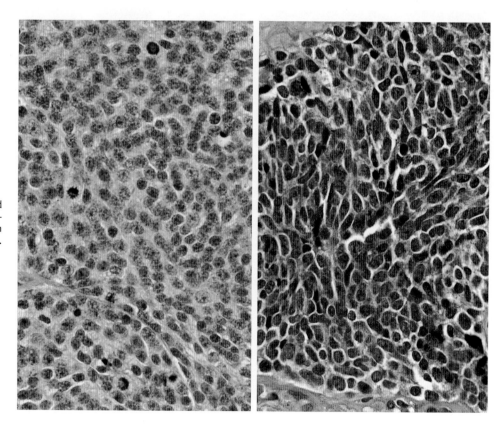

FIGURE 6-37

The tumor cells have uniformly round to oval nuclei with mild pleomorphism. Nuclear chromatin varies from delicate (*left*) to more coarse (*right*).

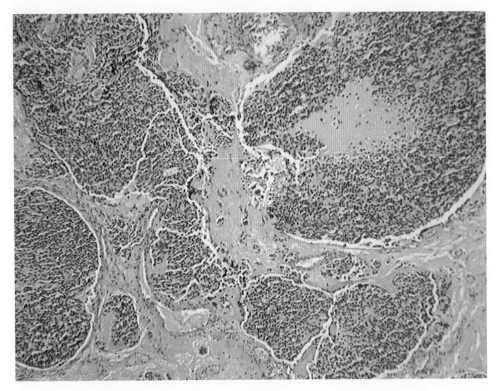

FIGURE 6-38

The lobules of tumor are separated by dense fibrosis. A large pseudorosette (Homer Wright) shows the central area of neurofibrillary matrix.

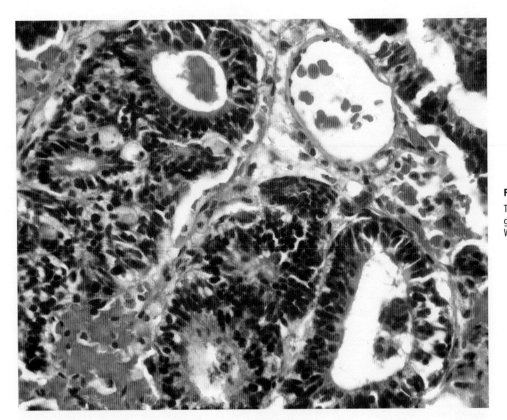

FIGURE 6-39

The columnar tumor cells form the glandular spaces of a true Flexner-Wintersteiner rosette.

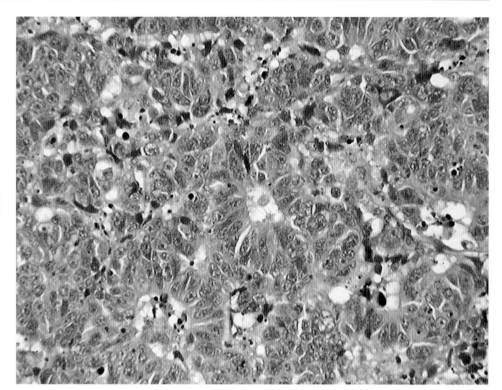

FIGURE 6-40

A grade III ONB showing a true Flexner-Wintersteiner rosette and increased mitotic figures.

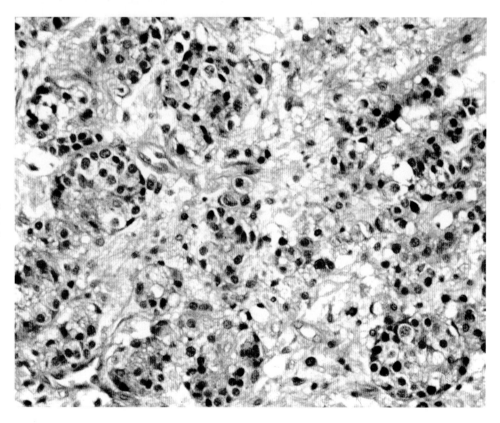

FIGURE 6-41

A grade IV ONB reveals bizarre tumor cells with increased mitotic activity. Notice the background fibrillar matrix.

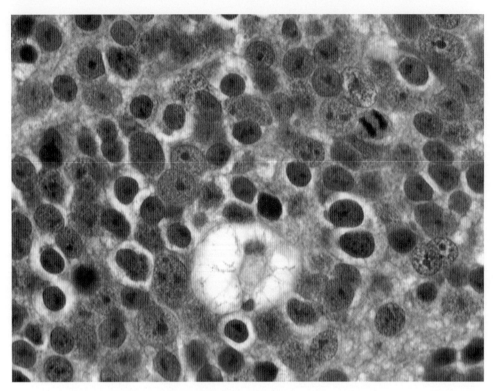

FIGURE 6-42
High power of a true Flexner-Wintersteiner rosette comprised of intermediate-sized cells with scant cytoplasm. A mitotic figure is present along with prominent nucleoli. Note the coarse chromatin distribution.

OLFACTORY NEUROBLASTOMA PATHOLOGIC FEATURES	
Gross findings	Polypoid, glistening, soft, vascular masses high in the nasal cavity and ethmoid region
Microscopic findings	Circumscribed lobule separated by vascularized stroma is maintained to some degree in all grades
	Tumor cells form solid nests, Homer Wright pseudorosettes with neurofibrillar matrix (30%), and Flexner-Wintersteiner–type true rosettes with glandular lumen (5%)
	Cells are uniform, small, with round nuclei and "salt-and-pepper" nuclear chromatin
	High-grade tumors have larger tumor cells, nuclear pleomorphism, and increased mitotic activity; neurofibrillary matrix is scent or absent
Ultrastructural features	Membrane-bound, dense core neurosecretory granules in the cytoplasm
	Neurite-like processes with neurofilaments and neurotubules
Immunohistochemical features	Neuron-specific enolase, chromogranin, synaptophysin, neurofilament protein positive in 80% of tumors
	S-100 protein positive cells confined to the periphery of tumor nests
Pathologic differential diagnosis	Sinonasal undifferentiated carcinoma, lymphoma, rhabdomyosarcoma, melanoma, neuroendocrine carcinoma

Chart 6-2
Hyams' grading system for olfactory neuroblastoma

Feature	Grade 1	Grade 2	Grade 3	Grade 4
Architecture	Lobular	Lobular	Lobular	Lobular
Mitotic activity	Absent	Present	Prominent	Marked
Nuclear pleomorphism	Absent	Moderate	Prominent	Marked
Fibrillary matrix	Prominent	Present	Minimal	Absent
Rosettes	Homer Wright	Homer Wright	Flexner-Wintersteiner	Flexner-Wintersteiner
Necrosis	Absent	Absent	±Present	Common

Tumors are graded based on the degree of differentiated, presence of neural stroma, mitotic figures, and necrosis from grade I to IV (Chart 6-2). The grade correlates with prognosis, although not as sensitively as tumor stage.

which additionally contain neurotubules and neurofilaments. The diameter of the granules is from 50 to 250 nm. Olfactory differentiation with olfactory vesicles and microvilli on apical borders may be seen in Flexner-Wintersteiner rosettes.

ANCILLARY STUDIES

ULTRASTRUCTURAL FEATURES

Membrane-bound dense core neurosecretory granules are present in the cytoplasm and in nerve processes,

IMMUNOHISTOCHEMICAL FEATURES

Neuron-specific enolase, chromogranin, synaptophysin and CD56 are expressed in a diffuse pattern in about 80% of tumors (Fig. 6-43). A small number of cells at the periphery of tumor nests react with the anti-

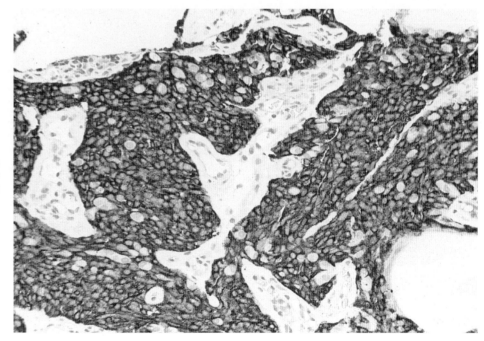

FIGURE 6-43

A diffuse expression of chromogranin in ONB. (Courtesy of Yao S. Fu, MD, Senior Pathologist, Providence St. Joseph Medical Center, Burbank, CA.)

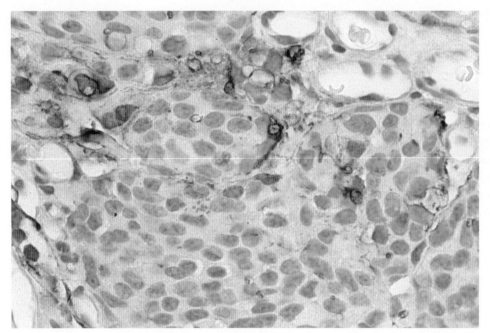

FIGURE 6-44
S-100 protein immunohistochemistry is only positive in cells at the periphery of tumor nests, indicative of Schwannian cell differentiation. (Courtesy of Yao S. Fu, MD, Senior Pathologist, Providence St. Joseph Medical Center, Burbank, CA.)

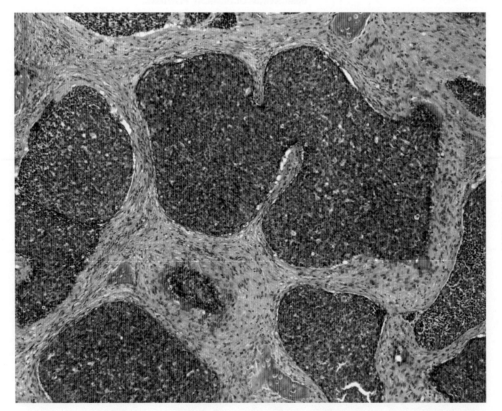

FIGURE 6-45
The solid, lobular pattern of growth in this adenoid cystic carcinoma can mimic an olfactory neuroblastoma. However, note the palisading at the periphery and the reduplicated basement membrane material.

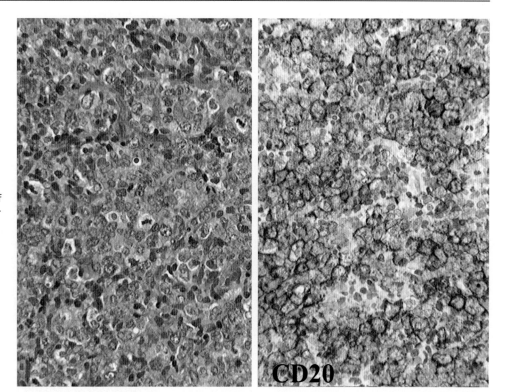

FIGURE 6-46

A diffuse large B cell lymphoma of the maxillary sinus with large, atypical lymphoid cells.

bodies against S-100 protein and glial filament acidic protein (GFAP) to suggest Schwann cell differentiation (Fig. 6-44). Keratins are rarely positive. The tumor cells are negative with CD45RB, HMB45, desmin, and MIC2 antigen (CD99).

DIFFERENTIAL DIAGNOSIS

The small, blue, round cell neoplasm group of the sinonasal tract includes sinonasal undifferentiated carcinoma, adenoid cystic carcinoma (Fig. 6-45), lymphoma, rhabdomyosarcoma, melanoma, neuroendocrine carcinoma, and ES/PNET (Chart 6-1). In a small biopsy with crush artifact, misinterpretation is common, especially as edge effect and diffuse artifacts with immunohistochemistry may not resolve the differential. Carcinomas tend to have higher mitotic activity, larger nucleoli, and obvious necrosis. A targeted immunohistochemistry panel may need to be expanded to encompass the differential, especially if the lesion is high in the nasal cavity.

PROGNOSIS AND THERAPY

The prognosis is both stage and grade dependent, with stage A tumors experiencing a 75% to 90% 5-year survival, while stage C has a 45% survival (see Appendix C). Likewise, low-grade tumors have an 80% survival, while high-grade tumors have a 40% survival. Recurrence is common (about 30%), usually within 2 years of the initial presentation. Metastasis develops in about

20% of cases, while distant metastasis occurs in up to 60% of patients. En bloc resection of the tumor and cribriform plate with clear margin via a trephination and craniofacial approach is the treatment of choice for these tumors. Postoperative radiation is given to most patients to improve local control. Patients with advanced tumor or poorly differentiated tumor usually receive multimodality treatment, including chemotherapy and bone marrow transplantation.

EXTRANODAL NK/T CELL LYMPHOMA, NASAL TYPE

Lymphoma is the most common malignant nonepithelial neoplasm found in the upper respiratory tract and most commonly involves the nasal cavity, the maxillary sinus, nasopharynx, and salivary gland. This discussion will be limited to extranodal NK/T cell lymphoma, nasal type (NK/T LNT), which is more common in the sinonasal region, although B cell lymphomas tend to be more common in the nasopharynx, Waldeyer's ring, and the sinuses (Fig. 6-46). Hodgkin lymphoma is uncommon in either location. Additionally, there are geographic differences, where Asian and South American patients have a much higher frequency of sinonasal tract lymphoma (about 7% of lymphomas), with the majority NT/T LNT, while in Western countries, sinonasal tract lymphomas account for <2% of lymphomas, with B cell-types predominating.

There are a number of differences between the types of lymphoid lesions which affect each of these locations, most closely related to the function of tissues affected.

For example, the sinonasal tract does not normally contain lymphoid tissue, therefore EBV associated NK/T LNT tends to be more common; the nasopharynx, by contrast, has a rich lymphoid tissue which can be affected by follicular hyperplasia or by B cell lymphomas, most specifically mantle cell lymphoma. The distinction of NK/T LNT from other diseases which give the clinical picture of midline destructive disease cannot be overstressed. The difference in treatment and patient outcome are diametrically opposite in many cases. Unfortunately, the diagnosis of NK/T LNT is often very challenging in the initial stages of presentation requiring very close clinical correlation between the pathologist, otorhinolaryngologist, oncologist, and radiation therapist.

Many different names have been used for this disorder in the past: angiocentric NK/T cell lymphoma, polymorphic reticulosis, lethal midline granuloma, Stewart's granuloma, and peripheral NK/T cell lymphoma, to name just a few. It is wisest to use the current WHO criteria since it incorporates clinical, histologic, immunophenotypic, molecular, and treatment considerations into the classification scheme.

CLINICAL FEATURES

All ages can be affecting, but patients usually present in the 5th–6th decades. Men are more commonly affected than women (3:1). The most frequent initial clinical presentation is nonspecific, with nasal discharge, sinusitis, headaches, facial and periorbital swelling, and epistaxis. As the tumor develops, the more destructive nature of the neoplasm is manifest through midline destruction, i.e., nasal cavity ulceration, paranasal sinuses (frequently bilaterally) necrosis, with palatal extension and fistula formation, orbital swelling, and a prominent edema (often with erythematous and "warm" skin overlying these structures). Pain and paresthesias develop with further destruction of the tissues. Systemic manifestations of weight loss, fever, fatigue, and profound night sweating can also be seen, especially if the stage of the lymphoma results in involvement of extra-sinonasal tract sites (skin, soft tissues, gastrointestinal tract). Most patients have stage IE or IIE disease at presentation (E: extranodal). Therefore, this particular type of lymphoma may be indolent or aggressive depending on the overall morphology and the stage of lymphoma. There is a very strong association with EBV in both the endemic and nonendemic populations.

PATHOLOGIC FEATURES

GROSS FINDINGS

A raised polypoid unilateral lesion in the early stage develops progressively into an ulcerated and necrotic mass, which may become bilateral. Cut surface reveals gray-white, friable, homogeneous tissue.

MICROSCOPIC FINDINGS

In contrast to the nasopharynx and tonsils, NK/T LNT are much more common than are B cell lymphomas in the nasal cavity. There is a development arc

EXTRANODAL NK/T CELL LYMPHOMA, NASAL TYPE DISEASE FACT SHEET	
Definition	Malignant NK/T cell lymphoma with the bulk of the disease in the sinonasal tract
Incidence and location	Most common nonepithelial malignancy of the sinonasal tract
	About 15% of all malignancies in sinonasal tract
	Nasal cavity and paranasal sinuses concurrently affected
Morbidity and mortality	Mortality in 50%–70% of patients
Gender, race, and age distribution	Male > Female (3 : 1)
	Endemic in Asians and Latin Americans
	Peak in 6th decade
Clinical features	Early disease difficult to detect with nonspecific symptoms
	Nasal obstruction, epistaxis, nasal discharge, and swelling
	Septal perforation and bone destruction later in course
	Uncommonly have fever and weight loss
	Most patients present with low-stage disease (stage I/II E)
Prognosis and treatment	Overall prognosis is 30%–50%
	Relapse/recurrences develops in up to 50%
	Advanced stage, bulky disease and systemic symptoms yield a worse prognosis
	Combined radiotherapy and chemotherapy, although chemotherapy is controversial

EXTRANODAL NK/T-CELL LYMPHOMA, NASAL TYPE PATHOLOGIC FEATURES	
Microscopic findings	Early disease difficult to detect in background reactive lymphoid infiltrate
	Diffuse infiltrate which is frequently angiocentric and angioinvasive associated with tumor necrosis
	Variable, large lymphoid cells, mixed small and large lymphoid cells
	May occasionally have extensive PEH of epithelium
Immunohistochemical features	Positive with CD2, cytoplasmic CD3e, CD56, perforin, TIA1, granzyme B, and EBER in situ hybridization
	CD5, CD16, CD57 are usually negative
Pathologic differential diagnosis	Reactive/inflammatory infiltrate, Wegener's granulomatosis, lymphomatoid granulomatosis, olfactory neuroblastoma, ES/PNET

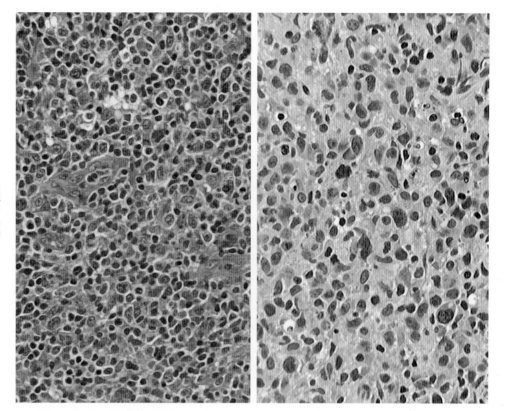

FIGURE 6-47

Left: A mixed population of inflammatory cells harboring the atypical lymphoid elements. *Right:* More cytologically atypical lymphoid cells, easier to identify after the disease has progressed.

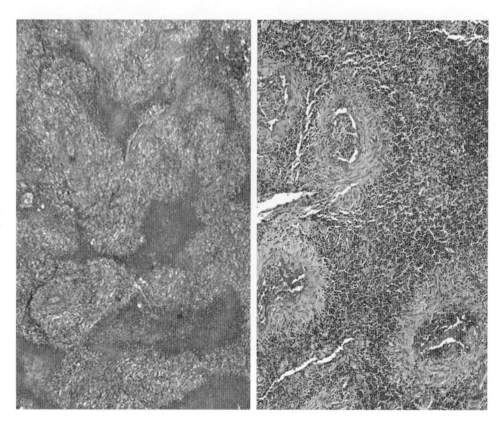

FIGURE 6-48

Left: Necrosis is noted between islands of atypical lymphoid cells and prominent arteries. *Right:* Arteries are invaded and surrounded by atypical lymphoid cells.

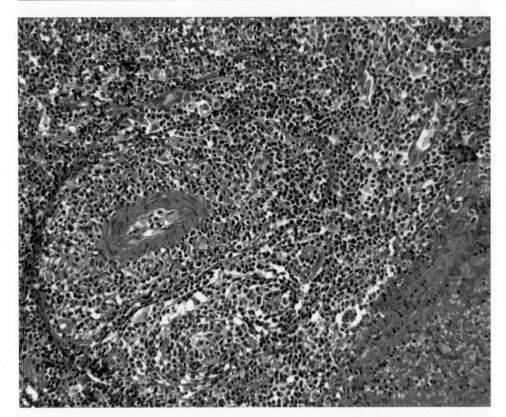

FIGURE 6-49

A vessel is surrounded and invaded by atypical cells; necrosis is present in the lower right.

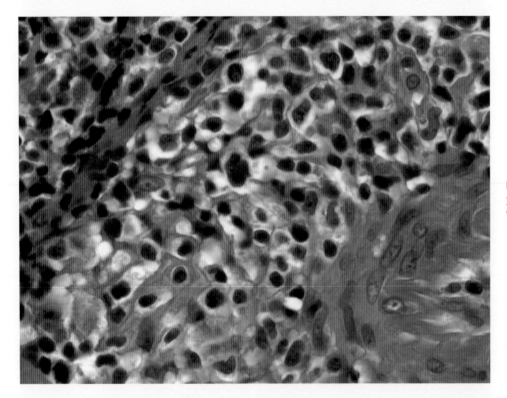

FIGURE 6-50

Infiltration of a vessel wall by atypical lymphoid cells.

associated with disease progression. Initially, there is a subepithelial, diffuse, and polymorphous cellular infiltrate composed of normal appearing lymphocytes, histiocytes, immunoblasts, eosinophils, and plasma cells. Within this milieu are a number of atypical lymphoid cells, increasing in number as the disease progresses.

This intermixed population of atypical NK/T cells interspersed throughout the specimen is often exceedingly difficult to identify, even with ancillary techniques (Fig. 6-47). The prominent background inflammatory component may completely obscure the underlying neoplasm, simulating a infectious or inflammatory condi-

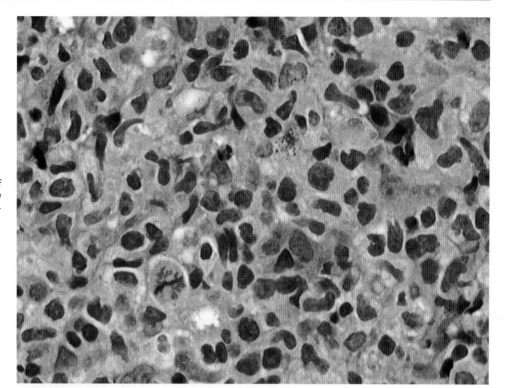

FIGURE 6-51

The atypical lymphoid cells consist of mixed small and large cells, many showing folded, cleaved, and irregular nuclei.

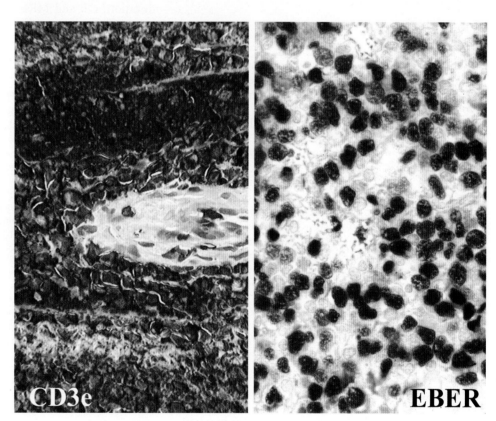

FIGURE 6-52

Left: The neoplastic cells within this vessel are strongly and diffusely immunoreactive with CD3e. *Right:* Nearly all of the cells are strongly and diffusely positive with EBER by in situ hybridization. (Courtesy of Dr. J.K.C. Chan.)

tion. When the vascular walls are invaded by the neoplastic cells to the point they occlude the lumen of the vessel, the presence of profound necrosis brings to mind the possibility of a neoplasm (Fig. 6-48). Angiocentricity and angioinvasion with necrosis is seen in about 50% to 60% of NK/T LNT cases (Figs. 6-49,

6-50). Due to the lack of ubiquitous angioinvasion and destruction, WHO proposed the term *extranodal NK/T cell lymphoma, nasal type,* instead of angiocentric NK-T cell lymphoma. Necrosis of the coagulative type may be widespread, further limiting interpretation, especially on small biopsies. Multiple and repeat biopsies are often required to render a definitive diagnosis—frequently in a patient who is deteriorating clinically! The neoplastic cells have a broad cytomorphologic spectrum, ranging in size from small to large, the latter usually remarkably atypical (Fig. 6-51). Tumor cell folding, cleaving, and grooving is characteristic for a NK/T cell lymphoma. Occasionally, pseudoepitheliomatous hyperplasia may simulate an epithelial malignancy.

ANCILLARY STUDIES

By in situ hybridization, nearly 100% of NK/T LNT have detectable EBER, better developed in Asian patients, but also present in Western patients (Fig. 6-52). The neoplastic cells are positive with T cell (CD3e [Fig. 6-51], CD2) and natural killer cell/cytotoxic-related markers (CD56, perforin, TIA1, granzyme B) (Fig. 6-51). CD43 and CD45RO may be positive. However, CD5, CD16, and CD57 are usually negative.

DIFFERENTIAL DIAGNOSIS

Inflammatory and infectious lesions and Wegener's granulomatosis are key considerations when faced with a lymphoid process. In benign conditions, nuclear atypia, and mitotic activity are absent or minimal. Immunohistochemical stains and in situ hybridization for EBER are helpful to confirm NK/T LNT. Separation from lymphomatoid granulomatosis (LYG) may be nearly impossible, as the latter diagnosis significantly overlaps the clinical, morphologic, and immunophenotype features of NK/T LNT. LYG may be a T cell rich EBV related B cell lymphoproliferative disease, in which T cells are abundant and reactive in nature. In contrast, NK/T LNT is a T-cell lymphoproliferative disorder, in which EBV occurs in T and NK cells. Separation from other "blue round cell tumors" can usually be achieved with pertinent immunohistochemistry (Chart 6-1).

PROGNOSIS AND THERAPY

The overall prognosis for NK/T LNT ranges from 30% to 50%, with relapses or recurrences developing in up to 50% of patients. Prognosis is determined by stage, bulky disease, and if systemic symptoms are present. Systemic disease development is common. Treatment for localized disease is radiotherapy with or without chemotherapy. It must be stressed again, that diffuse large B cell lymphomas are managed differently, although also showing a 5-year survival of 40% to 60%.

RHABDOMYOSARCOMA

About 40% of all rhabdomyosarcoma develop in the head and neck, about 20% of which involve the sinonasal tract and nasopharynx. The nasopharynx is more commonly affected than the sinonasal tract. Rhabdomyosarcoma is the most common childhood sarcoma. Rhabdomyosarcomas are subtyped into broad categories: embryonal, alveolar, and pleomorphic, with further subtypes within each category. Discussion will be limited to the most common types in the sinonasal tract: embryonal and alveolar.

CLINICAL FEATURES

Rhabdomyosarcoma has a peak incidence during the first and second decades of life, with a slight male predominance. Embryonal type predominates in childhood while the alveolar type predominates in adults. Difficulty breathing, epistaxis, facial swelling, visual disturbances, and sinusitis are present, often of a short duration. CT and MRI imaging delineate the size and extent of the tumour (Fig. 6-53).

RHABDOMYOSARCOMA DISEASE FACT SHEET	
Definition	Malignant neoplasm with skeletal muscle phenotype
Incidence and location	About 20% of rhabdomyosarcomas involve sinonasal tract
	Accounts for about 5%–10% of sinonasal nonepithelial malignancies
	Nasopharynx more commonly involved than sinonasal tract
Morbidity and mortality	Overall mortality of between 40%–60%, depending on age, histologic subtype, and stage
Gender, race, and age distribution	Slight male predilection
	Childhood and young adults (embryonal subtype)
	Adults (alveolar subtype)
Clinical features	Difficulty breathing, epistaxis, facial swelling, sinusitis
	Large, polypoid mass in the nasopharynx or nasal cavity
Prognosis and treatment	Prognosis is age, histologic subtype and clinical stage dependent
	Children have better prognosis than adults (60% vs 10% 5-yr survival)
	Prognosis best for botyroid, then embryonal, then alveolar
	Combined multimodality therapy (chemotherapy, radiotherapy, surgery)

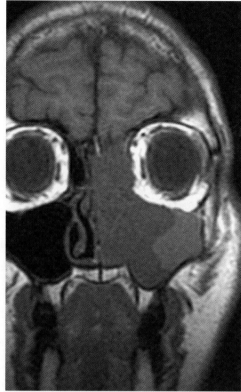
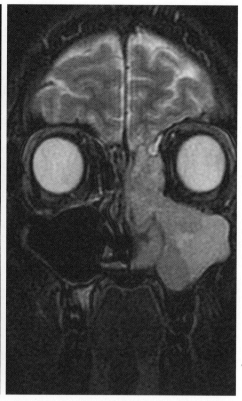

FIGURE 6-53

This MRI study shows the extent of the tumor within the maxillary and ethmoid sinuses on T1- and T2-weighted images.

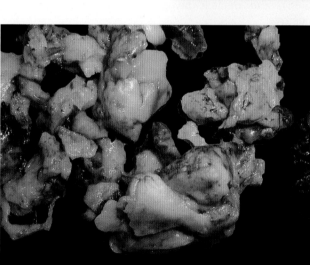

FIGURE 6-54

This macroscopic image demonstrates the similarity between sinonasal polyps and rhabdomyosarcoma.

RHABDOMYOSARCOMA PATHOLOGIC FEATURES	
Gross findings	Bulky, fleshy, polypoid, grape-like masses, simulating polyps
Microscopic findings	**Embryonal type (80%):**
	Round to spindled primitive mesenchymal cells with hyperchromatic nuclei
	Rhabdomyoblasts with cross-striations rare
	Myxoid stroma is common
	Botyroid variant has distinct submucosal hypercellular cambium layer, middle myxoid layer, and primitive cells in deep layers
	Alveolar type (20%):
	Fibrous septae separating loosely cohesive rhabdomyoblasts into alveolar spaces
	Multinucleated giant cells may be present
Ultrastructural features	Thick and thin myofilaments, incomplete sarcomeres, or well-formed Z-bands
Immunohistochemical features	Desmin, muscle-specific actin, myoglobin, myogenin, Myo-D1 positive
Pathologic differential diagnosis	Lymphoma, polyps with stromal atypia, undifferentiated carcinoma, ES/PNET, olfactory neuroblastoma, melanoma

PATHOLOGIC FEATURES

GROSS FINDINGS

When small, it has the appearance of solid nodule with a vascular pink-red smooth surface. With increasing size, these tumors produce bulky, fleshy, polypoid masses simulating multiple nasal polyps (Fig. 6-54). The botyroid variant has a "grape-like" appearance.

MICROSCOPIC FINDINGS

Rhabdomyosarcomas of the sinonasal tract are predominantly of the embryonal type (80%), and the remaining 20% alveolar or spindle cell variants. Sarcoma botryoides is a variant of embryonal rhabdomyosarcoma.

Embryonal Rhabdomyosarcoma

Made up of round to spindled cells with elongated to round hyperchromatic nuclei, the tumor has a distinct accumulation of primitive cells and rhabdomyoblasts beneath the squamous or respiratory mucosa, referred to as cambium layer (Figs. 6-55, 6-56). In the deeper parts of the tumor, primitive cells predominate and admix with a varying number of rhabdomyoblasts. Rhabdomyoblasts have many different appearances ranging from elongated strap-shaped cells to small round "tadpole" cells, both having densely eosinophilic cytoplasm. Cross-striations are rare (Fig. 6-57). A myxoid stroma may be present, occasionally abundant. The botyroid variant is polypoid with a submucosal hypercellular cambium layer, a myxoid hypocellular zone, and a deeper, cellular immature, primitive component (Fig. 6-58). The spindle cell variant is uncommon in the sinonasal tract.

Alveolar Rhabdomyosarcoma

The tumor cells are loosely cohesive groups of small to medium cells separated into clusters by fibrous septa, simulating a glandular neoplasm (Figs. 6-59, 6-60, 6-61). Multinucleated giant cells may be seen. While most rhabdomyoblasts have eosinophilic cytoplasm, some have vacuolated/cleared cytoplasm. A solid variant lacks septa. Mixtures of alveolar and embryonal patterns may occur.

ANCILLARY STUDIES

ULTRASTRUCTURAL FEATURES

Variable degrees of skeletal muscle differentiation, including thick and thin myofilaments with dense bodies or Z-band are seen by electron microscopy. Glycogen particles are usually present.

IMMUNOHISTOCHEMICAL FEATURES

Rhabdomyosarcomas express desmin, muscle specific actin, myoglobin, fast myosin, nuclear Myo-D1 (Fig. 6-62), and nuclear myogenin. CD99 may rarely be positive.

DIFFERENTIAL DIAGNOSIS

The differential diagnosis includes most of the small round cell tumors, such as lymphoma, leukemia, ES/PNET, olfactory neuroblastoma, melanoma, and undifferentiated carcinoma (Chart 6-1). These tumors can be excluded by the use of a panel of appropriate immunohistochemical stains. Sinonasal tract polyps with stromal atypia have inflammatory cells, lack the cellularity of a rhabdomyosarcoma, and usually have different clinical findings. The atypical spindle cells (Fig. 6-63) are myofibroblasts, so may have a similar immunoreactivity with actins.

PROGNOSIS AND THERAPY

The overall prognosis is determined by age, histologic subtype, and the clinical stage at presentation. A better prognosis is seen in children and in patients with the botyroid type. Overall survival is 44% to 69%, but can be 90% for stage I tumors; 60% versus 10% 5-year survival for children versus adults, respectively. Treatment encompasses a multimodality approach (chemotherapy, radiation, and surgery).

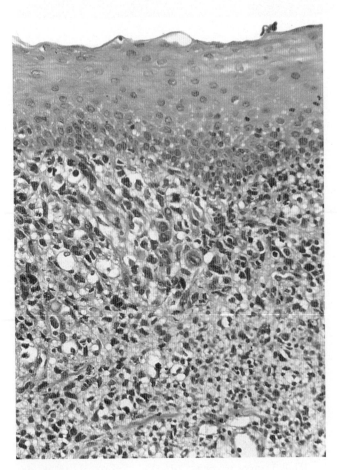

FIGURE 6-55

Beneath the squamous mucosa is a hypercellular cambium layer consists of primitive mesenchymal cells and rhabdomyoblasts. (Courtesy of Yao S. Fu, MD, Senior Pathologist, Providence St. Joseph Medical Center, Burbank, CA.)

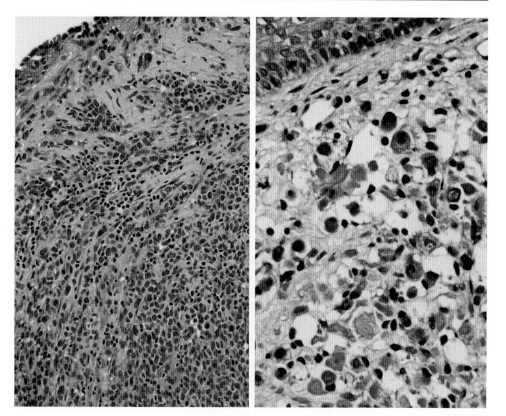

FIGURE 6-56

Left: A respiratory epithelium overlying a diffuse atypical proliferation. *Right:* A squamous mucosa overlying rhabdomyoblasts with eosinophilic cytoplasm.

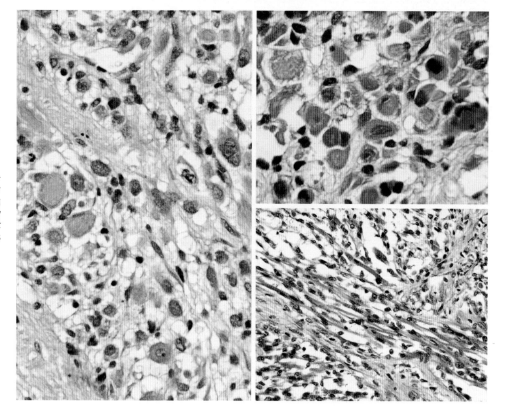

FIGURE 6-57

Left: Rhabdomyoblasts with elongated and spindled cells. *Right upper:* Predominantly primitive appearing cells with abundant, eccentrically placed eosinophilic cytoplasm. *Right lower:* Strap cells with cross striations are very uncommon.

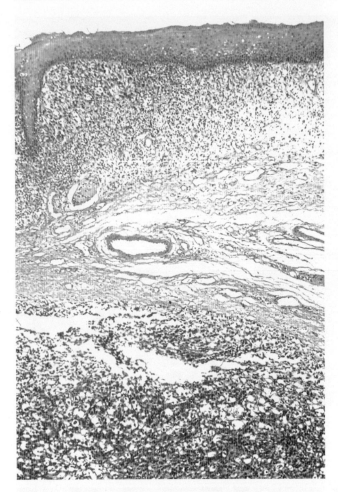

FIGURE 6-58

The sarcoma botyroid type is characterized by three distinct zones: hypercellular, cambium layer beneath the squamous mucosa; a second underlying zone of hypocellular myxoid stroma; and a third zone of predominantly primitive mesenchymal cells. (Courtesy of Yao S. Fu, MD, Senior Pathologist, Providence St. Joseph Medical Center, Burbank, CA.)

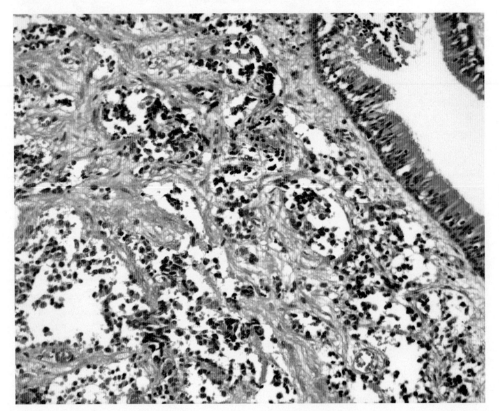

FIGURE 6-59

Alveolar rhabdomyosarcoma has tumor cells which form dilated alveolar spaces.

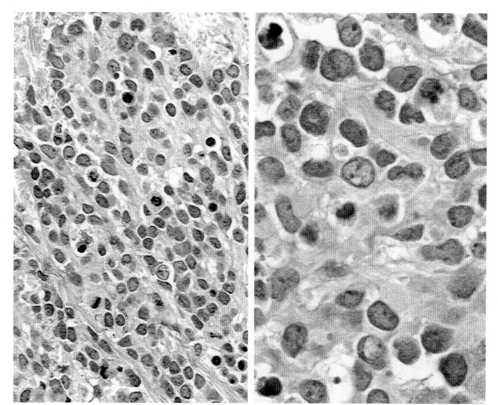

FIGURE 6-60

Left: Tumor cells are arranged around the periphery of this "alveolus." *Right:* The cells have small globules of strongly eosinophilic cytoplasm to suggest rhabdomyoblasts in this alveolar rhabdomyosarcoma.

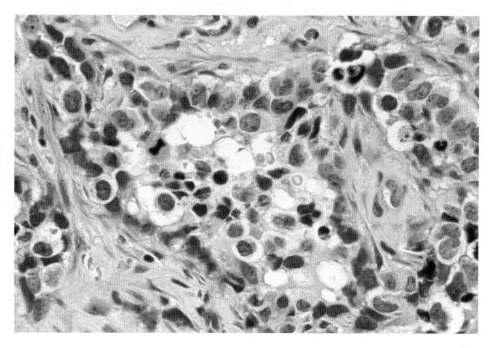

FIGURE 6-61

Not all rhabdomyoblasts have abundant cytoplasm, but instead have vacuolated cytoplasm to suggest glandular neoplasms. (Courtesy of Yao S. Fu, MD, Senior Pathologist, Providence St. Joseph Medical Center, Burbank, CA.)

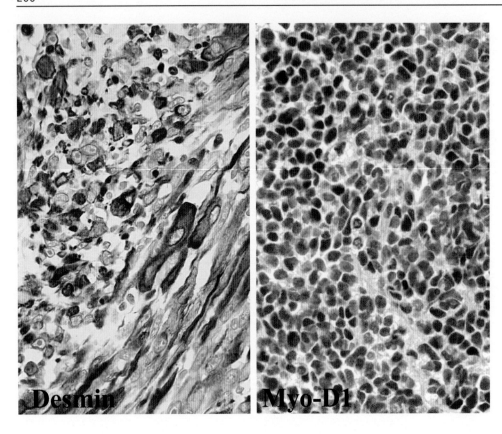

FIGURE 6-62
Left: Strong desmin immunoreaction is noted in the cytoplasm of this embryonal type rhabdomyosarcoma in both spindled and epithelioid areas. *Right:* Myo-D1 stains the nuclei of this rhabdomyosarcoma.

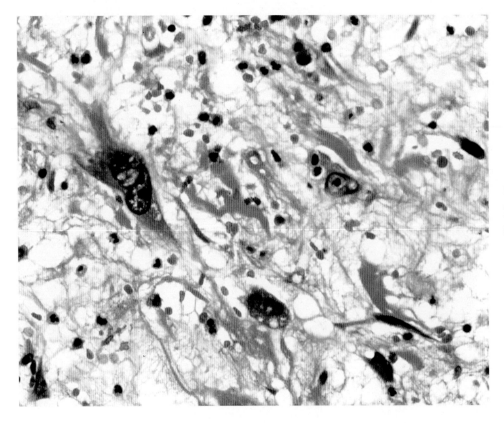

FIGURE 6-63
Atypical stromal cells are in isolation in this sinonasal polyp with myofibroblastic atypia.

EWING SARCOMA

Ewing sarcoma and primitive neuroectodermal tumor are closely related high-grade, round cell tumors with a neuroectodermal phenotype. These tumors are considered on a morphologic spectrum, with both expressing similar genetic alterations.

CLINICAL FEATURES

ES/PNET is uncommon in the head and neck. About 20% of affected children have ES/PNET in the head and neck, and 20% of these patients will have sinonasal tract involvement, most commonly in the maxillary sinus and nasal fossa. There is a slight male predominance. The tumor is most common in children and young adults who present with pain, mass, and obstruction.

PATHOLOGIC FEATURES

GROSS FINDINGS

The tumors, often polypoid, measure up to 6 cm, are gray-white and glistening, and often associated with ulceration and hemorrhage. Bone erosion is common. Tumors of the head and neck are much smaller at presentation than those of other anatomic sites.

MICROSCOPIC FINDINGS

Diffuse, densely cellular, sheets and nests of uniform, small- to medium-sized round cells with scant vacuolated cytoplasm make up this neoplasm. The nuclei are round with fine chromatin distribution and small nucleoli (Fig. 6-64). Mitotic figures are common. Coagulative necrosis is frequently identified (Fig. 6-65). Occasionally there is a greater degree of chromatin clumping, greater nuclear pleomorphism, and the presence of true rosettes and pseudorosettes (Fig. 6-66).

ANCILLARY STUDIES

HISTOCHEMICAL STUDIES

By PAS stains, glycogen is present in the cytoplasm.

IMMUNOHISTOCHEMICAL FEATURES

MIC2 (CD99) and vimentin is expressed in nearly all ES/PNET tumors (Fig. 6-64). NSE and synaptophysin are expressed less commonly. Uncommonly or rarely S100 protein, GFAP, and keratin will be expressed. FLI-1 (a portion of the gene fusion product of EWS/FLI1) can be detected by immunohistochemistry. The chromosomal translocation at t(11;22)(q24;q12) or t(21;22)(q22;q12) identified by PCR or fluorescent in situ hybridization (FISH) can confirm the diagnosis.

EWING SARCOMA
DISEASE FACT SHEET

Definition	High-grade, primitive neuroectodermal neoplasm (ES and PNET are considered a spectrum)
Incidence and location	Rare
	About 20% occur in head and neck with about 20% arising in sinonasal tract
	Maxillary sinus > nasal fossa
Morbidity and mortality	Better prognosis in head and neck, with about 30% mortality
Gender, race, and age distribution	Slight male predominance
	Most common in children and young adults
Clinical features	Pain, mass, and obstruction
	Polypoid mass occasionally
Prognosis and treatment	Size and stage dependent, although sinonasal tract location has better prognosis than thoracoabdominal disease
	Better prognosis when EWS/FLI1 fusion is present
	Overall 60%–70% 5-yr survival
	Multimodality therapy

EWING SARCOMA
PATHOLOGIC FEATURES

Gross findings	Often polypoid, grey, white glistening tumor with ulceration and hemorrhage
	Bone erosion/destruction is common
Microscopic findings	Dense, solid sheets of small to medium-sized monotonous cells
	High nuclear to cytoplasmic ratio with round nuclei
	Fine nuclear chromatin distribution, small nucleoli
	Mitotic activity is high with coagulative tumor necrosis common
	Occasionally may have neural differentiation
Immunohistochemical features	CD99, vimentin positive; rarely keratin positive
	FLI1 positive
	May react with other neural markers (NSE, synaptophysin, S-100 protein, NFP, GFAP, chromogranin)
Pathologic differential diagnosis	Lymphoma, rhabdomyosarcoma, olfactory neuroblastoma, melanotic neuroectodermal tumor of infancy, melanoma, undifferentiated carcinoma, pituitary adenoma

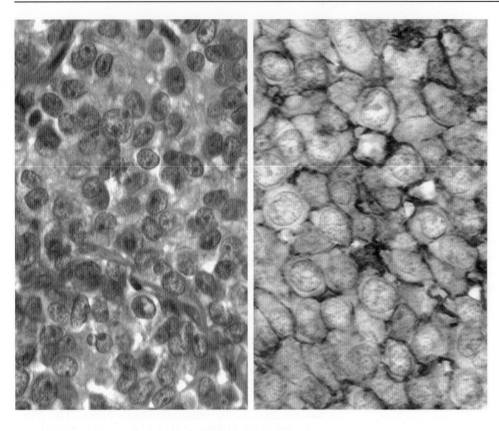

FIGURE 6-64

Left: Sheets of medium-sized cells with vacuolated cytoplasm. Fine chromatin and small nucleoli are noted. *Right:* The cells are strongly and diffusely reactive with CD99 (MIC2) immunohistochemistry.

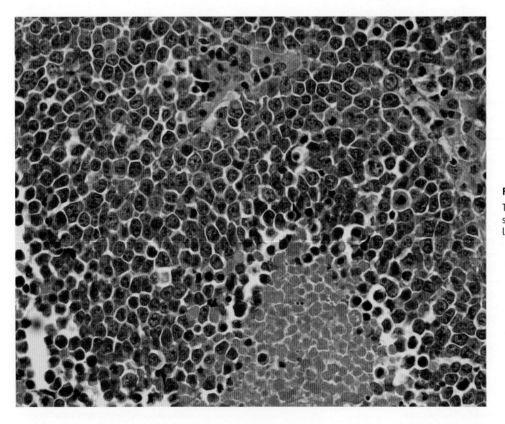

FIGURE 6-65

The sheets of medium cells with scant cytoplasm demonstrate coagulative necrosis.

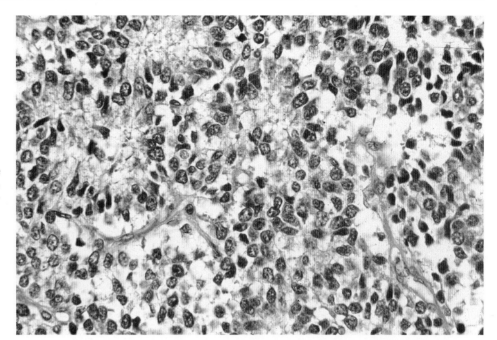

FIGURE 6-66

In some ES/PNET true rosettes are noted. (Courtesy of Yao S. Fu, MD, Senior Pathologist, Providence St. Joseph Medical Center, Burbank, CA.)

DIFFERENTIAL DIAGNOSIS

The differential diagnosis includes all the malignant small round cell tumors, such as lymphoma, rhabdomyosarcoma, olfactory neuroblastoma, melanotic neuroectodermal tumor, melanoma, small cell carcinoma, and pituitary adenoma (Chart 6-1). Different clinical presentation, patterns of growth, and immunohistochemistry allow for separation.

PROGNOSIS AND THERAPY

ES/PNET are considered to be highly aggressive neoplasms, often spreading into the adjacent paranasal sinuses. Staging according to the Clinical Groups of the Intergroup Rhabdomyosarcoma Study allows for a unified approach to the tumor. Sinonasal tract lesions tend to have a slightly better prognosis (60%–70% 5-yr survival) than their thoracoabdominal counterparts. Patients with the EWS/FLI1 fusion tend to have a better prognosis. Multimodality therapy achieves the best outcome.

FIBROSARCOMA

Carcinomas account for the majority of malignant tumors, followed by lymphomas. However, fibrosarcoma are considered the next most common malignancy of the sinonasal tract (rhabdomyosarcomas are more common in the head and neck, but not in the sinonasal tract).

Fibrosarcoma is defined as a malignant neoplasm, its differentiation limited to fibroblastic and myofibroblastic. Tumors with additional differentiation detected by ancillary techniques are excluded. Similarly, tumors having pleomorphic, bizarre cells are excluded from fibrosarcoma, and placed in the malignant fibrous histiocytoma category (Fig. 6-67).

CLINICAL FEATURES

Females are affected slightly more commonly than males (3:2), with a peak in the 5th–6th decades. Patients have

FIBROSARCOMA DISEASE FACT SHEET	
Definition	Malignant neoplasm with only fibroblastic and/or myofibroblastic differentiation
Incidence and location	Uncommon, but second most common nonepithelial sinonasal malignancy
	Usually paranasal sinus location
Morbidity and mortality	About 25% death in low-grade tumors
Gender, race, and age distribution	Female > Male (3 : 2)
	Peak, 5th–6th decades
Clinical features	Nasal obstruction and epistaxis most common
	Pain, sinusitis, nasal discharge, and swelling less common
Prognosis and treatment	Prognosis generally good with 75% survival
	Recurrences high (up to 60%) related to difficulty with complete extirpation
	Surgery is treatment of choice with adjuvant radiation

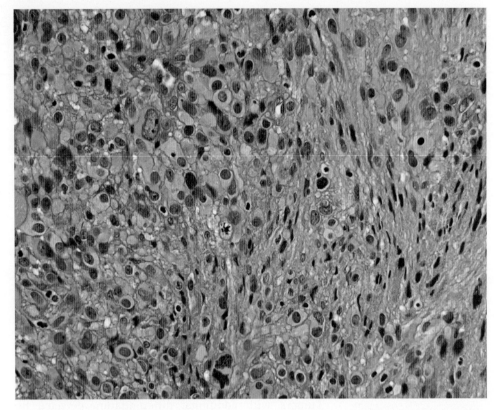

FIGURE 6-67

This highly pleomorphic neoplasm with increased mitotic figures and a storiform pattern would be placed in the malignant fibrous histiocytoma category.

nasal obstruction, often associated with epistaxis. Pain, sinusitis, nasal discharge, swelling, and anosmia are less common. Fibrosarcoma of the sinonasal tract occurs most frequently in the maxillary sinus, nasal cavity, and ethmoid region, uncommonly confined to the nasal cavity alone.

PATHOLOGIC FEATURES

GROSS FINDINGS

In the resection specimen, the tumor varies from 2–8 cm and has a smooth, polypoid, fleshy, white, homogeneous appearance. It grows by expansion with smooth borders or by infiltration. Necrosis and hemorrhage may be seen in higher grade tumors.

MICROSCOPIC FINDINGS

Tumors are unencapsulated, with infiltration into the bone and occasional surface ulceration. There is proliferation and entrapment of surface respiratory mucosa simulating inverted papilloma in up to one-third of fibrosarcomas (Fig. 6-68). The stroma may be vascular with scattered capillaries mimicking hemangiopericytoma, or may show delicate to dense bands of collagen. The cellularity is high, with the spindled cells arranged in a distinct herringbone pattern (Fig. 6-69). Occasionally a subtle fasciculation is noted, but not a storiform pattern. Although the elongated nuclei are relatively uniform in size and needle shape, there is evidence of nuclear atypia, altered chromatin patterns, small nucle-

FIBROSARCOMA PATHOLOGIC FEATURES	
Gross findings	Smooth, nodular, polypoid, fleshy mass
	2–8 cm with firm, homogenous cut surface
	Necrosis and hemorrhage in higher grade tumors
Microscopic findings	Unencapsulated, occasional with bone invasion
	Surface epithelial invagination common
	Spindle cells arranged in short, compact fascicles at acute angles (herringbone pattern)
	Cellularity is variable
	Fusiform cells with centrally placed hyperchromatic, needle-like nuclei with tapering cytoplasm
	Mitotic figures are variable
	Bizarre, pleomorphic cells are usually absent
Immunohistochemical features	Vimentin, and rarely, focal actin positivity
Pathologic differential diagnosis	Fibromatosis, glomangiopericytoma, inflammatory myofibroblastic tumor, solitary fibrous tumor, peripheral nerve sheath tumors, benign and malignant fibrous histiocytoma, synovial sarcoma, melanoma

oli, and usually increased mitotic activity in some part of the tumor (Fig. 6-70). A low mitotic activity combined with mild nuclear atypia contributes to the misdiagnosis of fibrosarcoma as fibromatosis and peripheral nerve sheath tumors. Poorly differentiated fibrosarcoma

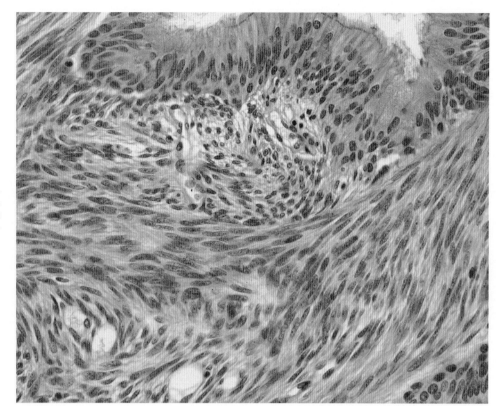

FIGURE 6-68

Sweeping fascicles of minimally pleomorphic spindled cells can occasionally be seen. The overlying surface epithelium is unremarkable, including the presence of cilia.

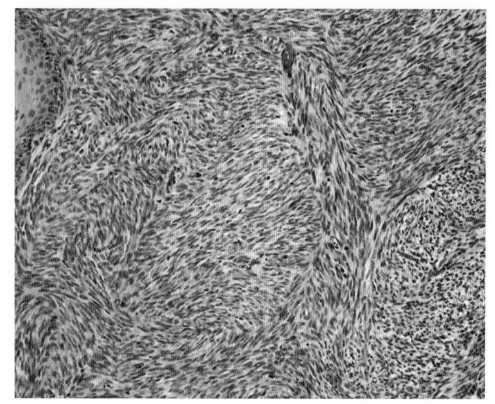

FIGURE 6-69

Short, angular intersections (herringbone or chevron) are most characteristic of a low-grade fibrosarcoma.

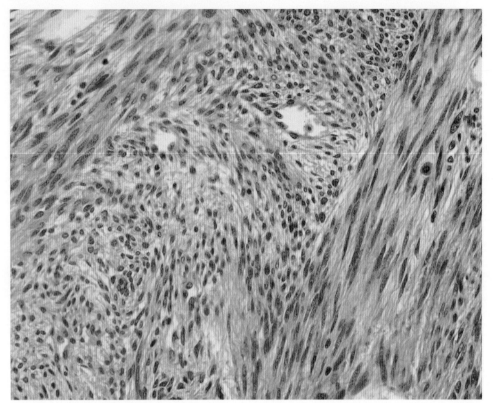

FIGURE 6-70
The tumor cells have uniform elongated nuclei showing mild nuclear atypia. The fibrous matrix is minimal in amount. Mitotic figures are inconspicuous.

is diagnosed when there is nuclear anaplasia, high mitotic activity, scant collagenous stroma, necrosis, and hemorrhage. The majority of sinonasal tract fibrosarcomas, however, are well differentiated.

ANCILLARY STUDIES

Fibrosarcoma by definition must be immunoreactive with vimentin only. Occasionally there is weak, focal actin reaction, but it must not be strong or diffuse.

DIFFERENTIAL DIAGNOSIS

The differential diagnosis includes malignant fibrous histiocytoma (Fig. 6-67), spindle cell squamous cell carcinoma, spindle cell melanoma, malignant peripheral nerve sheath tumor, synovial sarcoma, rhabdomyosarcoma, glomangiopericytoma, inflammatory myofibroblastic tumor, and fibromatosis (desmoid type). Fibromatosis usually affects children, lacks a metastatic potential, lacks infiltration, and is composed of mature fibroblasts that have uniform nuclei and indistinct nucleoli in a background of rich collagenous matrix (Fig. 6-71). Inflammatory myofibroblastic tumor has extensive inflammation and usually lacks the distinct pattern of a fibrosarcoma. Solitary fibrous tumor consists of plump fibroblasts in a mature collagenous stroma, sometimes rich in capillaries, resembling hemangiopericytoma. However, mitotic activity is rare and the strong CD34 reaction confirms the diagnosis. Distinction from other spindle cell sarcomas and melanoma is most effective with the use of immunohistochemical stains. Synovial sarcoma may have epithelial differentiation, but has the characteristic reciprocal translocation t(X;18)(p11.2; q11.2). Malignant peripheral nerve sheath tumors are much higher grade than fibrosarcomas, and express S-100 protein (Fig. 6-72). Rarely they may have rhabdomyoblastic elements, resulting in "Triton" tumors. Although reactive bone formation can occur in the periphery of fibrosarcoma, malignant osteoid or cartilage should not be seen in the substance of fibrosarcoma.

PROGNOSIS AND THERAPY

The majority of sinonasal tract fibrosarcomas are well differentiated and associated with favorable outcome (75% 5-yr survival). However, recurrences are common (up to 60%), probably due to difficulty with obtaining clear surgical margins in the anatomic complexity of the sinonasal tract. Distant metastasis is uncommon (15%), involving the lung and bones most commonly. A poor prognosis is related to large tumor size, high tumor stage (multiple sites involved), a high histologic grade, and positive surgical margins. The best prognosis is achieved with complete resection. Adjuvant radiation has been used with mixed results.

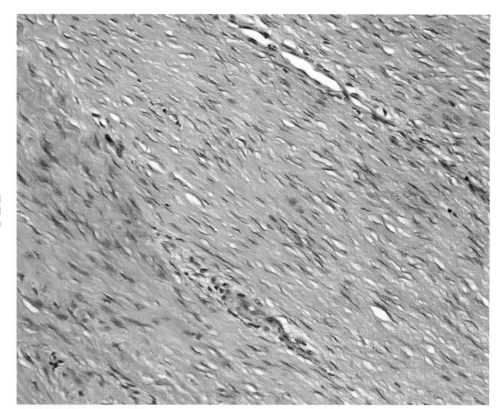

FIGURE 6-71

Heavy keloid-like collagen is deposited between the elongated and bland nuclei. Parallel vessels are noted in this fibromatosis.

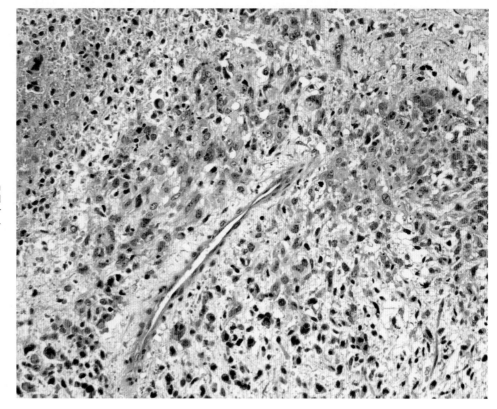

FIGURE 6-72

A malignant peripheral nerve sheath tumor is cellular, has necrosis, and will show epithelioid or fascicular growth. Mitotic activity and pleomorphism are readily identified.

TERATOCARCINOSARCOMA

This rare malignant neoplasm of sinonasal tract consists of various carcinomatous and sarcomatous elements, including immature epithelial, neuroepithelial, and mesenchymal tissues resembling immature teratoma.

CLINICAL FEATURES

Men are affected more commonly than women, with a mean age of 60 years at presentation. Similar to other malignant neoplasms, nasal obstruction, and epistaxis are the most common complaints, usually of a short duration. The tumor occurs most commonly high in the nasal cavity, ethmoid sinus, and maxillary sinus (Fig. 6-73).

TERATOCARCINOSARCOMA
DISEASE FACT SHEET

Definition	A complex malignant neoplasm with immature and malignant endodermal, mesodermal, and neuroepithelial elements
Incidence and location	Extremely rare Ethmoid and maxillary antrum
Morbidity and mortality	60% of patients die within 3 yr
Gender, race, and age distribution	Male >> Female Mean, 60 yr (adults)
Clinical features	Nasal obstruction and epistaxis of short duration
Prognosis and treatment	Poor prognosis with highly aggressive behavior Overall, 60% die within 3 yr Recurrences are common, with intracranial extension, usually in <3 yr Multimodality therapy does not seem to alter prognosis

PATHOLOGIC FEATURES

GROSS FINDINGS

Large, bulky, polypoid friable mass generally >4 cm or more with necrosis.

MICROSCOPIC FINDINGS

Teratocarcinosarcoma contains both carcinomatous and sarcomatous tissues, along with teratoma-like elements (Fig. 6-74). Elements from all three germ cell layers may be present, but the components are both benign and malignant. The carcinoma may be squamous or adenocarcinoma. The stromal elements include

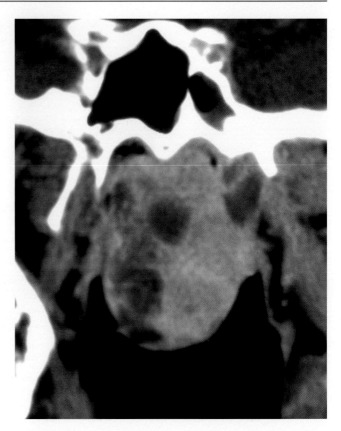

FIGURE 6-73
A CT scan demonstrating a complex mass in the nasal cavity with extension into the maxillary sinus.

TERATOCARCINOSARCOMA
PATHOLOGIC FEATURES

Gross findings	Large, bulky, polypoid friable masses
Microscopic findings	Carcinomatous and sarcomatous component mingled with multiple mature and immature tissues from all germ cell layers Carcinoma can be squamous or adenocarcinoma Neural elements show prominent rosettes and blastema-like cells Cartilage, bone, or muscle may form sarcoma
Immunohistochemical features	Neuroepithelial elements positive for neuron-specific enolase, chromogranin, synaptophysin, and MIC2 Spindle cell component positive with vimentin, GFAP, desmin, and/or actins Epithelial elements positive for cytokeratins and EMA
Pathologic differential diagnosis	Olfactory neuroblastoma, carcinomas, adenocarcinoma, rhabdomyosarcoma

hypercellular immature tissue with spindle cells embedded in a myxoid matrix, islands of cartilage and bone (Fig. 6-75), smooth muscle, and skeletal muscle in varying degrees of maturation (Fig. 6-76). Primitive neuroepithelial elements with rosettes, pseudorosettes,

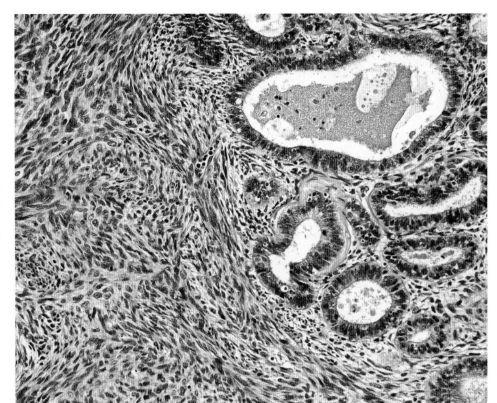

FIGURE 6-74

The adenocarcinoma is intimately associated with the sarcomatous portion, arranged in a "teratoma-like" distribution. Cytologic atypia is present in both constituents of the neoplasm.

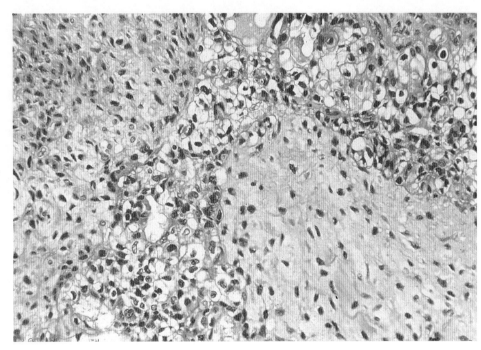

FIGURE 6-75

Immature cartilage and spindle cells in a teratocarcinosarcoma. (Courtesy of Yao S. Fu, MD, Senior Pathologist, Providence St. Joseph Medical Center, Burbank, CA.)

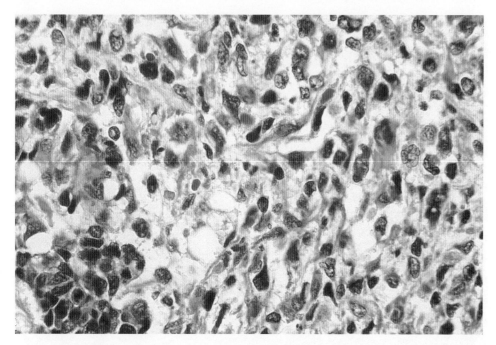

FIGURE 6-76
Rhabdomyoblasts have elongated nuclei and eosinophilic cytoplasm. (Courtesy of Yao S. Fu, MD, Senior Pathologist, Providence St. Joseph Medical Center, Burbank, CA.)

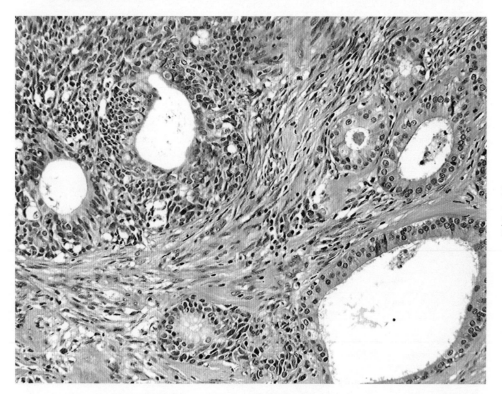

FIGURE 6-77
A primitive blastema-like component is immediately adjacent to a malignant glandular element that is juxtaposed with a malignant, cellular spindle cell constituent.

or neurofibrillary matrix often predominate in these tumors (Figs. 6-77, 6-78).

ANCILLARY STUDIES

Immunohistochemistry will highlight the various constituent elements accordingly: neuroepithelial elements are usually positive with NSE, chromogranin, synapto-

physin, and CD99 (MIC2); spindle cell elements are vimentin, GFAP, desmin, and/or actins; epithelial elements are positive for cytokeratins and EMA.

DIFFERENTIAL DIAGNOSIS

Depending on the cellular elements present in the biopsy, considerations includes olfactory neuroblas-

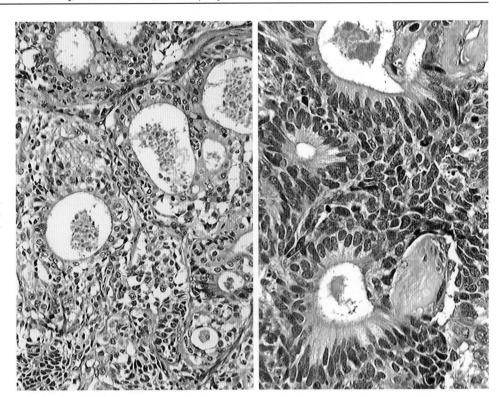

FIGURE 6-78

Left: An adenocarcinoma with primitive blastema-like cells. *Right:* The primitive cells can sometimes be arranged in a true rosette, similar to teratoma.

toma, rhabdomyosarcoma, and carcinoma. The presence of all three elements usually confirms the diagnosis.

PROGNOSIS AND THERAPY

This is a highly aggressive neoplasm with a poor prognosis. Most patients (60%) die within 3 years. Recurrences are common, often with intracranial extension, developing within 3 years of diagnosis. Lymph node metastasis occurs in about one-third of patients. Multimodality therapy does not seem to alter the prognosis.

SUGGESTED READING

Squamous Cell Carcinoma

1. Fu YS, Perzin KH: Chapter 6. Pathology of the nasal cavity, paranasal sinuses, and nasopharynx. In: Head and Neck Pathology with Clinical Correlations. Fu YS, Wenig BM, Abemayor E, and Wenig BL, eds. New York: Churchill Livingstone, 2001:137–230.
2. Hopkin N, McNicoll W, Dalley VM, Shaw HJ: Cancer of the paranasal sinuses and nasal cavities. Part I. Clinical features. J Laryngol Otol 1984;98:585–595.
3. Ishiyama A, Eversole LR, Ross DA, et al.: Papillary squamous neoplasms of the head and neck. Laryngoscope 1994;104:1446–1452.
4. Jackson RT, Fitz-Hugh GS, Constable WC: Malignant neoplasms of the nasal cavities and paranasal sinuses. Laryngoscope 1977;87:726–736.
5. Osborn DA: Nature and behavior of transitional tumors in the upper respiratory tract. Cancer 1970;25:50–60.
6. Pilch BZ, Bouquot J, Thompson LDR. Squamous cell carcinoma. In: Barnes EL, Eveson JW, Reichart P, Sidransky D, eds. Pathology and Genetics of Head and Neck Tumours. Kleihues P, Sobin LH, series eds. World Health Organization Classification of Tumours. Lyon, France: IARC Press, 2005:15–17.

Sinonasal Tract Adenocarcinoma

1. Alessi DM, Trapp TK, Fu YS, Calcaterra TC: Nonsalivary sinonasal adenocarcinoma. Arch Otolaryngol Head Neck Surg 1988;114:996–999.
2. Barnes L: Intestinal-type adenocarcinoma of the nasal cavity and paranasal sinuses. Am J Surg Pathol 1986;10:192–202.
3. Eveson JW. Salivary gland-type carcinomas. In: Barnes EL, Eveson JW, Reichart P, Sidransky D, eds. Pathology and Genetics of Head and Neck Tumours. Kleihues P, Sobin LH, series eds. World Health Organization Classification of Tumours. Lyon, France: IARC Press, 2005:24–25.
4. Franchi A, Gallo O, Santucci M: Clinical relevance of the histological classification of sinonasal intestinal-type adenocarcinoma. Hum Pathol 1999;30:1140–1145.
5. Franchi A, Santucci M, Wenig BM. Adenocarcinoma. In: Barnes EL, Eveson JW, Reichart P, Sidransky D, eds. Pathology and Genetics of Head and Neck Tumours. Kleihues P, Sobin LH, series eds. World Health Organization Classification of Tumours. Lyon, France: IARC Press, 2005:20–23.
6. Franquemont DW, Fechner RE, Mills SE: Histologic classification of sinonasal intestinal-type adenocarcinoma. Am J Surg Pathol 1991;15:368–375.
7. Heffner DK, Hyams VJ, Hauck KW, Lingeman C: Low-grade adenocarcinoma of the nasal cavity and paranasal sinuses. Cancer 1982;50:312–322.
8. Kleinsasser O, Schroeder HG: Adenocarcinoma of the inner nose after exposure to wood dust. Morphological findings and relationship between histopathology and clinical behavior in 79 cases. Arch Otorhinolaryngol 1988;245:1–15.
9. Wenig BM, Hyams VJ, Heffner DK: Nasopharyngeal papillary adenocarcinoma. A clinicopathologic study of a low-grade carcinoma. Am J Surg Pathol 1988;12:946–953.

Sinonasal Undifferentiated Carcinoma

1. Cerilli LA, Holst VA, Brandwein MS, et al.: Sinonasal undifferentiated carcinoma. Immunohistochemical profile and lack of EV association. Am J Surg Pathol 2001;25:156–163.
2. Franchi A, Moroni M, Massi D, et al.: Sinonasal undifferentiated carcinoma, nasopharyngeal-type undifferentiated carcinoma, and keratinizing and nonkeratinizing squamous cell carcinoma express

different cytokeratin patterns. Am J Surg Pathol 2002;26:1597–1604.

3. Frierson HF Jr, Mills SE, Fechner RE, et al.: Sinonasal undifferentiated carcinoma. An aggressive neoplasm derived from schneiderian epithelium and distinct from olfactory neuroblastoma. Am J Surg Pathol 1986;10:771–779.

4. Frierson HF Jr, Ross GW, Stewart FM, et al.: Unusual sinonasal small-cell neoplasms following radiotherapy for bilateral retinoblastomas. Am J Surg Pathol 1989;13:947–954.

5. Frierson HF Jr. Sinonasal undifferentiated carcinoma. In: Barnes EL, Eveson JW, Reichart P, Sidransky D, eds. Pathology and Genetics of Head and Neck Tumours. Kleihues P, Sobin LH, series eds. World Health Organization Classification of Tumours. Lyon, France: IARC Press, 2005:19.

6. Georgiou AF, Walker DM, Collins AP, et al.: Primary small cell undifferentiated (neuroendocrine) carcinoma of the maxillary sinus. Oral Surg Oral Med Oral Pathol Oral Radiol Endod 2004;98:572–578.

7. Helliwell TR, Yeoch LH, Stell PM: Anaplastic carcinoma of the nose and paranasal sinuses. Light microscopy, immunohistochemistry and clinical correlation. Cancer 1986;58:2038–2045.

8. Jeng YM, Sung MT, Fang DL, et al.: Sinonasal undifferentiated carcinoma and nasopharyngeal-type undifferentiated carcinoma. Two clinically, biologically, and histopathologically distinct entities. Am J Surg Pathol 2002;26:371–376.

9. Miyamoto RC, Gleich LL, Biddinger PW, Gluckman JL: Esthesioneuroblastoma and sinonasal undifferentiated carcinoma: Impact of histological grading and clinical staging on survival and prognosis. Laryngoscope 2000;110:1262–1265.

10. Smith SR, Som P, Fahmy A, et al.: A clinicopathological study of sinonasal neuroendocrine carcinoma and sinonasal undifferentiated carcinoma. Laryngoscope 2000;110:1617–1622.

Nasopharyngeal Carcinoma

1. Chan JKC, Bray F, McCarron P, et al: Nasopharyngeal carcinoma. In: Barnes EL, Eveson JW, Reichart P, Sidransky D, eds. Pathology and Genetics of Head and Neck Tumours. Kleihues P, Sobin LH, series eds. World Health Organization Classification of Tumours. Lyon, France: IARC Press, 2005:85–97.

2. Hawkins EP, Krischer JP, Smith BE, et al.: Nasopharyngeal carcinoma in children—a retrospective review and demonstration of Epstein-Barr viral genomes in tumor cell cytoplasm: a report of the pediatric oncology group. Hum Pathol 1990;21:805–810.

3. Hsu HC, Chen CL, Hsu MM, et al.: Pathology of nasopharyngeal carcinoma. Proposal of a new histologic classification correlated with prognosis. Cancer 1987;59:945–951.

4. Hsu MM, Tu SM: Nasopharyngeal carcinoma in Taiwan. Clinical manifestations and results of therapy. Cancer 1983;52:362–368.

5. Sham JST, Poon YF, Wei WI, Choi D: Nasopharyngeal carcinoma in young patients. Cancer 1990;65:2606–2610.

6. Kamino H, Huang SJ, Fu YS: Keratin and involucrin immunohistochemistry of nasopharyngeal carcinoma. Cancer 1988;61:1142–1148.

7. Shamugaratnam K, Sobin LH: Histological typing of upper respiratory tract tumor. International Histological Classification of Tumors, 2nd ed. Geneva, Switzerland: World Health Organization, 1991.

Malignant Melanoma

1. Billings KR, Wang MB, Sercarz JA, Fu YS: Clinical and pathologic distinction between primary and metastatic mucosal melanoma of the head and neck. Arch Otolaryngol Head Neck Surg 1995;112:700–706.

2. Franquemont DW, Mills SE: Sinonasal malignant melanoma. A clinicopathologic and immunohistochemical study of 14 cases. Am J Clin Pathol 1991;96:689–697.

3. Thompson LDR, Wieneke JA, Miettinen M: Sinonasal tract melanomas: a clinicopathologic study of 115 cases with a proposed staging system. Am J Surg Pathol 2003;27:594–611.

4. Wenig BM, Dulguerov P, Kapadia SB, Prasad ML, Fanburg-Smith JC, Thompson LDR. Neuroectodermal tumours. In: Barnes EL, Eveson JW, Reichart P, Sidransky D, eds. Pathology and Genetics of Head and Neck Tumours. Kleihues P, Sobin LH, series eds. World Health Organization Classification of Tumours. Lyon, France: IARC Press, 2005:65–75.

Olfactory Neuroblastoma

1. Argani P, Perez-Ordonez B, Xiao H, et al.: Olfactory neuroblastoma is not related to the Ewing family of tumors. Absence of EWS/FLI1 gene fusion and MIC2 expression. Am J Surg Pathol 1998;22:391–398.

2. Miller DC, Goodman ML, Pilch BZ, et al.: Mixed olfactory neuroblastoma and carcinoma. A report of two cases. Cancer 1984;54:2019–2028.

3. Mills SE, Frierson HF Jr.: Olfactory neuroblastoma. A clinicopathologic study of 21 cases. Am J Surg Pathol 1985;9:317–327.

4. Ordonez NG, Mackay B: Neuroendocrine tumors of the nasal cavity. Pathol Ann 1993;28(2):77–111.

5. Wenig BM, Dulguerov P, Kapadia SB, Prasad ML, Fanburg-Smith JC, Thompson LDR. Neuroectodermal tumours. In: Barnes EL, Eveson JW, Reichart P, Sidransky D, eds. Pathology and Genetics of Head and Neck Tumours. Kleihues P, Sobin LH, series eds. World Health Organization Classification of Tumours. Lyon, France: IARC Press, 2005:65–75.

Extranodal NK/T Cell Lymphoma, Sinonasal Type

1. Abbondanzo SL, Wenig BM: Non-Hodgkin's lymphoma of the sinonasal tract. A clinicopathologic and immunophenotypic study of 120 cases. Cancer 1995;75:1281–1291.

2. Chan ACL, Chan JKC, Cheung MMC, Kapadia SB. Haematolymphoid tumours. In: Barnes EL, Eveson JW, Reichart P, Sidransky D, eds. Pathology and Genetics of Head and Neck Tumours. Kleihues P, Sobin LH, series eds. World Health Organization Classification of Tumours. Lyon, France: IARC Press, 2005:58–64.

3. Cuadra-Garcia I, Proulx GM, Wu CL, et al.: Sinonasal lymphoma. A clinicopathologic analysis of 58 cases from the Massachusetts General Hospital. Am J Surg Pathol 1999;23:1356–1369.

4. Gaal K, Sun NCJ, Hernandez AM, Arber DA: Sinonasal NK/T-cell lymphoma in the United States. Am J Surg Pathol 2000;24:1511–1517.

5. Jaffe ES, Chan JKC, Su IJ, et al.: Report of the workshop on nasal and related extranodal angiocentric T/NK-cell lymphomas: definition, differential diagnosis and epidemiology. Am J Surg Pathol 1996;20:103–111.

6. Strickler JG, Meneses MF, Habermann TM, et al.: Polymorphic reticulosis: a reappraisal. Hum Pathol 1994;25:659–665.

7. van Gorp J, Weiping L, Jacobse K, et al.: Epstein-Barr virus in nasal T-cell lymphomas (polymorphic reticulosis/midline malignant reticulosis) in western China. J Pathol 1994;173:81–87.

8. Wilson WH, Kingma DW, Raffeld M, Wittes RE, Jaffe ES: Association of lymphomatoid granulomatosis with Epstein-Barr viral infection of B lymphocytes and response to interferon-alpha2b. Blood 1996;87:4531–4537.

Rhabdomyosarcoma

1. Callender TA, Weber RS, Janjan N, et al.: Rhabdomyosarcoma of the nose and paranasal sinuses in adults and children. Arch Otolaryngol Head Neck Surg 1995;112:252–257.

2. Cavazzana AO, Schmidt D, Ninfo V, et al.: Spindle cell rhabdomyosarcoma. A prognostically favorable variant of rhabdomyosarcoma. Am J Surg Pathol 1992;16:229–235.

3. Fu YS, Perzin KH: Non-epithelial tumors of the nasal cavity, paranasal sinuses and nasopharynx: A clinicopathologic study. V. Skeletal muscle tumors (rhabdomyoma and rhabdomyosarcoma). Cancer 1976;37:364–376.

4. Kapadia SB, Popek EJ, Barnes L: Pediatric otorhinolaryngic pathology: diagnosis of selected lesions. Pathology Annual 1994;29(Pt 1):159–209.

5. Thompson LDR, Fanburg-Smith JC. Malignant soft tissue tumours. In: Barnes EL, Eveson JW, Reichart P, Sidransky D, eds. Pathology and Genetics of Head and Neck Tumours. Kleihues P, Sobin LH, series eds. World Health Organization Classification of Tumours. Lyon, France: IARC Press, 2005:35–42.

Ewing Sarcoma

1. Csokonai LV, Liktor B, Arato G, Helffrich F: Ewing's sarcoma in the nasal cavity. Otolaryngol Head Neck Surg 2001;125:665–667.

2. Dehner LP. Primitive neuroectodermal tumor and Ewing's sarcoma. Am J Surg Pathol 1993;17:1–13.

3. Toda T, Atari E, Sadi AM, et al.: Primitive neuroectodermal tumor in sinonasal region. Auris Nasus Larynx 1999;26:83–90.
4. Wenig BM, Dulguerov P, Kapadia SB, Prasad ML, Fanburg-Smith JC, Thompson LDR. Neuroectodermal tumours. In: Barnes EL, Eveson JW, Reichart P, Sidransky D, eds. Pathology and Genetics of Head and Neck Tumours. Kleihues P, Sobin LH, series eds. World Health Organization Classification of Tumours. Lyon, France: IARC Press, 2005:65–75.

Fibrosarcoma

1. Fu YS, Perzin KH: Non-epithelial tumors of the nasal cavity, paranasal sinuses and nasopharynx: a clinicopathologic study. VI. Fibrous tissue tumors. Cancer 1976;37:2912–2928.
2. Gnepp DR, Henley J, Weiss S, Heffner D: Desmoid fibromatosis of the sinonasal tract and nasopharynx. A clinicopathologic study of 25 cases. Cancer 1996;78:2572–2579.
3. Heffner DK, Gnepp DR: Sinonasal fibrosarcomas, malignant schwannomas, and "Triton" tumors. A clinicopathologic study of 67 cases. Cancer 1992;70:1089–1101.
4. Thompson LDR, Fanburg-Smith JC. Malignant soft tissue tumours. In: Barnes EL, Eveson JW, Reichart P, Sidransky D, eds. Pathology and Genetics of Head and Neck Tumours. Kleihues P, Sobin LH, series eds.

World Health Organization Classification of Tumours. Lyon, France: IARC Press, 2005:35–42.
5. Zukerberg LR, Rosenberg AE, Randolph G, et al.: Solitary fibrous tumor of the nasal cavity and paranasal sinuses. Am J Surg Pathol 1991;15: 126–130.

Teratocarcinosarcoma

1. Cardesa A, Luna MA. Germ cell tumours. In: Barnes EL, Eveson JW, Reichart P, Sidransky D, eds. Pathology and Genetics of Head and Neck Tumours. Kleihues P, Sobin LH, series eds. World Health Organization Classification of Tumours. Lyon, France: IARC Press, 2005:76–79.
2. Heffner DK, Hyams VJ. Teratocarcinosarcoma (malignant teratoma?) of the nasal cavity and paranasal sinuses. A clinicopathologic study of 20 cases. Cancer 1984;53:2140–2154.
3. Pai SA, Naresh KN, Masih K, et al.: Teratocarcinosarcoma of the paranasal sinuses: a clinicopathologic and immunohistochemical study. Hum Pathol 1998;29:718–722.
4. Shimazaki H, Aida S, Tamai S: Sinonasal teratocarcinosarcoma: ultrastructural and immunohistochemical evidence of neuroectodermal origin. Ultrast Pathol 2000;24:115–122.

7 Non-Neoplastic Lesions of the Oral Cavity and Oropharynx

Susan Müller

FORDYCE GRANULES

CLINICAL FEATURES

Fordyce granules are considered benign ectopic sebaceous glands (not associated with hair follicles) that occur on the oral mucosa. A normal variant, they are reported in up to 80% of adults, most common on the upper and lower lip and the buccal mucosa. They present as multiple, uniform-sized yellow or yellow-white papules (Fig. 7-1), which may coalesce to form plaques. Usually asymptomatic, patients sometimes describe surface roughness.

PATHOLOGIC FEATURES

Biopsy reveals normal sebaceous glands near the surface epithelium without hair follicles (Fig. 7-2). A central duct sometimes connects the sebaceous lobules to the epithelial surface. The sebaceous cells are polygonal in shape with abundant foamy cytoplasm and a centrally placed nucleus.

FORDYCE GRANULES DISEASE FACT SHEET	
Definition	Benign ectopic sebaceous glands, considered to be a normal variant
Incidence and location	Reported in up to 80% of adults
	Present on the upper and lower lip and the buccal mucosa
Gender, race, and age distribution	Genders equally affected
	Less clinically evident in children and adolescents
Clinical features	Asymptomatic, multiple, small yellow papules
Prognosis and treatment	Considered a normal variant

FORDYCE GRANULES PATHOLOGIC FEATURES	
Microscopic findings	Normal sebaceous glands below the surface devoid of hair follicles

DIFFERENTIAL DIAGNOSIS

Superficial mucoceles, which can present as 1–3 mm papules on the lower lip, generally are blue to clear in color and spontaneously resolve.

PROGNOSIS AND THERAPY

No treatment is indicated, although laser ablation can be offered to patients for cosmesis.

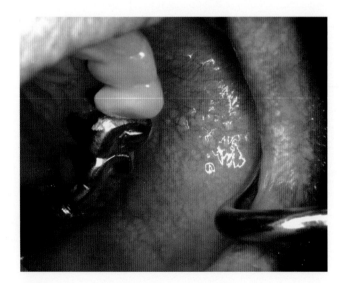

FIGURE 7-1
Clinical. Asymptomatic, multiple, small yellow papules on the buccal mucosa.

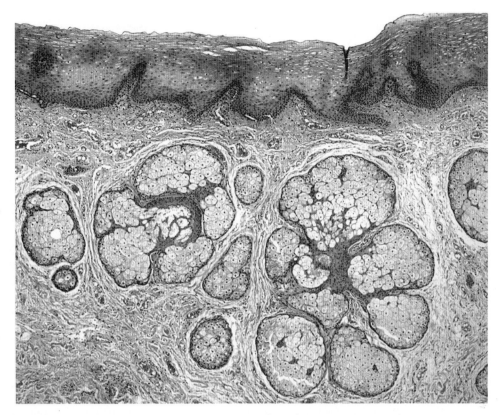

FIGURE 7-2
Multiple sebaceous glands in the superficial lamina propria.

AMALGAM TATTOO

CLINICAL FEATURES

Amalgam tattoo is a common localized area of blue, gray, or black pigmentation caused by amalgam that has been embedded into the oral tissues during dental procedures. Amalgam is a common material used for dental fillings and contains silver, tin, mercury, and other metals. Amalgam tattoos are most commonly located on the buccal mucosa and gingiva (Fig. 7-3), usually presenting as flat macules, anywhere from a few millimeters to larger, more diffuse areas of pigmentation.

AMALGAM TATTOO DISEASE FACT SHEET	
Definition	Localized pigmentation caused by amalgam which has been embedded in the oral tissues due to dental procedures
Incidence and location	Common
	Most common on the buccal mucosa and gingiva
Clinical features	Asymptomatic flat macules ranging from a few mm to more diffuse areas of blue, gray, or black pigmentation
Prognosis and treatment	No treatment necessary unless for cosmetic reasons

RADIOLOGIC FEATURES

Generally, amalgam tattoos are not visible on dental radiographs. Larger tattoos may be visible on radiographs and are densely radiopaque.

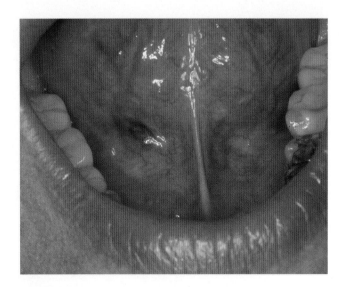

FIGURE 7-3
Clinical photograph of a blue-gray pigment present in the floor of mouth. The pigmented area is flat with no ulceration or induration and asymptomatic.

PATHOLOGIC FEATURES

An amalgam tattoo can demonstrate both discrete, fine black granules and scattered, irregular solid fragments (Fig. 7-4). Pigment granules are often arranged along collagen fibers, and around blood vessels and nerves. Most cases elicit no tissue reaction, although a foreign body giant cell reaction may be present.

DIFFERENTIAL DIAGNOSIS

Other exogenous pigmentations can mimic an amalgam tattoo. Melanin may also be present in pigmented nevi, oral melanotic macule, oral melanoacanthoma, and melanoma. Further investigation is suggested if amalgam tattoos occur in sites distant from dental work.

AMALGAM TATTOO PATHOLOGIC FEATURES	
Microscopic findings	Discrete, black granules, and/or solid fragments of pigment arranged along collagen fibers, around blood vessels and nerves
	Occasional foreign body reaction
Pathologic differential diagnosis	Other exogenous sources of pigmentation including pencil graphite, intentional tattoos, and coal dust

PROGNOSIS AND THERAPY

No treatment is generally required, unless for cosmetic reasons (surgery or laser treatment).

ECTOPIC THYROID

CLINICAL FEATURES

Ectopic thyroid is a result of the abnormal migration of the thyroglossal duct from the foramen cecum located at the junction of the anterior two-thirds and posterior one-third of the tongue to its normal prelarnygeal location. While uncommon, nearly 90 % of all ectopic thyroids are located on the tongue. In about 70 % of patients with lingual thyroid, this is the only functioning thyroid tissue. Females are affected 3–4 times as frequently as males. Symptoms, including dysphagia, dyspnea, globus sensation, and dysphonia, most often coincide with puberty onset, pregnancy, or menopause corresponding to elevated thyroid-stimulating hormone (TSH). Thyroid function tests should be evaluated as part of the workup. The endoscopic appearance at the base of the tongue is of a hyperemic mass (Fig. 7-5).

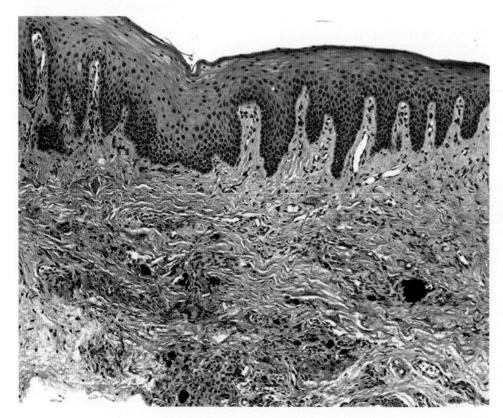

FIGURE 7-4

Black pigmented material is seen scattered in the lamina propria along collagen bundles and around blood vessels. The overlying epithelium is normal and scant inflammatory cells are present.

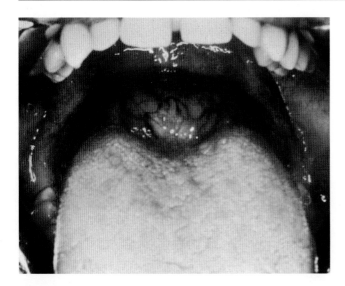

FIGURE 7-5
Clinical photograph of a lingual thyroid presenting as a midline nodular mass at the base of tongue. The surface is smooth and hyperemic.

RADIOLOGIC FEATURES

The iodine content of the thyroid tissue results in very high signal attenuation in relation to surrounding soft tissue using computed tomography.

PATHOLOGIC FEATURES

Immediately below the intact surface mucosa, ectopic thyroid follicles containing colloid and lined by cuboidal epithelium are identified insinuating between the tongue musculature (Fig. 7-6). Lymphocytic thyroiditis and adenomatoid nodules, as well as papillary carcinoma, have been reported.

ECTOPIC THYROID DISEASE FACT SHEET	
Definition	Rare developmental anomaly due to the abnormal migration of the thyroid gland from the base of the tongue
Incidence and location	Uncommon, with reported incidence of 1/100,000
	90% of ectopic thyroids are lingual thyroids
Morbidity and mortality	Larger lesions can cause airway obstruction
	Rare reports of carcinoma development
Gender, race, and age distribution	Female >> Male (3–4 : 1)
	All ages
Clinical features	Dysphagia, dyspnea, dysphonia, globus sensation
	One-third of patients are hypothyroid
	In 70%, ectopic tissue is only functional thyroid tissue
Prognosis and treatment	Suppression therapy with thyroxin to reduces size and symptoms
	Radioactive ^{131}I ablation
	Autotransplantation of lingual thyroid

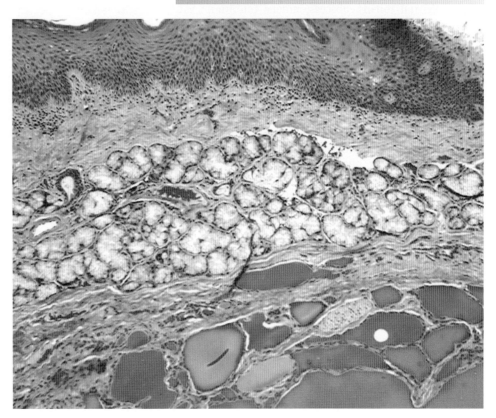

FIGURE 7-6
Normal stratified squamous epithelium overlying nonencapsulated collection of thyroid follicles.

ECTOPIC THYROID PATHOLOGIC FEATURES	
Microscopic findings	Nonencapsulated normal thyroid tissue insinuated through skeletal muscle
	Lymphocytic thyroiditis and adenomatoid nodules may develop
Pathologic differential diagnosis	Metastatic thyroid carcinoma

ANCILLARY STUDIES

RADIOISOTOPE STUDY

Radioisotopic studies (^{131}I and/or technetium-99m pertechnetate) may be needed to determine size, location, and activity of thyroid tissue.

FINE NEEDLE ASPIRATION

Fine needle aspiration biopsy can be utilized to confirm the diagnosis of ectopic thyroid or to rule out neoplastic changes.

DIFFERENTIAL DIAGNOSIS

There are a number of clinical differential diagnostic considerations (hemangioma, lymphangioma, hypertrophic lingual tonsils, abscess, mucus retention cyst, squamous cell carcinoma), but the histologic features of ectopic thyroid are pathognomonic.

PROGNOSIS AND THERAPY

Thyroxin suppresses TSH with a subsequent reduction in size. Surgery is employed if there is uncontrollable hemorrhage, airway obstruction, or inability to eat. Radioablation may be used in nonsurgical candidates. If no "normal" thyroid is identified in the anterior neck, autotransplantation can be performed. Malignancy is a rare complication (<1%), although more common in men.

ORAL LYMPHOEPITHELIAL CYSTS

CLINICAL FEATURES

Oral lymphoepithelial cysts develop within oral lymphoid tissue, usually along the posterior lateral border

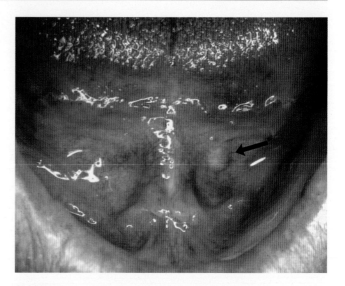

FIGURE 7-7
Clinical photograph showing a small round, yellow, soft mass in the left floor of mouth (*arrow*). The lesion was freely moveable and painless.

ORAL LYMPHOEPITHELIAL CYSTS DISEASE FACT SHEET	
Definition	Benign developmental keratin filled cyst surrounded by mature lymphoid tissue with germinal centers
Incidence and location	Unknown, but common incidental finding
	Usually located in the floor of mouth, ventral or posterolateral tongue
Gender, race, and age distribution	Equal gender distribution
	Usually in young adults
Clinical features	Asymptomatic, yellow or tan submucosal nodules <1 cm
Prognosis and treatment	Conservative excision if symptomatic or the diagnosis is uncertain

of the tongue or the anterior floor of mouth. Surface invaginations (crypts) may fill with keratin debris. If the crypt becomes obstructed or pinched off from the surface epithelium, a cyst within lymphoid tissue can develop. The cysts are generally asymptomatic, yellow or tan, submucosal masses measuring less than 1 cm (Fig. 7-7). The cyst is filled with cheesy keratinaceous material, and patients may complain of swelling or drainage. Oral lymphoepithelial cysts can occur at any age, but are most common in young adults.

PATHOLOGIC FEATURES

The cystic cavity is lined by parakeratinized stratified squamous epithelium, rarely containing mucus cells. The cyst lumen contains desquamated epithelial cells and keratin debris. The cyst wall contains reactive lymphoid tissue (Fig. 7-8).

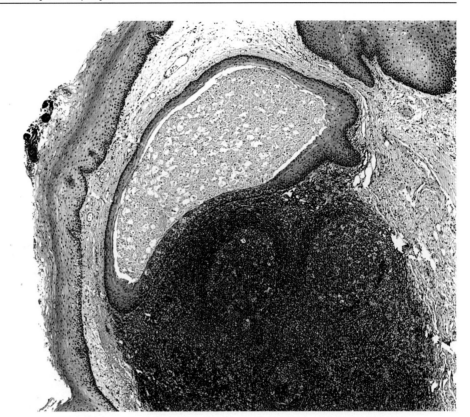

FIGURE 7-8
A keratin-filled cyst lined by parakeratotic, stratified squamous epithelium. The cyst wall has mature lymphoid tissue with germinal centers.

ORAL LYMPHOEPITHELIAL CYSTS PATHOLOGIC FEATURES	
Microscopic findings	Keratin filled cyst lined by a parakeratotic stratified squamous epithelium
	Cyst wall contains lymphoid tissue with germinal centers
Differential diagnosis	Benign lymphoid hyperplasia, bronchial cysts of the midline

DIFFERENTIAL DIAGNOSIS

The differential diagnosis is clinical, and includes lipoma, mucocele, granular cell tumor, and benign hyperplastic lymphoid tissue. Bronchial cysts may occur in the midline.

PROGNOSIS AND THERAPY

Most lesions are clinically obvious, but management, if necessary, is conservative surgical excision. The lesion seldom recurs after excision.

ORAL HAIRY LEUKOPLAKIA

CLINICAL FEATURES

Oral hairy leukoplakia (HL) is a benign epithelial disease associated with Epstein-Barr virus (EBV) and nearly always identified in immunocompromised

ORAL HAIRY LEUKOPLAKIA DISEASE FACT SHEET	
Definition	Benign, asymptomatic epithelial hyperplasia associated with Epstein-Barr virus nearly always in immunocompromised patients
Incidence and location	<10% of HIV-infected patients on HAART
	Primarily occurs on the lateral tongue
Gender, race, and age distribution	Increased particularly in HIV+ men
	No racial or age predilection
Clinical features	White patches that can have a corrugated or folded surface which cannot be rubbed off
	May be quite extensive
Prognosis and treatment	10% improve spontaneously
	No specific treatment, although secondary candida may need to be treated

patients. HL usually presents on the lateral border of the tongue as a white plaque, or vertical streaks, or with a corrugated surface (Fig. 7-9). The lesions can become quite extensive, and in some cases cover the entire lateral and dorsal tongue. The lesion is asymptomatic and cannot be rubbed off.

PATHOLOGIC FEATURES

HL is characterized by marked epithelial acanthosis with elongation of the rete ridges and prominent hyperkeratosis. In the superficial spinous layer, "balloon cells," characterized by intracellular ballooning degeneration, nuclear clearing and margination of the chromatin indicative of a viral cytopathic effect, are present (Fig. 7-10). These nonspecific findings require documentation of EBV within the lesion.

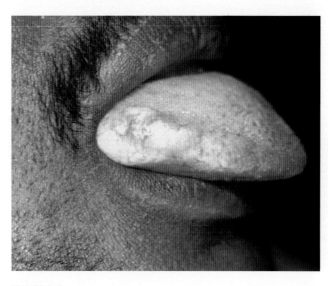

FIGURE 7-9

HIV+ patient with a white patch on the lateral border of the tongue exhibiting a corrugated appearance.

ORAL HAIRY LEUKOPLAKIA PATHOLOGIC FEATURES	
Microscopic findings	Epithelial hyperplasia, hyperparakeratosis, and acanthosis
	Balloon cells in the upper spinous layer
	Viral cytopathic effect can sometimes be seen
	Secondary candidal infection may be identified
Immunohistochemical features	Markers for Epstein-Barr virus antigens
Pathologic differential diagnosis	Frictional keratosis, candidiasis, leukoplakia

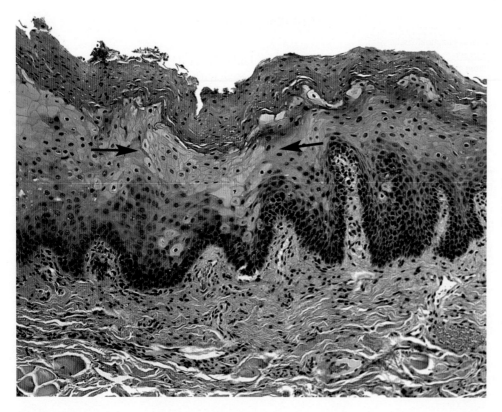

FIGURE 7-10

A corrugated hyperparakerotic epithelium and a layer of balloon cells in the upper spinous layer (*arrows*).

ANCILLARY STUDIES

IMMUNOHISTOCHEMICAL FEATURES

Immunomarkers for EBV latent antigens (EBNA, LMP), replicative antigens (EA, VCA), or regulatory antigens (BLZF1) can be performed on both touch preps and biopsy specimens. Depending on the immunostain used, latent versus replicative EBV infection can be determined.

MOLECULAR STUDIES

Quantitative polymerase chain reaction (PCR) and in situ hybridization assays can be useful when immunohistochemical studies fail to detect EBV, and especially when investigating EBV latent genes.

DIFFERENTIAL DIAGNOSIS

Clinically, HL can mimic frictional keratosis (tongue biting), oral leukoplakia, lichen planus, and lichenoid reactions. Oral candidiasis can be ruled out since HL cannot be rubbed off while candidiasis can. However, HL is frequently colonized by *Candida* species.

PROGNOSIS AND THERAPY

HL does not have any malignant potential. It reportedly improves spontaneously in 10 % of cases. The incidence in HIV-infected patients has decreased to <10 % with highly active anti-retroviral therapy (HAART). Treatment for concurrent candida may be necessary if "burning" is described by the patient.

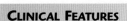

INFECTIONS

CLINICAL FEATURES

There are numerous infectious conditions that can involve the oral cavity including bacterial, fungal, viral, and protozoal infections. These infections can present as an acute, rapidly progressing infection with constitutional symptoms such as herpetic gingivostomatitis. Other infections can be chronic and slowly spreading, such as actinomycosis and leprosy. Sexually transmitted diseases, including syphilis and gonorrhea, can have oral manifestations. Deep fungal infections, including blastomycosis, coccidiomycosis, and histoplasmosis, can present as a nonspecific ulcer in the oral cavity. Since many infectious processes share clinical overlap, biopsy

and/or culture are necessary to obtain a diagnosis. Three of the more common oral infections are candidiasis, herpes simplex virus type I (HSV1), and actinomycosis.

The most common fungal infection in the oral cavity and oropharynx is candidiasis. *Candida albicans* is the most common type, but other species have been isolated.

INFECTIONS DISEASE FACT SHEET	
Definition	**Candidiasis:** The most common oral fungal infection manifested by a variety of clinical presentations and influenced by host immune status
	HSV1: A DNA virus transmitted via saliva or direct contact, with potential reactivation of latent disease
	Actinomycosis: Acute or chronic infection by a normal saprophytic oral flora gram-positive anaerobic bacteria
Incidence	**Candidiasis:** *Candida* species detected in up to 55% of healthy individuals
	HSV1: Up to 90% of adults have antibodies to HSV1
	Actinomycosis: Uncommon, exact incidence unknown
Morbidity and mortality	**Candidiasis:** Usually a mild and self-limiting disease, although recurrent infections may signify an underlying disease
	HSV1: Primary infection may be severely debilitating
	Actinomycosis: Periostitis, osteomyelitis, and fistula formation
Gender, race, and age distribution	**Candidiasis:** There is no gender or ethnic differences, but particularly in the very young and elderly
	HSV1: Prevalence increases with age and correlates with socioeconomic status (lower status has increased prevalence)
	Actinomycosis: No gender, ethnic, or age predilection
Clinical features	**Candidiasis:** Pseudomembranous, erythematous, median rhomboid glossitis, angular cheilitis, hyperplastic, and mucocutaneous types all have unique manifestations
	HSV1: Primary HSV1 may have fever, malaise, lymphadenopathy, multiple mucosal ulcerations, and painful erythematous gingiva
	Actinomycosis: Acute form presents with painful abscesses, while chronic form may be painless, hardened, and/or fistula formation with trismus
Prognosis and treatment	**Candidiasis:** Topical and/or systemic antifungal medication
	HSV1: Symptomatic or with topical/systemic antiviral drugs
	Actinomycosis: Prolonged high doses of antibiotics, with abscess drainage and excision of the fistula, if present

INFECTIONS PATHOLOGIC FEATURES		
Microscopic findings	**Candidiasis:** Fungal hyphae or pseudo-hyphae and ovoid spores (PAS positive) associated with neutrophilic microabscesses **HSV1:** Viral cytopathic effect includes acantholysis, ballooning degeneration, chromatin margination, and multinucleation **Actinomycosis:** Colonies of club-shaped filaments arranged in a rosette pattern surrounded by neutrophils	
Pathologic differential diagnosis	**Candidiasis:** Mucositis, leukoplakia, geographic tongue **HSV1:** Erythema multiforme, herpes zoster, EBV, HSV2, bacterial pharyngitis, acute necrotizing ulcerative gingivitis, traumatic ulcer **Actinomycosis:** Abscess, other bacterial infections	

Patients complain of a burning sensation, a foul or salty taste, or may be asymptomatic. In many infections, other factors play a role: antibiotic therapy, immunosuppression, including use of prednisone, xerostomia, and anemia. The clinical presentations are protean: pseudomembranous form (thrush); erythematous variant; median rhomboid glossitis presents as a red atrophic area on the midline of the dorsal tongue (Fig. 7-11), which may over time become nodular; angular cheilitis presents as red scaling, fissuring area at the corners of the mouth (Fig. 7-12), predisposed by drooling, parafunctional lip habits, and ill-fitting dentures; hyperplastic candidiasis presents as white plaques that are not removable, most often on the hard palate and anterior buccal mucosa; chronic mucocutaneous candidiasis presents as a chronic infection of the oral mucosa, nails, skin, and vagina, the familial form of which may present in early childhood and is associated with defects in cell-mediated immunity and endocrinopathies.

There are nearly ubiquitous antibodies (up to 90%) to the DNA HSV1 virus, transmitted via direct contact or through saliva. Prevalence increases with age and correlates with socioeconomic status. About 10% of patients when first exposed to HSV1 develop primary herpetic gingivostomatitis, while the remaining patients have subclinical symptoms. Symptoms include fever, lymphadenopathy, malaise, mucosal erythema, vesicles and ulcers, which resolve in 7 to 14 days. The virus remains latent within sensory and autonomic ganglion, reactivated in the trigeminal ganglion to result in infection of the vermilion border of the lip (herpes labialis), also called a "fever blister" or "cold sore" (Fig. 7-13). There is often a prodrome of burning, tingling or itching at the site of the eruption up to 24 hours before the outbreak. A cluster of fluid-filled vesicles form, which rupture, crust, and heal within 7 to 10 days. Recurrent HSV1 can also occur intraorally on the hard palate and gingiva (Fig. 7-14).

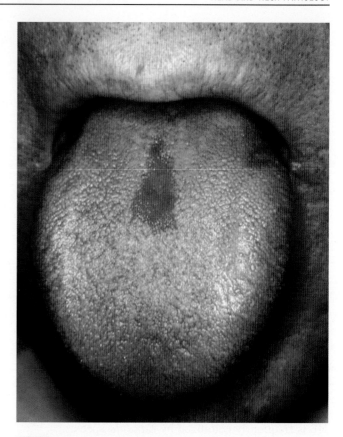

FIGURE 7-11

Clinical photograph of median rhomboid glossitis, with red atrophic area on the midline of the dorsal tongue, corresponding to lost of filiform papillae.

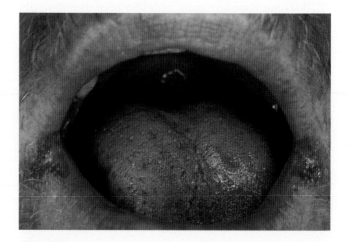

FIGURE 7-12

Clinical photograph of a patient with angular cheilitis; there is fissuring at the corners of the mouth, with painful red scaling areas.

Actinomyces are saprophytic, gram-positive anaerobic bacteria, part of normal oral flora. The primary pathogen is *A. israelii,* although other species can also cause infection. *Actinomyces* colonize tonsillar crypts, dental plaque, and gingival sulci. The presentation may be acute or chronic, with the bacteria entering through a site of trauma (tooth extraction site), infected tonsil, or soft tissue injury. In the acute suppurative phase, yellowish colonies of bacteria may be visible ("sulfur granules"), while the chronic form has extensive fibrosis, imparting a hard or "wooden" area of induration. A fistula may develop with extension to the surface, while periostitis and osteomyelitis may also develop.

PATHOLOGIC FEATURES

CANDIDA (INCLUDING MEDIAN RHOMBOID GLOSSITIS)

Candida can be seen on an exfoliative cytologic examination using either a periodic acid-Schiff (PAS; magenta stained hyphae) or KOH stain (normal cells are lysed, but hyphae remain). The 2 μm hyphae vary in length and can show branching along with ovoid spores or yeast forms (Fig. 7-15). In tissue sections, the organ-

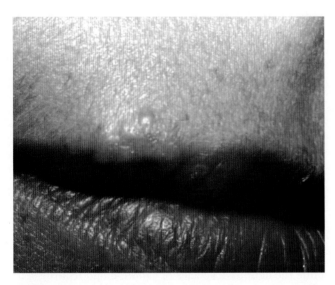

FIGURE 7-13
Clinical photograph of a cluster of fluid-filled vesicles of recurrent HSV1 on the vermilion border.

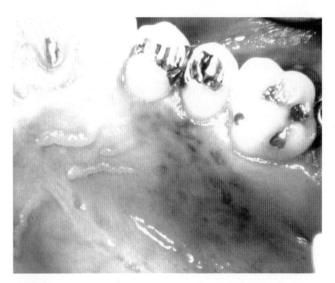

FIGURE 7-14
Clinical photograph of intraoral recurrent HSV on the hard palate. Intraoral vesicles rupture immediately, leaving red, eroded mucosa.

FIGURE 7-15
Exfoliative cytology with periodic acid-Schiff stain. The fungal hyphae, pseudo-hyphae and spores (at the terminal end, *arrow*) appear magenta.

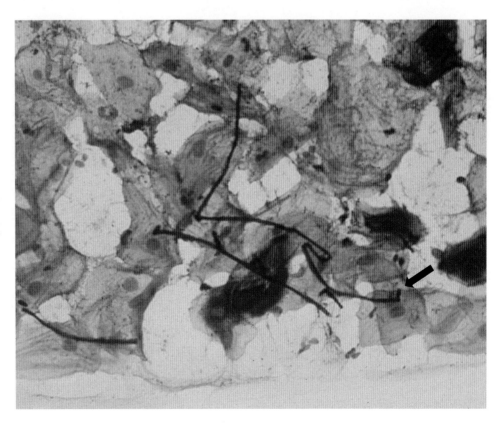

isms are seen in the parakeratin layer (Fig. 7-16), highlighted with a PAS stain, while neutrophilic microabscesses may be seen along with chronic inflammatory cells in the submucosa.

HERPES SIMPLEX VIRUS 1

Epithelial cells infected with HSV1 show marked acantholysis (Tzanck cells), nuclear enlargement (ballooning degeneration), and condensation of the chromatin around the periphery of the nucleus (Fig. 7-17). Infected epithelial cells can fuse to form multinucleated cells. The adjacent mucosa is edematous with secondary inflammation.

ACTINOMYCOSIS

Biopsies show granulation tissue, with a variable number of colonies of club-shaped, basophilic, filamentous organisms arranged in a radiating rosette pattern surrounded by neutrophils (Fig. 7-18). The diagnosis of *Actinomyces* can be confirmed by culture; however, due to the overgrowth of other bacteria or lack of anaerobic conditions, recovery rates are <30%.

DIFFERENTIAL DIAGNOSIS

Careful clinical history and familiarity with the clinical signs can often be sufficient for arriving at a diagnosis. However, overlap in clinical presentation and lack of resolution with appropriate management dictates

biopsy and/or culture. Mimics of candidiasis include severe mucositis, geographic tongue, lichen planus, leukoplakia, or squamous cell carcinoma.

Mimics of primary HSV1, especially in adults, include erythema multiforme, acute necrotizing ulcerative gingivitis (ANUG), pharyngotonsillitis of infectious mononucleosis, or streptococci pharyngitis. ELISA testing of a culture from a vesicle can be performed in 24 hours and is definitive for diagnosis, while serologic tests for HSV1 antibodies only document past exposure. Changing social mores have increased the incidence of HSV2, but the infections are clinically and microscopically identical. Herpes zoster lesions can affect both keratinized and nonkeratinized mucosa, whereas HSV1 affects only keratinized mucosa.

Cervicofacial actinomycosis can masquerade as abscesses and benign or malignant neoplasms. *Nocardia* species are separated by being acid-fast and stain well with a modified Ziehl-Neelsen, while *Actinomyces* species are not acid-fast.

PROGNOSIS AND THERAPY

Antimicrobial therapies are an area of constant change and improvement, so specific drug therapies will not be included here. However, if a patient does not respond to antifungal therapy, culture is recommended to determine the definitive species of *Candida* and its drug sensitivity. If an otherwise healthy patient develops chronic oral candidiasis then endocrine abnormalities and anemia studies should be evaluated. Any leukoplakic

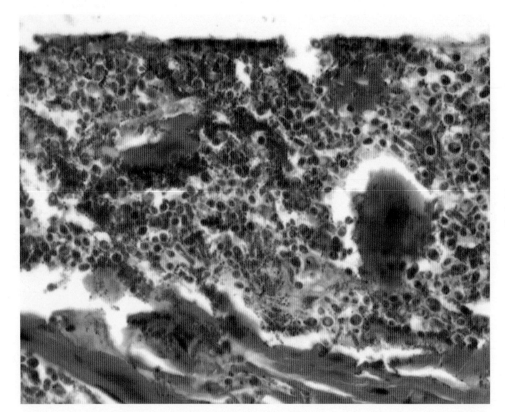

FIGURE 7-16

Yeast and hyphal forms noted within the parakeratin layer.

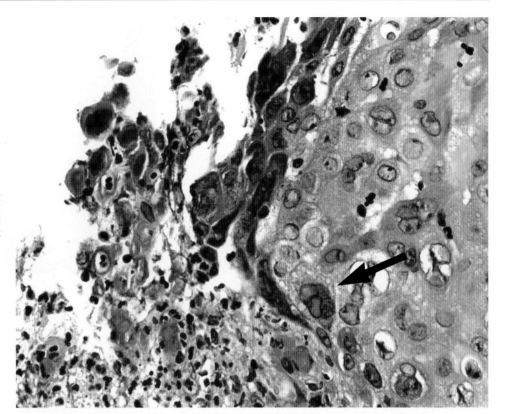

FIGURE 7-17
Acantholytic epithelial cell (Tzanck cells) and cells with nuclear enlargement. Multinucleated cells (*arrow*) also show chromatin condensation at the periphery.

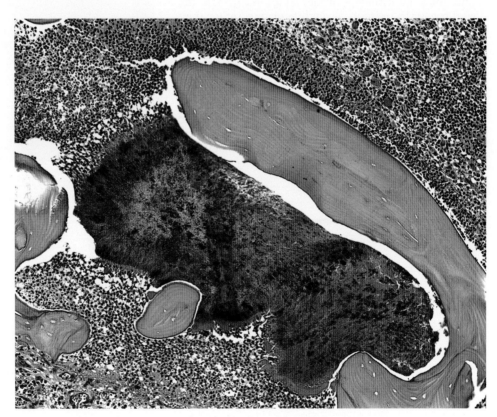

FIGURE 7-18
Colonies of club-shaped filamentous actinomycetes are arranged in a radiating rosette pattern surrounded by neutrophils and nonviable bone.

lesion that exhibits dysplasia with concomitant candidiasis should be treated with appropriate antifungals then reevaluated.

Primary HSV1, especially in pediatric patients, requires management of fever, hydration, nutritional intake, and oral pain. Topical antiviral medications are most effective when initiated during the prodrome period or within the first few hours of vesicle formation.

Chronic actinomycosis is best managed by long-term, high-dose, antibiotic therapy. Incision and drainage of any abscesses and excision of the sinus tracts is indicated.

ORAL LICHEN PLANUS

CLINICAL FEATURES

Lichen planus (LP) is a common mucocutaneous disease that can affect the skin, mucus membranes, nails, and eyes. Of patients with oral LP (OLP), only 15% to 35% develop cutaneous disease. LP is a self-limiting disease that affects mainly middle-aged adults, with women affected more often than men (2 : 1). OLP can manifest in various forms, most commonly reticular and erosive. The reticular variant is asymptomatic, presenting on the buccal mucosa with a lace-like network of fine white lines (Wickham's striae) (Fig. 7-19). On the dorsal tongue, it presents as a white plaque, rather than fine white striae. The erosive variant causes areas of erythema and superficial ulceration, often covered by a fibrinopurulent membrane, with symptoms of pain and burning which can interfere with speech and eating. At the periphery of the erythematous or eroded area, the more typical reticular form of OLP may be observed (Fig. 7-20). Approximately 10% of OLP is confined to the gingiva, commonly presenting with marked erythema resulting in desquamative gingivitis. The gingiva bleeds readily and can lead to gingival recession and periodontal disease.

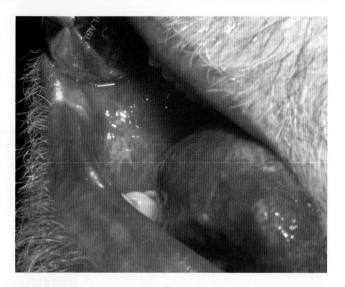

FIGURE 7-19
White lace-like striae (Wickham's striae) affecting the buccal mucosa and lateral tongue in a case of oral lichen planus.

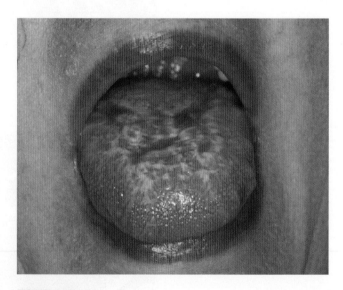

FIGURE 7-20
Clinical photograph of plaque-like erythema and erosions of the dorsal tongue in erosive lichen planus.

ORAL LICHEN PLANUS DISEASE FACT SHEET	
Definition	Common chronic, self-limited inflammatory mucocutaneous disorder of unknown etiology that can affect the skin, mucus membranes, nails, and eyes
Incidence and location	1%–2% of world population
Gender, race, and age distribution	Female > Male (1.4–2 : 1) Peak in middle-aged adults
Clinical features	Reticular variant: Fine white lace-like striae Erosive variant: Atrophic erythematous mucosa with ulceration
Prognosis and treatment	Symptomatic lesions controlled with topical corticosteroids

PATHOLOGIC FEATURES

While characteristic, the histology is not specific. OLP demonstrates hyperparakeratotic, acanthotic, stratified squamous epithelium with either absent rete or hyperplastic rete called saw-tooth rete. Basal cell liquefaction degeneration with an adjacent band-like lymphocytic infiltrate and occasional degenerating keratinocytes (colloid, cytoid, or Civatte bodies) are typical features (Fig. 7-21). Biopsies from an erosive area may have epithelial separation or absence. No dysplasia should be present.

ANCILLARY STUDIES

Direct immunofluorescence (DIF) of *perilesional* mucosa often demonstrates linear deposits of fibrin and fibrinogen at the basement membrane zone. Although this finding is nonspecific, it is especially useful in excluding other vesiculo-ulcerative diseases.

DIFFERENTIAL DIAGNOSIS

The clinical appearance is most important, but with more complex patterns, including the erosive pattern, biopsy is often needed to rule out other vesiculo-ulcerative diseases. These include mucous membrane pemphigoid (MMP), lupus erythematosus, pemphigus vulgaris, chronic graft-versus-host disease, linear immunoglobulin (Ig)A disease, a lichenoid reaction to dental materials, chronic ulcerative stomatitis, and lichenoid drug reactions. Both DIF and indirect immunofluorescence may help in delineating these disease processes. Furthermore, a solitary lesion should be biopsied to exclude a premalignant or malignant lesion, which will have cellular enlargement, nuclear pleomorphism, and increased or abnormal mitoses.

ORAL LICHEN PLANUS PATHOLOGIC FEATURES

Microscopic findings	Hyperkeratosis, acanthosis, "saw-tooth" rete
	Destruction of epithelial basal cell layer
	Band-like lymphocytic infiltrate
	Degenerating keratinocytes (cytoid, Civatte bodies)
	Erosive form may have epithelial separation from lamina propria
Immunofluorescence features	Direct immunofluorescence of *perilesional* tissue may show linear deposits of fibrin and fibrinogen at the basement membrane
Pathologic differential diagnosis	Mucous membrane pemphigoid, lichenoid drug reaction, lichenoid reaction to amalgam, dysplasia

PROGNOSIS AND THERAPY

OLP is a chronic disease with symptoms that wax and wane over the lifetime of the patient. No treatment is necessary for asymptomatic patients, but corticosteroids are used for erosive or erythematous OLP. If extensive, a short course of systemic prednisone can reduce the symptomatic areas sufficiently so that topical corticosteroids can manage symptoms. Occasionally, topical cyclosporine and tacrolimus are employed. Extended topical corticosteroid use places the patient at increased risk for developing oral candidiasis. While controversial,

FIGURE 7-21

Lichen planus demonstrates parakeratotic, acanthotic stratified squamous epithelium with absent rete. Interface inflammation with basal cell liquefaction and band-like, lymphoplasmacytic infiltrate is seen. A cytoid body (*arrow*) is noted.

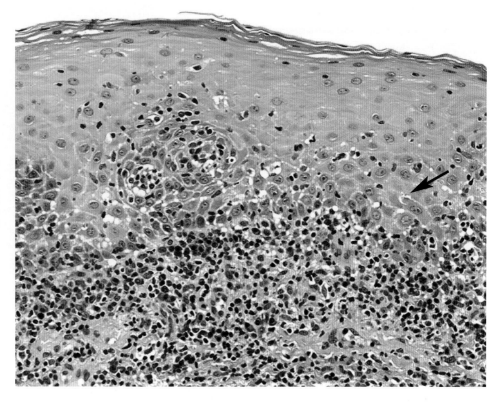

malignant transformation may rarely develop in the atrophic, erosive pattern of OLP, suggesting long-term clinical follow-up of patients with symptomatic OLP.

MUCOUS MEMBRANE PEMPHIGOID (CICATRICAL PEMPHIGOID)

CLINICAL FEATURES

Mucous membrane pemphigoid (MMP) is an autoimmune subepithelial blistering disease predominately affecting the mucus membranes. The underlying pathogenesis is autoantibodies (at least 10 different types identified) that target the basement membrane zone. Subglottic stenosis, airway obstruction, conjunctival scarring, and blindness are serious sequelae. The scarring in MMP is referred to as cicatrical pemphigoid. Middle-aged to elderly patients (50–70 years) are most commonly affected, with women more often than men (1.5–2 : 1). Almost 100% of patients with MMP have oral involvement, with the gingiva affected most commonly (Fig. 7-22). A positive Nikolsky sign, where clinically normal mucosa blisters upon induced trauma, is seen in MMP.

PATHOLOGIC FEATURES

Examination of *perilesional* mucosal tissue demonstrates a subepithelial cleft, with or without an inflammatory cell infiltrate containing lymphocytes and plasma cells in the superficial lamina propria (Fig. 7-23) with an intact basal cell layer. Occasionally neutrophils and eosinophils are seen.

ANCILLARY STUDIES

Direct immunofluorescence of perilesional mucosa demonstrates linear deposits along the basement membrane zone (BMZ) of IgA, IgG, and/or C3 (Fig. 7-24). These findings are not specific and require clinical correlation. Whereas indirect IF of patient's serum using salt-split skin can detect circulating antibodies to the BMZ, not all patients have detectable circulating

MUCOUS MEMBRANE PEMPHIGOID PATHOLOGIC FEATURES	
Microscopic findings	*Perilesional* tissue shows subepithelial cleft with intact basal cells with or without inflammatory cells
Immunofluorescence features	DIF demonstrates linear deposits along the basement membrane zone of IgG, IgA, and/or C3
Pathologic differential diagnosis	Lichen planus, erythema multiforme, linear IgA dermatoses, epidermolysis bullosa acquisita, paraneoplastic pemphigus

MUCOUS MEMBRANE PEMPHIGOID DISEASE FACT SHEET	
Definition	An autoimmune subepithelial blistering disease predominately affecting the mucus membranes associated with autoantibodies which target the basement membrane zone
Incidence and location	Incidence is unknown
Morbidity and mortality	Erosions heal with scarring, which can result in blindness, airway obstruction, and epistaxis
Gender, race, and age distribution	Female > Male (1.5–2 : 1) Mean, 50–70 yr
Clinical features	Blisters of the gingiva which collapse, resulting in red painful erosions Positive Nikolsky sign
Prognosis and treatment	Waxing-waning, long-term course is usual Disease progression despite appropriate therapy Treatment includes topical and/or systemic corticosteroids, immunosuppressive therapy, and intravenous immunoglobulin

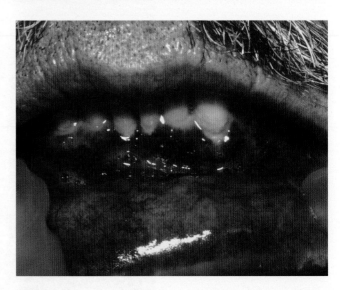

FIGURE 7-22

Mucous membrane pemphigoid presenting as desquamative gingivitis with a large area of red denuded mucosa resulting from sloughing of the epithelium.

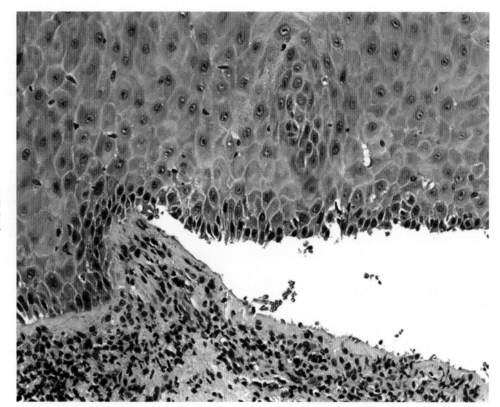

FIGURE 7-23

Perilesional tissue demonstrating subepithelial clefting and a sparse inflammatory cell infiltrate in the superficial lamina propria. No basal cell destruction.

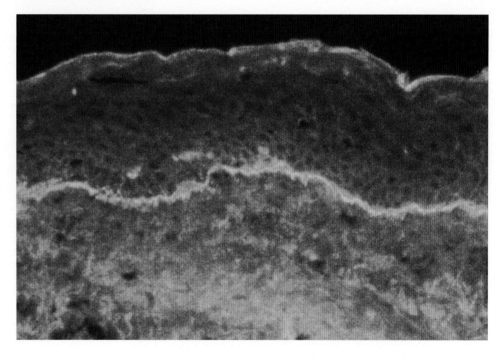

FIGURE 7-24

Direct immunofluorescence of perilesional mucosa from a patient with mucous membrane pemphigoid. A continuous linear band of IgG is seen at the basement membrane zone.

antibodies, and so indirect IF is not essential for the diagnosis. There is no correlation with circulating antibody titers and disease severity.

DIFFERENTIAL DIAGNOSIS

MMP must be separated from other blistering diseases of the oral cavity, including erosive lichen planus, erythema multiforme, pemphigus vulgaris, lupus erythematosus, linear IgA disease, epidermolysis bullosa acquisita, and pemphigoid-like drug reactions. Both DIF and indirect IF are essential in arriving at the correct diagnosis.

PROGNOSIS AND THERAPY

MMP confined to the oral cavity is more amenable to treatment and is rarely associated with scarring, as contrasted to the eye, genital, laryngeal, and esophageal areas. There is often disease progression despite appropriate therapy, which includes topical corticosteroids, systemic corticosteroids, azathioprine, dapsone, and cyclophosphamide. Intravenous immunoglobulin has been used with success in patients resistant to other treatment regimens.

PEMPHIGUS VULGARIS

CLINICAL FEATURES

Pemphigus vulgaris (PV) is an autoimmune mucocutaneous blistering disease. Circulating IgG antibodies to desmoglein 1 and 3 (Dsg1, Dsg3) adhesion molecules of squamous epithelial cells is the underlying defect causing loss of cell to cell adhesion. An uncommon disease, PV generally occurs between the 4th and 6th decades of life, but can be seen in all age groups. The genders are equally affected. The incidence of PV is higher in patients of Mediterranean descent and Ashkenazi Jews. About 50% of cases first present in the oral cavity with blisters that rupture leaving painful erosions that heal without scarring (Fig. 7-25). Mucosal PV may precede cutaneous PV by an average of 5 months, or may be the sole manifestation of the disease. PV can also affect other mucosal sites (esophagus, larynx, nasopharynx, conjunctiva, genitalia, anal mucosa). A flaccid blister on the upper trunk, head, neck, and intertriginous areas that readily rupture is the clinical presentation. After rupture, large areas of painful, denuded epithelium remain. A positive Nikolsky sign and Asboe-Hansen sign are seen (lateral pressure on a bullae extends it into uninvolved mucosa).

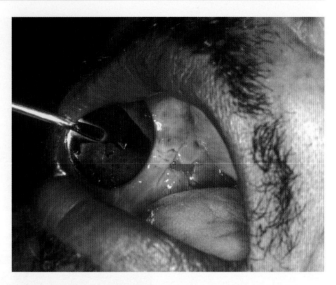

FIGURE 7-25
Large, irregularly shaped ulcer of the buccal mucosa from a patient with oral, oropharyngeal, esophageal, and laryngeal lesions.

PEMPHIGUS VULGARIS DISEASE FACT SHEET	
Definition	Autoimmune mucocutaneous blistering disease associated with autoantibodies to adhesion molecules of squamous epithelium
Incidence and location	Incidence ranges .08 to 3.2/100,000-population
	50% of cases first present with oral disease
Morbidity and mortality	Morbidity related to disease severity
	Mortality rate up to 10%, due to prolonged immunosuppression
Gender, race, and age distribution	Peak incidence between 4th–6th decades
	Higher incidence in Ashkenazi Jews and people of Mediterranean descent
Clinical features	Bullae/blisters readily rupture leaving irregularly shaped, painful ulcerations and erosions, which may be quite extensive
	Skin lesions are flaccid, fluid filled blisters which rupture leaving painful ulcers
Prognosis and treatment	Steroid and immunosuppressive therapy
	Plasmapheresis or IV immunoglobulins
	Long-term therapy may achieve remission, especially if mild disease and rapid response to therapy

PATHOLOGIC FEATURES

A biopsy taken from the edge of a blister will show an intraepithelial blister above the basal layer of the epithelium. Intercellular edema, acantholysis, and loss of adhesion between epithelial cells are observed (Fig. 7-26). The basal cells remain attached to the basement membrane, giving a "tombstone" appearance. The superficial lamina propria may contain a mild inflammatory cell infiltrate.

ANCILLARY STUDIES

Direct immunofluorescence of perilesional tissue demonstrates intercellular deposits of IgG throughout the epithelium (Fig. 7-27). C3 and IgM can sometimes be noted, but less frequently than IgG. Indirect immuno-

fluorescence using monkey esophagus as a substrate, detects circulating IgG autoantibodies in 80% to 90% of patients with PV. The titer of circulating antibody correlates to disease activity. A specific enzyme-linked immunosorbent assays (ELISA) can detect Dsg3 and Dsg1 autoantibodies, which correlates with disease severity.

DIFFERENTIAL DIAGNOSIS

The clinical differential includes many desquamative-blistering disorders, with biopsy of perilesional tissue for histopathologic examination and DIF, as well as patient's serum for indirect IF considered essential for the diagnosis. Paraneoplastic pemphigus (PNP) affects both mucosal and cutaneous sites and is associated with malignancies (lymphoma, chronic lymphocytic leukemia, bronchogenic carcinoma). There is histologic and DIF overlap between PV and PNP, but more specific tests for PNP include indirect IF, using transitional epithelium of rat bladder and immunoprecipitation assays for the specific autoantibodies in the sera of patients with PNP.

PROGNOSIS AND THERAPY

Mortality from PV is up to 10%, mainly due to complications from the long-term immunosuppressive therapy,

PEMPHIGUS VULGARIS PATHOLOGIC FEATURES	
Microscopic findings	Intraepithelial blister above the basal cell layer
	Intercellular edema, acantholysis, and loss of adhesion
	Basal cells remain attach to the basement membrane
	Mild inflammatory cell infiltrate
Immunofluorescence features	Direct immunofluorescence: Intercellular deposits of IgG throughout the epithelium. C3 and IgM infrequent finding
	Indirect immunofluorescence: IgG autoantibodies detect on monkey esophagus substrate
Pathologic differential diagnosis	Paraneoplastic pemphigus, pemphigus-like drug eruption, erythema multiforme, Grover disease, Hailey-Hailey disease

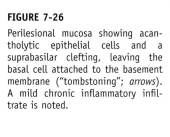

FIGURE 7-26

Perilesional mucosa showing acantholytic epithelial cells and a suprabasilar clefting, leaving the basal cell attached to the basement membrane ("tombstoning"; *arrows*). A mild chronic inflammatory infiltrate is noted.

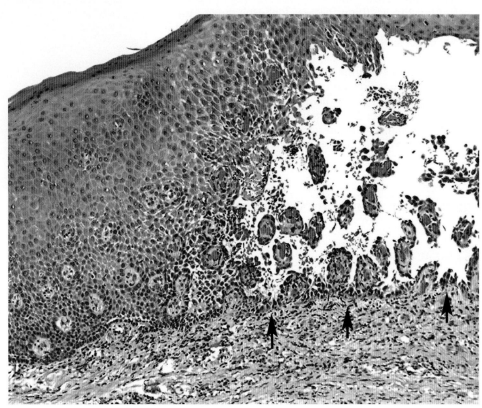

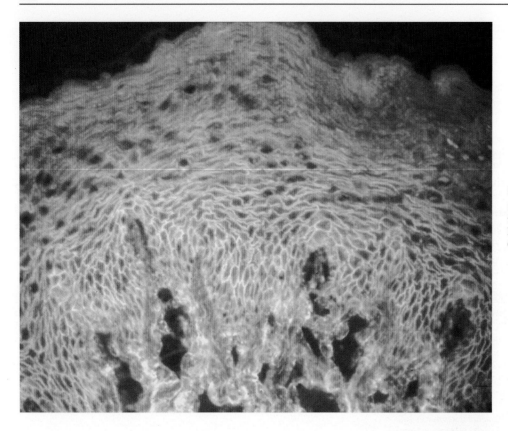

FIGURE 7-27
Perilesional mucosa depicting direct immunofluorescence with deposits of IgG in the intercellular areas of the epithelium.

although mortality was much higher before the implementation of systemic corticosteroid therapy. Treatment consists of local and systemic therapy depending on the disease location and severity. Adjuvant immunosuppressants are used for their steroid-sparing effect (methotrexate, azathioprine, cyclophosphamide, and cyclosporine). Drugs which also have an anti-inflammatory effect such as minocin, dapsone, or tetracycline, have also been used. Plasmapheresis or high-dose intravenous immunoglobulins are used in patients resistant to other therapies. The duration of treatment is variable, with the average time to achieve complete remission ranging from 2 to 10 years. Complete remission is highest in patients who present with mild disease and have a rapid response to treatment.

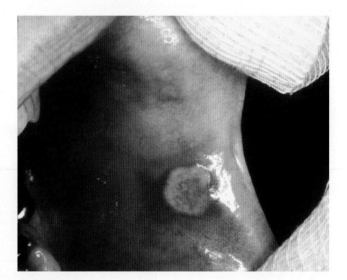

FIGURE 7-28
Clinical photograph of an aphthous ulcer present on the buccal mucosa. The ulcer is covered by a fibrinous membrane and surrounded by an erythematous halo.

RECURRENT APHTHOUS STOMATITIS

CLINICAL FEATURES

Recurrent aphthous stomatitis (RAS), also known as canker sores, are common oral ulcers estimated to affect up to 30% to 35% of the population. These painful ulcers generally last from 10 to 30 days, and range in size from a few millimeters to several centimeters. Minor aphthae, accounting for 80% of all aphthae, are characterized by <1 cm ulcers with a white, gray, or yellow fibrinopurulent membrane surrounded by an erythematous halo present on nonkeratinized oral mucosa (buccal mucosa, labial mucosa, soft palate, floor of mouth, and lateral and ventral tongue; Fig. 7-28). These ulcers typically heal within 10–14 days without scarring. Major aphthae, >1 cm often take longer to heal and may heal with scarring. Herpetiform aphthous ulcers present as numerous pinpoint ulcers that can coalesce into a larger ulcer.

The etiology of RAS is thought to be multifactorial, including allergens, stress, anxiety, local mechanical trauma, and hormones. Reported allergens include cinnamon, cereal products, tomatoes, nuts, citrus fruits, and chocolates. A familial association has been observed in about 40% of cases. No known bacterial or viral infections are associated with RAS.

PATHOLOGIC FEATURES

The microscopic findings are of a nonspecific ulcer, covered by a fibrinopurulent membrane. The underlying connective tissue contains an acute and chronic inflammatory cell infiltrate (Fig. 7-29).

DIFFERENTIAL DIAGNOSIS

The clinical differential diagnosis is wide, although the microscopic differential of nonspecific inflammation is limited. The clinical differential includes herpes simplex virus, herpangina, traumatic ulcer, pyostomatitis vegetans, and Behçet's disease (ocular and orogenital ulcers). RAS typically develops on freely moveable

RECURRENT APHTHOUS STOMATITIS DISEASE FACT SHEET	
Definition	Common, noninfectious ulcers occurring on nonkeratinzed oral mucosa of multifactorial etiology
Incidence and location	Up to 35% of the population
Gender, race, and age distribution	Ulcers usually start in childhood and persist through adulthood
Clinical features	Minor or major aphthae present as ulcers with a white-gray or yellow fibrinopurulent membrane with an erythematous halo on the nonkeratinized oral mucosa (buccal and labial mucosa, floor of mouth, soft palate, lateral and ventral tongue)
Prognosis and treatment	Treatment goals include reducing pain and promote healing with the judicious use of topical/systemic corticosteroids, and identifying specific triggers to prevent future ulcer development

RECURRENT APHTHOUS STOMATITIS PATHOLOGIC FEATURES	
Microscopic findings	Nonspecific ulcer with a fibrino-purulent membrane overlying edematous granulation tissue that contains a mixed inflammatory cell infiltrate
Pathologic differential diagnosis	Traumatic ulcer, pyostomatitis vegetans, HSV

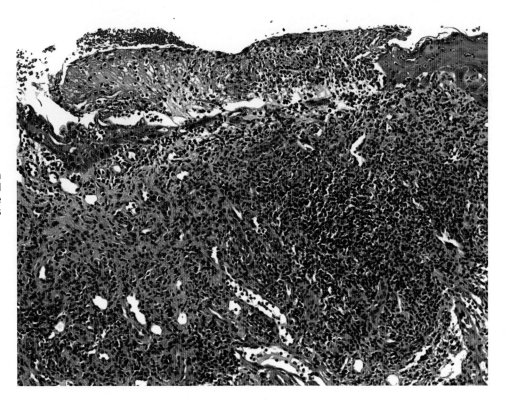

FIGURE 7-29

An aphthous ulcer exhibiting a fibrinopurulent membrane admixed with neutrophils. Granulation tissue beneath the ulcer bed contains inflammatory cells.

mucosa, while herpes develops on bound down mucosa (hard palate, gingiva). Pyostomatitis vegetans is an uncommon pustular disorder which develops in patients with ulcerative colitis and is composed of microabscesses in the spinous layer. Lesions that fail to heal or respond to appropriate treatment, usually within 2 weeks, should be biopsied to exclude other diseases.

PROGNOSIS AND THERAPY

The treatment of aphthous ulcer includes both over-the-counter products and prescription medications. Topical corticosteroids (triamcinolone, fluocinonide, and clobetasol) are effective in reducing the pain and decrease healing time. Oral systemic corticosteroids can be administered to patients with severe RAS. An important part of therapy is to detect and reduce local factors that trigger RAS. Elimination diets and patch testing may help in isolating the triggering agent. Patients who have more than four or five outbreaks a year should also be evaluated for systemic causes, including iron anemia, pernicious anemia, celiac disease, and Crohn's disease.

GEOGRAPHIC TONGUE (BENIGN MIGRATORY GLOSSITIS, ERYTHEMA MIGRANS)

CLINICAL FEATURES

Geographic tongue (GT) is a benign, inflammatory condition of unknown etiology, although a hypersensitivity

reaction is suspected. The reported prevalence of GT ranges up to 15%. Adult women are affected more common than men or children. The anterior two-thirds of the dorsal tongue is the most common location, but infrequently GT can be identified on the buccal mucosa, soft palate, and labial mucosa. GT has a characteristic appearance, presenting as well-demarcated zones of erythema, surrounded by a white, circinate, or scalloped border (Fig. 7-30). The erythema represents atrophy of the filiform papillae. The lesions can increase in size and shape and then resolve, only to appear on another area of the tongue. GT is usually asymptomatic, but hot spicy food, acidic food, certain flavoring agents, or oral hygiene products may produce a burning sensation.

PATHOLOGIC FEATURES

The histologic findings of GT are similar to psoriasis, with spongiosis, hyperparakeratosis, and elongation of the rete ridges. Neutrophilic microabscesses are observed in the superficial spinous layer of the epithelium (Fig. 7-31). The lamina propria usually contains both lymphocytes and neutrophils.

GEOGRAPHIC TONGUE PATHOLOGIC FEATURES	
Microscopic findings	Hyperparakeratosis, spongiosis and elongation of the rete ridges Neutrophilic microabscesses in the superficial spinous layers
Pathologic differential diagnosis	Oral candidiasis, psoriasis, inflammatory papillary hyperplasia

GEOGRAPHIC TONGUE DISEASE FACT SHEET	
Definition	A benign, usually asymptomatic inflammatory disorder of the tongue characterized by atrophic erythematous mucosa surrounded by a white scalloped border
Incidence and location	Up to 15% Nearly all cases occur on the tongue
Gender, race, and age distribution	Female > Male (2 : 1) Adults are generally affected more than children
Clinical features	Multifocal, circinate erythematous patches surrounded by a white border Lesions can change size, location, or pattern over a period of days (benign *migratory* glossitis)
Prognosis and treatment	Benign condition managed by symptomatic relief with judicious use of topical corticosteroids

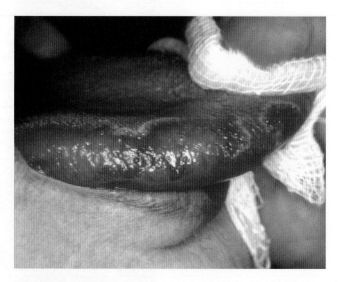

FIGURE 7-30

Clinical photograph of geographic tongue exhibiting irregular erythematous atrophic tongue papillae surrounded by a slightly raised white circinate border.

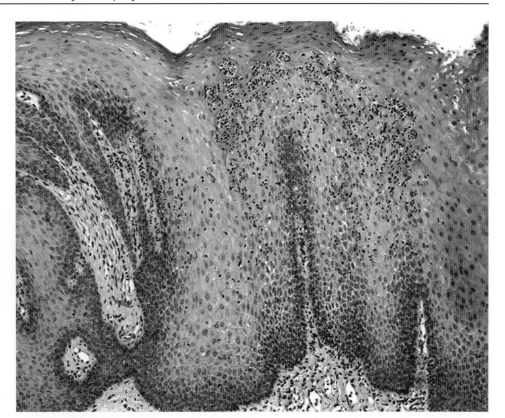

FIGURE 7-31
Hyperparakeratosis, spongiosis, and elongation of the rete. Neutrophilic microabscesses are seen in the superficial spinous layer of the epithelium.

DIFFERENTIAL DIAGNOSIS

Because of the characteristic clinical appearance, GT is usually not confused with other entities. Erosive lichen planus usually has more severe symptoms and lesions usually are seen elsewhere in the oral cavity.

PROGNOSIS AND THERAPY

Asymptomatic lesions do not need to be treated. Patients with complaints of burning or tenderness may benefit from judicious use of topical corticosteroids. Avoidance of any known aggravating factor(s) is the best long-term therapy.

HAIRY TONGUE

CLINICAL FEATURES

Hairy tongue results from the failure of the filiform papillae to desquamate. There are a number of precipitating factors including poor oral hygiene, medications (especially broad-spectrum antibiotics), radiation therapy of the head and neck and xerostomia. Tobacco smoking and coffee and tea drinking can also contribute

HAIRY TONGUE DISEASE FACT SHEET	
Definition	Failure of the filiform papillae to desquamate resulting in elongation, precipitated by numerous factors including poor oral hygiene and medications
Incidence and location	Approximately 0.5% of adults
Gender, race, and age distribution	No sex or race predilection
	Generally seen in adults, but can be present in children
Clinical features	Elongated filiform papillae seen of the dorsal tongue anterior to the circumvallate papillae
	The papillae are different colors depending on etiology or growth of pigment-producing bacteria
Prognosis and treatment	Desquamation of the elongated papillae by scraping or brushing the tongue

to the hairy tongue. The filiform papillae appear elongated, and retain pigment from food, tobacco, beverages, candies, and mouthwash (Fig. 7-32), with the tongue appearing black, yellow, brown, green, or other colors depending on the etiology. Hairy tongue generally is asymptomatic, although some patients complain of a gagging sensation. Symptomatic hairy tongue (burning sensation) usually results from secondary candidal infection.

PATHOLOGIC FEATURES

Elongated filiform papillae with associated bacterial colonies and occasional inflammatory cells can be seen microscopically (Fig. 7-33). Candidal overgrowth may be demonstrated with a PAS stain.

DIFFERENTIAL DIAGNOSIS

Other entities that can involve the dorsal surface of the tongue include lichen planus, leukoplakia, and candidiasis. However, none of these entities are associated with elongated filiform papilla.

HAIRY TONGUE PATHOLOGIC FEATURES	
Microscopic findings	Elongation and marked hyperparakeratosis of the filiform papillae, usually associated with numerous bacterial colonies
Pathologic differential diagnosis	Oral candidiasis, oral leukoplakia

PROGNOSIS AND THERAPY

Mechanical debridement with a tongue scraper or toothbrush aids in removing the elongated papillae. If the precipitating factor was antibiotics, the tongue returns to normal after the antibiotic therapy is discontinued. If the patient has xerostomia, therapies to increase saliva are of benefit. Patients who have candidiasis associated with hairy tongue require antifungal therapy.

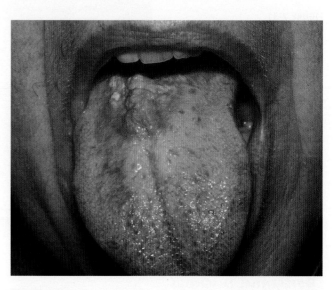

FIGURE 7-32
Clinical photograph of hairy tongue with marked elongated filiform papillae on the midline of the tongue.

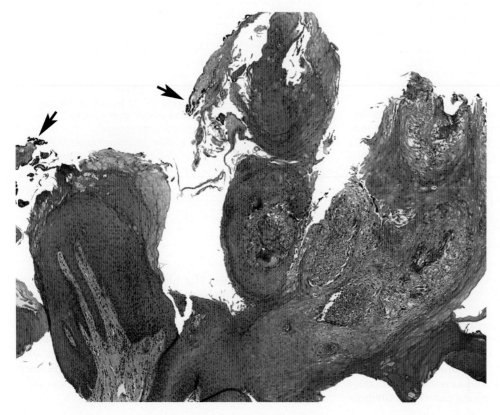

FIGURE 7-33
Hairy tongue showing elongation and marked parakeratosis of the filiform papillae. Numerous bacterial colonies are present on the epithelial surface (*arrows*).

MELANOTIC MACULE

CLINICAL FEATURES

Oral or labial melanotic macule is a term used to describe a benign pigmented lesion of the oral cavity. Up to 85% of diagnosed cases are reported in females, and the average age at presentation is 40 years. The vermilion border of the lower lip is the most common location, followed by gingiva, buccal mucosa, and palate. The melanotic macule is a solitary, flat, well-delineated area of uniform pigmentation that can range in color from black to brown, blue or gray, although tan to dark brown is the most common color (Fig. 7-34). The lesion is typically <1 cm in size, remaining stable.

MELANOTIC MACULE DISEASE FACT SHEET	
Definition	Benign pigmented lesion of the oral cavity with increased melanin pigmentation along the basal cell layer of the epithelium
Incidence and location	Exact incidence unknown
	Majority of cases occur on the vermilion border of the lip
Gender, race, and age distribution	Female >> Male (7–8 : 1)
	Mean, 40 yr
Clinical features	Usually solitary, flat, well delineated, uniformly pigmented, asymptomatic, <1 cm macule
Prognosis and treatment	Unsightly lesions can be removed by short-pulsed laser for aesthetic reasons
	Excise any pigmented lesion of recent onset, large size, change in size or uneven pigmentation

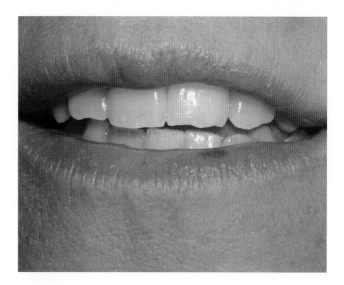

FIGURE 7-34
Clinical photograph of a melanotic macule on the vermilion border of the lower lip presenting as an asymptomatic brown macule.

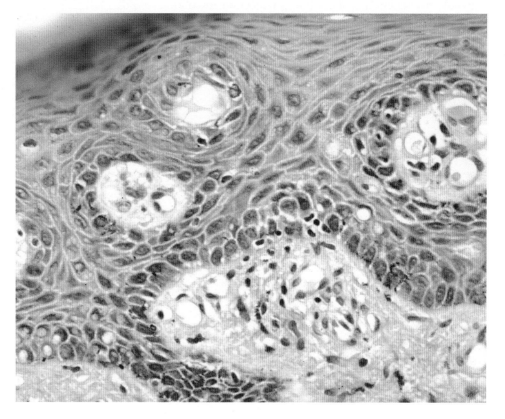

FIGURE 7-35
Normal stratified squamous epithelium with melanin pigmentation in the basal and parabasal cell layer. Incontinent melanin pigment in the lamina propria.

MELANOTIC MACULE PATHOLOGIC FEATURES	
Microscopic findings	Increased melanin pigmentation in the basal cell layer Melanin pigment present in the lamina propria There may or may not be increase in melanocytes
Pathologic differential diagnosis	Postinflammatory pigmentation, drug-induced pigmentation

PATHOLOGIC FEATURES

Increase melanin pigmentation in the basal and parabasal layers is present within normal stratified squamous mucosa (Fig. 7-35), although the number of melanocytes is generally not affected. Incontinent melanin pigment can be noted in the superficial lamina propria along with occasional melanophages.

DIFFERENTIAL DIAGNOSIS

The differential diagnosis for melanotic macules, include amalgam tattoo, intraoral nevi, postinflammatory hyperpigmentation, drug-induced pigmentation, and melanoma. Most intraoral nevi are raised. Blue nevi generally are <1 cm macule with a predilection for the hard palate. Postinflammatory and drug-induced pigmentation will appear more diffuse than melanotic macule. The amalgam tattoo is blue-gray, and is seen adjacent to an area of dental work. Clinical history and clinical appearance are key to arriving at the correct diagnosis.

PROGNOSIS AND THERAPY

The melanotic macule does not undergo malignant transformation and requires no treatment. Unsightly melanotic macules can be removed with short-pulsed lasers for aesthetic reasons. Any pigmented lesion of recent onset, large size or changing size or uneven pigmentation should be excised.

SUGGESTED READING

Fordyce Granules

1. Alawi F, Siddiqui A: Sebaceous carcinoma of the oral mucosa: case report and review of the literature. Oral Surg Oral Med Oral Pathol Oral Radiol Endod 2005;99:79–84.
2. Daley TD: Intraoral sebaceous hyperplasia. Diagnostic criteria. Oral Surg Oral Med Oral Pathol 1993;75:343–347.

3. Verbin RS, Guggenheimer J, Appel BN: Fordyce granules. In: Barnes L, ed. Surgical Pathology of the Head and Neck, 2nd ed. New York: Marcel Dekker, 2001:240–241.

Amalgam Tattoo

1. Aoyagi H, Katagiri M: Long-term effects of Ag-containing alloys on mucous tissue present in biopsy samples. Dent Mater J 2004;23: 340–347.
2. Buchner A, Hansen LS: Amalgam pigmentation (amalgam tattoo) of the oral mucosa. A clinicopathologic study of 268 cases. Oral Surg Oral Med Oral Pathol 1980;49:139–147.
3. Buchner A: Amalgam tattoo (amalgam pigmentation) of the oral mucosa: clinical manifestations, diagnosis and treatment. Refuat Hapeh Vehashinayim 2004;21:25–28, 92.
4. Owens BM, Johnson WW, Schuman NJ: Oral amalgam pigmentations (tattoos): a retrospective study. Quintessence Internat 1992;23: 805–810.
5. Seward GR: Amalgam tattoo. Br Dent J 1998;184:470–471.
6. Shah G: Treatment of an amalgam tattoo with a Q-switched alexandrite (755 nm) laser. Dermatol Surg 2002;28:1180–1181.

Ectopic Thyroid

1. Atiyeh BS, Abdelnour A, Haddad FF, et al.: Lingual thyroid: tongue-splitting incision for transoral excision. J Laryngol Otol 1995;109: 520–524.
2. Barnes TW, Olsen KD, Morgenthaler TI: Obstructive lingual thyroid causing sleep apnea: a case report and review of the literature. Sleep Med 2004;5:605–607.
3. Batsakis JG, El-Naggar AK, Luna MA: Thyroid gland ectopias. Ann Otol Rhinol Laryngol 1996;105:996–1000.
4. Baughman RA: Lingual thyroid and lingual thyroglossal tract remnants. A clinical and histopathologic study with review of the literature. Oral Surg Oral Med Oral Pathol 1972;34:781–799.
5. Douglas PS, Baker AW: Lingual thyroid. Brit J Oral Maxillofac Surg 1994;32:123–124.
6. Emmanouil-Nikoloussi EN, Kerameos-Foroglou C: Developmental malformations of human tongue and associated syndromes (review). Bull Group Int Rech Sci Stomatol Odontol 1992;35:5–12.
7. Turgut S, Murat OK, Celikkanat S, et al.: Diagnosis and treatment of lingual thyroid: a review. Rev Laryngol Otol Rhinol (Bord) 1997;118:189–192.
8. Verbin RS, Guggenheimer J, Appel BN: Ectopic thyroid tissue. In: Barnes L, ed. Surgical Pathology of the Head and Neck, 2nd ed. New York: Marcel Dekker, 2001:251–254.

Oral Lymphoepithelial Cysts

1. Alpaslan G, Oygur T, Saracgil S: Lymphoepithelial cyst. J Marmara Univ Dent Fac 1993;1:333–336.
2. Buchner A, Hansen LS: Lymphoepithelial cysts of the oral cavity. A clinicopathologic study of thirty-eight cases. Oral Surg Oral Pathol Oral Med 1980;50:441–449.
3. Kumara GR, Gillgrass TJ, Bridgman JB: A lymphoepithelial cyst (branchial cyst) in the floor of the mouth. N Z Dent J 1995;91:14–15.
4. Schiodt M: HIV-associated salivary gland disease: a review. Oral Surg Oral Med Oral Pathol 1992;73:164–167.
5. Seifert G: Lymphoid lesions of the oral cavity. Pathol Res Pract 1980;167:179–203.

Oral Hairy Leukoplakia

1. de Faria PR, Vargas PA, Saldiva PH, et al.: Tongue disease in advanced AIDS. Oral Dis 2005;11:72–80.
2. Marcus M, Maida CA, Freed JR, et al.: Oral white patches in a national sample of medical HIV patients in the era of HAART. Community Dent Oral Epidemiol 2005;33:99–106.
3. Patton LL, Phelan JA, Ramos-Gomez FJ, et al.: Prevalence and classification of HIV-associated oral lesions. Oral Dis 2002;8 Suppl 2:98–109.
4. Ranganathan K, Umadevi M, Saraswathi TR, et al.: Oral lesions and conditions associated with human immunodeficiency virus infection in 1,000 South Indian patients. Ann Acad Med Singapore 2004;33:37–42.

5. Shiboski CH, Hilton JF, Neuhaus JM, et al.: Human immunodeficiency virus-related oral manifestations and gender. A longitudinal analysis. The University of California, San Francisco, Oral AIDS Center Epidemiology Collaborative Group. Arch Intern Med 1996;156:2249–2254.
6. Walling DM, Etienne W, Ray AJ, et al.: Persistence and transition of Epstein-Barr virus genotypes in the pathogenesis of oral hairy leukoplakia. J Infect Dis 2004;190:387–395.

Infections

1. Belmont MJ, Behar PM, Wax MK: Atypical presentations of actinomycosis. Head Neck 1999;21:264–268.
2. Brandwein M: Actinomycoses. In: Barnes L, ed. Surgical Pathology of the Head and Neck, 2nd ed. New York: Marcel Dekker, 2001:2024–2123.
3. Eisen D: The clinical characteristics of intraoral herpes simplex virus infection in 52 immunocompetent patients. Oral Surg Oral Med Oral Pathol Oral Radiol Endod 1998;86:432–437.
4. Kessler HR: Herpes virus infections: a review for the dental practitioner. Tex Dent J 2005;122:150–165.
5. Odell EW: Median rhomboid glossitis. In: Barnes EL, Eveson JW, Reichart P, Sidransky D, eds. Pathology and Genetics of Head and Neck Tumours. Kleihues P, Sobin LH, series eds. World Health Organization Classification of Tumours. Lyon, France: IARC Press, 2005:189.
6. Sciubba JJ: Herpes simplex and aphthous ulcerations: presentation, diagnosis and management—an update. Gen Dent 2003;51:510–516.
7. Sitheeque MA, Samaranayake LP: Chronic hyperplastic candidosis/candidiasis (candidal leukoplakia). Crit Rev Oral Biol Med 2003;14:253–267.
8. Vazquez J, Sobel JD: Mucosal candidiasis. Infect Dis Clin North Am 2002;16:793–820.

Oral Lichen Planus

1. DeRossi SS, Ciarrocca KN: Lichen planus, lichenoid drug reactions, and lichenoid mucositis. Dent Clin North Am 2005;49:77–89, viii.
2. Eisen D: The clinical manifestations and treatment of oral lichen planus. Dermatol Clin 2003;21:79–89.
3. Scully C, Beyli M, Ferreiro MC, et al.: Update of oral lichen planus: etiopathogenesis and management. Crit Rev Oral Biol Med 1998;9:86–122.
4. Sugerman PB, Savage NW, Walsh LJ, et al.: The pathogenesis of oral lichen planus. Crit Rev Oral Biol Med 2002;13:350–365.
5. Sugerman PB, Savage NW: Oral lichen planus: causes, diagnosis and management. Aust Dent J 2002;47:290–297.

Mucous Membrane Pemphigoid (Cicatrical Pemphigoid)

1. Bagan J, Lo ML, Scully C: Mucosal disease series. Number III. Mucous membrane pemphigoid. Oral Dis 2005;11:197–218.
2. Chan LS, Ahmed AR, Anhalt GJ, et al.: The first international consensus of mucous membrane pemphigoid. Arch Dermatol 2002;138:370–379.
3. Sami N, Yeh SW, Ahmed AR: Blistering diseases in the elderly: diagnosis and treatment. Dermatol Clin 2004;22:73–86.
4. Sollecito TP, Parisi E: Mucous membrane pemphigoid. Dent Clin North Am 2005;49:91–106, viii.

Pemphigus Vulgaris

1. Bystryn JC, Rudolph JL: Pemphigus. Lancet 2005;366:61–73.
2. Castellano Suarez JL: Gingival disorders of immune origin. Med Oral 2002;7:271–283.

3. Challacombe SJ, Setterfield J, Shirlaw P, et al.: Immunodiagnosis of pemphigus and mucous membrane pemphigoid. Acta Odontol Scand 2001;59:226–234.
4. Ettlin DA: Pemphigus. Dent Clin North Am 2005;49:107–125.
5. Grando S: New approaches to the treatment of pemphigus. J Investig Dermatol Symp Proc 2004;9:84–91.
6. Scully C, Challacombe SJ: Pemphigus vulgaris: update of etiopathogenesis, oral manifestations, and management. Crit Rev Oral Biol Med 2002;13:397–408.
7. Weinberg MA, Insler MS, Campen RB: Mucocutaneous features of autoimmune blistering diseases. Oral Med Oral Pathol Oral Radiol Endod 1997;84:517–534.

Recurrent Aphthous Stomatitis

1. Akintoye SO, Greenberg MS: Recurrent aphthous stomatitis. Dent Clin North Am 2005;49:31–47.
2. Natah SS, Konttinen YT, Enattah NS, et al.: Recurrent aphthous ulcers today: a review of the growing knowledge. Int J Oral Maxillofac Surg 2004;33:221–234.
3. Porter S, Scully C: Aphthous ulcers (recurrent). Clin Evid 2004;1687–1694.
4. Scully C, Gorsky M, Lozada-Nur F: The diagnosis and management of recurrent aphthous stomatitis: a consensus approach. J Am Dent Assoc 2003;134:200–207.
5. Zunt SL: Recurrent aphthous stomatitis. Dermatol Clin 2003;21:33–39.

Geographic Tongue (Benign Migratory Glossitis, Erythema Migrans)

1. Assimakopoulos D, Patrikakos G, Fotika C, Elisaf M: Benign migratory glossitis or geographic tongue: an enigmatic oral lesion. Am J Med 2002;113:751–755.
2. Espelid M, Bang G, Johannessen AC, et al.: Geographic stomatitis: report of 6 cases. J Oral Pathol Med 1991;20:425–428.
3. Hume WJ: Geographic stomatitis: a critical review. J Dent 1975;3:25–43.

Hairy Tongue

1. Salonen L, Axell T, Hellden L: Occurrence of oral mucosal lesions, the influence of tobacco habits and an estimate of treatment time in an adult Swedish population. J Oral Pathol Med 1990;19:170–176.
2. Winzer M, Gilliar U, Ackerman AB: Hairy lesions of the oral cavity. Clinical and histopathologic differentiation of hairy leukoplakia from hairy tongue. Am J Dermatopathol 1988;10:155–159.

Melanotic Macule

1. Buchner A, Merrell PW, Carpenter WM: Relative frequency of solitary melanocytic lesions of the oral mucosa. J Oral Pathol Med 2004;33:550–557.
2. Gaeta GM, Satrino RA, Baroni A: Oral Pigmented lesions. Clin Dermatol 2002;20:286–288.
3. Gupta G, Williams RE, Mackie RM: The labial melanotic macule: a review of 79 cases. Br J Dermatol 1997;136:772–775.
4. Ho KK, Dervan P, O'Loughlin S, et al.: Labial melanotic macule: a clinical, histopathologic, and ultrastructural study. J Am Acad Dermatol 1993;28:33–39.
5. Weathers DR, Corio RL, Crawford BE, et al.: The labial melanotic macule. Oral Surg Oral Med Oral Pathol 1976;42:196–205.

Benign Neoplasms of the Oral Cavity and Oropharynx

William Westra

FIBROMA

The term fibroma, unless further qualified (e.g., ossifying fibroma, ameloblastic fibroma, etc.) refers to a localized proliferation of fibrous connective tissue in response to tissue irritation. As such, oral fibromas are reactive in nature; some advocate use of the alternative designation "localized fibrous hyperplasia," as it more fittingly captures the true reactive nature of this lesion.

CLINICAL FEATURES

Fibroma is the most common "tumor" encountered in the oral cavity. It occurs more often in women than in men by a 2 : 1 ratio, and it usually presents during the 4th to 6th decades of life. There is no racial predilection. Distribution within the oral cavity, not surprisingly, reflects those sites most prone to trauma. There is a par-

tiality for the buccal mucosa along the bite line and the lateral border of the tongue, but they commonly involve the lips and gingiva as well. The classic clinical appearance is that of an elevated sessile nodule with a smooth mucosal-lined surface (Fig. 8-1). Most are only a few millimeters, and only the rare lesion reaches a diameter of 1 to 2 cm. Fibromas are painless.

PATHOLOGIC FEATURES

GROSS FINDINGS

Oral fibroma is seen as a round nodule with a smooth mucosal surface. The cut surface is solid and gray with a consistency that ranges from soft to firm.

MICROSCOPIC FINDINGS

The histologic picture is dominated by the nodular deposition of submucosal collagen (Fig. 8-2). Spindled fibroblasts and small blood vessels are dispersed among the pink and dense bands of collagen (Fig. 8-3). The periphery of the nodule may be rounded and sharply demarcated or it may blend imperceptibly with the sur-

FIBROMA DISEASE FACT SHEET	
Definition	A localized proliferation of fibrous connective tissue in response to tissue irritation
Incidence and location	Most common "tumor" encountered in the oral cavity
	Most common in oral sites prone to irritation (e.g., buccal mucosa along the bite line, lateral tongue)
Gender, race, and age distribution	Female > Male (F : M = 2 : 1)
	Most common between 30–50 yr
Clinical features	Painless and asymptomatic
	Submucosal nodules with limited growth potential (usually a few millimeters in diameter)
Prognosis and treatment	Conservative surgical resection is curative
	Potential for recurrence if inciting trauma persists

FIBROMA PATHOLOGIC FEATURES	
Gross findings	Dome-shaped nodule ranging from a few millimeters to 2 centimeters
	Smooth surface unless secondarily ulcerated
Microscopic findings	Histologic picture dominated by submucosal collagen
	Inconspicuous spindled fibroblasts sparsely dispersed among collagen bundles
	Squamous epithelium is usually unremarkable, but may demonstrate varying degrees of rete atrophy, hyperkeratosis, and/or superficial ulceration
Pathologic differential diagnosis	Not easily confused with other oral submucosal nodules at the histologic level

rounding fibrous connective tissues. The covering squamous lining may be thin with flattening of its rete ridges as if it were being tightly stretched over the nodular mass. Trauma to the nodule can incite secondary changes ranging from friction-induced hyperkeratosis to ulceration.

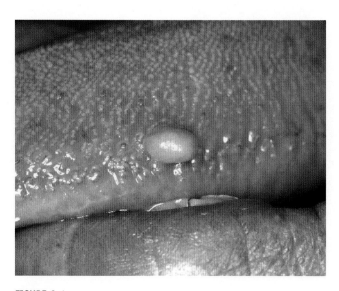

FIGURE 8-1

This fibroma occurs along the lateral border of the tongue, and is seen as a raised sessile nodule with a smooth surface.

The fibroblasts of irritation fibromas are spindled and inconspicuous. The presence of larger stellate fibroblasts with large and multiple nuclei is more defining of the *giant cell fibroma* (Fig. 8-4). In contrast to the more mundane irritation fibroma, the giant cell fibroma is not associated with trauma, and it tends to occur in a younger group of patients.

DIFFERENTIAL DIAGNOSIS

Although fibromas are common and clinically inconsequential, surgical removal with microscopic examination is prudent to rule out various benign and malignant neoplasms that can simulate the clinical appearance of fibromas such as schwannomas, neurofibromas, granular cell tumors, and salivary gland neoplasms. This clinical differential diagnosis is easily resolved at the light microscopic level.

PROGNOSIS AND THERAPY

As a reactive non-neoplastic process, fibromas have no malignant potential. Simple surgical resection is curative. If the source of inciting trauma has not been adequately addressed, the lesion may rarely recur.

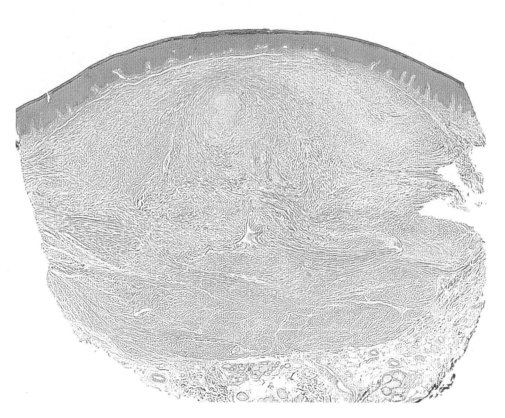

FIGURE 8-2

At low power, the deposition of connective tissue forms a discrete submucosa nodule.

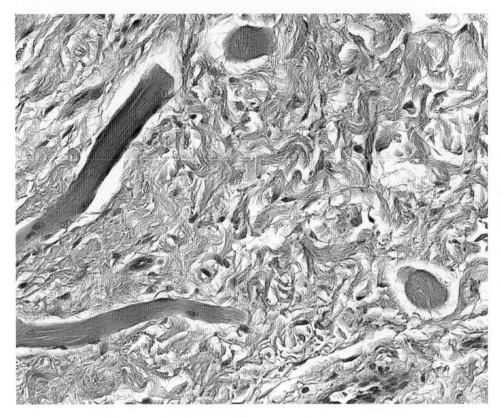

FIGURE 8-3

At higher power, the nodule is comprised of inconspicuous fibroblasts in a collagen-rich stroma.

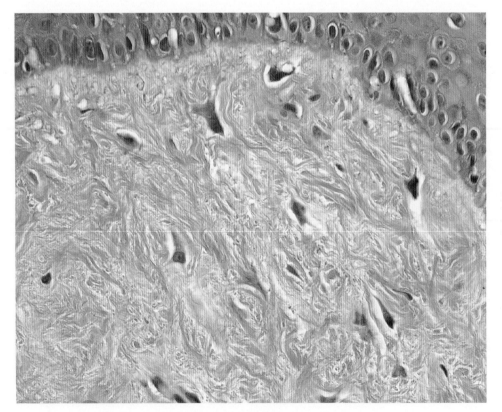

FIGURE 8-4

In contrast to the conventional (i.e., irritation) fibroma, the giant cell fibroma features stellate fibroblasts with large hyperchromatic nuclei.

SQUAMOUS PAPILLOMA (INCLUDING VERRUCA AND CONDYLOMA)

Squamous papilloma of the oral cavity is a localized benign exophytic proliferation of the squamous epithelium. Its signature microscopic feature is the presence of papillary fronds. It is one of several neoplastic processes of the oral cavity where squamous proliferation is driven in part by the human papillomavirus (HPV). Other HPV-driven proliferations of the oral mucosa include verruca vulgaris (common wart) and condyloma acuminatum (venereal wart). The nononcogenic HPV subtypes 6 and 11 are most consistently detected in oral squamous papillomas and condyloma; while the HPV subtypes 2 and 4 are associated with verruca vulgaris.

CLINICAL FEATURES

Squamous papillomas represent the most common benign neoplasm originating from the oral mucosa. They occur across a broad age range, affecting both children and adults. Most lesions, however, are diagnosed in individuals 30 to 50 years of age. Some large studies indicate that males are affected more commonly than females and whites more than blacks. They can arise from any intraoral mucosal location, but they show a definite predilection for the hard and soft palate and uvula.

Squamous papillomas are clinically observed as soft, white pedunculated nodules that usually measure less than 1 cm (Fig. 8-5). Their hallmark frond-like projections give rise to surface irregularities that range from granular, to spiny, to convoluted (i.e., "cauliflower-like"). Most papillomas of the oral cavity are solitary lesions.

PATHOLOGIC FEATURES

GROSS FINDINGS

The squamous papilloma tends to be exophytic, warty, friable, and white to gray. The degree of its

SQUAMOUS PAPILLOMA (INCLUDING VERRUCA AND CONDYLOMA) DISEASE FACT SHEET	
Definition	A localized benign exophytic warty proliferation of the squamous epithelium driven in part by human papillomavirus, particularly by the nononcogenic subtypes 6 and 11
Incidence and location	Most common benign neoplasm originating from the surface epithelium May originate from any intraoral mucosal site, but with a preference for the hard and soft palate and uvula
Morbidity and mortality	Benign proliferations with little potential to undergo malignant transformation
Gender, race, and age distribution	May affect males slightly more often than females May affect whites slightly more often than blacks Occur over a broad range of ages, but most commonly present between 30–50 yr
Clinical features	Painless and asymptomatic Warty exophytic growth Usually solitary and small (<1 cm)
Prognosis and treatment	Conservative surgical resection or laser ablation is curative

SQUAMOUS PAPILLOMA (INCLUDING VERRUCA AND CONDYLOMA) PATHOLOGIC FEATURES	
Gross findings	Exophytic, warty, friable and white to gray Surface irregularities ranging from granular, to spiny, to convoluted
Microscopic findings	Fibrovascular cores lined by mature, stratified squamous epithelium The cells of the prickle layer may show koilocytic change (nuclear condensation and cytoplasmic clearing) Hyperplasia of the basal cell layer is common and should not be mistaken as a premalignant (i.e., dysplastic) change
Pathologic differential diagnosis	Other HPV-driven squamous proliferations (verruca vulgaris, condyloma acuminatum), reactive papillary hyperplasia, proliferative verrucous leukoplakia, papillary squamous cell carcinoma

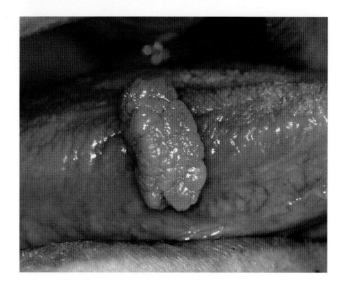

FIGURE 8-5

This squamous papilloma occurs along the lateral aspect of the tongue, and is seen as an exophytic cauliflower-like mass having a convoluted surface.

surface irregularities reflects the length and complexity of the papillae.

MICROSCOPIC FINDINGS

The trademark feature of squamous papilloma, namely its papillary extensions, is histologically characterized by multilayered squamous epithelium supported by a central core of fibrovascular tissue (Fig. 8-6). The squamous layer is often thickened, but it demonstrates normal maturation (Fig. 8-7). Hyperplasia of the basal cell layer with increased mitotic figures is not uncommon and should not be interpreted as a premalignant (i.e., dysplastic) change. HPV-induced cytopathic changes can sometimes be appreciated in cells within the prickle cell layer. These altered cells are referred to as koilocytes, and they are characterized by dark condensed nuclei with a surrounding zone of cytoplasmic clearing (Fig. 8-8, inset).

ANCILLARY STUDIES

In situ hybridization analysis using type-specific HPV probes is a fairly reliable method of documenting the presence of HPV 6 or 11 in oral squamous papillo-

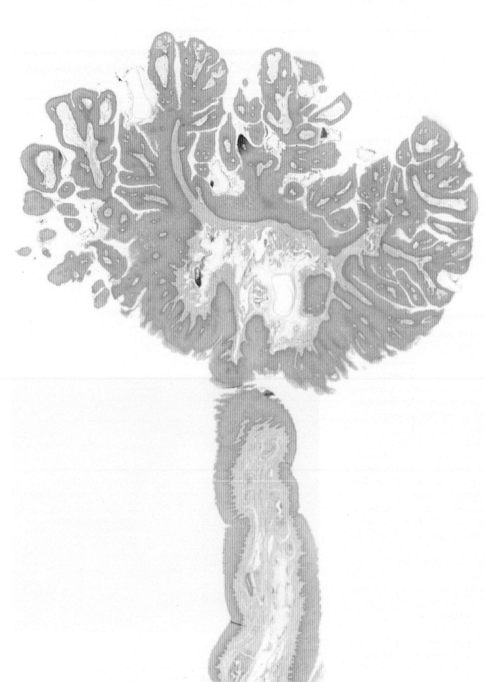

FIGURE 8-6

A low-power view demonstrates the complex branching papillary structures of a squamous papilloma.

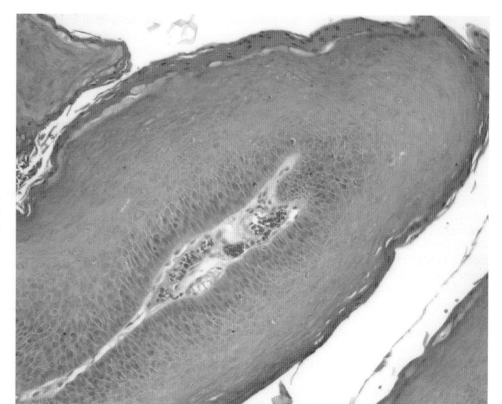

FIGURE 8-7

A higher power view highlights the papillary frond comprised of a fibrovascular core that supports a layer of squamous epithelium.

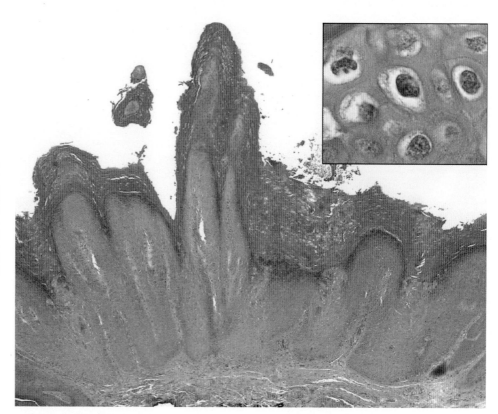

FIGURE 8-8

Low-power view of verruca vulgaris. In contrast to the squamous papilloma, verruca has a broad flat base, a prominent granular layer and extensive hyperkeratosis. The inset demonstrates cells with dark condensed nuclei surrounded by a zone of cytoplasmic clearing. These koilocytic changes are viral-induced and are characteristic of HPV-related lesions of the oral cavity.

mas, but this technique plays no practical role in diagnosing squamous papilloma, determining treatment, or predicting clinical behavior.

DIFFERENTIAL DIAGNOSIS

Squamous papillomas can be distinguished from other HPV-driven exophytic squamous proliferations of the oral cavity on clinical and histopathologic grounds. Verruca vulgaris usually occurs as warty excrescences located along the vermilion border, labial mucosa, and/or the anterior tongue of children. At the microscopic level, verruca lesions tend to have a broad flat base, a prominent granular layer, and spires of hyperkeratosis and parakeratosis (Fig. 8-8). Oral condyloma is considered a sexually transmitted disease. It is most commonly seen in young adults at sites of sexual contact (e.g., labial mucosa, soft palate). It is clinically seen as clusters of pink nodules that coalesce into broad-based exophytic masses. Microscopically, its papillary fronds are broader and more blunted than the papillary projections of squamous papilloma (Fig. 8-9).

Other oral lesions that may be confused with squamous papilloma owing to a papillary growth include reactive papillary hyperplasia, progressive verrucous leukoplakias and papillary squamous cell carcinoma. The distinction between papilloma and papillary hyperplasia is best made on clinical grounds. Papillary hyperplasia is seen clinically as multiple small papillary projections that occur along points of contact with ill-fitting dentures. Progressive verrucous leukoplakias may appear histologically indistinguishable from the simple oral papilloma, but over time it manifests its true nature as a multifocal, widespread, and histologically variable process with an inexorable resolve for malignant progression. In papillary squamous cell carcinoma, the papillae are lined by overtly malignant cells.

PROGNOSIS AND THERAPY

As a benign neoplasm with a limited growth potential, the oral papilloma is cured by local excision or laser ablation. Local recurrence is uncommon and malignant transformation is exceedingly rare. Importantly, they do not share with juvenile laryngeal papillomas the penchant for multifocality, widespread growth, and rapid recurrence.

FOCAL EPITHELIAL HYPERPLASIA

Focal epithelial hyperplasia (Heck's disease) is a viral-driven benign proliferation of the oral squamous epithelium that mostly affects children and adolescents. It

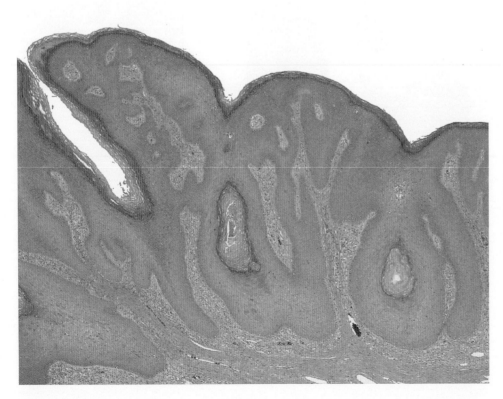

FIGURE 8-9
Oral condyloma exhibits papillary fronds that are broader and more blunted than the papillary projections of squamous papilloma.

occurs with ethnic incidence, but it is not as restricted to certain populations as was once supposed: Originally reported in American Indians and Inuits, cases involving populations from around the world are now well documented. HPV is the responsible agent, with HPV 13 and 32 being the subtypes most consistently identified.

CLINICAL FEATURES

Overall focal epithelial hyperplasia is not common, but incidence rates vary widely as a function of age and ethnicity: In certain ethnic groups, nearly 40 % of children are affected. Initially described in American Indians and Inuits, the ethic incidence of focal epithelial hyperplasia is broader than initially anticipated. It has been reported in populations from South and Central America, Africa, the Middle East, and elsewhere. In some ethnic populations, females are affected more frequently than males by a 2 : 1 ratio. Most cases involve children and adolescents, but it can sometimes occur in adults. Focal epithelial hyperplasia has been reported among adults who are HIV positive.

FOCAL EPITHELIAL HYPERPLASIA DISEASE FACT SHEET	
Definition	A localized benign simple hyperplasia of the squamous epithelium driven in part by human papillomavirus, particularly by the nononcogenic subtypes 13 and 32
Incidence and location	Very uncommon overall, but disproportionately affects certain ethnic groups
	Predilection for the labial, lingual, and buccal mucosa
Morbidity and mortality	Benign squamous proliferation with no potential for malignant progression
	Spontaneous regression is common
Gender, race, and age distribution	Female > Male (2 : 1) in some ethnic groups
	First reported in American Indians and Inuits, but now recognized in broader range of ethnic groups
	Generally considered a childhood condition
	Sometimes involves HIV-positive adults
Clinical features	Painless and asymptomatic
	Multifocal slightly raised flat papules and rounded nodules
	Individual lesions are small (<1 cm) but may coalesce to form large patches of mucosal involvement
Prognosis and treatment	Harmless lesions that often spontaneously regress
	Treatment is not necessary, but conservative surgical resection or laser ablation for cosmetic purposes is optional when lesions are few in number

FOCAL EPITHELIAL HYPERPLASIA PATHOLOGIC FEATURES	
Gross findings	Tan, soft nodules with a sessile base and smooth surface
Microscopic findings	Abrupt acanthosis (simple squamous hyperplasia) with orderly maturation
	Expansion, clubbing and fusion of the rete ridges
	Viral-induced alterations include koilocytes and a peculiar form of nuclear fragmentation resembling a mitotic figure ("mitosoid cell")

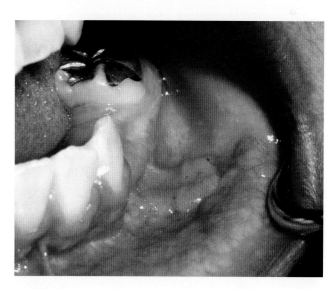

FIGURE 8-10
Focal epithelial hyperplasia involving the labial mucosa. Small, tightly packed papules merge to form larger confluent lesions.

Focal epithelial hyperplasia has a distinct clinical appearance. It is seen as multiple clustered flat-topped papules and rounded nodules that have a site predilection for the labial, lingual and buccal mucosa (Fig. 8-10). Individual papules are discrete and small (a few millimeters to 1 cm), but tightly clustered papules can merge to form large confluent lesions. The papules tend to be soft and painless.

PATHOLOGIC FEATURES

GROSS FINDINGS

Focal epithelial hyperplasia is grossly seen as tan, soft nodules with a sessile base and a smooth surface.

MICROSCOPIC FINDINGS

The hallmark histologic feature is acanthosis of the squamous epithelium (Fig. 8-11). The rete ridges are

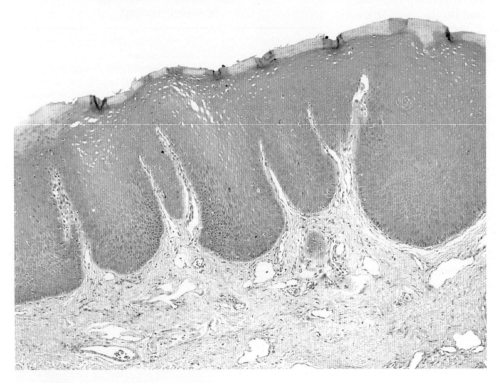

FIGURE 8-11
Low-power view showing acanthosis of the squamous epithelium with expansion and clubbing of rete ridges.

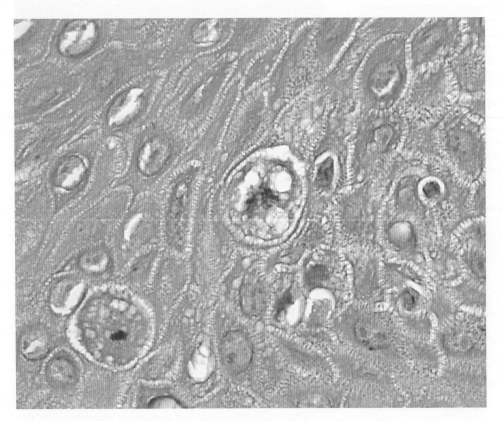

FIGURE 8-12
A high-power view of a "mitosoid cell": the pattern of nuclear fragmentation in this keratinocyte has the appearance of a mitotic figure.

expanded and often fused. The keratinocytes show orderly maturation without atypia. Parakeratosis is a common finding. Viral-induced cellular alterations are sometimes present in the superficial keratinocytes. These alterations include koilocytic changes typical of HPV infection, and a more unique type of alteration characterized by fragmentation of the nuclei in a way that resembles a mitotic figure (the so-called "mitosoid cell") (Fig. 8-12).

ANCILLARY STUDIES

The presence of HPV can be documented using a variety of detection methods ranging from electron microscopy to type-specific DNA in situ hybridization. Viral detection, however, is a matter more of academic interest than of diagnostic relevance; these techniques do not play any significant role in diagnosing focal epithelial hyperplasia or predicting its clinical behavior.

DIFFERENTIAL DIAGNOSIS

Careful correlation of the clinical and pathologic features should allow ready distinction of focal epithelial hyperplasia from other papular eruptions of the oral cavity. Condyloma acuminatum, for example, can clinically present as multifocal coalescent nodules of the oral mucosa. At the microscopic level, however, condyloma acuminatum and its family of HPV-related oral warts are characterized by a papillary growth as opposed to the simple squamous hyperplasia of focal epithelial hyperplasia.

PROGNOSIS AND THERAPY

Focal epithelial hyperplasia is a benign epithelial proliferation that often undergoes spontaneous regression. Removal of individual lesions by surgical excision or laser ablation for cosmetic purposes is feasible when a few lesions are present, but impractical when lesions are more numerous and widespread.

PYOGENIC GRANULOMA (LOBULAR CAPILLARY HEMANGIOMA)

Pyogenic granuloma is a benign acquired polypoid form of capillary hemangioma of the oral cavity that is histologically characterized by a lobular arrangement of proliferating small blood vessels. The time-honored term

pyogenic granuloma draws attention to common secondary changes including ulceration and inflammation, but the lesion is neither an infectious or granulomatous process. The alternative designation of "lobular capillary hemangioma" better reflects its true essence.

CLINICAL FEATURES

Pyogenic granuloma occurs in all age groups. Although it occurs equally in both sexes overall, some have noted an unequal gender distribution across different age groups: Patients younger than 18 years are predominantly male, patients between 18 and 39 years are predominantly female, and patients over 39 years are more evenly divided. The proportional increase in females during reproductive years reflects the contribution of hormonally driven lesions that occur during early stages of pregnancy. There is no race predominance.

The most frequently involved oral sites are the lips, gingiva, cheek, and tongue. Those lesions that arise during pregnancy almost exclusively involve the gingiva. About one-third develop following minor trauma. Bleeding is the most common clinical complaint. Lesions of the oral cavity are almost always solitary. The clinical presentation is that of a nonpainful, purple-red polypoid mass that is friable and bleeds easily (Fig. 8-13). The surface is often ulcerated and sometimes covered with an exudate. Most lesions range in size from a few millimeters to a few centimeters.

PYOGENIC GRANULOMA (LOBULAR CAPILLARY HEMANGIOMA) DISEASE FACT SHEET

Definition	An acquired polypoid form of capillary hemangioma that is histologically characterized by a lobular arrangement of proliferating vessels
Incidence and location	Common
	In the oral cavity the most frequently involved sites are the lips, gingiva, cheek, and tongue
Morbidity and mortality	Benign with no potential for invasive growth or malignant progression
Gender, race, and age distribution	Equal gender distribution
	A hormonally driven form affects a small percentage (1%) of pregnant women
	Occurs in all ages
Clinical features	Nonpainful, purple-red, polypoid mass that is friable and bleeds easily
Prognosis and treatment	Conservative local excision is usually curative, but a small percentage may locally recur if incompletely excised
	Pregnancy-associated lesions usually regress following parturition

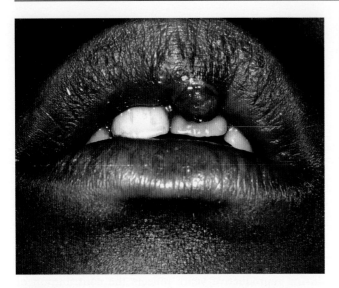

FIGURE 8-13
This pyogenic granuloma of the lip is seen as a purple polypoid nodule.

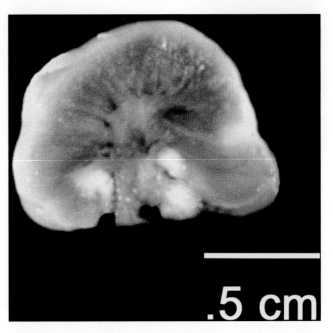

FIGURE 8-14
The cut surface of a pyogenic granuloma. An expanded cap of exuberant granulation tissue positioned on a stalk gives rise to a mushroom-like appearance.

PYOGENIC GRANULOMA (LOBULAR CAPILLARY HEMANGIOMA) PATHOLOGIC FEATURES	
Gross findings	Smooth, polypoid, pedunculated gray-tan mass
Microscopic findings	Lobular arrangement of compact capillaries around a central larger feeding vessel
	Surface ulceration with varying degrees of stromal edema, inflammation and fibrosis
Immunohistochemical features	Positive for endothelial markers including factor VIII-related antigen and CD31
Pathologic differential diagnosis	Granulation tissue, nasopharyngeal angiofibroma, aggressive vascular neoplasms (e.g., Kaposi's sarcoma, angiosarcoma, hemangiopericytoma)

PATHOLOGIC FEATURES

GROSS FINDINGS

The pyogenic granuloma is grossly seen as a polypoid often pedunculated gray-tan mass. The surface is usually ulcerated, and the presence of an underlying exuberant granulation tissue often forms a prominent cap on a narrower stalk (Fig. 8-14).

MICROSCOPIC FINDINGS

At low magnification, pyogenic granuloma is an obvious exophytic growth connected to the oral mucosa by a broad stalk that is often collared by hyperplastic squamous epithelium (Fig. 8-15). The fundamental microscopic makeup is that of a lobulated capillary hemangioma. Each lobule consists of a compact proliferation of capillaries around a central larger feeding vessel (Fig. 8-16). In the presence of ulceration, the

stroma becomes inflamed and edematous, particularly in the superficial aspect of the lesion. When these secondary stromal changes are pronounced, the lobular pattern is lost and the distinction between a lobulated capillary hemangioma and an exuberant granulation tissue is obscured. The endothelial cells lining the capillaries are often plump with an epithelioid appearance. Mitotic activity is highly variable.

ANCILLARY STUDIES

The vascular component of pyogenic granuloma is immunoreactive with endothelial markers including factor VIII-related antigen and CD31; it is not immunoreactive for epithelial markers (e.g., cytokeratin) or melanocytic markers (e.g., S-100 and HMB45). Immunohistochemical documentation of its vascular nature has diagnostic utility when the epithelioid appearance of some cellular pyogenic granulomas causes confusion with an epithelial or melanocytic neoplasm.

DIFFERENTIAL DIAGNOSIS

Pyogenic can be confused with various benign and malignant processes, particularly when there has been distortion of its typical lobular pattern. Inflammation with prominent stromal edema can be dismissed as exuberant granulation tissue. In these instances, histologic

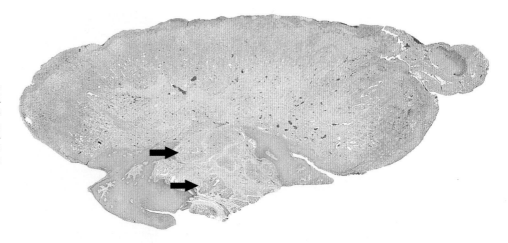

FIGURE 8-15

Low-power view showing the characteristic zonal panel. The superficial aspect of this pyogenic granuloma is ulcerated, edematous, and inflamed. The lobular proliferation of small blood vessels is best appreciated in the deeper portion of the lesion (*arrows*).

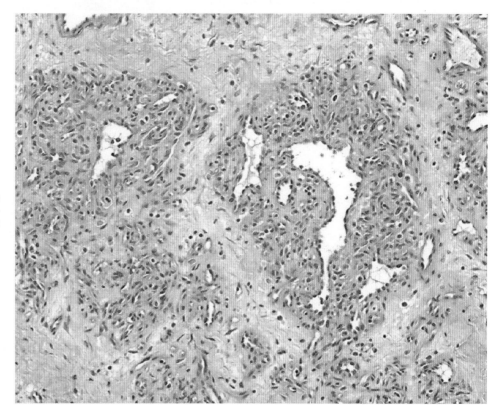

FIGURE 8-16

A high-power view of a lobule shows the compact proliferation of capillaries around a central larger feeding vessel.

examination of the deeper aspect of the lesion represents the best prospect for identifying a preserved lobular arrangement of the vessels. Prominent stromal fibrosis with separation of the blood vessels can resemble a juvenile angiofibroma. Juvenile angiofibroma, however, presents as a nasopharyngeal mass, and it lacks the capillary proliferation of pyogenic granuloma. Pyogenic granulomas with a predominant solid growth pattern and brisk mitotic activity can be mistaken for more aggressive vascular lesions, such as angiosarcoma, Kaposi's sarcoma, and hemangiopericytoma. When the endothelial cells in these solid areas take on a more epithelioid appearance, the lesion can mimic epithelioid hemangioma, angiolymphoid hyperplasia with eosinophilia, and even carcinoma or melanoma. Unlike

malignant vascular, epithelial and melanocytic tumors, pyogenic granuloma is exophytic and circumscribed without infiltration of surrounding structures.

PROGNOSIS AND THERAPY

Pyogenic granuloma is a benign vascular neoplasm with no potential for locally invasive tumor growth or metastatic spread. Conservative local excision is usually curative, but a small percentage may locally recur if incompletely excised. Pregnancy-associated lesions usually regress following parturition.

PERIPHERAL OSSIFYING FIBROMA

Peripheral ossifying fibroma is a reactive non-neoplastic proliferation of fibrous tissue with focal mineralization forming a gingival mass (*peripheral* implies non-osseous, soft tissue involvement, while *central* implies within bone).

CLINICAL FEATURES

Peripheral ossifying fibroma is a common lesion that occurs almost exclusively on the gingiva. They more commonly affect the maxilla than the mandible, and they tend to arise from the interdental papilla of the incisor/cuspid region. In some cases, a source of chronic irritation (e.g., ill-fitting dentures, orthodontics, trauma) is identified. They occur over a broad age range but cases are concentrated in teenagers and young adults. Females are affected more commonly than males at a ratio of 1.7 : 1. Peripheral ossifying fibroma appears clinically as a sessile or pedunculated nodule that ranges in size from a few millimeters to 2 cm (Fig. 8-17). The surface is ulcerated in the majority of cases.

PATHOLOGIC FEATURES

GROSS FINDINGS

The pyogenic granuloma is grossly seen as a polypoid sometimes pedunculated nodule. The surface may be intact or ulcerated.

MICROSCOPIC FINDINGS

The fundamental makeup of the peripheral ossifying fibroma is fibroblastic tissue with randomly distributed

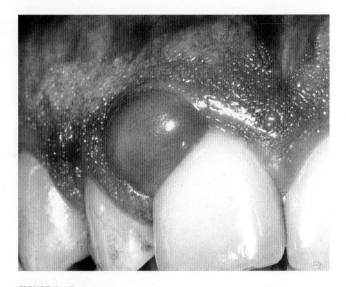

FIGURE 8-17
This peripheral ossifying fibroma is arising from the interdental papilla as a smooth, rounded, sessile nodule.

PERIPHERAL OSSIFYING FIBROMA PATHOLOGIC FEATURES	
Gross findings	Polypoid sometimes pedunculated gray-tan mass
Microscopic findings	Fibroblast proliferation with randomly distributed deposits of mineralized material (e.g., dystrophic calcifications, cementum, bone)
Pathologic differential diagnosis	Pyogenic granuloma, peripheral giant cell granuloma

deposits of mineralized material (Fig. 8-18). Variation in cellularity, extent of mineralization and type of mineralization as a result of lesion maturation gives rise to some inconstancy in its histopathologic appearance. The fibroblastic proliferation is covered by a stratified squamous epithelium, but this epithelium is often ulcerated and replaced by an inflammatory exudate. The overall cellularity of the fibroblastic component varies according to the relative proportion of plump fibroblasts and stromal collagen. The nature of the mineralized material varies from dystrophic calcification to cementum-like material to well-formed bone (Fig. 8-19). Multinucleated giant cells may be present, but they are never numerous.

DIFFERENTIAL DIAGNOSIS

Peripheral ossifying fibroma can be confused with other fibrous lesions of the gingiva. Ulcerated lesions without conspicuous mineralization may be confused with pyogenic granuloma. A thorough microscopic examination

PERIPHERAL OSSIFYING FIBROMA DISEASE FACT SHEET	
Definition	A reactive, non-neoplastic proliferation of fibrous tissue with mineralized material forming a gingival mass
Incidence and location	Common
	Almost exclusively involve the gingiva, usually arising from the interdental papilla
Morbidity and mortality	Reactive process with no malignant potential
Gender, race, and age distribution	More common in females
	Peak incidence in the 2nd decade
Clinical features	Sessile or pedunculated nodule that ranges in size from a few millimeters to 2 cm
	Surface ulceration is common
Prognosis and treatment	Local surgical excision down to periosteum
	Can recur locally

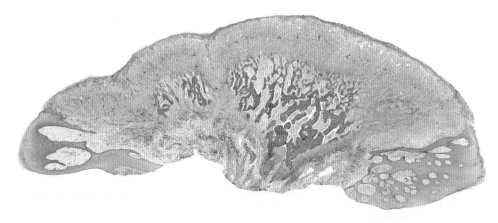

FIGURE 8-18

A low-power view demonstrates an exophytic mass of exuberant fibro-connective tissue emanating from a central nidus of mineralization. There is ulceration of the overlying epithelium.

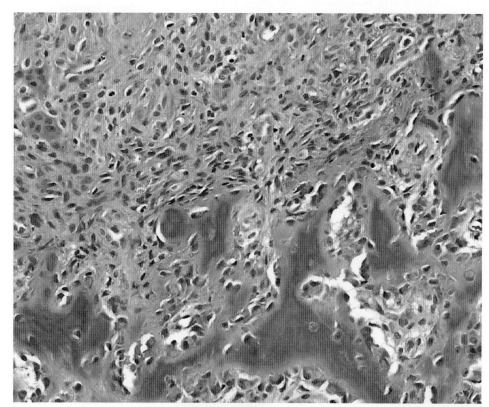

FIGURE 8-19

A higher power view shows the mineralized component to be made up of reactive newly formed bone.

is usually sufficient in establishing a diagnosis of peripheral ossifying fibroma by demonstrating the presence of focal mineralized deposits and the absence of a lobular proliferation of capillaries. Individual or clustered multinucleated giant cells are present in a subset of peripheral ossifying fibromas, but they are not nearly as numerous as the multinucleated giant cells of peripheral giant cell granuloma.

PROGNOSIS AND THERAPY

Even though a reactive non-neoplastic process, approximately 16% of peripheral ossifying fibromas recur following local surgical excision. Aggressive excision down to periosteum along with the removal of any chronic

irritant is recommended as a means of minimizing the risk of local recurrence.

PERIPHERAL GIANT CELL GRANULOMA

Peripheral giant cell granuloma is a reactive proliferation caused by chronic irritation of the gingival mucosa. It is microscopically seen as an exuberant proliferation of multinucleated giant cells. The traditional term, *peripheral giant cell reparative granuloma,* is inaccurate as the multinucleated giant cells have little if any capacity for local tissue reparation. *Peripheral* implies soft tissue involvement, while *central* implies an intraosseous location.

CLINICAL FEATURES

Peripheral giant cell granuloma is a relatively common exophytic lesion of the oral cavity. They occur over a broad age range, but most patients are between 40–60 years. Females are affected slightly more often than males. The peripheral giant cell granuloma presumably arises from the periodontal ligament, and thus occurs exclusively on the gingiva, usually between the permanent molars and incisors. The mandible and maxilla are involved at an almost equal frequency. Peripheral giant cell granuloma classically presents as solitary broad-based reddish-blue polypoid nodule (Fig. 8-20). The surface epithelium is frequently ulcerated. It varies in size, but it generally does not exceed 2–3 centimeters.

PERIPHERAL GIANT CELL GRANULOMA DISEASE FACT SHEET

Definition	An exuberant reactive proliferation of multinucleated giant cells forming a gingival mass
Incidence and location	Relatively common
	Almost exclusively involves the gingiva
Morbidity and mortality	Reactive process with no malignant potential
Gender, race, and age distribution	More common in females
	Most patients 40–60 yr
Clinical features	Reddish-blue rubbery nodules that range in size from a few millimeters to 2 cm
	Surface ulceration is common
Prognosis and treatment	Local surgical excision down to bone
	Can recur locally

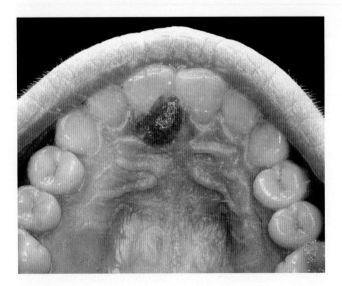

FIGURE 8-20

This peripheral giant cell granuloma is arising from the gingiva as a broad-based reddish-blue polypoid nodule.

RADIOLOGIC FEATURES

Unlike central giant cell granuloma, the peripheral giant cell granuloma does not arise within the craniofacial bones. Nonetheless, the peripheral giant cell granuloma can occasionally induce focal resorption of underlying alveolar bone giving rise to a superficial cup-shaped radiolucency.

PATHOLOGIC FEATURES

GROSS FINDINGS

The peripheral giant cell granuloma grossly appears as a soft to rubbery broad-based polypoid nodule that measures a few millimeters up to 3 cm. Its surface tends to be smooth.

MICROSCOPIC FINDINGS

The eye-catching feature on microscopic examination is the multinucleated giant cells (Figs. 8-21, 8-22). They are abundantly present and dominate the microscopic picture. The relationship of these cells to true osteoclasts is unclear, but they certainly are osteoclast-like in their appearance having an abundant cytoplasm that houses up to 100 nuclei (Fig. 8-23). The multinucleated giant cells are interspersed among spindled to oval mononuclear cells. Secondary background features include hemorrhage, hemosiderin deposition, chronic inflammation, and islands of metaplastic bone.

DIFFERENTIAL DIAGNOSIS

There are a handful of lesions that closely resemble the peripheral giant cell granuloma in their histologic

PERIPHERAL GIANT CELL GRANULOMA PATHOLOGIC FEATURES

Gross findings	Broad-based rubbery polypoid nodule with smooth surface
Microscopic findings	Histologic picture dominated by multinucleated giant cells admixed with mononuclear stromal cells
	Background features include hemorrhage, hemosiderin deposition, chronic inflammation, and islands of metaplastic bone
Pathologic differential diagnosis	Other giant cell rich tumors include central giant cell tumor, brown tumor of hyperparathyroidism, and cherubism

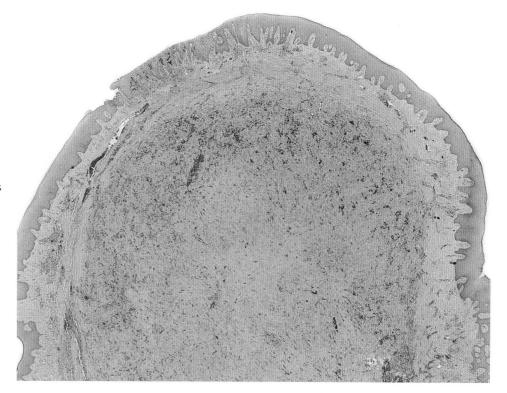

FIGURE 8-21

The proliferation of giant cells forms a submucosal nodule.

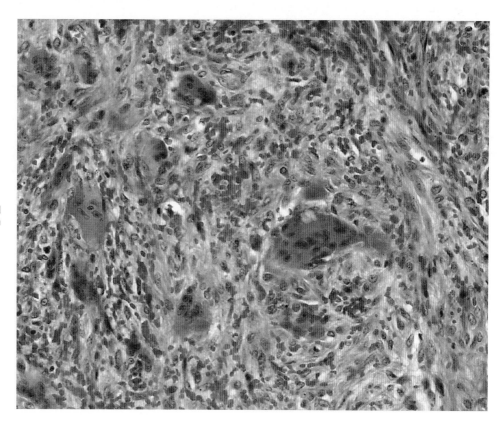

FIGURE 8-22

The giant cells are interspersed among stromal mononuclear cells in a hemorrhagic background.

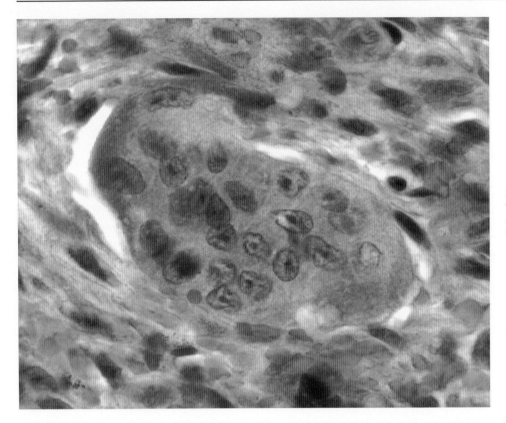

FIGURE 8-23
The giant cells have an abundant cytoplasm that houses numerous nuclei.

appearance. These include central giant cell granuloma, brown tumor of hyperparathyroidism, and cherubism. In contrast to peripheral giant cell granuloma, these occur within the craniofacial bones. Thus, the radiographic features and clinical findings are essential when it comes to sorting out the various giant cell-rich lesions of the oral cavity.

PROGNOSIS AND THERAPY

The standard treatment of the peripheral giant cell granuloma is excision down to bone. Failure to include the periosteum or periodontal ligament is believed to risk local recurrence, which occurs in about 10% of lesions. Efforts should be taken to identify and remove any source of chronic irritation.

CONGENITAL GRANULAR CELL EPULIS

Congenital granular cell epulis is a rare benign mesenchymal tumor comprised of large cells with coarse granular cytoplasm. It classically arises from the anterior alveolar ridge of the newborn. Its cell of origin remains elusive, and it is not to be regarded as the congenital counterpart of the Schwann cell-derived adult granular cell tumor.

CLINICAL FEATURES

Congenital granular cell epulis is a rare tumor that occurs almost exclusively in newborns. Females are

CONGENITAL GRANULAR CELL EPULIS DISEASE FACT SHEET	
Definition	A benign mesenchymal tumor arising from the anterior alveolar ridge of the newborn and comprised of large cells with course granular cytoplasm
Incidence and location	Rare
	Almost exclusively involve the alveolar ridge with a distinct preference for gingiva overlying the future canine and lateral incisor teeth
	The maxilla is involved more commonly than the mandible
Morbidity and mortality	Obstructive masses may cause difficulty with respiration and feeding
Gender, race, and age distribution	Female >>> Male (F : M = 9 : 1)
	Newborns
Clinical features	Smooth nonulcerated polypoid masses with a broad-based attachment to the alveolar ridge
Prognosis and treatment	Stop growing at birth and often regress over time
	Local conservative resection is curative
	Do not recur

affected much more commonly than males at a ratio of about 9 : 1. Congenital granular cell epulis is a lesion of the alveolar ridge with a particular predilection for the gingiva overlying the future canine and lateral incisor teeth. The maxilla is involved more commonly than the mandible. They tend to be seen as smooth nonulcerated polypoid masses with a broad-based attachment to the alveolar ridge (Fig. 8-24). The bone and teeth are un-involved. Most lesions measure about 1 cm, but they can achieve sizes over 5 cm. Affected newborns often present with a mass protruding from the oral cavity. Mechanical obstruction can cause problems with feeding and respiration.

PATHOLOGIC FEATURES

GROSS FINDINGS

Congenital granular cell epulis is typically seen as a tan-pink polypoid mass with a smooth nonulcerated surface. The cut surface is homogenous, firm, and tan to yellow.

MICROSCOPIC FINDINGS

The congenital granular cell epulis is composed of the unique granular cell (Fig. 8-25). These cells are charac-terized by an abundance of eosinophilic granular cyto-plasm. The granular cells grow in a sheet-like pattern supported by delicate fibrovascular septa (Fig. 8-26). Incorporation of odontogenic epithelium is sometimes seen. The overlying surface epithelium is usually intact without hyperplastic changes.

CONGENITAL GRANULAR CELL EPULIS PATHOLOGIC FEATURES	
Gross findings	Tan-pink polypoid mass with a smooth nonulcerated surface
Microscopic findings	Submucosal proliferation of cells with abundant eosinophilic granular cytoplasm.
Immunohistochemical features	Absence of S-100 protein staining, in contrast to adult granular cell tumors
Pathologic differential diagnosis	Adult granular cell tumor, alveolar soft part sarcoma, rhabdomyoma

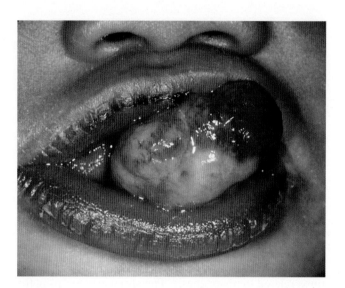

FIGURE 8-24
This congenital granular cell epulis arises from the alveolar ridge of the maxilla and emanates from the oral cavity as a large polypoid mass.

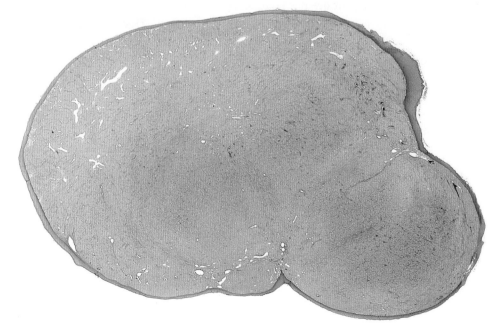

FIGURE 8-25
Low-power view showing sheets of granular cells filling the submucosa.

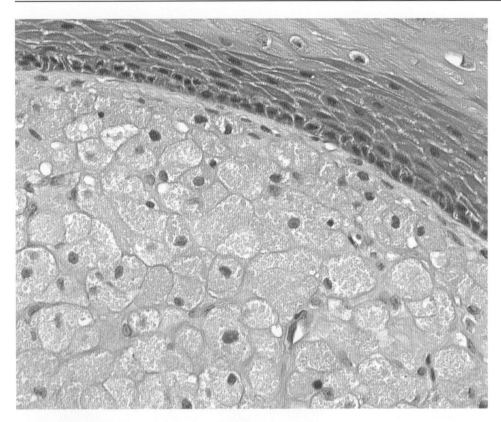

FIGURE 8-26
Higher power view demonstrating the abundant pink granular cytoplasm of the granular cells.

ANCILLARY STUDIES

Immunohistochemical studies have focused on questions related to histogenesis. The absence of staining for muscle markers, epithelial markers, and neural markers points to origin from some uncommitted mesenchymal cell. Notably, the lack of S-100 protein staining has supported the argument that, histologic similarities aside, the congenital granular epulis, and the Schwann cell-derived granular cell tumor are not related.

DIFFERENTIAL DIAGNOSIS

The granular cells in congenital granular cell epulis and granular cell tumor are microscopically identical, but they should not be regarded as equivalent tumors. In contrast to congenital granular cell epulis, granular cell tumors usually affect adults, have a site predilection for the tongue, are immunoreactive for S-100 protein, and are associated with hyperplasia of the overlying epithelium (i.e., pseudoepitheliomatous hyperplasia). Other pink cell tumors that can involve the oral cavity include alveolar soft part sarcoma and rhabdomyoma, but these rarely cause diagnostic confusion when the histologic picture is considered together with the age of the patient and location of the mass.

PROGNOSIS AND THERAPY

The tumor stops growing at birth and regresses over time. Complete regression without therapy has been reported. Most tumors are surgically excised. As they do not recur even following incomplete removal, surgical excision should be conservative.

TERATOMA

Teratoma is a neoplasm comprised of an admixture of tissue types reflecting contributions from all three germ cell layers. Oral teratomas presumably arise from pluripotential cells displaced during embryogenesis.

CLINICAL FEATURES

Less than 5% of teratomas involve head and neck sites. Of these head and neck teratomas, the cervical soft tissues and nasopharynx are the most commonly targeted sites. Teratomas of the oral cavity and oropharynx tend to arise from the tongue, palate and palatine tonsils. The vast majority of oral and oropharyngeal teratomas are present at birth, and most can be detected in the prenatal period. Common prenatal findings include

TERATOMA DISEASE FACT SHEET	
Definition	A benign neoplasm of the newborn and infant that is comprised of an admixture of tissue types reflecting contributions from all three germ cell layers
Incidence and location	Very rare
	Only about 5% of teratomas involve head and neck sites
	In the head and neck, teratomas of the nasopharynx and cervical soft tissues are more common than those arising in the oral cavity and oropharynx
Morbidity and mortality	Obstructive masses may cause difficulty with feeding and respiration
	Death, when it occurs, is usually related to airway obstruction
Gender, race, and age distribution	Equal gender distribution
	Newborns and infants
Clinical features	Prenatal: Elevated maternal α-fetoprotein, polyhydramnios, fetal facial mass
	Perinatal: Bosselated tumor mass projecting from oral cavity and ranging in size from 1–13 cm
Radiographic findings	Heterogeneous and multiloculated mass with calcifications
Prognosis and treatment	Benign in the pediatric population
	The exceptional teratoma that occurs in an adult should be regarded as malignant
	Prenatal detection is critical in a planned delivery that includes protection of the airway
	Complete resection is curative

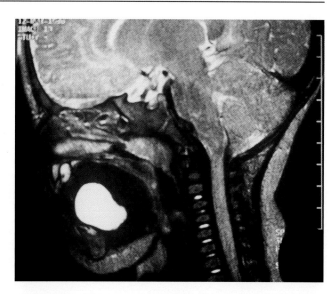

FIGURE 8-27
This teratoma of the tongue is seen by T2-weighted MRI as a rounded mass of high-signal intensity.

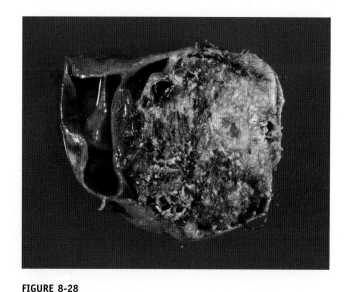

FIGURE 8-28
The cut surface of a teratoma reveals a solid and cystic mass. Abundant hair and sebaceous material is evident.

an elevated maternal α-fetoprotein, polyhydramnios, and a heterogeneous solid and cystic facial mass by ultrasound. There is an equal sex distribution. Tumor size is highly variable ranging from a few centimeters to 13 cm. Morbidity and mortality is primarily a function of size and location. Teratomas of the oral cavity and oropharynx are often associated with feeding difficulty. Large bulky tumors can cause airway obstruction resulting in respiratory distress and even death.

RADIOLOGIC FEATURES

Teratomas of the oral cavity and oropharynx have the same radiographic appearance as teratomas arising in nonoral sites. Imaging studies demonstrate a rounded, often lobulated heterogeneous mass containing soft tissue elements with fluid and fat attenuation (Fig. 8-27). Calcification is a frequent finding. Computed tomography is most suitable for demonstrating its intrinsic elements including soft tissue, fat, fluid, and calcification.

PATHOLOGIC FEATURES

GROSS FINDINGS

Like teratomas in other sites, teratomas of the head and neck are often bulky masses with smooth and bosselated external surfaces. On cut section, the common presence of hemorrhage, necrosis, calcification, cyst formation, and multiloculations gives rise to a highly complex and variegated appearance (Fig. 8-28).

MICROSCOPIC FINDINGS

The histologic composition of teratomas is highly variable and includes somatic tissue derivatives from all three germ cell layers (i.e., ectoderm, endoderm, and mesoderm). A teratoma can harbor any combination of cartilage, bone, fat, muscle, neural tissue, adnexal structures, gastrointestinal epithelium, respiratory epithelium, and other assorted tissue types (Figs. 8-29, 8-30). These tissues may appear mature (i.e., adult-like) or immature (i.e., embryo-like). The presence of immature elements does not signify malignant transformation. Hemorrhage and necrosis may be seen.

DIFFERENTIAL DIAGNOSIS

Developmental errors resulting in an oral mass is not restricted to teratomas. Lingual thyroid, dermoid cysts, hairy polyps, and heterotopic glial tissue are also characterized by abnormally placed somatic tissues within the oral cavity and oropharynx. The absence of derivatives from all three germ cell layers is critical in distinguishing these developmental inclusions from teratomas.

PROGNOSIS AND THERAPY

Teratomas in the pediatric population are uniformly benign, even those tumors that harbor immature elements. Although they have no malignant potential, morbidity may be high depending on the size and location of the mass. Death is usually related to airway obstruction, a complication that is more likely with cervical and nasopharyngeal teratomas than with oral teratomas. Prenatal diagnosis has vastly improved perinatal outcome by permitting a coordinated delivery with emphasis on airway management. Surgical resection is curative, and tumors do not recur when removal is complete.

On very rare occasions, a teratoma may arise in the head and neck region of an adult. Unlike teratomas of newborns and infants, these are biologically aggressive tumors that are usually malignant.

TERATOMA PATHOLOGIC FEATURES	
Gross findings	External surface: Smooth, bosselated, multilobated
	Cut surface: Solid and cystic with hemorrhage, necrosis, and calcification
Microscopic findings	Haphazard admixture of mature and/or immature tissue types from all three germ cell layers (ectoderm, mesoderm, endoderm)
Pathologic differential diagnosis	Developmental inclusions including lingual thyroid, glial heterotopia, hairy polyps, and dermoid cysts

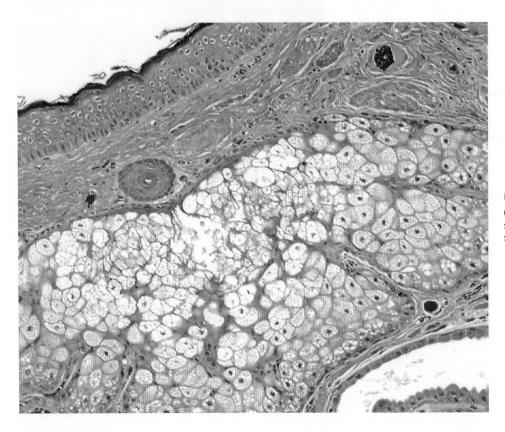

FIGURE 8-29

Cysts are lined by hair follicles and sebaceous glands resembling normal skin.

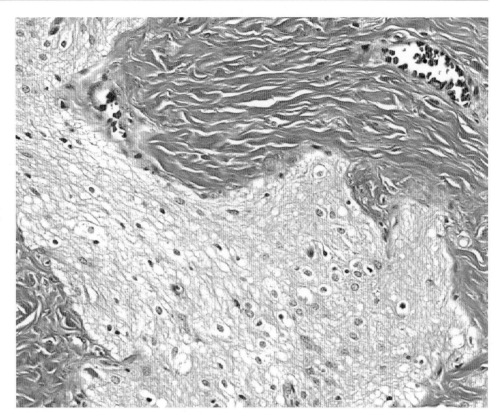

FIGURE 8-30
Additional somatic tissues including glial tissue were present in other areas of the teratoma.

SUGGESTED READING

Fibroma

1. Neville BW, Damm DD, Allen CM, Bouquot JE: Soft tissue tumors. In: Neville BW, Damm DD, Allen CM, Bouquot JE. Oral and Maxillofacial Pathology, 2nd ed. New York: WB Saunders, 2002:437–479.
2. Regezi, JA, Sciubba JJ, Jordan RCK: Connective tissue lesions. In: Regezi, JA, Sciubba JJ, Jordan RCK. Oral Pathology: Clinical Pathologic Correlations, 4th ed. St. Louis: Saunders, 2003:157–181.
3. Yeatts D, Burns JC: Common oral mucosal lesions in adults. Am Fam Physician 1991;44:2043–2050.

Squamous Papilloma (Including Verruca and Condyloma)

1. Abbey LM, Page DG, Sawyer DR: The clinical and histopathologic features of a series of 464 oral squamous cell papillomas. Oral Surg Oral Med Oral Pathol 1980;49:419–428.
2. Garlick JA, Taichman LB: Human papillomavirus of the oral mucosa. Am J Dermatopathol 1991;13:386–395.
3. Greer R, Goldman H: Oral papillomas. Oral Surg Oral Med Oral Pathol 1974;38:435–440.
4. Odell EW: Papilloma. In: Barnes EL, Eveson JW, Reichart P, Sidransky D, eds. Pathology and Genetics of Head and Neck Tumours. Kleihues P, Sobin LH, series eds. World Health Organization Classification of Tumours. Lyon, France: IARC Press, 2005:182–184.
5. Regezi, JA, Sciubba JJ, Jordan RCK: Connective tissue lesions. In: Regezi, JA, Sciubba JJ, Jordan RCK. Oral Pathology: Clinical Pathologic Correlations, 4th edition. St. Louis: Saunders, 2003:157–181.

Focal Epithelial Hyperplasia

1. Archard HO, Heck JW, Stanley HR: Focal epithelial hyperplasia: an unusual oral mucosal lesion found in Indian children. Oral Surg Oral Med Oral Pathol 1965;20:201–212.
2. Carlos RB, Sedano HO: Multifocal papilloma virus epithelial hyperplasia. Oral Surg Oral Med Oral Pathol 1994;77:631–635.
3. Moerman M, Danielides VG, Nousia CS, et al.: Recurrent focal epithelial hyperplasia due to HPV13 in an HIV-positive patient. Dermatology 2001;203:339–341.

4. Odell EW: Papillary hyperplasia. In: Barnes EL, Eveson JW, Reichart P, Sidransky D, eds. Pathology and Genetics of Head and Neck Tumours. Kleihues P, Sobin LH, series eds. World Health Organization Classification of Tumours. Lyon, France: IARC Press, 2005:189.
5. Padayachee A, van Wyk CW: Human papillomavirus (HPV) DNA in focal epithelial hyperplasia by in situ hybridization. J Oral Pathol Med 1991;20:210–214.

Pyogenic Granuloma (Lobular Capillary Hemangioma)

1. Bhaskar SN, Jacoway JR: Pyogenic granuloma: clinical features, incidence, histology and result of treatment—report of 242 cases. J Oral Surg 1966;24:391–398.
2. Kapadia SB, Heffner DK: Pitfalls in the histopathologic diagnosis of pyogenic granuloma. Eur Arch Otorhinolaryngol 1992;249:195–200.
3. Mills SE, Cooper PH, Fechner RE: Lobular capillary hemangioma: the underlying lesion of pyogenic granuloma: a study of 73 cases from the oral and nasal membranes. Am J Surg Pathol 1980;4:471–479.

Peripheral Ossifying Fibroma

1. Buchner A, Hansen LS: The histomorphologic spectrum of peripheral ossifying fibroma. Oral Surg Oral Med Oral Pathol 1987;63:452–461.
2. Gardner DG: The peripheral odontogenic fibroma: an attempt at clarification. Oral Surg Oral Med Oral Pathol 1982;54:40–48.
3. Kendrick F, Waggoner WF: Managing a peripheral ossifying fibroma. ASDC J Dent Child 1996;63:135–138.
4. Zain RB, Fei YJ: Fibrous lesions of the gingiva: a histopathologic analysis of 204 cases. Oral Surg Oral Med Oral Pathol 1990;70:466–470.

Peripheral Giant Cell Granuloma

1. Katsikeris N, Kakarantza-Angelopoulou E, Angelopoulos AP: Peripheral giant cell granuloma. Clinicopathologic study of 224 cases and review of 956 reported cases. Int J Oral Maxillofac Surg 1988;17:94–99.
2. Neville BW, Damm DD, Allen CM, Bouquot JE: Soft tissue tumors. In: Neville BW, Damm DD, Allen CM, Bouquot JE. Oral and Maxillofacial Pathology, 2nd ed. New York: WB Saunders, 2002:437–479.

Congenital Granular Cell Epulis

1. Filie AC, Lage JM, Azumi N: Immunoreactivity of S100 protein, alpha-1-antitrypsin, and CD68 in adult and congenital granular cell tumors. Mod Pathol 1996;9:888–892.
2. Lack EE, Worsham GF, Callihan MD, et al.: Gingival granula cell tumors of the newborn (congenital "epulis"): a clinical and pathologic study of 21 patients. Am J Surg Pathol 1981;5:37–46.
3. Lapid O, Shaco-Levy R, Krieger Y, et al.: Congential epulis. Pediatrics 2001;107:E22.
4. Speight PM: Granular cell tumour. In: Barnes EL, Eveson JW, Reichart P, Sidransky D, eds. Pathology and Genetics of Head and Neck Tumours. Kleihues P, Sobin LH, series eds. World Health Organization Classification of Tumours. Lyon, France: IARC Press, 2005:185–186.
5. van der Waal I: Congenital granular cell epulis. In: Barnes EL, Eveson JW, Reichart P, Sidransky D, eds. Pathology and Genetics of Head and Neck Tumours. Kleihues P, Sobin LH, series eds. World Health Organization Classification of Tumours. Lyon, France: IARC Press, 2005:198.
6. Zuker RM, Buenechea R: Congenital epulis: review of the literature and case report. J Oral Maxillofac Surg 1993;51:1040–1043.

Teratoma

1. Lalwani AK, Engel TL: Teratoma of the tongue: a case report and review of the literature. Int J Pediatr Otorhinolaryngol 1992;24:261–268.
2. McMahon MJ, Chescheir NC, Kuller JA, et al.: Perinatal management of a lingual teratoma. Obstet Gynecol 1996;87:848–851.
3. Mills SE, Gaffey JM, Frierson HF: Germ cell tumors. In: Mills SE, Gaffey JM, Frierson HF. Atlas of Tumor Pathology: Tumors of the Upper Aerodigestive Tract and Ear, 3rd series. Washington, DC: Armed Forces Institute of Pathology, 1997:313–318.
4. Sharma AK, Sharma CS, Gupta AK, et al.: Teratomas in pediatric age group: experience with 75 cases. Indian Pediatr 1993;30:689–694.

9 Malignant Neoplasms of the Oral Cavity and Oropharynx

William Westra

SQUAMOUS CELL CARCINOMA

Squamous cell carcinoma (SCC) of the oral cavity and oropharynx is a malignant neoplasm that arises from the surface epithelium lining this region. It is a heterogeneous disease with distinct patterns of exposure, presentation, and behavior. From an epidemiological and clinicopathologic viewpoint, "oral cancer" can be divided into squamous cell carcinoma of the lip vermilion, the oral cavity proper, and the oropharynx.

CLINICAL FEATURES

Squamous cell carcinoma is by far the most common form of carcinoma to involve the oral cavity and oropharynx, accounting for more than 90% of the 28,900 cases of oral cancer that are diagnosed in the United States each year. Most occur in patients older than 50 years. Men are more commonly affected than women at a ratio of about 3 : 1. The incidence of oral cancer is higher among blacks than whites.

Carcinogen exposure, diet, infectious agents, and preexisting medical conditions may all play a role, individually or in combination, in the development of oral cancer (i.e., SCC of the oral cavity and oropharynx). Tobacco is the most important risk factor. Depending on the number of cigarettes smoked, the risk of developing oral cancer is 5 to 17 times greater for smokers than for nonsmokers. Though less substantial, snuff and chewing tobacco have also been associated with an increased risk for oral cancer. In some parts of the world, chronic use of betel quid takes the place of cigarettes as the most relevant risk factor. The association of marijuana use and oral cancer among young adults awaits further clarification. Alcohol consumption is an independent risk factor, but it is most significant for the way in which it potentiates the carcinogenic activity of tobacco. There is an inverse association between consumption of fruits and vegetables and the incidence of oral cancer, likely reflecting the protective effects of dietary carotenoids. Chronic sun exposure is strongly associated with the development of carcinoma at the lip vermilion. The human papillomavirus (HPV), particularly the tumorogenic 16 subtype, plays a causative role

SQUAMOUS CELL CARCINOMA DISEASE FACT SHEET	
Definition	A malignant neoplasm arising from the squamous epithelium lining the oral cavity and oropharynx
Incidence and location	The most common malignancy of the oral cavity and oropharynx
	Over 25,000 cases diagnosed in the United States each year
	For the oral cavity proper, squamous cell carcinoma most commonly arise from the lip, followed by the tongue, floor of mouth, gingiva, palate, and buccal mucosa
	For the oropharynx, most squamous cell carcinomas from the tonsils followed by the base of the tongue
Morbidity and mortality	Although anatomic site, tumor stage and many other factors affect outcome, the overall 5-yr survival rate for oral cancer as a group is 50%–55%
Gender, race, and age distribution	Male > Female (~3 : 1)
	Most patients > 50 yr
	Higher incidence among blacks than whites
Clinical features	Early premalignant changes are visible as white (leukoplakia) or red (erythroplakia) mucosal patches
	Invasive carcinomas range from depressed ulcerated lesions to fungating masses
	30% of patients have metastatic spread to regional lymph nodes at the time of initial evaluation
Prognosis and treatment	Tumor stage has a dramatic impact on outcome and therapy
	Surgery and/or radiation therapy is standard treatment for limited stage cancers
	Surgery with adjuvant radiation therapy is standard therapy for more advanced stage disease
	Patients with advanced stage disease may also benefit from the addition of chemotherapy

in the development of most oropharyngeal carcinomas, but in only a small percentage of head and neck carcinomas arising in nonoropharyngeal sites. Patients with underlying medical conditions causing immunosuppression (e.g., AIDS), chromosomal fragility or defects

263

in chromosomal repair (e.g., Fanconi's anemia) are at increased risk of developing oral cancer.

Carcinoma of the oral cavity most commonly arise from the lip, followed by the tongue, floor of mouth, gingiva, palate, and buccal mucosa. Oropharyngeal carcinomas usually arise from the tonsils and the base of the tongue. The clinical presentation is largely dependent on tumor site and stage. Invasive oral cancers are generally preceded by clinically visible but asymptomatic premalignant alterations of the oral mucosa known as leukoplakia and erythroplakia. During cancer progression, these patches of mucosal alterations may evolve into expanding nonhealing ulcers. Tumor invasion is heralded by bleeding, loosening of teeth, dysphagia, dysarthria, odynophagia, or a palpable neck mass.

Leukoplakia is a clinical term that refers to a white patch in the oral cavity (Fig. 9-1). Leukoplakia varies in thickness, and its surface features range from granular, to nodular to fissured. Erythroplakia is a clinical term that refers to a red patch of the oral mucosa (Fig. 9-2). It tends to have a soft and velvety appearance. These white and red lesions are sometimes, but not always, associated with histologic evidence of premalignant or malignant changes. Erythroplakia is much more likely than leukoplakia to be associated with dysplasia or carcinoma.

The clinical appearance of invasive carcinomas is highly variable, ranging from depressed ulcerated lesions to fungating masses (Fig. 9-3). The presence of a neck mass ominously points to metastatic spread to regional lymph nodes. Approximately 30% of patients with oral cancers have regional spread at the time of initial evaluation. Metastases most frequently involve the ipsilateral cervical lymph nodes; but advanced tumors, tumors near the midline, and some base of tongue tumors can involve contralateral or bilateral cervical lymph nodes. Involved lymph nodes tend to be

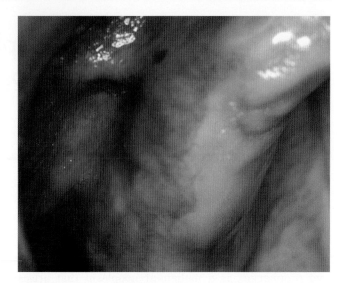

FIGURE 9-2
This patch of erythroplakia is seen as a subtle red lesion of the buccal mucosa. (Courtesy of Dr. J. Sciubba.)

enlarged, firm, and nontender. Fixation to the skin and surrounding soft tissues indicates tumor extension beyond the capsule of the lymph node.

RADIOLOGIC FEATURES

Radiologic evaluation is primarily used for staging purposes. Either computed tomography or magnetic resonance imaging is routinely performed to determine the extent of local invasion (Fig. 9-4) and the presence of metastatic spread to regional lymph nodes.

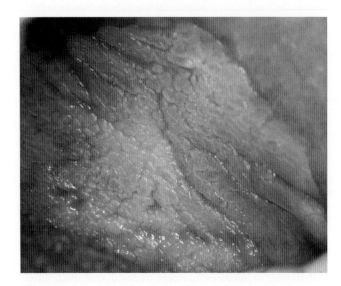

FIGURE 9-1
This patch of leukoplakia is seen as a white cobblestone thickening of the buccal mucosa. (Courtesy of Dr. J. Sciubba.)

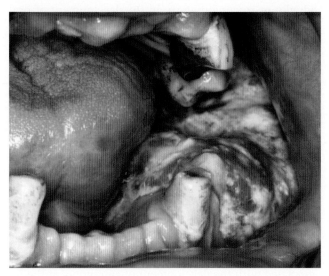

FIGURE 9-3
A large fungating mass of the alveolar ridge and floor of mouth.

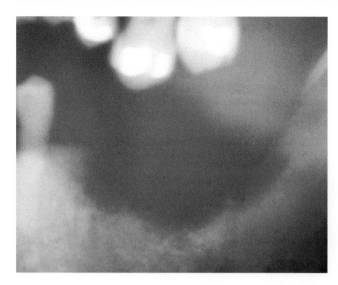

FIGURE 9-4
A radiograph helps discern the depth of invasion. In this case, there is invasion of the mandible.

PATHOLOGIC FEATURES

GROSS FINDINGS

Surgically excised specimens range from small mucosal biopsies of leukoplakia and erythroplakia to large and complex composite resections of high-stage SCC. The gross appearance, in turn, varies from subtle grayish white thickening of the mucosa to large ulcerative, flat, or fungating masses with infiltration of local structures (Fig. 9-5). Depending on the degree of desmoplasia and tumor necrosis, the cut surface of invasive tumors ranges from solid and firm to cystic and friable.

MICROSCOPIC FINDINGS

Oral dysplasia refers to neoplastic alterations of the surface epithelium prior to invasion of the subepithelial connective tissues. These changes include abnormal cellular organization, increased mitotic activity, and nuclear enlargement with pleomorphism. These alterations are typically graded on a scale of 1 to 3 based on the severity of the atypia. Although terminology varies, atypia limited to the lower one-third of the epithelium is generally referred to as mild dysplasia (Fig. 9-6), atypia limited to the lower two-thirds of the epithelium as moderate dysplasia (Fig. 9-7), and atypia involving the full thickness of the epithelium as severe dysplasia/carcinoma in situ (Fig. 9-8).

With progression, the carcinoma in situ breaks through the basement membrane and infiltrates the subepithelial connective tissue as cohesive nests and cords. With advanced tumor growth, nests of invasive tumor invade skeletal muscle, craniofacial bones, and facial skin (Fig. 9-9). Invasion may be associated with tumor extension along nerves (i.e., perineural invasion) and involvement of lymphatic spaces. Tumor grade

SQUAMOUS CELL CARCINOMA PATHOLOGIC FEATURES	
Gross findings	Subtle grayish white thickening of the mucosa to large ulcerative, flat, or fungating masses
Microscopic findings	**Premalignant (noninvasive) stage (dysplasia):** Atypical epithelial alterations limited to the surface squamous epithelium and including abnormal cellular organization, increased mitotic activity, and nuclear enlargement with pleomorphism **Malignant (invasive) stage:** Infiltrating nests and cords of cells showing varying degrees of squamous differentiation (pink cytoplasm, intercellular bridges and keratin pearl formation) Desmoplastic stromal reaction including stromal fibrosis and chronic inflammation Variants characterized by a verrucous pattern of growth (verrucous carcinoma), a papillary pattern of growth (papillary variant), spindling of the tumor cells (spindle cell variant) and a prominent basaloid appearance of the tumor cells (basaloid squamous cell carcinoma)
Fine needle aspiration	Atypical squamous cells in a background of keratinaceous debris and necrotic cystic debris
Immunohistochemical features	Immunoreactivity for epithelial markers (e.g., cytokeratin)
Pathologic differential diagnosis	Pseudoepitheliomatous hyperplasia, necrotizing sialometaplasia, malignant melanoma, verrucous hyperplasia, sarcomas, squamous papilloma, solid variant of adenoid cystic

varies from well differentiated to moderately differentiated to poorly differentiated. Well-differentiated carcinomas usually demonstrate obvious squamous differentiation in the form interconnecting nests of cells with pink cytoplasm, intercellular bridges and keratin pearl formation. At the other extreme, poorly differentiated tumors demonstrated little or no apparent squamous differentiation. Regardless of tumor grade, nests of infiltrating SCC tend to elicit a prominent host reaction in the form of fibrosis and chronic inflammation.

Certain variants of SCC depart from the typical appearance of conventional SCC.

1. *Verrucous carcinoma* is seen clinically as an exophytic mass with a warty or papillary surface, and histologically as a markedly thickened squamous epithelium with "church spires" of parakerototic squamous cells (Fig. 9-10). In contrast to conventional SCC, verrucous carcinoma invades as a burrowing mass with broad pushing borders, it lacks any significant atypia, and it has little to no potential to metastasize.

2. The *papillary variant* is characterized by a prominent exophytic component of papillary growth

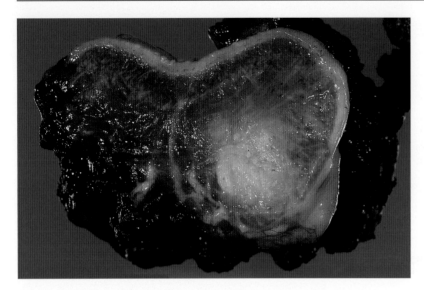

FIGURE 9-5

A base of tongue squamous cell carcinoma results in a large mass infiltrating into the muscle of the tongue. (Courtesy of Dr. J. Ohara.)

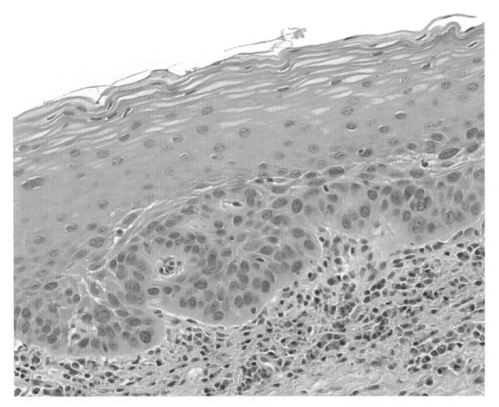

FIGURE 9-6

Dysplasia of the oral cavity are graded: in mild dysplasia, the atypical changes are limited to the lower one-third of the epithelium.

FIGURE 9-7

Dysplasia of the oral cavity are graded: in moderate dysplasia, the alterations are limited to the lower two-thirds of the epithelium.

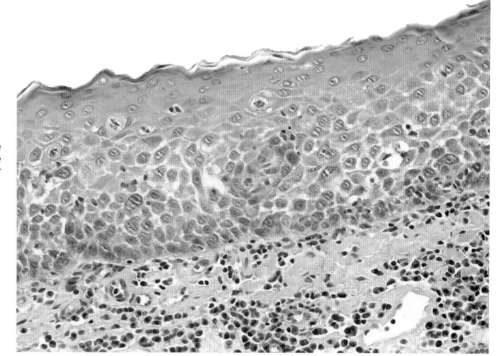

FIGURE 9-8

Dysplasia of the oral cavity are graded: in severe dysplasia/carcinoma in situ, the atypical changes involve the full thickness of the epithelium.

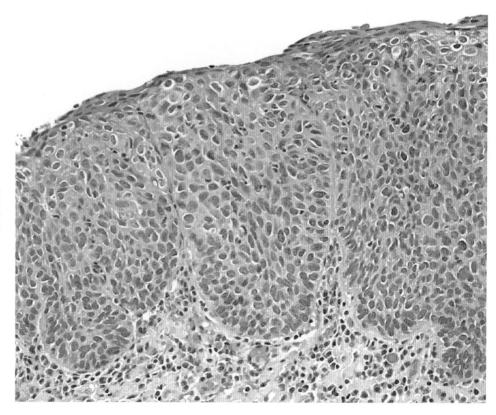

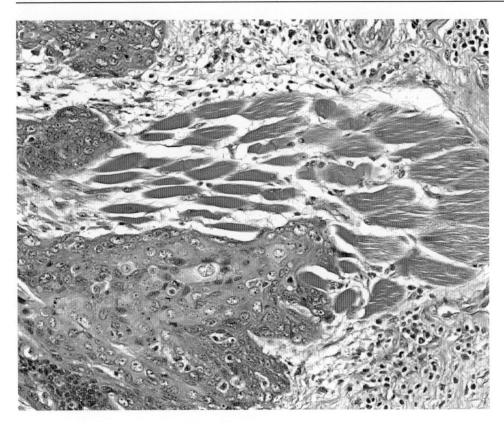

FIGURE 9-9
Irregular nests of squamous cell carcinoma infiltrate deep skeletal muscle of the tongue.

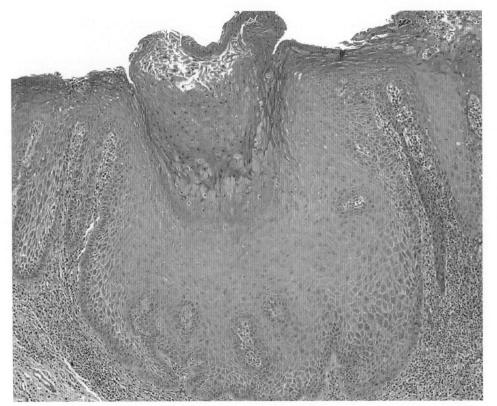

FIGURE 9-10
Verrucous carcinoma invades as a burrowing mass with broad pushing borders. It lacks the overtly malignant cytologic features of conventional squamous cell carcinoma.

(Fig. 9-11). In contrast to the benign squamous papilloma, the papillary fronds are lined by overtly malignant squamous cells.

3. The *spindle cell variant* is characterized by the proliferation of noncohesive spindle cells. Its microscopic appearance more closely resembles a sarcoma than a carcinoma (Fig. 9-12).

4. *The basaloid squamous variant* is characterized by expanding lobules of hyperchromatic basaloid cells, which have areas of squamous differentiation somewhere in the neoplasm (Fig. 9-13).

ANCILLARY STUDIES

FINE NEEDLE ASPIRATION

Up to 30% of patients with oral cancer have cervical metastases at the time of initial presentation, and in some of these patients the primary tumor site is not obvious on clinical grounds. Fine needle aspiration is an effective means of establishing a diagnosis of metastatic SCC. Cytologic smears are often cellular with both, syncytial fragments of large pleomorphic cells as well as single dispersed tumor cells. The cells characteristically have enlarged nuclei, prominent nucleoli, and cytoplasm with squamoid or keratinizing features. Common background changes include necrotic cystic debris, keratinaceous debris, and multinucleated giant cells (see Chapter 21).

IMMUNOHISTOCHEMICAL FEATURES

Immunohistochemistry may play a useful role in the diagnosis of poorly differentiated SCC that do not display overt squamous differentiation by routine light microscopy. Most SCC of the oral cavity are immunoreactive for wide spectrum cytokeratins; they are not immunoreactive for lymphoid markers (CD45RB, CD20), melanocytic markers (S-100, HMB45, melanin A) or mesenchymal markers (actin, desmin, FVIII-RAg).

DIFFERENTIAL DIAGNOSIS

At the one extreme, SCC can be mistaken for reactive non-neoplastic squamous proliferations of the oral cavity such as pseudoepitheliomatous hyperplasia, radiation-induced stromal atypia, and necrotizing sialometaplasia—a proliferation of metaplastic squamous cells within the ducts and acini of minor salivary glands. These reactive processes are generally preceded by an inciting event (e.g., ulceration, radiation); and in contrast to SCC, they do not display the combination of infiltrative growth, desmoplastic stromal reaction, and overtly malignant cytologic atypia. At the other extreme, poorly differentiated nonkeratinizing squamous cell carcinoma may be confused with various nonepidermoid malignancies such as malignant melanoma, sarcoma, or lymphoma. In this setting, immunohistochemistry may

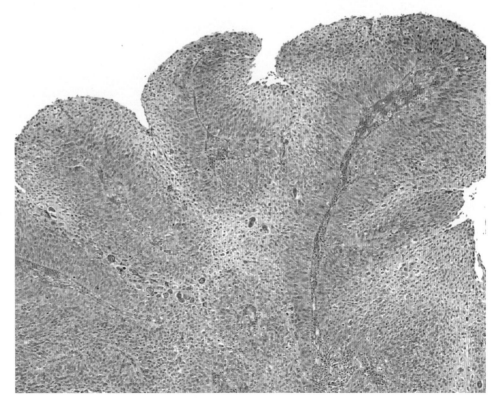

FIGURE 9-11

The papillary variant is characterized by papillary fronds lined by a cytologically malignant squamous epithelium.

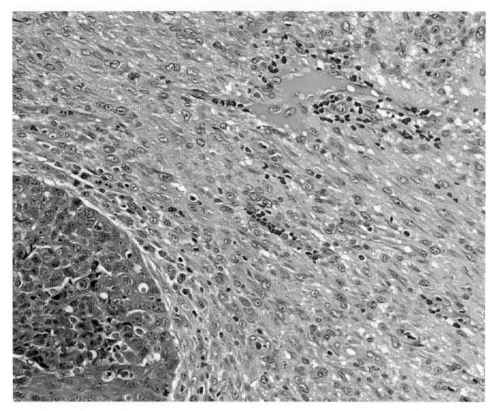

FIGURE 9-12

In the spindle cell variant, the spindled cells are easily mistaken for a sarcoma. In this example, a component of conventional squamous carcinoma is visible on the lower left.

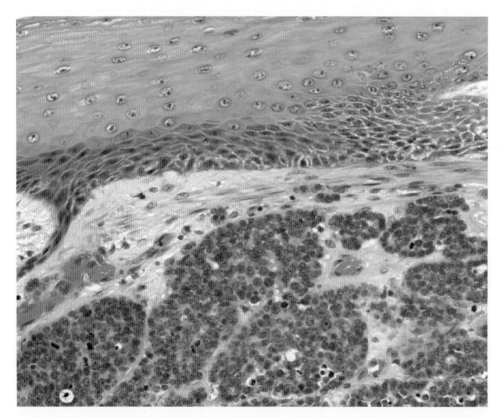

FIGURE 9-13

In basaloid squamous cell carcinoma, the carcinoma infiltrates as lobules of tumor cells having a high nuclear to cytoplasmic ratio.

play a useful role in establishing the diagnosis of carcinoma by demonstrating positive staining for cytokeratin, and negative staining for a panel of lymphoid markers, melanocytic markers, and mesenchymal markers.

PROGNOSIS AND THERAPY

Although prognosis varies by anatomic site, the overall 5-year survival rate for oral cancer as a group remains at 50% to 55%. Tumor stage has a dramatic impact on outcome: stage I squamous carcinomas of the oral cavity are associated with survival rates of 80% to 90%, but fewer than 30% of patients with local or regionally advanced disease (stage III or IV) are cured. The frustrating inability to improve survival rates largely reflects a persistent failure to diagnosis oral cancer during its early stages.

Treatment options are highly variable and depend on many factors, including size and location of the primary tumor, spread of the primary tumor to regional lymph nodes and distant sites, the patient's ability to tolerate treatment, and the patient's wishes. In general, surgery and/or radiation therapy is the standard treatment for limited stage cancers. Surgery with adjuvant radiation therapy is often used for more advanced stage disease. Patients with advanced stage disease may also benefit from the addition of chemotherapy. Certain cytotoxic agents may also be used to reduce tumor volume and control symptoms in patients with incurable, recurrent or metastatic disease.

KAPOSI'S SARCOMA

Kaposi's sarcoma (KS) is proliferation of spindle cells showing endothelial differentiation. Its pathogenesis has long been in dispute, but it is now generally regarded as a malignant neoplasm as opposed to a multicentric hyperplastic process. The human herpes virus (HHV8) is believed to be a necessary factor in disease development. Once regarded as an oddity that was rarely encountered in the oral cavity, an AIDS-related form of KS has resulted in a dramatic increase in oral KS among the population of HIV-infected individuals.

CLINICAL FEATURES

Four epidemiologically and biologically distinct forms of KS are recognized: A classic form that occurs primarily in older men of Eastern European (especially Ashkenazi Jew) or Mediterranean descent; an endemic form that is common to regions of Africa and is particularly prevalent among young Bantu children of South Africa; a

KAPOSI'S SARCOMA DISEASE FACT SHEET	
Definition	An unusual vascular-type neoplasm that occurs in certain patient populations, most notably in individuals infected with HIV
Incidence and location	Non-AIDS related forms of KS are rare and mostly confined to older men of Eastern European or Mediterranean descent; individuals in certain regions of Africa, and transplant recipients
KS is common in patients with AIDS (~15%–20%)
The palate is the most commonly involved intraoral site followed by the gingiva and dorsum of the tongue
Morbidity and mortality	Lesions of oral KS may become ulcerated, painful and interfere with eating and speaking
Mortality is dependent on patient's immunologic status
Gender, race, and age distribution	In the HIV-infected population, oral KS is most commonly encountered in homosexual men with a peak incidence in 4th decade
Clinical features	Oral lesions are commonly multifocal
Early lesions tend to be flat, red, and asymptomatic
As the lesions age, they become larger, darker, nodular, and ulcerated
Prognosis and treatment	Mortality rates dependent on patient's immunologic status, presence of opportunistic infections, stage of disease and other factors
General treatment: Highly active antiretroviral therapy (HAART), radiation, chemotherapy
Local treatment of problematic oral lesions: Surgery, cryotherapy, laser ablation, intralesional injections of chemotherapeutic or sclerosing agents

transplant associated form that occurs in transplant recipients that receive high doses of immunosuppressive therapy; and an AIDS-associated form that is particularly prevalent among HIV-infected homosexual males. Approximately 15% to 20% of patients with AIDS develop KS. The clinical presentation and course varies widely across these subtypes, yet all KS lesions are consistently infected with the HHV8, a gamma-herpesvirus closely related to the Epstein-Barr virus. Immunosuppression appears to be an important cofactor in the pathogenesis and clinical expression of disease.

The AIDS-associated form is by far the most likely subtype of KS to be encountered in the oral cavity. KS represents the most frequent oral malignancy seen in association with HIV infection, and it may be the first manifestation of this condition. In the HIV-infected population, oral KS is most commonly encountered in homosexual men with a peak incidence in the 4th decade. The palate is the most commonly involved intra-

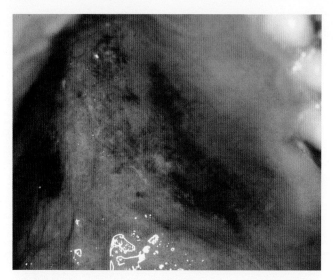

FIGURE 9-14
An early stage of oral KS seen as a flat red discoloration of the palatal mucosa.

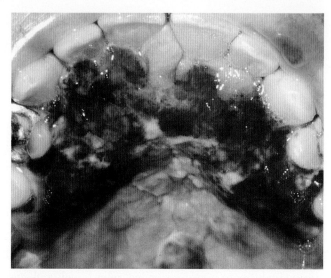

FIGURE 9-15
A more advanced stage of oral KS seen as diffuse reddish-purple nodules of the palate.

oral site followed by the gingiva and dorsum of the tongue. Multiple oral lesions are common often with concurrent involvement of cutaneous sites and visceral organs. The clinical appearance changes with lesion progression. Early lesions tend to be flat, red and asymptomatic (Fig. 9-14). As the lesions age, they become larger, darker, and raised (Fig. 9-15). With continued growth, large nodular lesions may become ulcerated and painful, and they may interfere with eating and speaking.

PATHOLOGIC FEATURES

GROSS FINDINGS

Early lesions are small, flat, and red. Advanced lesions are larger, deep-red to purple, and nodular.

MICROSCOPIC FINDINGS

KS is a nonencapsulated infiltrative lesion. The histologic picture varies with stage of progression. The histologic findings in early stages of KS (patch stage) are subtle. The submucosa may show nothing more specific than an ill-defined proliferation of dilated, irregular, angulated blood vessels with an interspersed infiltrate of chronic inflammatory cells (Fig. 9-16). As the lesions progress over time (plaque stage), the dilated vascular channels become surrounded by aggregates of spindle cells (Fig. 9-17). In advanced lesions, the histologic picture is dominated by a highly cellular proliferation of spindle cells separated by slit-like vascular spaces containing red blood cells (Fig. 9-18). The spindle cells are elongated with minimal cytologic atypia, and mitotic figures are not abundant. The presence of pleomorphism and high mitotic activity is unusual, and their presence generally portends a more aggressive form

KAPOSI'S SARCOMA PATHOLOGIC FEATURES	
Gross findings	Early lesions: Small, red, and flat
	Advanced lesions: Large, deep-red to purple, and nodular
Microscopic findings	Early lesions (patch stage): Proliferation of dilated, irregular, angulated blood vessels
	Maturing lesions (plaque stage): Dilated vascular channels surrounded by aggregates of spindle cells
	Advanced lesions (nodular stage): Cellular proliferation of spindle cells, slit-like vascular spaces, extravasated blood cells, hemosiderin deposits and hyaline globules
Immunohistochemical features	Variable immunoreactivity for endothelial markers (e.g., CD31, CD34, FVIII-RAg)
Pathologic differential diagnosis	Reactive vascular ectasia, bacillary angiomatosis, lobular capillary hemangioma, well-differentiated angiosarcoma, fibrosarcoma

of KS. This cellular background is admixed with extravasated red blood cells, hemosiderin, and small eosinophilic hyaline bodies that likely represent fragmented erythrocytes (Fig. 9-18, inset). Dilated vessels and chronic inflammatory cells are noted at the periphery of the lesion.

ANCILLARY STUDIES

In most cases, the spindle cells of KS are immunoreactive for FVIII-RAg, CD34, CD31, and other endothelial

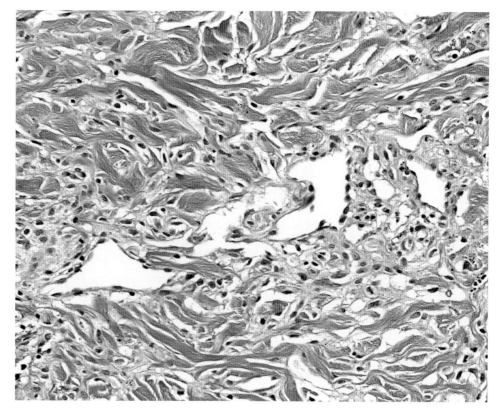

FIGURE 9-16

In the early (patch) phase, irregular dilated blood vessels dissect between collagen bundles.

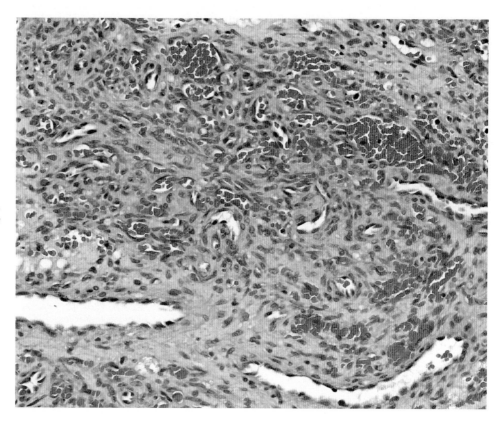

FIGURE 9-17

In the maturing (plaque) phase, vascular channels are surrounded by aggregates of spindle cells.

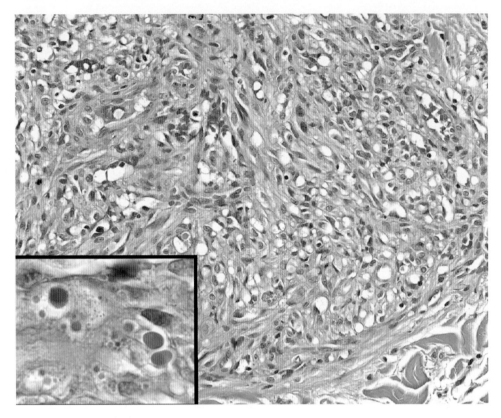

FIGURE 9-18

In the advanced (nodular) phase, the submucosa is infiltrated by cellular nodular aggregates of spindled cells forming slit-like spaces. The background is littered by extravasated blood cells and hyaline globules (*inset*).

markers. As the differential diagnosis is mostly comprised of other vascular proliferations, immunohistochemical confirmation of endothelial differentiation is often not helpful in establishing a diagnosis. However, HHV8 antibodies may assist in separation, although the immunohistochemistry can be difficult to interpret.

DIFFERENTIAL DIAGNOSIS

The differential diagnosis is contingent on the stage of histologic progression. Due to the subtlety of microscopic alterations, early lesions may be easily dismissed as reactive vascular ectasia. As the proliferation of small irregular vessels become more apparent, KS may cause confusion with lobular capillary hemangioma (pyogenic granuloma), bacillary angiomatosis, and even well-differentiated angiosarcoma. If bacillary angiomatosis is a consideration, a Warthin-Starry stain should be performed to look for the bacteria present in bacillary angiomatosis. In advanced stages, the highly cellular proliferation of spindle cells may be mistaken for fibrosarcoma. Unlike KS, the spindle cells of fibrosarcoma are not immunoreactive for FVIII-RAg, CD34, or CD31.

PROGNOSIS AND THERAPY

The behavior of KS is variable and related to clinical subtype, degree of dissemination, and immunologic competence of the patient. KS runs a much more aggressive course in immunocompromised patients such as those with AIDS. Even in this particular subgroup, overall mortality rates are highly dependent on a number of interrelated parameters, such as the presence of opportunistic infections, stage of disease, and presence of systemic symptoms.

The preferred treatment for KS in general is radiation and/or chemotherapy. For problematic lesions of the oral cavity, local symptoms (pain, bleeding or functional impairment) can be relieved by intralesional injection of chemotherapeutic or sclerosing agents, or by removal via surgery, cryotherapy, or laser therapy. The use of highly active antiretroviral therapy has improved the length and quality of life for HIV-infected individuals and has dramatically decreased the incidence and morbidity of oral KS.

SUGGESTED READING

Squamous Cell Carcinoma

1. Gale N, Pilch BZ, Sidransky D, El Naggar A, Westra W, Califano J, Johnson N, MacDonald DG: Epithelial precursor lesion. In: Barnes EL, Eveson JW, Reichart P, Sidransky D, eds. Pathology and Genetics of Head and Neck Tumours. Kleihues P, Sobin LH, series eds. World Health Organization Classification of Tumours. Lyon, France: IARC Press, 2005:177–179.
2. Gillison ML, Koch WM, Capone RB, et al.: Evidence for a causal association between human papillomavirus and a subset of head and neck cancers. J Natl Cancer Inst 2000;92:709–720.
3. Johnson N, Franceschi S, Ferlay J, Ramadas K, Schmid S, MacDonald DG, Bouquot JE, Slootweg PJ: Squamous cell carcinoma. In: Barnes EL, Eveson JW, Reichart P, Sidransky D, eds. Pathology and Genetics of Head and Neck Tumours. Kleihues P, Sobin LH, series eds. World Health Organization Classification of Tumours. Lyon, France: IARC Press, 2005:168–175.

4. Mills SE, Gaffey JM, Frierson HF: Squamous cell carcinoma: diagnostically problematic variants. In: Mills SE, Gaffey JM, Frierson HF. Atlas of Tumor Pathology: Tumors of the upper aerodigestive tract and ear, 3rd series. Washington, DC: Armed Forces Institute of Pathology, 1997:71–106.
5. Neville BW, Day TA: Oral cancer and precancerous lesions. CA Cancer J Clin 2002;52:184–189.
6. Vokes EE, Weichselbaum RR, Lippman SM, Hong WK: Head and neck cancer. N Engl J Med 1993;328:184–194.
7. Wenig BM: Squamous cell carcinoma of the upper aerodigestive tract: precursors and problematic variants. Mod Pathol 2002;15:229–254.

Kaposi's Sarcoma

1. Cherry-Peppers G, Daniels CO, Meeks V, et al.: Oral manifestations in the era of HAART. J Natl Medical Assoc 2003;95:21S–30S.
2. Greenspan D, Greenspan JS: HIV-related oral disease. Lancet 1996;348: 729–733.
3. Regezi JA, MacPhail LA, Daniels TE, et al.: Oral Kaposi's sarcoma: a 10-year retrospective histopathologic study. J Oral Pathol Med 1993;22:292–297.
4. Schwartz RA: Kaposi's sarcoma: an update. J Surg Oncol 2003;87: 146–151.
5. van der Waal I, Lamovec J, Knuutila S: Kaposi sarcoma. In: Barnes EL, Eveson JW, Reichart P, Sidransky D, eds. Pathology and Genetics of Head and Neck Tumours. Kleihues P, Sobin LH, series eds. World Health Organization Classification of Tumours. Lyon, France: IARC Press, 2005:193–194.

10 | Non-Neoplastic Lesions of the Salivary Glands

Mary S. Richardson

DEVELOPMENTAL, INCLUDING HETEROTOPIA AND ONCOCYTOSIS

CLINICAL FEATURES

Salivary glands are composed of three paired major glands—the parotid, the submandibular, and the sublingual, and roughly a thousand minor seromucus glands that are distributed throughout the sinonasal tract, oral cavity, larynx, and lower respiratory tree. All the glands develop from ingrowth of surface epithelium,

have common architecture, and are vulnerable to the same disorders.

Lesions of salivary gland, although uncommon, are a heterogeneous group of disorders. Enlargement of salivary glands is most often due to non-neoplastic or inflammatory conditions that include cysts, inflammatory diseases, and developmental abnormalities.

Heterotopia of salivary gland is the existence of salivary gland tissue in locations external to the major and minor salivary glands. In contrast, accessory salivary glands exist as isolated lobules of glands situated along a major salivary duct.

Ectopic or heterotopic salivary gland tissue has been reported in a myriad of anatomic locations (Table 10-1). The most common sites for heterotopic salivary gland are the middle ear, the neck, the mandible, and pituitary gland. Removal of these salivary gland tissue deposits may occur for cosmetic reasons, intervention for a congenital abnormality, or neoplasia. In the latter instance, if the tumor is malignant, there may be confusion as to whether the tumor is primary in heterotopic salivary gland tissue or metastatic from a different salivary gland.

The occurrence of oncocytic cells in salivary gland can be categorized as oncocytic metaplasia, nodular, or diffuse oncocytosis and oncocytoma. Oncocytes are characterized by abundant granular eosinophilic cytoplasm surrounding a round nucleus which contains a single nucleolus. The granular cytoplasm is due to an overabundance of mitochondria. The number of oncocytic cells in salivary gland varies as does the growth pattern. Oncocytic metaplasia involves the change of acinar and ductal structures to oncocytes. Oncocytic metaplasia is uncommon before the age of 50 and increases with advancing age. The metaplasia is usually seen focally and may be found in conjunction with salivary gland neoplasms (pleomorphic adenoma, mucoepidermoid carcinoma). Oncocytosis is a focal collection of oncocytes in the salivary gland tissue.

DEVELOPMENTAL, INCLUDING HETEROTOPIA AND ONCOCYTOSIS DISEASE FACT SHEET	
Definition	Heterotopia: salivary gland tissue in a location external to the major and minor salivary glands
	Oncocytes are transformed acinar or ductal cells with finely granular eosinophilic cytoplasm, categorized as oncocytic metaplasia, oncocytosis (nodular or diffuse), and oncocytoma
Incidence and location	Heterotopia most commonly involves the parotid and cervical lymph nodes
	Oncocytic tumors of salivary gland are rare (<1%)
Gender, race, and age distribution	Salivary gland heterotopia has no known age or gender predilection
	Oncocytic lesions are uncommon in patients <50 yr, peak incidence is 7th to 9th decade
Clinical features	Heterotopia is usually found incidentally or as a mass secondary to an inflammatory or neoplastic process
	Oncocytic lesions (oncocytosis/ oncocytoma) may be multifocal within the gland, unilateral or bilateral
Prognosis and treatment	Simple excision if clinically indicated for heterotopia
	Oncocytic lesions have about 30% recurrence rate; tumors may require surgery

PATHOLOGIC FEATURES

GROSS FINDINGS

On gross and microscopic examination the heterotopic salivary gland tissue has the characteristic spec-

276

trum of features of normal salivary gland tissue (mucus, seromucus, or serous acini, and excretory ducts). There is no specific gross for oncocytosis.

MICROSCOPIC FINDINGS

Histologic examination of an oncocytic lesion shows polygonal cells with abundant finely granular eosinophilic cytoplasm. The oncocytic transformation can involve acinar and ductal cells (Fig. 10-1). The nuclei are usually uniformly round with granular chromatin and contain a single nucleolus. Mitotic figures are absent or rare. The presence of a fibrous capsule surrounding a nodule may aid in the distinction between an oncocytoma and nodular oncocytic hyperplasia. Oncocytes may grow as a solid nodule of cells with or without focal cystic areas. The architectural growth pattern of the cells within the nodule is often organoid or forming cords in a hepatoid pattern. The individual cells show a variable eosinophilic staining quality (Fig. 10-2), and on a rare occasion, may contain focal or diffuse clear cells.

ANCILLARY STUDIES

Although not necessary for the diagnosis, the following may be useful in demonstrating the presence of mitochondria within oncocytic lesions.

DEVELOPMENTAL, INCLUDING HETEROTOPIA AND ONCOCYTOSIS PATHOLOGIC FEATURES

Gross findings	Oncocytic nodules may measure up to 7 cm, with small, cystic areas
Microscopic findings	Oncocytic cells are characterized by finely granular, eosinophilic cytoplasm
	There is a single round nucleus with nucleolus
	Architectural growth patterns are usually organoid with variable areas showing cording and prominent capillaries
	Oncocytes may undergo "clear cell" change
Ancillary studies	Phosphotungstic acid hematoxylin (PTAH) stain accentuates granules
Pathologic differential diagnosis	When clear cell oncocytes are present, metastasis from clear cell mucoepidermoid carcinoma, clear cell acinic cell, and renal cell carcinoma

---

TABLE 10-1

Reported Sites of Heterotopic Salivary Tissues

Middle ear	Mediastinum
External auditory canal	Pituitary gland
Neck	Cerebellopontine angle
Thyroglossal duct cyst	Stomach
Mandible (intraosseous)	Rectum
Cervical and paraparotid lymph nodes	Prostate gland

FIGURE 10-1

At medium power, the tinctorial difference between the basophilic acinar cells and the eosinophilic oncocytes is easily noted. Oncocytic metaplasia may be seen in acinar and ductal cells.

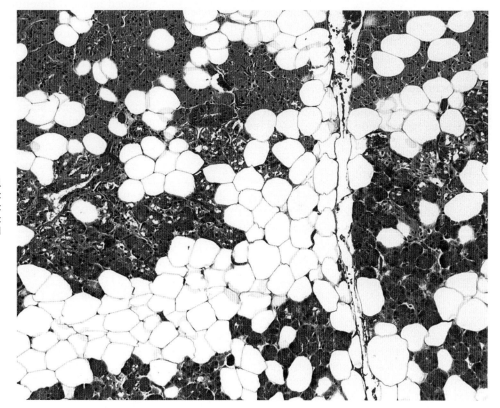

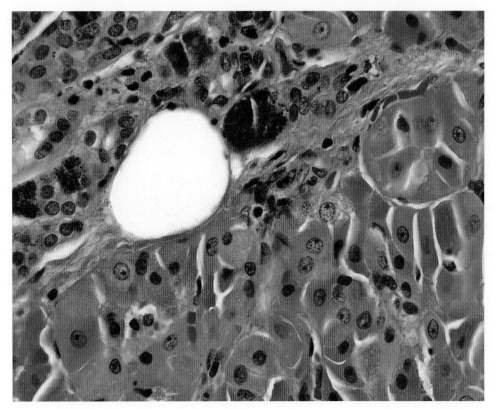

FIGURE 10-2
At high power, the finely granular eosinophilic cytoplasm and round nucleus with a single nucleolus is seen. Note the variability in eosinophilic staining of the onco-cytic cytoplasm.

ULTRASTRUCTURAL FEATURES

On ultrastructural evaluation, abundant mitochon-dria may completely fill the cytoplasmic compartment. The mitochondria show some variability in their shape ranging from round to irregular and elongate. Desmo-somal cell attachments are identified.

HISTOCHEMICAL FEATURES

A phosphotungstic acid hematoxylin stain (PTAH) will stain mitochondria. The results of this stain, however, are not always consistent.

FINE NEEDLE ASPIRATION

On fine needle aspiration, oncocytes are easily iden-tified. Distinguishing oncocytic metaplasia from onco-cytomas, however, is done primarily on excised lesions.

DIFFERENTIAL DIAGNOSIS

Distinguishing between nodular hyperplasia and nodular oncocytosis from an oncocytoma may be prob-lematic. One publication defines an oncocytoma as a single nodule while others require the presence of a partial capsule. The distinction between the oncocytic hyperplasia and neoplasia is still not well defined. Onco-cytic metaplasia and a variety of clear cell neoplasms are included in the differential diagnosis with oncocytoma. Areas of oncocytic metaplasia may be found in pleo-morphic adenomas and within mucoepidermoid carci-nomas. These areas of oncocytic metaplasia are usually isolated. In contrast, oncocytomas lack the architectural patterns of these two neoplasms. Mucus cell differ-entiation and squamous metaplasia are rare within oncocytomas and help distinguish oncocytoma from mucoepidermoid carcinoma. Oncocytomas do not have myxoid or chondroid differentiation which is charac-teristic of pleomorphic adenoma.

Acinic cell carcinoma may be difficult to distinguish from a multinodular oncocytic hyperplasia; however, the microcystic and papillary follicular growth pat-terns of acinic cell carcinoma are not seen in oncocytic hyperplasia.

PROGNOSIS AND THERAPY

Oncocytic metaplasia and oncocytosis are usually present in a gland removed for another reason. No therapy is necessary for these benign reactions. Hetero-topias are excised, with an excellent prognosis.

MUCUS RETENTION CYST, MUCOCELE, SIALOTHIASIS

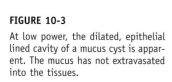

CLINICAL FEATURES

The most common non-neoplastic lesion of salivary gland tissue is the mucocele. The mucocele is defined as the pooling of mucin in a cystic cavity. Two types of mucoceles are described: (a) the retention type (Fig. 10-3), mucin pooling confined within a dilated excretory duct (Fig. 10-4); and (b) extravasation type (Fig. 10-5), escape of salivary secreted mucin from the duct system into connective tissue (Figs. 10-6 and 10-7). The extravasated type is the most common mucocele and its peak incidence is in the 3rd decade. The lower lip is the most common site followed by the tongue, floor of mouth, palate, and buccal mucosa. A large mucocele that may arise in the floor of the mouth from the sublingual or minor salivary gland and descend into the soft tissues of the floor of the mouth is called a ranula. The mucus retention cyst is more common in the parotid and submandibular glands and the peak incidence is in the 7th to 8th decades.

A sialolith is a collection of concretions which form a stone within the salivary gland excretory duct system. Sialothiasis most frequently involves the submandibular gland and may cause a chronic sclerosing sialadenitis distal to the stone (Fig. 10-8). The stone will cause dis-

MUCUS RETENTION CYST, MUCOCELE, SIALOTHIASIS DISEASE FACT SHEET	
Definition	The pooling of salivary mucus within a cystic cavity resulting from blockage/rupture of a salivary gland duct
Incidence and location	Most common non-neoplastic lesion of salivary glands
	Lower lip is the most common site followed by tongue, floor of mouth, palate, and buccal mucosa
	Mucoceles in the floor of mouth are called "ranula"
Gender, race, and age distribution	Equal gender distribution
	Peak incidence in 3rd decade
	Most common intra-oral lesion in the first two decades of life
Clinical features	Soft, fluctuant, semitranslucent, painless swelling that may be noted to occur after a traumatic event
	The lesion may fluctuate with meals or when ruptured secondary to trauma
	Lesion may be recurrent to the same site
Prognosis and treatment	Complete excision, including minor salivary gland, usually is adequate
	Recurrence is usually seen with inadequate excision

FIGURE 10-3

At low power, the dilated, epithelial lined cavity of a mucus cyst is apparent. The mucus has not extravasated into the tissues.

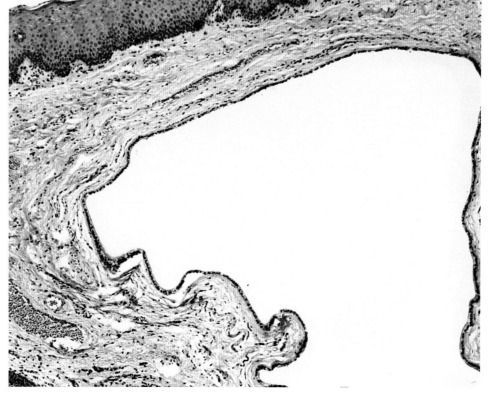

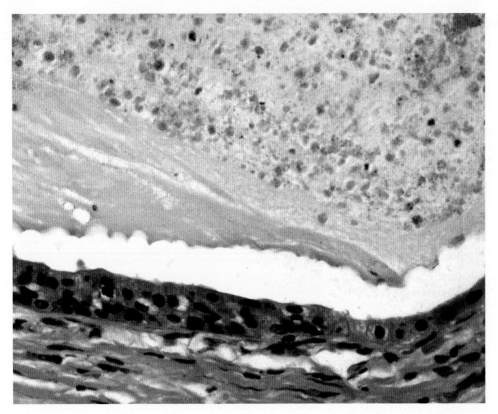

FIGURE 10-4

At high power, the low cuboidal lining of the cyst is seen and very little inflammatory response in the subjacent connective tissue is noted.

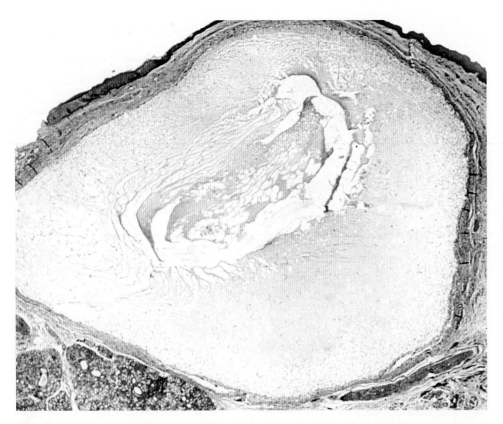

FIGURE 10-5

At low power, the circumscribed extravasated mucus is identified.

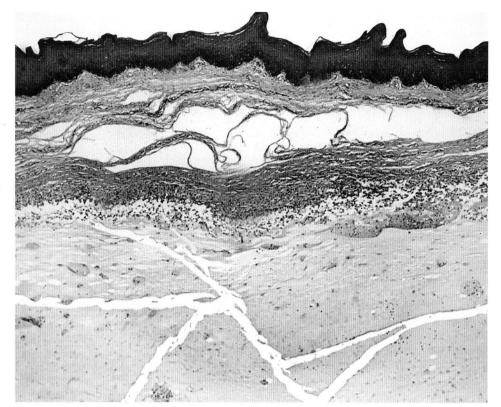

FIGURE 10-6

At medium power, the absence of an epithelial lining and mixed inflammatory infiltrate is noted at the mucus and connective tissue interface.

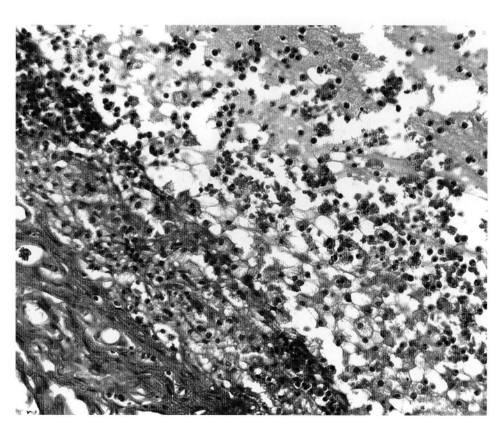

FIGURE 10-7

At high power, a prominent inflammatory infiltrate and foamy, mucin-laden macrophages are noted within the connective tissue and within the mucin. No epithelium is identified.

tention of the duct system and retention of secreted fluids causing glandular swelling and pain.

RADIOLOGIC FEATURES

Sialoliths are always visible on radiographic examination. The most common site for a sialolith is Wharton's duct of the submandibular gland which can be visualized easily on a radiograph (Fig. 10-9).

PATHOLOGIC FEATURES

Histologically, the retention cyst captures the mucus within the epithelial-lined lumen. There is usually scant to no inflammatory infiltrate within the wall (Fig. 10-4) unless there is adjacent rupture. In contrast, the lesions of extravasated mucin (mucocele) show compression of the adjacent connective tissue with a brisk inflammatory reaction circumscribing the mucin pool (Fig. 10-6). Also within the infiltrate of the mucocele wall are

numerous foamy macrophages that contain phagocytized mucin (Fig. 10-7). As the lesion progresses, granulation tissue from the wall becomes more prominent and may organize to obliterate the lumen of the mucocele. In a primarily granulation tissue laden lesion, a mucicarmine stain will highlight the residual mucin containing macrophages.

A sialolith will frequently demonstrate a nidus of cellular debris found in the center of the concentric laminated calcium deposits (Fig. 10-10).

MUCUS RETENTION CYST, MUCOCELE, SIALOTHIASIS PATHOLOGIC FEATURES	
Gross findings	Cystic cavity within connective tissue containing glistening fluid
Microscopic findings	Circumscribed mucin with inflammation within the wall
	Retention cyst has epithelial lining of the lumen
Ancillary studies	PAS and mucicarmine stains mucin
Pathologic differential diagnosis	Organizing hematoma

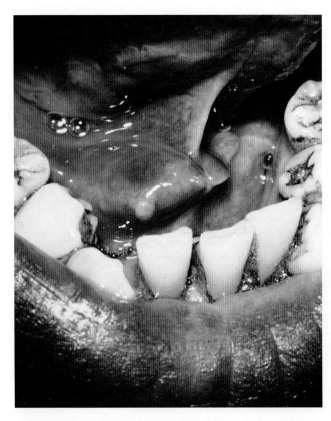

FIGURE 10-8
A sialolith present at orifice of Wharton's duct is just beginning to protrude from lumen of the duct.

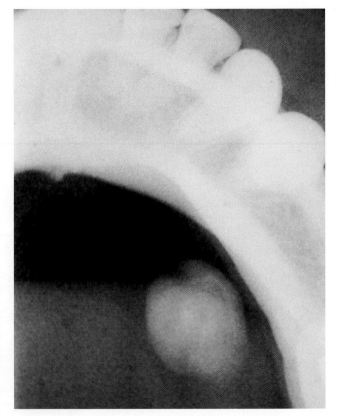

FIGURE 10-9
Sialoliths are common in Wharton's duct of the submandibular gland. The lamination of the sialolith can be appreciated on this radiograph.

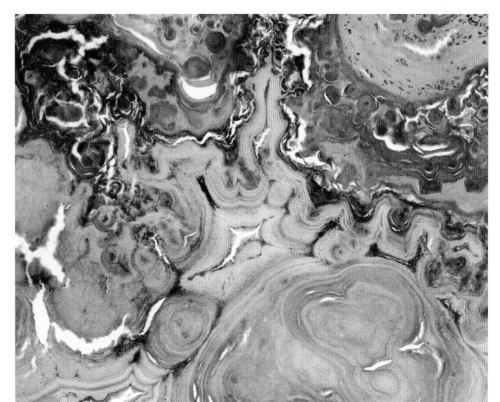

FIGURE 10-10

At low power, the laminated concretions around nidi of cellular debris are seen in this section of a sialolith.

DIFFERENTIAL DIAGNOSIS

Few entities enter into the differential diagnosis of an extravasated type mucocele. Certainly, the extravasated mucocele, with just remaining granulation tissue, could be considered a small hematoma or a thrombus. The use of mucicarmine, however, would illustrate the presence of mucin-laden macrophages and aid in this distinction. The mucus retention cyst is lined by a thin layer of cuboidal epithelium with little to no inflammatory cell infiltrate. Mucoepidermoid carcinoma could enter the differential diagnosis of a mucus retention cyst. Mucoepidermoid carcinoma, however, contains three cell types: mucus goblet cells, intermediate cells, and squamous cells. Within mucus retention cysts, the epithelium is attenuated and lacks papillary projections that protrude into the lumen.

PROGNOSIS AND THERAPY

Surgical excision to include the minor mucoserous gland is suggested, as clinically indicated by the patient's condition. Alginate has been used by some with variable results. Recurrence is seen in patients with inadequate excision.

NECROTIZING SIALOMETAPLASIA

CLINICAL FEATURES

Necrotizing sialometaplasia is an uncommon destructive reactive inflammatory process of the salivary gland. The clinical and histologic characteristics resemble

NECROTIZING SIALOMETAPLASIA DISEASE FACT SHEET	
Definition	Ischemic necrosis of salivary gland tissue which maintains a lobular distribution
Incidence and location	Palate is most frequent site of involvement
Gender, race, and age distribution	Male predominance
	All ages affected
Clinical features	Rapid swelling of the mucosa with ulceration in a few days
	Lesion slowly heals over several weeks
	Patients complain of pain or numbness which simulates malignancy
Prognosis and treatment	No therapy is necessary for this self-healing process

malignant neoplasms and can lead to misdiagnosis and inappropriate therapy. The age range of reported patients with necrotizing sialometaplasia is from 1.5–83 years, with the average age of approximately 46 years. The lesion has a 2 : 1 predominance in men. The vast majority of these lesions are seen in the hard palate or at the junction of the hard and soft palate. Lesions are most commonly unilateral; however, occasional bilateral or midline lesions develop. Other common sites for this lesion are oral cavity, lower lip, retromolar trigone, tongue, and buccal mucosa, although the entire upper aerodigestive tract can be affected. Occurrence of this lesion in major salivary glands, primarily the parotid gland, is uncommon, representing 8.5% of necrotizing sialometaplasia cases.

Clinically, the lesion appears in the palate as a deep, sharply defined, crater-like ulcer which develops rapidly over a few days and fails to heal for an extended period of time. Duration of healing of this lesion can range up to 6 months; however, most heal within 1 month. All such lesions that fail to resolve are usually biopsied. Other symptoms associated with this lesion (pain or numbness) may simulate malignancy.

PATHOLOGIC FEATURES

GROSS FINDINGS

On gross examination, there is only a slight suggestion of softening of these submucosal tissues with a glis-tening cut surface. Usually there is no distinguishing mass.

MICROSCOPIC FINDINGS

Microscopically, the characteristic feature of necro-tizing sialometaplasia is ischemic necrosis or infarction which is thought to be the pathogenesis of this lesion. The key histologic features in identifying this lesion are (a) lobular coagulative necrosis of the salivary gland acini (Figs. 10-11 and 10-12), (b) prominent and prolif-

NECROTIZING SIALOMETAPLASIA PATHOLOGIC FEATURES	
Gross findings	Usually the overlying mucosa shows ulceration
	Ulcer may be up to 3 cm
Microscopic findings	Lobular coagulative necrosis of glandular acinae
	Prominent squamous metaplasia of salivary gland ducts
	Inflammation is present
	Pseudoepitheliomatous hyperplasia of the overlying mucosal epithelium may be seen
Pathologic differential diagnosis	Squamous cell carcinoma, mucoepidermoid carcinoma

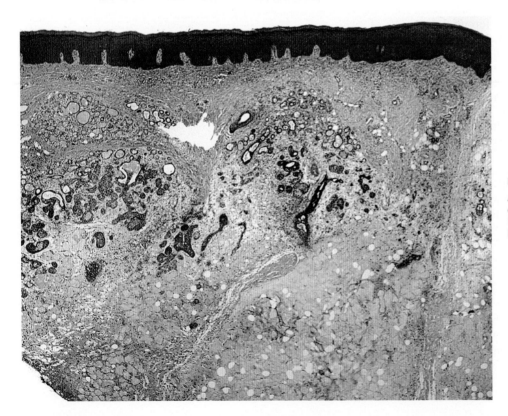

FIGURE 10-11

An intact epithelium overlies lobules of acinar degeneration and necrosis. Fibrosis is noted between the lobules.

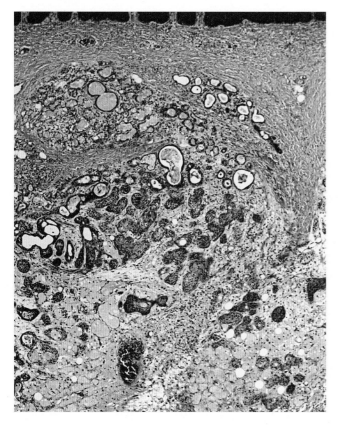

FIGURE 10-12

At low power, acinar alteration is noted; however, fibrous septa and ducts define the retained lobular architecture.

erative squamous metaplasia of the excretory ducts, (c) pseudoepitheliomatous hyperplasia of the overlying mucosa, and (d) prominent inflammatory infiltrate. The most prominent and useful features histologically are the coagulative necrosis and ductal metaplasia (Fig. 10-13). The lobular architecture of the salivary gland is preserved and the mucin acini show the ghosted outline of coagulative necrosis which are replaced with metaplastic squamous mucosa (Fig. 10-14).

DIFFERENTIAL DIAGNOSIS

The diagnosis of necrotizing sialometaplasia can be problematic if the biopsy is not adequate or oriented properly. The chief differential diagnoses for this lesion are mucosal squamous cell carcinoma and mucoepidermoid carcinoma. In an adequately oriented biopsy, it is easy to distinguish these lesions based on the maintenance of the salivary gland lobular architecture. The cytologic features within necrotizing sialometaplasia are bland and the inflammatory infiltrate is prominent. Squamous cell carcinoma and mucoepidermoid carcinoma are frequently associated with inflammatory infiltrate; however, it is not nearly as intense as the inflammatory infiltrate accompanying necrotizing sialometaplasia and these two malignancies infiltrate the gland.

FIGURE 10-13

At medium power, there is extensive degeneration and necrosis with islands of squamous metaplasia are evident.

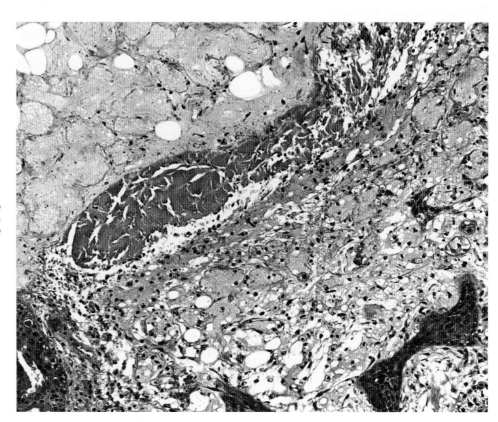

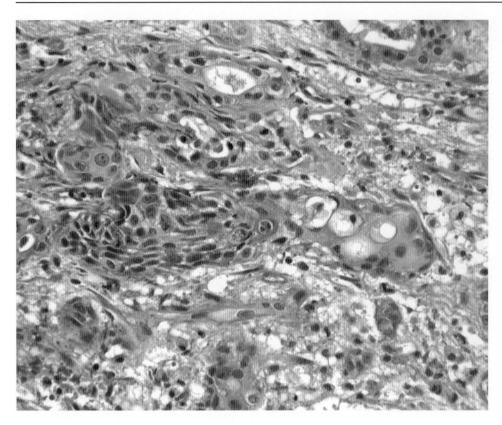

FIGURE 10-14
At high power, islands of squamous metaplasia are cytologically bland, not to be confused with malignancy. There is inflammation surrounding the outlines of the acini and ducts.

PROGNOSIS AND THERAPY

No specific therapy is required for necrotizing sialometaplasia. These lesions are self-healing.

BENIGN LYMPHOEPITHELIAL LESION

Benign lymphoepithelial lesion is used to describe a characteristic lymphocytic infiltrate in salivary glands. The term does not commit to an etiologic cause but refers to histologic findings.

CLINICAL FEATURES

Clinically, the lesions present as unilateral, bilateral or diffuse enlargement of salivary glands (usually parotid) or lacrimal glands. This lesion may occur in children and adults of either gender. Most cases of benign lymphoepithelial lesion present in women in the 4th and 5th decade and is associated with or a precursor to the autoimmune disease Sjögren's syndrome. In some cases this is a precursor lesion to salivary MALT lymphoma. Patients experience facial swelling with or without pain, dry mouth, and keratoconjunctivitis.

BENIGN LYMPOEPITHELIAL LESION DISEASE FACT SHEET	
Definition	Salivary gland tissue with an intense lymphocytic infiltrate with associated epimyoepithelial islands
Incidence and location	Uncommon lesion
Morbidity and mortality	Increased risk of lymphoma
Gender, race, and age distribution	Female predominance Mean age, 50 yr
Clinical features	85% of cases occur in the parotid gland Diffuse swelling of the affected gland
Prognosis and treatment	Prognosis relates to development of lymphoma which is usually a low-grade extranodal marginal zone B-cell lymphoma (MALT lymphoma) Surgery

PATHOLOGIC FEATURES

GROSS FINDINGS

On gross examination the benign lymphoepithelial lesion may be seen as diffuse enlargement of the gland or present as discrete tan micronodules. The gross appearance can be mistaken for a neoplastic process due to the multinodularity; however, the capsule in major salivary glands is intact.

MICROSCOPIC FINDINGS

Irregular, multifocal islands of epithelial proliferations surrounded by a dense lymphocytic infiltrate characterize benign lymphoepithelial lesions. The extent of the lymphocytic infiltrate can vary within a lobule and ultimately progresses to total acinar atrophy with only remaining ducts (Fig. 10-15). The remaining excretory ducts are usually infiltrated by intermediate-sized lymphocytes. Similar changes to those seen in the major salivary glands can occur in the minor salivary glands of patients with Sjögren's syndrome. The changes in minor glands are a chronic lymphocytic sialadenitis usually without epithelial hyperplasia. The changes seen in a labial minor salivary gland biopsy is supportive but not pathognomonic evidence for the diagnosis of Sjögren's syndrome (Fig. 10-16). Numeric grading systems are employed based on the number of aggregates (50 lymphocytes comprise an aggregate) present in salivary gland lobules, but clinical and serologic confirmation are required for a definitive diagnosis.

BENIGN LYMPOEPITHELIAL LESION PATHOLOGIC FEATURES	
Gross findings	Small tan nodules to diffuse replacement of gland by creamy tan tissue
Microscopic findings	Heavy lymphocytic infiltrate associated with destruction of salivary acini
	Proliferating epimyoepithelial islands
Pathologic differential diagnosis	Lymphoma

ANCILLARY STUDIES

The lymphoid infiltrate that is present in these lesions is a mixture of T and B lymphocytes similar to those seen in hyperplastic lymph nodes. Plasma cells, eosinophils, and polymorphonuclear leukocytes are not usually present. Use of immunohistochemistry for CD3 (T cell marker) or CD20 (B cell marker) can reveal a mixed population of T and B lymphocytes. Fresh tissue at the time of biopsy may be submitted for flow cytometry analysis and gene rearrangement studies to exclude a lymphoma.

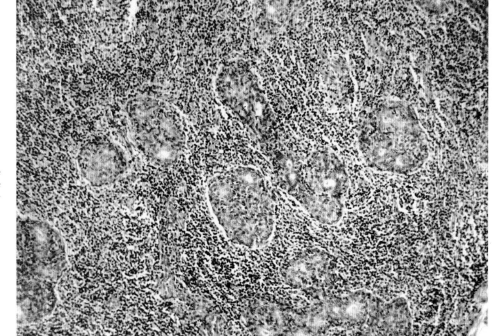

FIGURE 10-15

At high power, the proliferative ductal epithelium is evident. The epimyoepithelial islands show infiltration by the lymphocytic infiltrate.

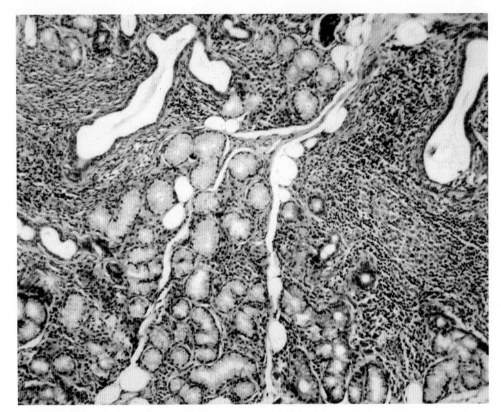

FIGURE 10-16
Focal lymphocytic sialadenitis is adjacent to normal-appearing acini. Germinal center formation in the lymphocytic infiltrate is noted. This biopsy specimen is from a patient with Sjögren's syndrome.

DIFFERENTIAL DIAGNOSIS

The differential diagnosis includes malignant lymphoma, metastatic carcinoma, chronic sialadenitis, and sarcoidosis. The following are helpful in distinguishing lymphoma from a benign lymphoepithelial lesion: the infiltrate remaining within the normal lobular architecture of the gland, lack of invasion of capsule and paraglandular tissue, lack of infiltrated epithelial islands and lack of the atypical nuclear features of malignant lymphocytes. Metastatic carcinoma can be excluded by the benign appearance of the cells within the myoepithelial islands. The distinction between chronic sialadenitis and sarcoidosis is often not quite as clear. Chronic sialadenitis is composed of a mixed chronic inflammatory infiltrate containing plasma cells and neutrophils with prominent fibrosis. Sarcoidosis is characterized by noncaseating granulomas.

PROGNOSIS AND THERAPY

Lymphomas arising in benign lymphoepithelial lesions are most frequently characterized as low grade B cell lymphomas similar to lymphomas of other mucosal associated lymphoid tissue (MALT lymphoma). Any salivary gland being biopsied for Sjögren's syndrome or for a persistent mass, should have material submitted for flow cytometry analysis, immunohistochemical techniques, and gene arrangements to exclude the possibility of lymphoma.

Malignant lymphoepithelial lesions, though rare, may arise in a setting of benign lymphoepithelial lesion. These lesions have only been reported in major salivary glands, usually the parotid gland, and women seem to be affected more often than men. There are, however, two subgroups who are affected: Eskimos and Chinese. These carcinomas may present with regional lymph node metastasis. Within Eskimos, this lesion has more commonly been reported in parotid, while within Chinese it is more common in the submandibular gland with less frequent regional lymph node disease.

LYMPHOEPITHELIAL CYST

CLINICAL FEATURES

The benign cystic salivary gland lesions known as lymphoepithelial cysts occur most commonly in the parotid glands and oral cavity. The name reflects the two histologic components that constitute the lesions: lymphoid tissue and epithelial-lined cysts. These lesions are seen in a small minority of HIV-positive individuals, although they may be present at birth, and may not

LYMPHOEPITHELIAL CYST DISEASE FACT SHEET	
Definition	A cyst lined by epithelium that is surrounded by a dense lymphoid infiltrate
Incidence and location	Uncommon lesion
	Parotid gland most commonly affected
Morbidity and mortality	There may be facial nerve dysfunction with compression when involving the parotid gland
Gender, race, and age distribution	Male > Female (3 : 1)
	Peak incidence 4th decade
	HIV-associated lymphoepithelial cysts are more common in children
Clinical features	Lesions are usually asymptomatic with occasional associated pain or tenderness and rarely facial nerve dysfunction
	Unilateral or bilateral (HIV-related) parotid enlargement
	Small nodules may be located in minor salivary glands (floor of mouth, lateral tongue) or tonsillar tissues
Prognosis and treatment	Usually treated by surgical excision and are not known to recur

LYMPHOEPITHELIAL CYST PATHOLOGIC FEATURES	
Gross findings	Well-demarcated nodule or mass which varies in size by location from 0.1 cm (intra-oral sites) to 8 cm (parotid)
Microscopic findings	Epithelial lined cysts composed of stratified squamous, cuboidal, columnar, or pseudostratified-ciliated type
	Lymphoid tissue within the cyst wall which may show follicular hyperplasia
	The lumen may be filled with desquamated cells
	In HIV associated cysts, proliferating epimyoepithelial islands may be seen
Fine-needle aspiration	Composed of lymphocytes and desquamated squamous cells
Pathologic differential diagnosis	Warthin's tumor, cystic metastatic squamous carcinoma, metastatic nasopharyngeal carcinoma

become clinically obvious until later in adult life. They frequently present as a unilateral painful swelling. Pain may occur, however, due to secondary infection or nerve compression.

PATHOLOGIC FEATURES

GROSS FINDINGS

On gross examination the cysts measure 0.5 to 7 cm. The cyst contents are usually a straw-colored serous fluid.

MICROSCOPIC FINDINGS

Microscopically the cyst lining is composed of either squamous, columnar, or cuboidal epithelium (Fig. 10-17). Occasionally, there may be goblet cells or oncocytic metaplasia identified within the cyst lining. The cyst wall is composed of lymphoid tissue which will contain germinal centers. Depending on the location of the cyst, it may be within an intraparotid lymph node or cervical lymph node.

ANCILLARY STUDIES

Due to the accessibility of lymphoepithelial cysts, they frequently undergo fine needle aspiration. Findings on

aspiration are fairly nonspecific. There can be a predominance of lymphoid cells with some squamous cells. The differential diagnosis of an aspirate from these lesions may include cystadenoma and Warthin's tumor.

DIFFERENTIAL DIAGNOSIS

These cysts are frequently misdiagnosed as tumors. They may be mistaken histologically for cystic low-grade mucoepidermoid carcinomas or metastatic cystic squamous cell carcinoma. The lining of the lymphoepithelial cyst is a benign squamous lining with no pleomorphism or atypia (Fig. 10-18). Generally, lymphoepithelial cysts lack mucin cells with micro- and macrocystic structures, contain no papillary projections, and have no intermediate cells.

PROGNOSIS AND THERAPY

Surgical excision is curative. If a fistulous tract is present, then it is necessary to remove the sinus tract or fistula to prevent recurrence. There are alternative treatments to surgery for HIV-positive patients. Frequently, the only purpose for removing the cyst is for cosmetic reasons.

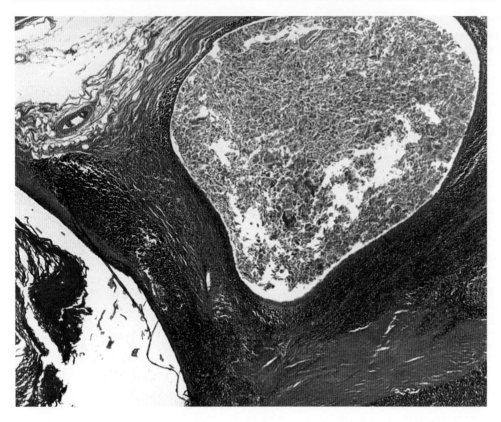

FIGURE 10-17
The dilated squamous lined cysts are surrounded by a lymphocytic infiltrate within the parotid. Fine needle aspirate findings of squamous cells and lymphocytes are easily explained by the above tissue architecture.

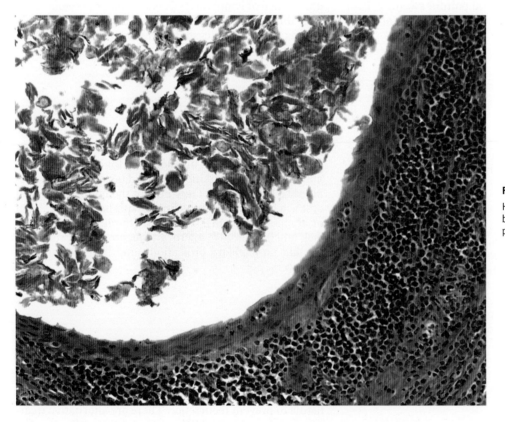

FIGURE 10-18
High power shows the attenuated benign squamous lining of a lymphoepithelial cyst.

SARCOIDOSIS

Sarcoidosis is a multisystem granulomatous disorder of unknown etiology. This disease process is world wide in its distribution. In the United States, the disease is 12 times more common in blacks than whites. There is a slight female predominance and peak incidence between the 2nd and 4th decades.

CLINICAL FEATURES

Sarcoidosis usually appears suddenly with common symptoms of dyspnea, dry cough, chest pain, fever, malaise, fatigue, arthralgias, and weight loss. One-fifth of patients have no symptoms and disease is picked up on a routine chest radiograph.

Although any organ system may be involved, it most commonly involves lung, lymph nodes, skin, eyes, and salivary glands. The mediastinal and paratracheal lymph nodes are most commonly involved, thus providing the radiographic findings of bilateral hilar lymph adenopathy.

PATHOLOGIC FEATURES

GROSS FINDINGS

Salivary gland involvement usually presents as diffuse enlargement of major and minor salivary gland tissues. Frequently, an increased incidence of mucoceles may be noted.

MICROSCOPIC FINDINGS

The disease is characterized by tight noncaseating granulomas typically composed of epithelioid macrophages and multinucleated giant cells (Fig. 10-19). A variable lymphoid infiltrate surrounds the granulomas (Fig. 10-20). Occasionally, asteroid bodies (Fig. 10-21), Schaumann bodies (calcified laminated concretions within multinucleated giant cells) and Hamazaki-Wesenberg (coccoid, golden-brown, acid-fast) cytoplasmic inclusions can be seen in sarcoidosis. Long-standing granulomas may undergo fibrosis and eventual hyalinization. If necrosis is associated with the granulomas it is fibrinoid type. Biopsy of salivary gland tissue has been suggested as a diagnostic aid in suspected cases of sarcoidosis. Some investigators have documented success rates around 45 % with this technique.

ANCILLARY STUDIES

The diagnosis of granulomatous inflammation generally precipitates the use of special stains to exclude common infectious etiologies. Special stains for fungus and bacteria, particularly mycobacterium, are negative in cases of sarcoidosis.

DIFFERENTIAL DIAGNOSIS

The differential diagnosis of sarcoidosis in salivary glands is chronic sialadenitis and benign

SARCOIDOSIS DISEASE FACT SHEET	
Definition	Multisystem granulomatous disorder of unknown etiology
Incidence and location	Uncommon disorder
	Any organ may be affected but most commonly lung, lymph nodes, skin, eyes, and salivary glands
Morbidity and mortality	About 10%–20% do not respond to therapy
Gender, race, and age distribution	Female predominance (slight)
	Black >>> White (12 : 1)
	Peak incidence 2nd – 4th decades
Clinical features	Major and minor salivary gland enlargement with xerostomia
	Mucoceles may form secondary to granulomatous inflammation
	Elevated angiotensin-converting enzyme levels
	Heerfordt syndrome (uveoparotid fever) may be seen in patients with symptoms of parotid enlargement, anterior uveitis, facial paralysis, and fever
Prognosis and treatment	Approximately 60% of patients resolve within 2 years without treatment
	About 10% may die with disease as a result of respiratory or central nervous system complications

SARCOIDOSIS PATHOLOGIC FEATURES	
Gross findings	Diffuse enlargement of salivary glands
	Salivary gland cut surface may appear normal or show speckled areas of gray homogeneous tissue
Microscopic findings	Noncaseating granulomas with multinucleated giant cells and/or epithelioid histiocytes
	Variable number of lymphocytes
	Occasionally may have asteroid bodies, Schaumann bodies, or Hamazaki-Wesenberg inclusions
Ancillary studies	Special stains for organisms (fungus and bacteria, particularly mycobacterium), must be negative
Pathologic differential diagnosis	Chronic sialadenitis, infectious disease, benign lymphoepithelial lesion, Sjögren's syndrome

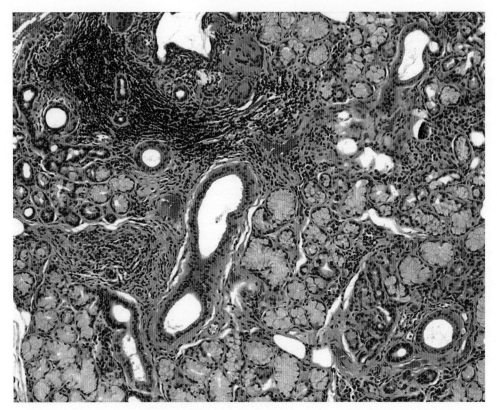

FIGURE 10-19

At medium power, periductal non-caseating granulomas are seen. Note the thin cuff of lymphocytes and the adjacent normal acini.

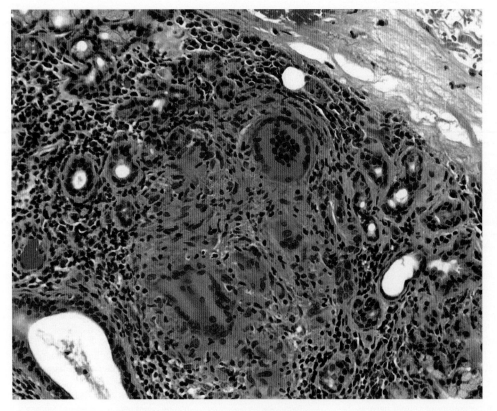

FIGURE 10-20

At high power, the multinucleated giant cells, epithelioid histiocytes, and Langerhans-type giant cells can be seen in this salivary gland biopsy from a patient with sarcoidosis.

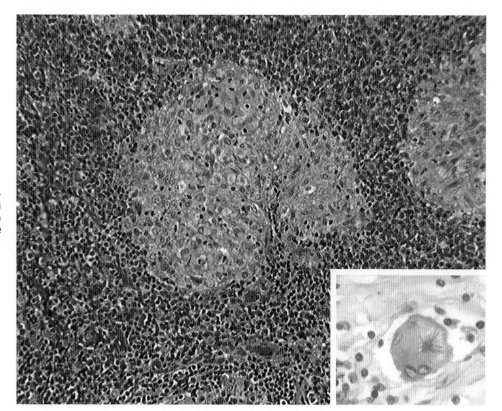

FIGURE 10-21

Tight granuloma surrounded by lymphocytes. The inset demonstrates an asteroid body which can be seen in sarcoid, although not specific for the disease.

lymphoepithelial lesion. The characteristic histologic finding for chronic sialadenitis is a mixture of chronic inflammatory cells and fibrosis. Benign lymphoepithelial lesion is characterized by epithelial/myoepithelial islands and hyperplastic lymphoid tissue. The misdiagnosis of Sjögren's syndrome from minor salivary gland biopsies has also been reported in patients with sarcoidosis.

PROGNOSIS AND THERAPY

In 60% of patients with sarcoidosis, the symptoms resolve within 2 years without therapy. Patients requiring medication have a variable response rate. In approximately 15% of patients affected with sarcoidosis, resolution does not occur even with treatment, and a minority of individuals may experience a progressive downward and possible fatal course, usually from respiratory or central nervous system complications.

SUGGESTED READING

Developmental, Including Heterotopia and Oncocytosis

1. Bouquot JE, Gnepp DR, Dardick I, Hietanen JHP: Intraosseous salivary tissue: Jawbone examples of choristomas, hamartomas, embryonic rests, and inflammatory entrapment. Oral Surg Oral Med Oral Pathol Oral Radiol Endod 2000;90:205–217.
2. Brandwein MS, Huvos AG: Oncocytic tumors of major salivary glands. A study of 68 cases with follow-up of 44 patients. Am J Surg Pathol 1991;15:514–528.

3. Lassaletta-Atienza L, Lopez-Rios F, Martin G, et al.: Salivary gland heterotopia in the lower neck: a report of five cases. Int J Ped Otorhinolaryngol 1998;43:153–161.
4. Scott J, Burns J, Flower EA: Histological analysis of parotid and submandibular glands in chronic alcohol abuse: a necropsy study. J Clin Pathol 1988;41:837–840.
5. Toh H, Kodama J, Fujuda J, et al.: Incidence and histology of human accessory parotid glands. Anat Rec 1993;236:589–590.
6. Zajtchuk JT, Patow CA, Hyams VJ: Cervical heterotopic salivary gland neoplasms: a diagnostic dilemma. Otolaryngol Head Neck Surg 1982;90:178–181.

Mucus Retention Cyst, Mucocele, Sialothiasis

1. Eveson JW: Superficial mucoceles: pitfall in clinical and microscopic diagnosis. Oral Surg Oral Med Oral Pathol 1988;66:318–322.
2. Gnepp DR, Brandwein MS, Henley JD: Salivary and lacrimal glands. In: Gnepp DR, ed. Diagnostic Surgical Pathology of the Head and Neck. Philadelphia: WB Saunders; 2001:332–334.
3. Peel RL: Diseases of the salivary glands. In: Barnes L, ed. Surgical Pathology of the Head and Neck, 2nd ed. New York: Marcel Dekker; 2001:642–644.
4. Raymond AK, Batsakis JG: Angiothiasis and sialothiasis in the head and neck. Ann Otol Rhinol Laryngol 1992;101:455–457.

Necrotizing Sialometaplasia

1. Abrams AM, Melrose RJ, Howell FV: Necrotizing sialometaplasia. A disease of simulating malignancy. Cancer 1973;32:130–135.
2. Brannon RB, Fowler CB, Hartman KS: Necrotizing sialometaplasia. Oral Surg Oral Med Oral Pathol 1991;72:317–325.
3. Gnepp DR, Brandwein MS, Henley JD: Salivary and lacrimal glands. In: Gnepp DR, ed. Diagnostic Surgical Pathology of the Head and Neck. Philadelphia: WB Saunders; 2001:336–349.

Benign Lymphoepithelial Lesion

1. Cleary KR, Batsakis JG: Undifferentiated carcinoma with lymphoid stroma of the major salivary gland. Ann Otol Rhinol Laryngol 1990;99:236–238.
2. DiGiuseppe JA, Corio RL, Westra WH: Lymphoid infiltrates of the salivary glands: pathology, biology, and clinical significance. Curr Opin Oncol 1996;8:232–237.
3. Falzon M, Isaacson PG: The natural history of benign lymphoepithelial lesion of the salivary gland in which there is a monoclonal population of B cells. Am J Surg Pathol 1991;15:59–65.
4. Godwin JT: Benign lymphoepithelial lesion of the parotid gland (adenolymphoma, chronic inflammation, lymphoepithelioma, lymphocytic tumor, Mikulicz disease): report of eleven cases. Cancer 1952;5:1089–1093.
5. Saw D, Lau WH, Ho JH, et al.: Malignant lymphoepithelial lesion of the salivary gland. Hum Pathol 1986;17:914–923.
6. Wallace AC, MacDougall JT, Hildes JA, Lederman JM: Salivary gland tumors in Canadian eskimos. Cancer 1963;16:1338–1353.

Lymphoepithelial Cyst

1. d'Agay MF, de Roquanacourt A, Peuchmaur M, et al.: Cystic benign lymphoepithelial lesion of the salivary glands in HIV-positive patients. Virchows Arch A Pathol Anat 1990;417:353–356.
2. Cleary KR, Batsakis JG: Lymphoepithelial cysts of the parotid region: a "new face" on an old lesion. Ann Otol Rhinol Laryngol 1990;99:162–164.
3. Huang RD, Perlman S, Friedman WH, Loree T: Benign cystic vs. solid lesions of the parotid gland in HIV patients. Head Neck 1991;13:522–527.
4. Layfield LJ, Gopez V: Cystic lesions of the salivary glands: cytologic features in fine needle aspiration biopsies. Diagn Cytopathol 2002;27:197–204.

Sarcoidosis

1. Batsakis JG: Granulomatous sialadenitis. Ann Otol Rhinol Laryngol 1991;100:166–169.
2. van der Walt D, Leake J: Granulomatous sialadenitis of the major salivary glands. A clinicopathological study of 57 cases. Histopathology 1987;11:131–144.
3. Weinberger SE: Sarcoidosis. In: Goldman L, Ausiello D, eds. Cecil Textbook of Medicine, 22nd ed. Philadelphia: WB Saunders; 2004:547–551.

11 Benign Neoplasms of the Salivary Glands

Kevin Torske

PLEOMORPHIC ADENOMA

Pleomorphic adenoma (aka: benign mixed tumor; mixed tumor) is a benign salivary gland neoplasm composed of ductal epithelial and myoepithelial cell proliferations set within a mesenchymal stroma. This tumor displays remarkable histomorphologic diversity, including varying cellularity, cell morphology, matrix type, and encapsulation.

CLINICAL FEATURES

Pleomorphic adenoma (PA) is the most common neoplasm within the salivary glands, accounting for 54% to 76% of all neoplasia. The vast majority of pleomorphic adenomas are diagnosed in the parotid gland, followed by the minor salivary glands (especially the palate), and the submandibular gland. In adults, females are affected more often than males, with a wide age range peaking in the 4th to 5th decade. In children and adolescents, the incidence peaks between 5–15 years of age, and males are affected more frequently.

Presentation usually consists of a painless, slowly growing firm mass. Mucosal ulceration or paresthesia due to nerve compression are rare findings. Nodules tend to be singular and mobile, and may become very large if neglected.

PATHOLOGIC FEATURES

GROSS FINDINGS

The surgical specimen of a pleomorphic adenoma typically is a well-circumscribed, smooth to slightly lobular, round to oval mass. Encapsulation is highly variable, ranging from thick to nonexistent. The cut surface is white to tan and often shiny to translucent.

PLEOMORPHIC ADENOMA DISEASE FACT SHEET	
Definition	A benign neoplasm composed of ductal epithelial cells and myoepithelial cells set within a mesenchymal stroma
Incidence and location	Most common salivary gland neoplasm
	Comprises approximately 60% of parotid, submandibular, and minor salivary gland tumors
Gender, race, and age distribution	Female > Male
	Peak incidence in 4th to 5th decades
Clinical features	Asymptomatic, slow growing mass
	May become very large if neglected
Prognosis and treatment	20%–45% recurrence rate with enucleation
	Multinodular recurrences with potential for malignant transformation
	Superficial or total parotidectomy, submandibular gland resection, or wide excision

PLEOMORPHIC ADENOMA PATHOLOGIC FEATURES	
Gross findings	Well-circumscribed, round-oval, variably encapsulated mass
	White-tan, possibly shiny or translucent cut surface
Microscopic findings	Epithelial glandular ductal structures
	Myoepithelial cells in spindle, plasmacytoid, epithelioid, stellate, or basaloid morphologies
	Mesenchymal stroma either myxoid, mucochondroid, hyalinized, osseous, and/or fatty
Immunohistochemical features	Cytokeratin cocktail, S-100 protein, smooth muscle actin, glial fibrillary acidic protein reactive
Pathologic differential diagnosis	Myoepithelioma, adenoid cystic carcinoma, polymorphous low-grade adenocarcinoma

Recurrent tumors are commonly multifocal, ranging in size from <1 mm to several centimeters.

Microscopic Findings

The histologic range of appearances of pleomorphic adenoma is enormously varied. However, all mixed tumors display epithelial ductal structures, myoepithelial cells, and a mesenchymal stroma (Fig. 11-1). Three main groups of tumors may be found: myxoid ("stroma-rich"; = 80 % stroma), cellular ("cell-rich"; "myoepithelial predominant"; = 80 % cellular), and mixed (classic), with the stroma-rich variant being more prone to recurrence.

Encapsulation is highly variable in pleomorphic adenoma, ranging from thick to nonexistent. Lack of encapsulation is particularly evident in tumors of the minor salivary glands (especially the palate) or those stroma-rich, with direct interface between the tumor and the surrounding gland or connective tissues (Fig. 11-2).

Ductal epithelial cells comprise the minority of the cell population, forming variably sized ductal or cystic structures. The remainder of the cellularity is myoepithelial, with a wide range of cytomorphology, including spindled, plasmacytoid, squamoid, stellate, or basaloid. Neoplastic myoepithelial cells may be abluminal, individual and scattered, or in nests, solid sheets, or trabeculae.

Mucochondroid stromal changes are most frequent. However, the amount of collagenation is variable, with stroma appearing from loose and myxoid to dense and hyalinized. Chondroid, osteoid, and adipose-like tissues may also occur.

Multinodular growth, although rare in primary mixed tumors, is very common in recurrent disease. The nodules tend to be stroma-rich, widely scattered in the prior surgical area, and number up to over 100 (Fig. 11-3).

Pleomorphic adenomas which display mild-to-moderate pleomorphism, prominent nucleoli, or numerous mitotic divisions may be termed *atypical*. If malignant features such as tumor necrosis, atypical mitoses, and profound nuclear pleomorphism are present, but limited to the interior of the neoplasm (i.e., without capsular invasion), the diagnosis ***carcinoma ex mixed tumor in situ*** is appropriate. Other than indicating a stronger need for close clinical follow-up, these features do not appreciably alter the prognosis.

Ancillary Studies

Immunohistochemical Features

Cytokeratin cocktail is strongly reactive in ductal epithelial and squamoid myoepithelial cells, and variably reactive in other myoepithelial forms. Vimentin, S-100 protein, glial fibrillary acidic protein (GFAP), and smooth muscle actin (SMA) decorate the myoepithelial component. However, the staining patterns are irregular, with strongest reactivity for GFAP in the myxoid areas and SMA in the spindle cells.

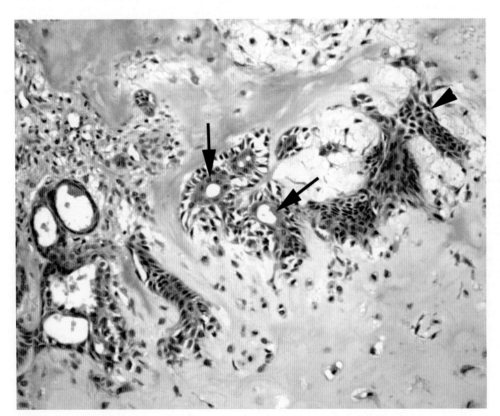

FIGURE 11-1

Pleomorphic adenoma, medium power. Ductal structures (*arrows*) are surrounded by abluminal myoepithelial cells, which are also present in sheets (*arrowhead*) and singly scattered. Hyalinized, myxoid, and chondromyxoid stroma types are evident.

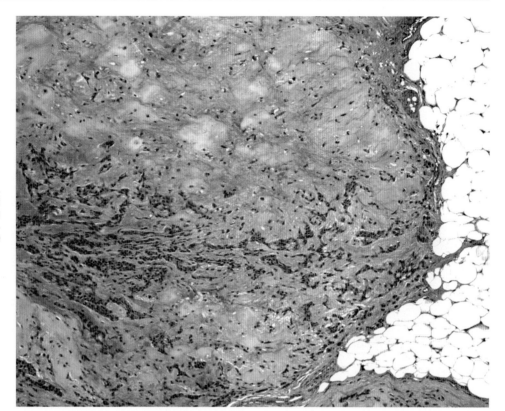

FIGURE 11-2

Pleomorphic adenoma, low power. Unencapsulated myxoid (stroma-rich) variant showing direct apposition with the adjacent adipose tissue. Note the small tumor extensions into the fat.

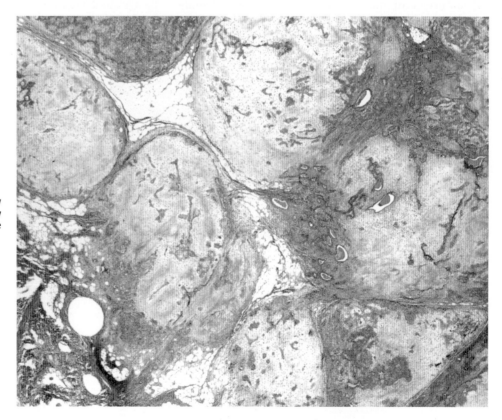

FIGURE 11-3

Recurrent pleomorphic adenoma, low power. Note the numerous, variably sized nodules which characterize recurrent disease.

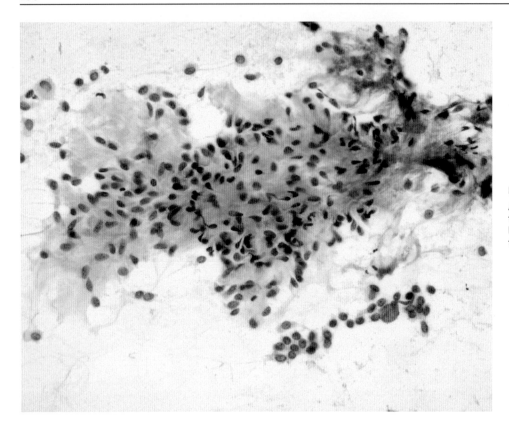

FIGURE 11-4

A Papanicolau-stained FNA preparation shows small glands with a fibrillar matrix material intermixed with the epithelial component.

FINE NEEDLE ASPIRATION

Aspirates are variably cellular, with a biphasic appearance of luminal (ductal) epithelial cells and abluminal myoepithelial cells. The ductal cells display ample cytoplasm with round-oval nuclei and small nucleoli.

Myoepithelial cells may be single or clustered, and plasmacytoid, spindle-shaped, or stellate (Fig. 11-4). Mucoid background material may also be present, taking on a bright, fibrillar, magenta quality with Wright stained material (Fig. 11-5).

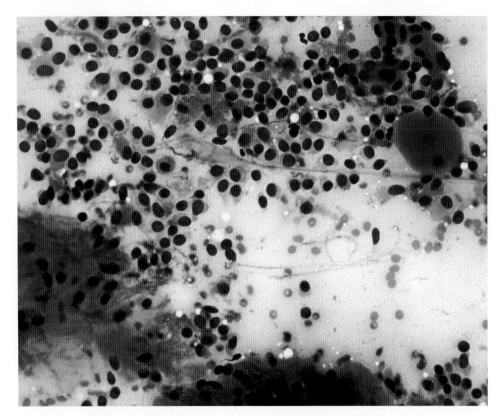

FIGURE 11-5

A May-Grunwald-Giemsa FNA preparation stains the mucochondroid material bright magenta. It is intimately interspersed with the epithelial component.

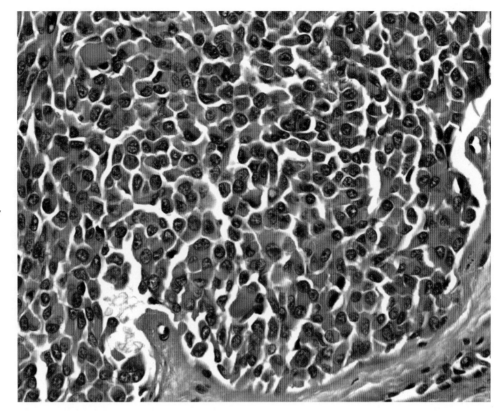

FIGURE 11-6
Myoepithelioma, plasmacytoid variant, high power.

DIFFERENTIAL DIAGNOSIS

The differential includes myoepithelioma, a benign epithelial salivary gland neoplasm composed predominantly or entirely of myoepithelial cells. This neoplasm may represent one end of the spectrum of mixed tumor in which ductal structures are extremely rare to absent. Plasmacytoid (Fig. 11-6) or spindled (Fig. 11-7) myoepithelial cells predominate, although any myoepithelial form may be present.

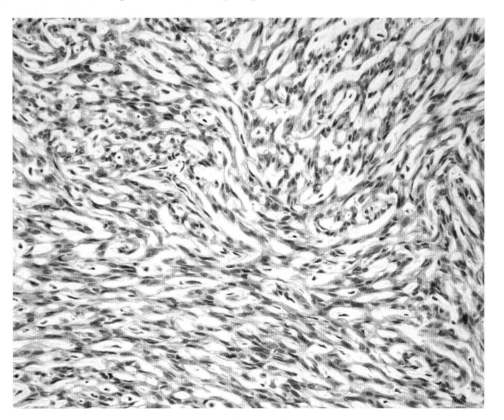

FIGURE 11-7
Myoepithelioma, spindle cell variant, medium power.

Basal cell adenoma may also be included in the differential. Unencapsulated tumors, especially those of the palate, may appear infiltrative, mimicking malignancies such as polymorphous low-grade adenocarcinoma or adenoid cystic carcinoma.

PROGNOSIS AND THERAPY

Recurrence rate after simple tumor enucleation approaches 45%. This is due to lack of encapsulation, leading to tumor rupture with spillage or incomplete removal. Therefore, superficial or total parotidectomy, resection, or excision with a rim of uninvolved tissue are the treatments of choice for parotid, submandibular, or minor salivary gland tumors, respectively. Recurrence rate with such treatment is up to 2.5%, with most occurring in less than 10 years. Recurrent disease tends to include multiple nodules, with a resultant higher degree of surgical difficulty and risk of further recurrences.

Malignant change transpires in 2% to 7%. Influencing factors include multiple recurrences, age >40 years, male sex, nodule >2 cm in diameter, and deep lobe tumors.

BASAL CELL ADENOMA

Basal cell adenoma is a benign salivary gland epithelial neoplasm composed of a proliferation of small basaloid cells in solid, tubular, trabecular, or membranous patterns. Histogenesis is most likely from intercalated ducts or the basal cells of striated ducts.

CLINICAL FEATURES

Basal cell adenoma represents approximately 2% of salivary gland neoplasms. Usual presentation is of an asymptomatic, solitary, slow growing mass, with almost 75% arising within the parotid gland. Females are affected slightly more commonly than males.

The membranous pattern of basal cell adenoma, however, has a different presentation. Males are affected more frequently and the tumor has a propensity for multicentricity. In addition, the membranous-type (aka: *dermal anlage tumor*) may be part of the "skin/salivary gland tumor diathesis," a rare complex that includes concomitant skin neoplasms such as dermal cylindroma, trichoepithelioma, or eccrine spiradenoma.

BASAL CELL ADENOMA DISEASE FACT SHEET

Definition	Benign epithelial salivary gland neoplasm composed of small basaloid cells in solid, trabecular, tubular, or membranous growth patterns
Incidence and location	Represents 2% of salivary gland neoplasms 75% within parotid gland, remainder in submandibular and minor salivary glands
Gender, race, and age distribution	Female > Male (solid and tubulo-trabecular); Male > Female in membranous Peak incidence in 6th decade
Clinical features	Asymptomatic, slow growing mass Multifocality; membranous variant is associated with skin adnexal tumors
Prognosis and treatment	25% recurrence rate and small chance of malignant transformation for membranous type Low recurrence rate for other forms Surgical excision with possible parotidectomy

PATHOLOGIC FEATURES

GROSS FINDINGS

Grossly, the tumor is well circumscribed, pink-brown and smooth in texture, simulating an enlarged lymph node. Size may be large, but is generally <3 cm in diameter.

MICROSCOPIC FINDINGS

Basal cell adenoma is a well-circumscribed, usually encapsulated epithelial tumor that classically displays two cell morphologies. Peripheral cells line the outer surface of tumor nodules, often in a palisade-like fashion. The basaloid cells are small, with scant cytoplasm and dense basophilic nuclei. Central cells form the bulk of the nodules and solid sheets. Polygonal or angular in shape, they are larger with more abundant cytoplasm, and pale round nuclei (Fig. 11-8). Small ductal structures or squamous metaplasia, including keratinization, may be observed.

Four basic architectural patterns are seen: solid, tubular, trabecular (Fig. 11-9), and membranous (Fig. 11-10). A single tumor may display all patterns, but a single form usually predominates. The membranous-type is characterized by a "jig-saw" puzzle pattern, with nodules surrounded and separated by a dense, periodic acid-Schiff positive hyaline band (Fig. 11-11). The hyaline material may also form small round globules within the cellular islands. The membranous type may be multifocal or unencapsulated, with limited infiltration into the surrounding parenchyma.

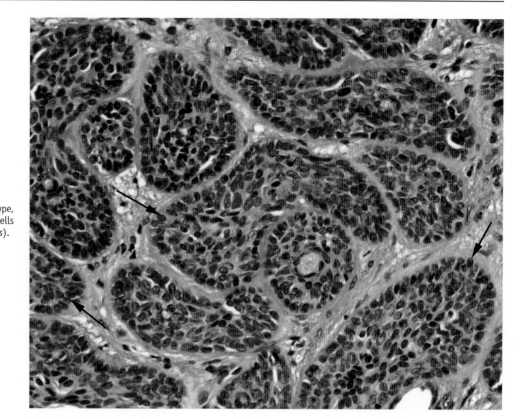

FIGURE 11-8

Basal cell adenoma, solid type, medium power. Nests of basaloid cells with peripheral palisading (*arrows*).

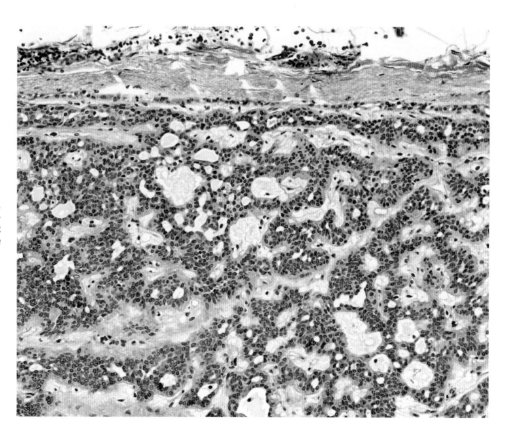

FIGURE 11-9

Basal cell adenoma, trabecular type, medium power. Encapsulated neoplasm composed of variably thick chains of basaloid cells in a loose fibrous stroma.

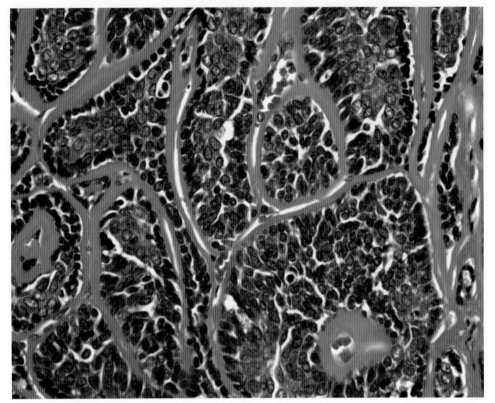

FIGURE 11-10
Basal cell adenoma, membranous type, medium power. Nests of basaloid cells are surrounded by a distinct hyaline band.

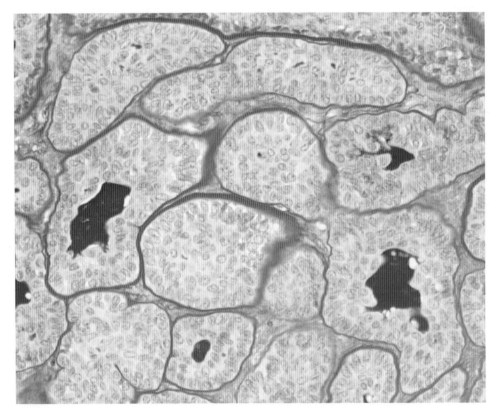

FIGURE 11-11
Basal cell adenoma, membranous type, medium power. The periodic acid-Schiff special stain accentuates the hyaline bands surrounding the basaloid cell nests.

BASAL CELL ADENOMA PATHOLOGIC FEATURES	
Gross findings	Well-circumscribed, encapsulated, pink-brown mass
Microscopic findings	Solid, trabecular, tubular, and membranous patterns
	Small basaloid cells with peripheral palisading around sheets and islands
	Focal squamous metaplasia with keratinization
Immunohistochemical features	Cytokeratin, S-100 protein, and smooth muscle actin reactive
Pathologic differential diagnosis	Basal cell adenocarcinoma, canalicular adenoma

ANCILLARY STUDIES

IMMUNOHISTOCHEMICAL FEATURES

Cytokeratin cocktail is reactive in all tumors, albeit with variable distribution and density. S-100 protein, smooth muscle actin, and muscle-specific actin may display focal reactivity in the basal aspect of the peripheral epithelial cells.

FINE NEEDLE ASPIRATION

Aspirates consist of sheets or syncytial fragments of bland oval cells with scanty cytoplasm and round-to-oval nuclei. Nests or groups may be surrounded by a bright green (Papanicolau) or pale magenta (May-Grunwald-Giemsa) hyaline band.

DIFFERENTIAL DIAGNOSIS

The differential diagnosis may include malignancies such as basal cell adenocarcinoma or adenoid cystic carcinoma. However, cytologic atypia, infiltration, and perineural invasion are seen in carcinoma but not in adenoma. Benign entities such as canalicular adenoma, pleomorphic adenoma or myoepithelioma may also be considered, but usually have different patterns of growth.

PROGNOSIS AND THERAPY

Surgical excision, to possibly include parotidectomy, is the treatment of choice. Although very low for most forms, the recurrence rate for membranous type is up to 25%, possibly due to capsular infiltration or multifocality. In addition, malignant degeneration or concomitant skin lesions are possible with this variant.

CANALICULAR ADENOMA

Canalicular adenoma is a benign epithelial salivary gland neoplasm characterized by chains of columnar cells and preference for the minor salivary glands. An excretory duct origin is favored.

CLINICAL FEATURES

Canalicular adenoma is almost invariably associated with minor salivary glands, especially those of the upper lip, with occasional cases in the buccal mucosa or the palate. Indeed, it is the second most common salivary gland neoplasm of the upper lip, just behind pleomorphic adenoma. It typically presents as an asymptomatic, firm-to-fluctuant, slow growing, 1–2 cm submucosal nodule in the 7th decade of life. Although usually solitary, multifocal tumors may occur. Females are more commonly affected, as are blacks.

PATHOLOGIC FEATURES

GROSS FINDINGS

Canalicular adenomas are well circumscribed yet nonencapsulated. Cut surface is pinkish-brown to tan, with a solid or cystic consistency.

CANALICULAR ADENOMA DISEASE FACT SHEET	
Definition	Benign epithelial salivary gland neoplasm characterized by chains of columnar cells and a loose connective tissue stroma
Incidence and location	1% of all salivary gland neoplasms; 4% of all minor salivary gland neoplasms
	Minor salivary glands: especially upper lip
Gender, race, and age distribution	Female > Male
	Black > White
	Peak incidence in 7th decade
Clinical features	Asymptomatic, potentially multinodular mass
Prognosis and treatment	Recurrence rare
	Simple excision with clear margins

MICROSCOPIC FINDINGS

Canalicular adenoma is commonly composed of long single-layered strands or tubules of epithelial cells within a loose, lightly collagenized stroma (Fig. 11-12). The strands may run parallel to one another with a thin "canal-like" space in between, then attach to one another and separate, creating a "beaded" appearance (Fig. 11-13). Cystic degeneration is common. The tumor may be multifocal, with possible small, unencapsulated "incipient" tumors evident within surrounding minor salivary glands.

Usually columnar, the cells may vary from cuboidal to basaloid, with eosinophilic cytoplasm and basophilic, oval nuclei (Fig. 11-14). Pleomorphism is minimal and mitotic figures are rare.

ANCILLARY STUDIES

The cells are reactive for cytokeratin cocktail and S-100 protein, while nonreactive for actin myofilaments, and calponin. GFAP reactivity is rare and focal.

DIFFERENTIAL DIAGNOSIS

The differential includes benign neoplasms pleomorphic adenoma and basal cell adenoma. Malignancies commonly affecting the minor salivary glands, predominantly adenoid cystic carcinoma and polymorphous low-grade adenocarcinoma, may also be considered.

PROGNOSIS AND THERAPY

Simple local excision to include a rim of normal surrounding tissue is the treatment of choice. Although true recurrence is rare, the presence of multiple lesions may set the stage for possible clinical reappearance.

CANALICULAR ADENOMA PATHOLOGIC FEATURES	
Gross findings	Well-circumscribed, nonencapsulated, solid or cystic, pink-tan mass
Microscopic findings	Long chains of columnar cells that may join then separate
	Tubules, duct-like forms, and rare solid groups
	Loose, lightly collagenous stroma
Immunohistochemical features	Cytokeratin and S-100 protein reactive
Pathologic differential diagnosis	Basal cell adenoma, polymorphous low-grade adenocarcinoma

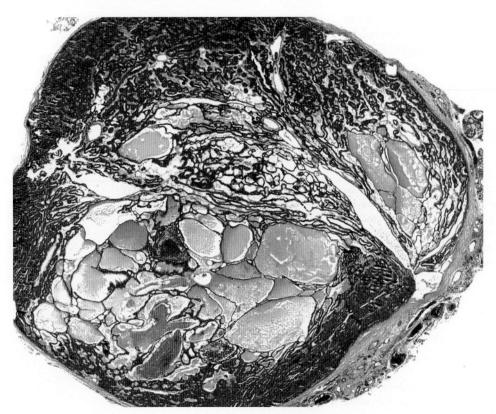

FIGURE 11-12

Canalicular adenoma, low power. Well-circumscribed neoplasm displaying chains of cells in a loose fibrous stroma. Note the numerous cystically dilated spaces.

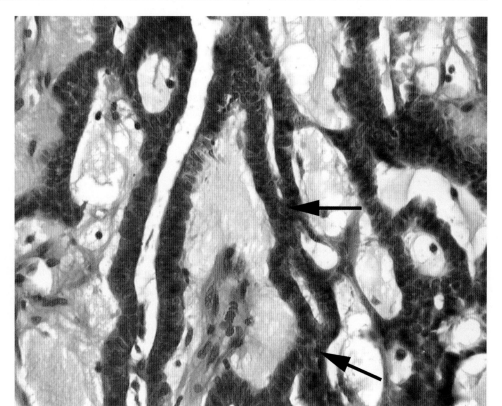

FIGURE 11-13

A high power of the basaloid cells of a canalicular adenoma are arranged in a palisaded architecture with central lumens. "Beading" is noted where the cells come together and then separate (*arrows*).

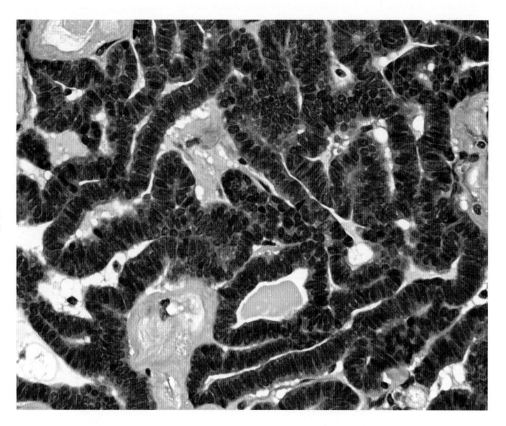

FIGURE 11-14

Canalicular adenoma, medium power. Single file chains of columnar cells with oval nuclei characterize this entity.

ONCOCYTOMA

Oncocytoma (oncocytic adenoma) is a putative neoplastic proliferation of oncocytically altered cells. Histogenesis may be associated with therapeutic radiation exposure.

CLINICAL FEATURES

Oncocytoma typically presents as an asymptomatic, slow-growing mass in the 7th–8th decade of life. It affects the parotid gland in 80% to 90% of cases, and represents about 1% of all parotid gland neoplasms. A slight female predominance is noted. Approximately 7% of tumors have a bilateral presentation. Caucasoid patients are affected much more commonly than other races.

PATHOLOGIC FEATURES

GROSS FINDINGS

Oncocytoma presents as a soft, well-circumscribed, tan-brown nodule. Usually solitary, size may range from 1–7 cm.

MICROSCOPIC FINDINGS

Oncocytes are polygonal cells with abundant eosinophilic, finely granular cytoplasm, and uniform, round, centrally placed nuclei, with or without nucleoli (Fig. 11-15). Oncocytes may accumulate copious amounts of intracytoplasmic glycogen, and due to processing, artifacts appear "clear" and devoid of cytoplasmic staining (Fig. 11-16).

Oncocytic metaplasia is identified as solitary or small groups of acinar cells that become oncocytes, a process practically universal after 70 years of age. A distinct and immediate transformation of one cell type to another occurs, without alteration of the glandular architecture.

Oncocytosis (oncocytic hyperplasia) includes multiple areas of oncocytic change, ranging from isolated variably sized cellular groupings (*nodular form*), to a diffuse process affecting a majority of the gland (*diffuse form*). An intimate, unencapsulated relationship between the glandular parenchyma and the oncocytic nodule is present, and may include normal acini intermixed with oncocytes (Fig. 11-17).

Oncocytoma is well circumscribed with variably thick encapsulation (Fig. 11-18). Architectural patterns include monotonous solid sheets, acinar, trabecular, papillary-cystic, or follicular. Slight nuclear pleomorphism may be identified, including prominent nucleoli. Significant stromal hyalinization or vascularity is possible. It is common to appreciate focal areas of oncocytosis in conjunction with an oncocytoma. *Clear cell oncocytosis/oncocytoma* may be applied if the majority of the oncocytes display cleared cytoplasm.

ANCILLARY STUDIES

HISTOCHEMICAL FEATURES

Phosphotungstic acid-hematoxylin highlights the abundant mitochondria, seen as deep blue cytoplasmic granularity, ranging from focal and patchy to diffuse. Striated duct epithelial cells may act as a positive internal control.

ELECTRON MICROSCOPY

The organelles are shifted by an overwhelming number of mitochondria, many of which will show abnormal cristae (Fig. 11-19).

FINE NEEDLE ASPIRATION

Aspirates contain polygonal epithelial cells in papillary fragments, sheets, acinar-like structures, or singly.

ONCOCYTOMA
DISEASE FACT SHEET

Definition	Neoplasm composed of large polygonal cells containing abundant, abnormal mitochondria
Incidence and location	Approximately 1% of all parotid gland neoplasms
	Parotid >> submandibular gland
Gender, race, and age distribution	Female ≥ Male
	Predominantly affects whites
	7th to 8th decades
Clinical features	Asymptomatic, slow growing mass
Prognosis and treatment	Minimal recurrence with adequate excision
	Parotidectomy

ONCOCYTOMA
PATHOLOGIC FEATURES

Gross findings	Single, soft, well-circumscribed tan-brown nodule
Microscopic findings	Large polygonal cells with abundant eosinophilic granular cytoplasm
	Solid, acinar, trabecular, or follicular patterns
	Clear cell change can be seen
Ancillary studies	Cytokeratin and PTAH reactive
Pathologic differential diagnosis	Nodular oncocytic hyperplasia, metastatic renal cell carcinoma

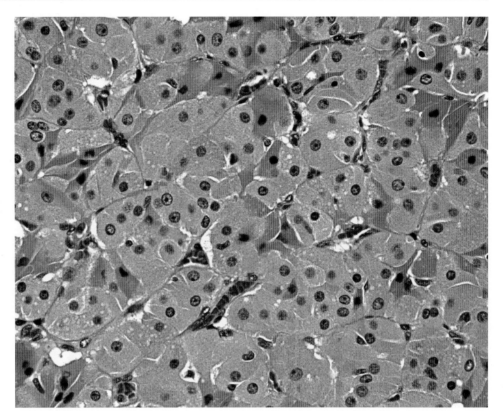

FIGURE 11-15

Oncocytoma, high power. Oncocytes are polygonal cells with abundant granular eosinophilic cytoplasm and round, centrally placed nuclei, with or without nucleoli.

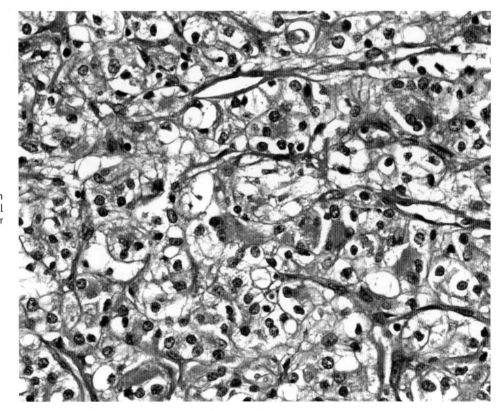

FIGURE 11-16

Oncocytoma, clear cell variant, high power. Note scattered cells still possessing eosinophilic granular cytoplasm.

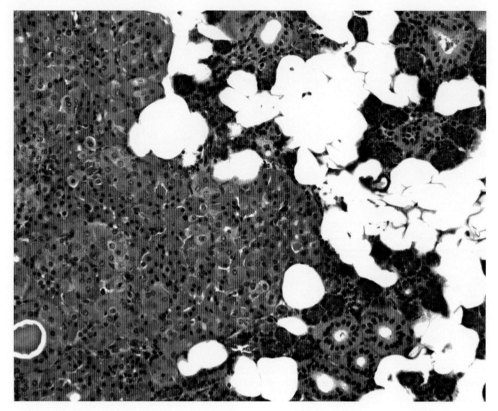

FIGURE 11-17
Oncocytosis, medium power. Sheets of oncocytes (*left*) with an intimate association with the salivary gland parenchyma.

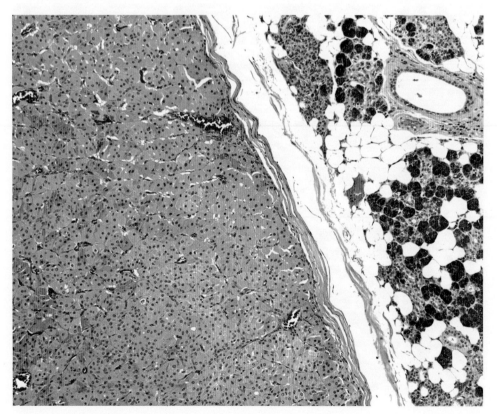

FIGURE 11-18
Oncocytoma, low power. Well-encapsulated neoplasm composed of sheets of oncocytically altered cells.

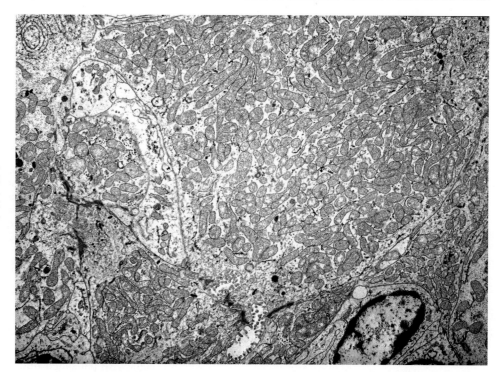

FIGURE 11-19

The cytoplasm is laden with mitochondria identified by this electron microscopic image of an oncocytoma. A small lumen is noted along with tight junctions and short microvilli. (Courtesy of Dr. I. Dardick.)

Prominent nucleoli may be noted, but mitoses are rare to nonexistent. There is no background lymphoid component.

DIFFERENTIAL DIAGNOSIS

The benign differential includes Warthin tumor and a dominant nodule within oncocytic hyperplasia. Warthin tumor has lymphoid elements and oncocytic hyperplasia often blends with the surrounding parenchyma. Malignancies may include acinic cell adenocarcinoma or metastatic renal cell carcinoma, especially if clear cells predominate. Special studies usually help to resolve this differential. Oncocytic carcinoma is invasive with profound pleomorphism and necrosis.

PROGNOSIS AND THERAPY

Superficial parotidectomy for lateral tumors, or total parotidectomy for deep lobe tumors, is the treatment of choice. Recurrence is minimal, but may occur due to multifocality or incomplete removal. The rare tumors of the minor salivary glands require complete excision with a small margin of uninvolved tissue.

PAPILLARY CYSTADENOMA LYMPHOMATOSUM (WARTHIN TUMOR)

Warthin tumor is a relatively common lesion composed of a double layer of oncocytic epithelium, a papillary and cystic architectural pattern, and a dense lymphoid stroma. It possibly arises from entrapped salivary tissue in intraparotid or periparotid lymph nodes.

CLINICAL FEATURES

Warthin tumor is the second most common benign salivary gland tumor and characteristically presents in the lower portion of the lateral lobe of the parotid gland. With slight caucasoid male predominance, presentation normally occurs in the 6th–7th decades as an asymptomatic, slowly growing 1–4 cm mass. Bilaterality or multifocality occurs more frequently than with any other salivary gland tumor, and it is synchronously identified with other tumors more frequently than any other tumor type (i.e., if there are two tumors, one is likely to be a Warthin tumor). Cigarette smoking is a likely etiologic factor.

PAPILLARY CYSTADENOMA LYMPHOMATOSUM (WARTHIN TUMOR) DISEASE FACT SHEET	
Definition	Biphasic tumor composed of bilayered oncocytic cells forming cysts and papillary fronds set within a dense lymph node-like stroma
Incidence and location	Second most common salivary gland tumor Parotid gland
Gender, race, and age distribution	Male ≥ Female White > Black 6th–7th decade
Clinical features	Asymptomatic, slow growing mass Most common "second" and bilateral tumor
Prognosis and treatment	Recurrence rate 4%–25% Lumpectomy to parotidectomy

PAPILLARY CYSTADENOMA LYMPHOMATOSUM (WARTHIN TUMOR) PATHOLOGIC FEATURES	
Gross findings	Circumscribed, firm to cystic, brown, yellow, or red mass
Microscopic findings	Double layer of oncocytic epithelium with cuboidal basal cell and overlying columnar luminal cell Numerous cysts with papillary infoldings Dense lymph node-like stroma with possible reactive germinal centers
Immunohistochemical features	Epithelial component CK reactive Lymphoid component reactive with B and T cell markers
Pathologic differential diagnosis	Sebaceous lymphadenoma

PATHOLOGIC FEATURES

GROSS FINDINGS

Macroscopically, Warthin tumor is circumscribed, solid, papillary, or cystic, and brown, yellow, or red. Cysts may contain yellow-brown fluid.

MICROSCOPIC FINDINGS

The name "papillary cystadenoma lymphomatosum," while cumbersome, correctly describes the overall microscopic appearance (Fig. 11-20). Papillary fronds and cystic spaces are lined by oncocytic epithelium, con-

sisting of cuboidal basal cells supporting tall columnar cells with palisaded nuclei (Fig. 11-21), often creating a "tram-tracking" nuclear appearance. The cystic spaces may be filled with fluid, desquamated epithelial cells, or lymphoid cells. Intimately associated with the epithelial component is a dense lymph node-like stroma, including reactive germinal centers. The proportion of the three elements is variable.

Trauma may lead to cyst rupture and subsequent foreign body giant cell reaction, fibrosis, squamous metaplasia, or necrosis. Such findings may occur after fine needle aspiration biopsy.

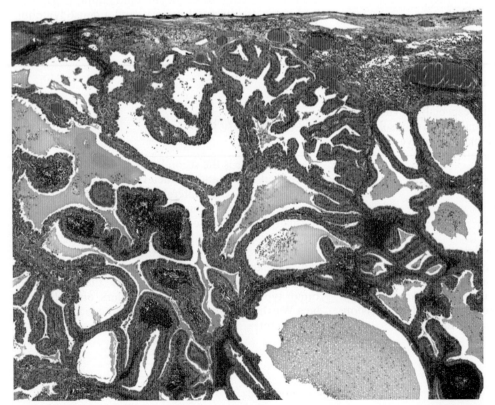

FIGURE 11-20

Warthin tumor, low power. Papillary-cystic tumor associated with a dense lymphoid stroma.

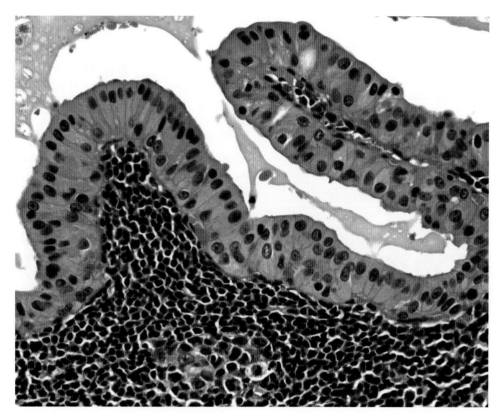

FIGURE 11-21

Warthin tumor, high power. Papillary fronds and cystic spaces lined by a double cell layer of oncocytes. A small germinal center is evident in the bottom center.

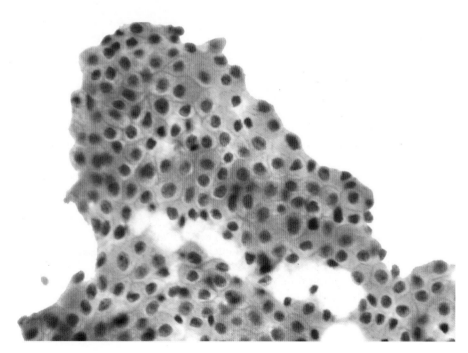

FIGURE 11-22

A Papanicolau-stained smear demonstrates a cohesive cluster of epithelial cells in a honeycomb pattern with well-defined cell borders.

ANCILLARY STUDIES

IMMUNOHISTOCHEMICAL FEATURES

The epithelial component is reactive for cytokeratin cocktail. The lymphoid portion is similar to a reactive lymph node, including kappa and lambda light-chain polyclonality.

FINE NEEDLE ASPIRATION

Aspirates display small collections of epithelial cells surrounded by lymphocytes. The epithelial islands demonstrate a "honeycomb" pattern, with well-defined cell borders and relatively large, centrally placed nuclei (Fig. 11-22). Squamoid cells may also be evident. Background lymphoid elements are easily identified. The cytoplasm appears opacified and "blue" with air-dried preparations (Fig. 11-23).

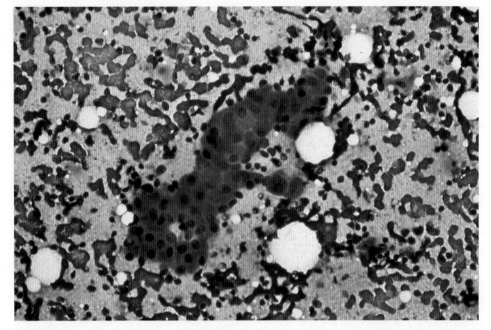

FIGURE 11-23
A May-Grunwald-Giemsa preparation stains the papillary frond epithelium a light blue. Lymphocytes are noted in the bloody background. Histiocytes may be seen within the background as part of the cyst fluid.

DIFFERENTIAL DIAGNOSIS

The differential diagnosis includes lymphatic metastasis or sebaceous lymphadenoma. The cytologically bland, bilayered, oncocytic epithelial element mitigates against both. Cystadenomas may be oncocytic, but do not have the lymphoid stroma and usually have small, multilocular cystic spaces.

PROGNOSIS AND THERAPY

The recurrence rate after excision is 4% to 25%, likely associated with multifocality or incomplete excision. Treatment may range from lumpectomy to total parotidectomy, depending on size and location. A low malignant transformation rate of 1% is recognized, usually being squamous cell carcinoma or a low-grade B cell lymphoma.

SEBACEOUS ADENOMA/LYMPHADENOMA

Sebaceous adenoma is a benign epithelial neoplasm composed of proliferating, incompletely differentiated sebaceous glands. Sebaceous lymphadenoma is a rare variant in which the epithelial proliferation is supported by a dense lymphoid stroma, and possibly arises from entrapped salivary gland tissue within intraparotid or periparotid lymph nodes.

CLINICAL FEATURES

The clinical presentations of both neoplasms are similar and therefore discussed together. Both represent <1% of all salivary gland neoplasms, and are rarely reported outside of the parotid gland. Males and females are affected equally, with most lesions presenting in the 6th–7th decades of life as an asymptomatic, slow-growing mass.

SEBACEOUS ADENOMA/LYMPHADENOMA DISEASE FACT SHEET	
Definition	Benign epithelial neoplasms composed of proliferating, incompletely differentiated sebaceous glands set within a fibrous (*s. adenoma*) or dense lymphoid (*s. lymphadenoma*) stroma
Incidence and location	Approximately 0.1% of all salivary gland neoplasms
	Parotid gland
Gender, race, and age distribution	Equal gender distribution
	6th–7th decades
Clinical features	Slow growing, asymptomatic mass
Prognosis and treatment	Minimal recurrence rate
	Surgical excision with rim of normal tissue

PATHOLOGIC FEATURES

GROSS FINDINGS

Both sebaceous adenoma and lymphadenoma are firm, well-circumscribed masses. Cut section is pinkish-gray to white or yellow, and may be solid or cystic.

MICROSCOPIC FINDINGS

Sebaceous adenoma is a well-circumscribed neoplasm composed of solid and cystic epithelial structures surrounded by a dense fibrous stroma (Fig. 11-24). Epithe-

lial nests are squamoid, displaying peripheral basaloid cells maturing inwardly into sebaceous cells (Fig. 11-25). Sebaceous cells, either singly or in groups, may also be found within cyst walls.

Sebaceous lymphadenoma is composed of a similar epithelial component which is evenly distributed throughout the tumor. However, instead of a fibrous background, the stroma consists of a dense population of lymphocytes, to perhaps include reactive germinal centers (Fig. 11-26). A histologically similar tumor, devoid of sebaceous differentiation, is termed *lymphadenoma*.

ANCILLARY STUDIES

IMMUNOHISTOCHEMICAL FEATURES

Cytokeratin cocktail and epithelial membrane antigen are reactive in the epithelial proliferation. S-100 protein and smooth muscle actin are nonreactive. As with Warthin tumor, the lymphoid component in sebaceous lymphadenoma is similar to a reactive lymph node.

FINE NEEDLE ASPIRATION

Aspirates of sebaceous adenoma demonstrate aggregates of large cells with foamy cytoplasm and central crenated nuclei, consistent with sebaceous cells. Less mature squamoid forms with dense cytoplasm and round-to-oval nuclei are also present. Sebaceous

SEBACEOUS ADENOMA/LYMPHADENOMA PATHOLOGIC FEATURES	
Gross findings	Well-circumscribed, solid or cystic, pink-gray mass
Microscopic findings	Solid nests or cystic structures
	Mature sebaceous differentiation in center of nodules or wall of cysts
	Fibrous stroma (*s. adenoma*) or dense lymph node-like stroma (*s. lymphadenoma*)
Immunohistochemical features	Epithelial component is cytokeratin and EMA reactive
Pathologic differential diagnosis	Sebaceous carcinoma, mucoepidermoid carcinoma, Warthin tumor

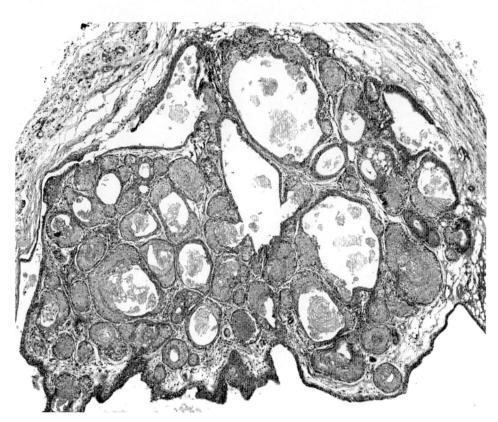

FIGURE 11-24

Sebaceous adenoma, low power. Numerous solid and cystically dilated nests of squamoid cells.

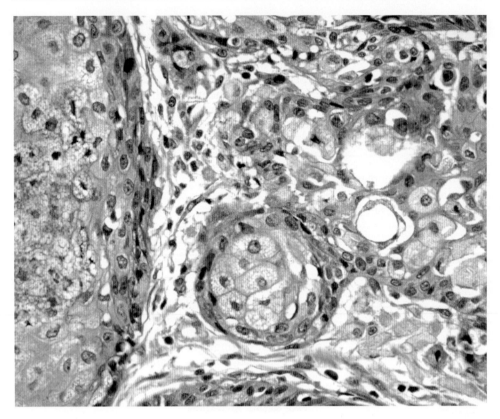

FIGURE 11-25
Sebaceous adenoma, medium power.
Nests of squamoid cells displaying
central sebaceous cell differentiation.

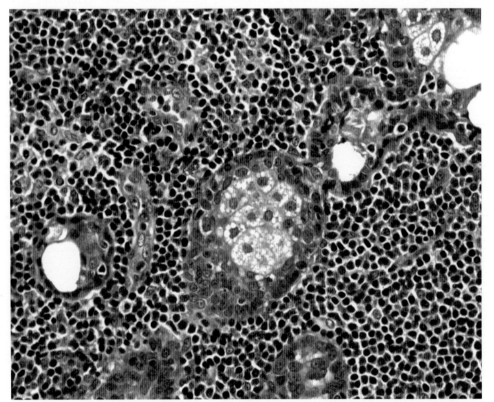

FIGURE 11-26
Sebaceous lymphadenoma, medium
power. Solid and cystic nests of
squamoid cells with sebaceous differentiation within a dense lymphoid
stroma.

lymphadenoma is similar, but also displays a background of small mature lymphocytes.

DIFFERENTIAL DIAGNOSIS

The sebaceous adenoma differential includes mucoepidermoid carcinoma and sebaceous adenocarcinoma. Sebaceous lymphadenoma may be confused with metastatic squamous cell carcinoma.

PROGNOSIS AND THERAPY

Treatment includes surgical excision to include a rim of normal surrounding tissue. Recurrence rate is minimal following complete removal.

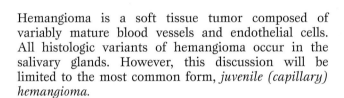

HEMANGIOMA

Hemangioma is a soft tissue tumor composed of variably mature blood vessels and endothelial cells. All histologic variants of hemangioma occur in the salivary glands. However, this discussion will be limited to the most common form, *juvenile (capillary) hemangioma*.

CLINICAL FEATURES

Juvenile (capillary) hemangioma (JH) affects the very young, arising at birth or shortly thereafter, and is the most common salivary gland neoplasm to arise in this time frame. Females predominate, and the parotid gland is the affected site in a vast majority of cases. Bilateral-

ity is found in approximately 25%. A rapid growth phase is followed by a very slow involutional phase. The tumor may become large, affecting greater than half of the face, and extend into the ear, lip, subglottis, or nose. Usually asymptomatic, complications such as cutaneous ulceration, bleeding, airway compression, or rarely congestive heart failure may arise.

PATHOLOGIC FEATURES

GROSS FINDINGS

Macroscopically, parotid JH is hemorrhagic, lobular, and red-to-brown. As opposed to a discreet mass, the lesion diffusely affects the lobes of the gland.

MICROSCOPIC FINDINGS

JH appears as a diffuse replacement of the salivary gland parenchyma. The lobular architectural pattern and anatomic boundaries of the salivary gland are maintained, with replacement of the serous acini by sheets of small endothelial cells and immature capillaries (Fig. 11-27). Striated ducts and peripheral nerves, however, seem unaffected.

The endothelial cells are small with indistinct cell borders. Nuclei are oval or irregular, with possible grooves and occasional inconspicuous nucleoli. Mitotic figures, normal in morphology, may be numerous. Dense cellularity may mask the vascular differentiation (Fig. 11-28). Erythrocytes are noted within the lumens.

ANCILLARY STUDIES

IMMUNOHISTOCHEMICAL FEATURES

The endothelial cells are reactive with CD31, CD34, and FVIII-RAg. Reticulin accentuates the vascularity. Cytokeratin cocktail highlights the residual ductal structures.

HEMANGIOMA (JUVENILE) DISEASE FACT SHEET

Definition	Soft tissue tumor composed of variably mature blood vessels and endothelial cells
Incidence and location	Rare Parotid gland
Gender, race, and age distribution	Female > Male Perinatal or neonatal
Clinical features	Rapid growth followed by slow involution Usually asymptomatic
Prognosis and treatment	Majority with spontaneous resolution over time Pharmacologic therapy if required

---

HEMANGIOMA (JUVENILE) PATHOLOGIC FEATURES

Gross findings	Hemorrhagic, lobular, red-brown
Microscopic findings	Interdigitation between salivary acini and intercalated ducts by immature endothelial cells and small capillaries Lobular architecture of gland intact
Immunohistochemical features	Endothelial cells are CD31, CD34, and Factor VIII reactive
Pathologic differential diagnosis	Angiosarcoma

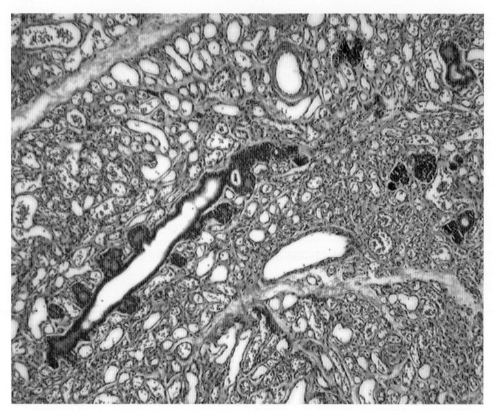

FIGURE 11-27

Juvenile capillary hemangioma, low power. Salivary gland lobules replaced by endothelial cells and small blood vessels. Note that the glandular architecture and excretory ducts are still intact.

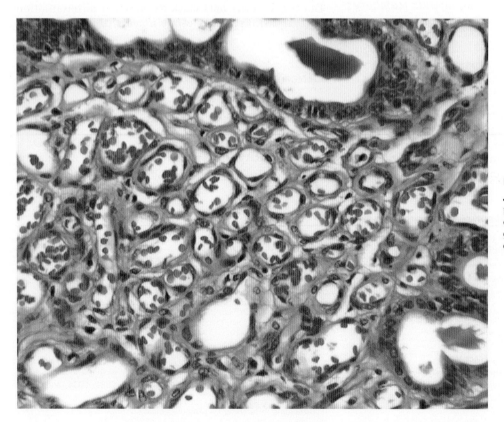

FIGURE 11-28

Juvenile capillary hemangioma, high power. Small uniform endothelial cells and small capillaries replace the glandular acini. Note the residual excretory duct.

FINE NEEDLE ASPIRATION

Aspirates consist of a spindle cell proliferation, including cohesive groups of bland cells in a bloody background, or hypercellular groups arranged in compact, three-dimensional coils. The cells have scant-to-moderate cytoplasm and oval nuclei. Needless to say, FNA is not recommended if the clinical differential includes a vascular neoplasm.

DIFFERENTIAL DIAGNOSIS

Angiosarcoma is very rare in this age group, yet is at the top of the differential. Bland cytomorphology and maintenance of glandular architecture favors JH.

PROGNOSIS AND THERAPY

Most JH involute over time, with 75% to 95% displaying spontaneous regression by 7 years. However, pharmacologic therapy, including corticosteroids and/or interferon (α-2a or α-2b), may be required if complications develop. Resection is not advised due to blood loss or possible injury to the facial nerve.

SIALOBLASTOMA

Sialoblastoma is an extremely rare benign to low-grade malignant epithelial and myoepithelial neoplasm reminiscent of the embryonic stage of major salivary gland development. Other names used to describe this entity include embryoma, congenital basal cell adenoma, and congenital hybrid basal cell adenoma–adenoid cystic carcinoma.

CLINICAL FEATURES

Sialoblastoma arises in the perinatal to neonatal period, with most cases involving the parotid gland. There is significant variability in the clinical course, local aggressiveness, and growth rate. Lesions may become large, leading to surface skin ulceration and airway compromise. Sialoblastoma has been reported arising in conjunction with other congenital anomalies, including nevus sebaceus and hepatoblastoma.

PATHOLOGIC FEATURES

GROSS FINDINGS

Excision specimens typically display a lobular, partially circumscribed mass, which is gray, yellow, or white. Focal necrosis and hemorrhage may be appreciated.

MICROSCOPIC FINDINGS

Basaloid cells predominate, with scanty cytoplasm, round-to-oval nuclei with fine chromatin and small nucleoli. Cuboidal cells with eosinophilic cytoplasm, and spindle-shaped myoepithelial forms may also occur. Architecturally, patterns may include solid nests with variable central necrosis (comedonecrosis), cribriform, or nodules of basaloid cells with peripheral palisading resembling basal cell adenoma. Ductal structures may also be observed. Background tissue is typically loose and myxoid (Fig. 11-29).

Mitotic rate may be high, being up to or surpassing 20/10 HPF (Fig. 11-30). Significant nuclear pleomorphism and invasion into surrounding parenchyma,

---

SIALOBLASTOMA DISEASE FACT SHEET	
Definition	Benign to low-grade malignant epithelial and myoepithelial neoplasm recapitulating the embryonic stage of salivary gland development
Incidence and location	Very rare
	Parotid gland
Gender, race, and age distribution	Equal gender distribution
	Perinatal or neonatal
Clinical features	Slow to rapidly growing mass
	Skin ulceration or airway compromise possible
Prognosis and treatment	Local recurrence of 30%; metastasis unusual
	Complete excision (parotidectomy) with rim of normal tissue

SIALOBLASTOMA PATHOLOGIC FEATURES	
Gross findings	Lobular, partially circumscribed, gray-white mass
	Possible focal necrosis and hemorrhage
Microscopic findings	Solid, nested with peripheral palisading, or cribriform architectural patterns
	Basaloid cells with scanty cytoplasm
	Potentially high mitotic rate and comedonecrosis
Immunohistochemical features	S-100 protein in basaloid cells
Pathologic differential diagnosis	Basal cell adenoma, adenoid cystic carcinoma

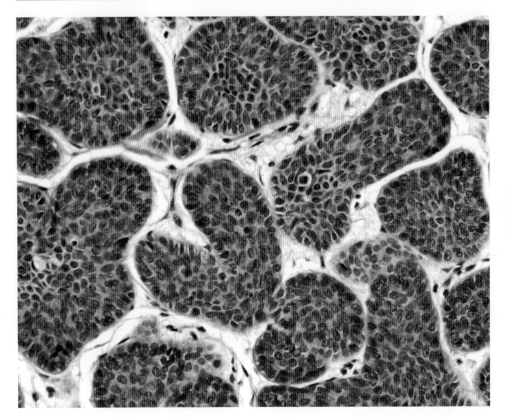

FIGURE 11-29
Sialoblastoma, medium power. Nests of basaloid cells in a loose fibrous stroma.

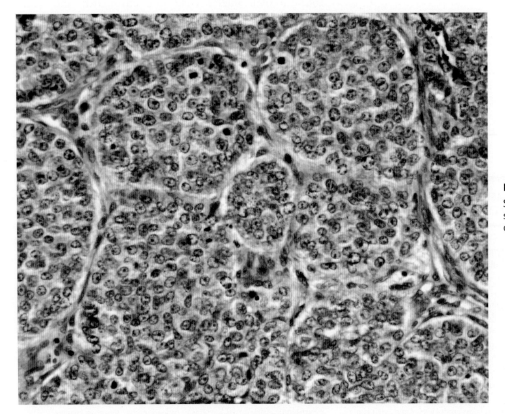

FIGURE 11-30
Sialoblastoma, high power. Nests and sheets of basaloid cells with numerous scattered mitotic figures.

nerves, or blood vessels may be present. Although highly indicative of malignancy, these features do not necessarily correlate with untoward clinical behavior or distant metastasis.

ANCILLARY STUDIES

S-100 protein is reactive in the basaloid and surrounding spindle cells. Cytokeratin cocktail accentuates the ductal structures.

DIFFERENTIAL DIAGNOSIS

Pleomorphic adenoma, basal cell adenoma, and malignancies such as mucoepidermoid carcinoma, basal cell adenocarcinoma, and acinic cell adenocarcinoma may be entertained. However, all of these entities are exquisitely rare in this age group, and therefore the differential diagnosis is usually limited.

PROGNOSIS AND THERAPY

Complete surgical excision is the treatment of choice. Adjuvant therapy should be avoided due to the young age of patients and the potential for long-term sequelae.

Local recurrence is the primary concern with sialoblastoma, occurring in approximately 30% of reported cases. Metastasis, however, is unusual, with only one reported case to regional cervical lymph nodes, no reports of distant spread or casualties related to disease. These findings suggest that sialoblastoma is a low-grade malignancy, despite aggressive clinical presentations or high-grade malignant cytomorphologic features. Since the number of reported cases is limited, the exact behavior of this rare lesion is still uncertain.

SUGGESTED READING

Pleomorphic Adenoma

1. Alves FA, Perez DEC, Almeida OP, et al.: Pleomorphic adenoma of the submandibular gland: clinicopathologic and immunohistochemical features of 60 cases in Brazil. Arch Otolaryngol Head Neck Surg 2002;128:1400–1403.
2. Buenting JE, Smith TL, Holmes DK: Giant pleomorphic adenoma of the parotid gland: case report and review of the literature. Ear Nose Throat J 1998;77:634–640.
3 Cardesa L, Alos L: Myoepithelioma. In: Barnes EL, Eveson JW, Reichart P, Sidransky D, eds. Pathology and Genetics of Head and Neck Tumours. Kleihues P, Sobin LH, series eds. World Health Organization Classification of Tumours. Lyon, France: IARC Press, 2005:259–260.
4. Dardick I: Myoepithelioma: definitions and diagnostic criteria. Ultrastruct Pathol 1995;19:335–345.
5. Eveson JW, Kusafuka K, Stenman G, Nagao T: Pleomorphic adenoma. In: Barnes EL, Eveson JW, Reichart P, Sidransky D, eds. Pathology and Genetics of Head and Neck Tumours. Kleihues P, Sobin LH, series eds.

World Health Organization Classification of Tumours. Lyon, France: IARC Press, 2005:254–259.
6. Glas AS, Vermey A, Hollema H, et al.: Surgical treatment of recurrent pleomorphic adenoma of the parotid gland: a clinical analysis of 52 patients. Head Neck 2001;23:311–316.
7. Guntinas-Lichius O, Kick C, Klussmann JP, et al.: Pleomorphic adenoma of the parotid gland: a 13-year experience of consequent management by lateral or total parotidectomy. Eur Arch Otorhinolaryngol 2004;261:143–146.
8. Kawahara A, Harada H, Kage M, et al.: Characterization of the epithelial components in pleomorphic adenoma of the salivary gland. Acta Cytol 2002;46:1095–1100.
9. Marioni G, Marino F, Stramare R, et al.: Benign metastasizing pleomorphic adenoma of the parotid gland: a clinicopathologic puzzle. Head Neck 2003;25:1071–1076.
10. Nishimura T, Furukawa M, Kawahara E, Miwa A: Differential diagnosis of pleomorphic adenoma by immunohistochemical means. J Laryngol Otol 1991;105:1057–1060.
11. Simpson RHW, Jones H, Beasley P: Benign myoepithelioma of the salivary glands: a true entity? Histopathology 1995;27:1–9.
12. Stennert E, Guntinas-Lichius O, Klussmann JP, Arnold G: Histopathology of pleomorphic adenoma in the parotid gland: a prospective unselected series of 100 cases. Laryngoscope 2001;111:2195–2200.
13. Stennert E, Wittekindt C, Klussmann JP, et al.: Recurrent pleomorphic adenoma of the parotid gland: a prospective histopathological and immunohistochemical study. Laryngoscope 2004;114:158–163.
14. Valentini V, Fabiani F, Perugini M, et al.: Surgical techniques in the treatment of pleomorphic adenoma of the parotid gland: our experience and review of the literature. J Craniofac Surg 2001;12:565–568.

Basal Cell Adenoma

1. Batsakis JG, Luna MA, El-Naggar AK: Basaloid monomorphic adenomas. Ann Otol Rhinol Laryngol 1991;100:687–690.
2. Dardick I, Lytwyn A, Bourne AJ, Byard RW: Trabecular and solid-cribriform types of basal cell adenoma: a morphologic study of two cases of an unusual variant of monomorphic adenoma. Oral Surg Oral Med Oral Pathol 1992;73:75–83.
3. de Araujo VC: Basal cell adenoma. In: Barnes EL, Eveson JW, Reichart P, Sidransky D, eds. Pathology and Genetics of Head and Neck Tumours. Kleihues P, Sobin LH, series eds. World Health Organization Classification of Tumours. Lyon, France: IARC Press, 2005:261–262.
4. Ferreiro JA: Immunohistochemistry of basal cell adenoma of the major salivary glands. Histopathol 1994;24:539–542.
5. Galed-Placed I, Yebra-Pimentel MT: Synchronous, double parotid tumor: fine needle aspiration cytology diagnosis of the membranous basal cell adenoma component. Acta Cytol 2000;44:1120–1122.
6. Jungehulsing M, Wagner M, Damm M: Turban tumor with involvement of the parotid gland. J Laryngol Otol 1999;113:779–783.
7. Sahu K, Pai RR, Pai KP: Basal cell adenoma, solid variant, diagnosed by fine needle aspiration cytology. Acta Cytol 1999;43:1198–1200.
8. Yu GY, Ubmuller J, Donath K: Membranous basal cell adenoma of the salivary gland: a clinicopathologic study of 12 cases. Acta Otolaryngol 1998;118:588–593.
9. Yu GY, Ussmueller J, Donath K: Histogenesis and development of membranous basal cell adenoma. Oral Surg Oral Med Oral Pathol 1998;86:446–451.
10. Zarbo RJ, Prasad AR, Regezi JA, et al.: Salivary gland basal cell and canalicular adenomas: immunohistochemical demonstration of myoepithelial participation and morphogenetic considerations. Arch Pathol Lab Med 2000;124:401–405.

Canalicular Adenoma

1. Ferreiro JA: Canalicular adenoma. In: Barnes EL, Eveson JW, Reichart P, Sidransky D, eds. Pathology and Genetics of Head and Neck Tumours. Kleihues P, Sobin LH, series eds. World Health Organization Classification of Tumours. Lyon, France: IARC Press, 2005:267.
2. Furuse C, Tucci R, de Souza SOM, et al.: Comparative immunoprofile of polymorphous low-grade adenocarcinoma and canalicular adenoma. Ann Diagnos Pathol 2003;7:278–280.
3. Harmse, Saleh HA, Odutoye T, et al.: Recurrent canalicular adenoma of the minor salivary glands in the upper lip. J Laryngol Otol 1997;111:985–987.

4. Neville BW, Damm DD, Weir JC, Fantasia JE: Labial salivary gland tumors. Cancer 1988;61:2113–2116.
5. Rousseau A, Mock D, Dover DG, Jordan RCK: Multiple canalicular adenomas: a case report and review of the literature. Oral Surg Oral Med Oral Pathol 1999;87:346–350.
6. Suarez P, Hammond HL, Luna MA, Stimson PG: Palatal canalicular adenoma: report of 12 cases and review of the literature. Ann Diagn Pathol 1998;2:224–228.
7. Waldron CA, El-Mofty SK, Gnepp DR: Tumors of the intraoral minor salivary glands: a demographic and histologic study of 426 cases. Oral Surg Oral Med Oral Pathol 1988;66:323–333.

Oncocytoma

1. Brandwein MS, Huvos AG: Oncocytic tumors of major salivary glands: a study of 68 cases with follow-up of 44 patients. Am J Surg Pathol 1991;15:514–528.
2. Capone RB, Ha PK, Westra WH, et al.: Oncocytic neoplasms of the parotid gland: a 16-year institutional review. Oto Head Neck Surg 2002;126:657–662.
3. Dardick I, Birek C, Lingen MW, Rowe PE: Differentiation and the cytomorphology of salivary gland tumors with specific reference to oncocytic metaplasia. Oral Surg Oral Med Oral Pathol 1999;88:691–701.
4. Davy CL, Dardick I, Hammond E, Thomas MJ: Relationship of clear cell oncocytoma to mitochondrial-rich (typical) oncocytomas of parotid salivary gland. Oral Surg Oral Med Oral Pathol 1994;77:469–478.
5. Ellis GL: "Clear cell" oncocytoma of salivary gland. Hum Pathol 1988;19:862–867.
6. Huvos AG: Oncocytoma. In: Barnes EL, Eveson JW, Reichart P, Sidransky D, eds. Pathology and Genetics of Head and Neck Tumours. Kleihues P, Sobin LH, series eds. World Health Organization Classification of Tumours. Lyon, France: IARC Press, 2005:266.
7. Kanazawa H, Furuya T, Murano A, Yamaki M: Oncocytoma of an intraoral minor salivary gland: report of a case and review of the literature. J Oral Maxillofac Surg 2000;58:894–897.
8. McLoughlin PM, Barrett AW, Speight PM: Oncocytoma of the submandibular gland. Int J Oral Maxillofac Surg 1994;23:294–295.
9. Palmer TJ, Gleeson MJ, Eveson JW, Cawson RA: Oncocytic adenomas and oncocytic hyperplasia of salivary glands: a clinicopathological study of 26 cases. Histopathology 1990;16:487–493.
10. Verma K, Kapila K: Salivary gland tumors with a prominent oncocytic component: cytologic findings and differential diagnosis of oncocytomas and Warthin tumor on fine needle aspirates. Acta Cytol 2003;47:221–226.

Papillary Cystadenoma Lymphohomatosum (Warthin Tumor)

1. Batsakis JG, El-Naggar AK: Warthin tumor. Ann Otol Rhinol Laryngol 1990;99:588–591.
2. Gallo O: New insights into the pathogenesis of Warthin tumor. Oral Oncol Eur J Cancer 1995;31B:211–215.
3. Seven H, Calis AB, Basak T, Senvar A: Multifocal synchronous Warthin tumor: a case report. Am J Oto 1999;20:346–349.
4. Shikhani AH, Shikhani LT, Kuhajda FP: Warthin tumor-associated neoplasms: report of two cases and review of the literature. Ear Nose Throat J 1993;72:264–273.
5. Simpson RHW, Eveson JW: Warthin tumour. In: Barnes EL, Eveson JW, Reichart P, Sidransky D, eds. Pathology and Genetics of Head and Neck Tumours. Kleihues P, Sobin LH, series eds. World Health Organization Classification of Tumours. Lyon, France: IARC Press, 2005:263–265.
6. Skálová A, Michal M: Cystadenoma. In: Barnes EL, Eveson JW, Reichart P, Sidransky D, eds. Pathology and Genetics of Head and Neck Tumours. Kleihues P, Sobin LH, series eds. World Health Organization Classification of Tumours. Lyon, France: IARC Press, 2005:273–274.
7. To EWH, Tsang WM, Leung CY, Lee KL: Warthin tumor with multiple sarcoid-like granulomas: a case report. J Oral Maxillofac Surg 2002;60:585–588.
8. Vories AA, Ramirez SG: Warthin tumor and cigarette smoking. South Med J 1997;90:416–418.
9. Yoo GH, Eisele MD, Askin FB, et al.: Warthin tumor: a 40-year experience at the Johns Hopkins hospital. Laryngoscope 1994;104:799–803.

Sebaceous Adenoma/Lymphadenoma

1. Batsakis JG, El-Naggar AK: Sebaceous lesions of salivary glands and oral cavity. Ann Otol Rhinol Laryngol 1999;99:416–418.
2. Derias NW, Chong WH, Pambakian H: Sebaceous adenoma of parotid gland—a rare tumor diagnosed by fine needle aspiration cytology. Cytopathology 1994;5:392–395.
3. Firat P, Hosal S, Tutar E, Ruacan S: Sebaceous lymphadenoma of the parotid gland. J Otol 2000;29:114–116.
4. Gnepp DR: Sebaceous adenoma. In: Barnes EL, Eveson JW, Reichart P, Sidransky D, eds. Pathology and Genetics of Head and Neck Tumours. Kleihues P, Sobin LH, series eds. World Health Organization Classification of Tumours. Lyon, France: IARC Press, 2005:268.
5. Gnepp DR, Brannon R: Sebaceous neoplasms of salivary gland origin: report of 21 cases. Cancer 1984;53:2155–2170.
6. Gnepp DR, Cheuk W, Chan JKC, Nagao T: Lymphadenomas: sebaceous and non-sebaceous. In: Barnes EL, Eveson JW, Reichart P, Sidransky D, eds. Pathology and Genetics of Head and Neck Tumours. Kleihues P, Sobin LH, series eds. World Health Organization Classification of Tumours. Lyon, France: IARC Press, 2005:269.
7. Iezzi G, Rubini C, Fioroni M, Piattelli A: Sebaceous adenoma of the cheek. Oral Oncol 2002;38:111–113.
8. Izutsu T, Kumamoto H, Kimizuka S, Ooya K: Sebaceous adenoma in the retromolar region: report of a case with a review of the English literature. Int J Oral Maxillofac Surg 2003;32:423–426.

Hemangioma

1. Childers ELB, Furlong MA, Fanburg-Smith LC: Hemangioma of the salivary glands: a study of ten cases of a rarely biopsied/excised lesion. Ann Diag Pathol 2002;6:339–344.
2. Damiani S, Corti B, Neri F, Collina G: Primary angiosarcoma of the parotid gland arising from benign congenital hemangioma. Oral Surg Oral Med Oral Pathol Oral Radiol Endod 2003;96:66–69.
3. Greene AK, Rogers GF, Mulliken LB: Management of parotid hemangioma in 100 children. Plast Recon Surg 2004;113:53–60.
4. Khurana KK, Mortelliti AJ: The role of fine-needle aspiration biopsy in the diagnosis and management of juvenile hemangioma of parotid gland and cheek. Arch Pathol Lab Med 2001;125:1340–1343.
5. Odell E: Haemangioma. In: Barnes EL, Eveson JW, Reichart P, Sidransky D, eds. Pathology and Genetics of Head and Neck Tumours. Kleihues P, Sobin LH, series eds. World Health Organization Classification of Tumours. Lyon, France: IARC Press, 2005:276.

Sialoblastoma

1. Alverez-Mendoza A, Calderon-Elvir C, Carrasco-Daza D: Diagnostic and therapeutic approach to sialoblastoma: report of a case. J Pediatr Surg 1999;34:1875–1877.
2. Brandwein-Gensler MS: Sialoblastoma. In: Barnes EL, Eveson JW, Reichart P, Sidransky D, eds. Pathology and Genetics of Head and Neck Tumours. Kleihues P, Sobin LH, series eds. World Health Organization Classification of Tumours. Lyon, France: IARC Press, 2005:253.
3. Brandwein M, Al-Naeif NS, Manwani D, et al.: Sialoblastoma–clinicopathological/immunohistochemical study. Am J Surg Pathol 1999;23:342–348.
4. Luna MA: Sialoblastoma and epithelial tumors in children: their morphologic spectrum and distribution by age. Adv Anat Pathol 1999;6:287–292.
5. Siddiqi SH, Solomon MP, Haller JO: Sialoblastoma and hepatoblastoma in a neonate. Pediatr Radiol 2000;30:349–351.
6. Siefert G, Donath K: The congenital basal cell adenoma of the salivary glands. Virchows Arch 1997;430:311–319.
7. Taylor GP: Congenital epithelial tumor of the parotid–sialoblastoma. Pediatr Pathol 1988;8:447–452.

12 Malignant Neoplasms of the Salivary Glands

John W. Eveson

ADENOCARCINOMA, NOT OTHERWISE SPECIFIED

CLINICAL FEATURES

Adenocarcinoma, not otherwise specified [AC (NOS)], is a diagnosis by exclusion with variable reporting of these tumors, making the interpretation of published data difficult and inconsistent. However, it represents approximately 17% of all salivary gland carcinomas. There is a slight female preponderance and the peak age incidence is in the 6th decade. These tumors are rare in children. About 60% arise in the major glands, predominantly the parotid. The most common intraoral sites are the junction of the hard and soft palates, buccal mucosa, and lips. Tumors usually present as a slow growing, painless mass with a duration varying from 1 to 10 years. About 20% of patients, however, have evidence of facial nerve involvement or pain, and the latter is more common in tumors in the submandibular gland. Tumors involving minor glands may ulcerate and extend into underlying bone.

PATHOLOGIC FEATURES

GROSS FINDINGS

The tumor can be well defined or have an irregular, infiltrative margin. There may be areas of intratumoral hemorrhage and necrosis.

ADENOCARCINOMA, NOT OTHERWISE SPECIFIED
DISEASE FACT SHEET

Definition	Adenocarcinoma, not otherwise specified, is a malignant salivary gland tumor which shows ductal differentiation but lacks the histomorphologic features that characterize other specific types of salivary carcinoma
Incidence and location	Represents up to 17% of salivary gland carcinomas
	60% of cases involve major glands, mostly the parotid
	40% seen in minor glands: palate, buccal mucosa, and lips
Morbidity and mortality	15-yr survival rate 54%–3% depending on grade (low grade–high grade)
Gender, race, and age distribution	Slight female predominance
	Peak incidence in 6th decade
	Very rare in children
Clinical features	Usually forms a slow growing mass
	Pain or facial nerve involvement seen in 20% cases
	Tumors of minor glands may ulcerate and involve underlying bone
Prognosis and treatment	Prognostic factors include tumor grading, stage, and location
	Tumors involving minor glands have better prognosis than major glands
	Surgery is the treatment of choice, supplemented by radiotherapy in advanced or recurrent cases

---

ADENOCARCINOMA, NOT OTHERWISE SPECIFIED
PATHOLOGIC FEATURES

Gross findings	May be well defined or show irregular outline
	Hemorrhage and necrosis common in high-grade tumors
Microscopic findings	Duct-like structures showing infiltrative growth
	Patterns include ducts, theques, sheets, and trabeculae
	Cytological variability used to grade the tumors into low-, intermediate-, and high-grade types
	Perineural and lymph-vascular invasion may be seen
Fine needle aspiration	Cellular smears with loose cohesion
	Obvious features of malignancy include cytologic variability, nuclear pleomorphism and occasional mucus cells
Pathologic differential diagnosis	Diagnosis of exclusion, metastatic adenocarcinoma, undifferentiated carcinoma

MICROSCOPIC FINDINGS

AC (NOS) all show duct-like structures with evidence of an infiltrative growth pattern (Fig. 12-1). By definition, they lack the characteristic features of more specific tumor types. There is wide variability in growth patterns, which can include ductal configurations, theques, sheets, and trabeculae (Fig. 12-2).

Cytological variability can be used to grade these tumors into low-, intermediate, and high-grade types. In most tumors the cells are cuboidal or oval; and in low-grade AC (NOS), there is minimal cytological atypia and infrequent mitotic figures. Ductal differentiation is typically a conspicuous feature of these tumors. Intermediate and high-grade tumors show increasing cellular atypia with hyperchromatism, high nuclear to cytoplasmic ratio, frequent and abnormal mitoses, and foci of hemorrhage and necrosis (Fig. 12-3). The stroma is often fibrous and cellular in low-grade tumors but more scanty in higher-grade tumors, which often have a solid growth pattern with minimal ductal differentiation. There may be evidence of lymph-vascular and nerve involvement (Fig. 12-4).

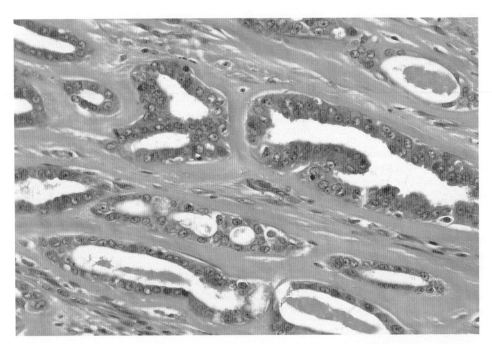

FIGURE 12-1
Heavy desmoplastic stroma separates these atypical epithelial cells arranged in glands.

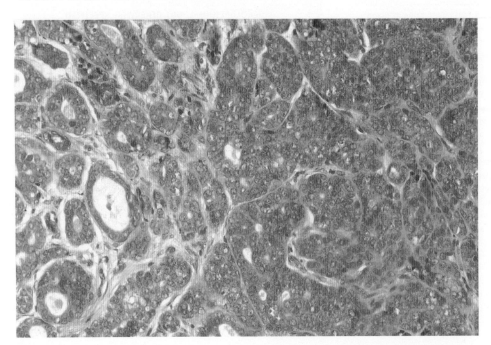

FIGURE 12-2
Trabeculae and tubules of atypical epithelial cells in this adenocarcinoma (NOS).

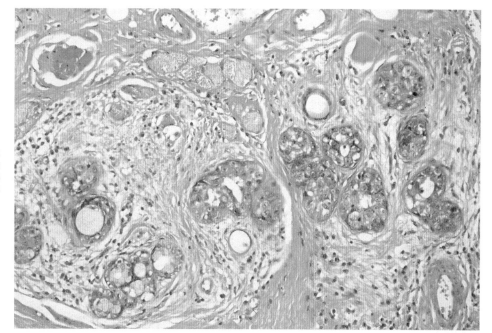

FIGURE 12-3
Glandular differentiation within a fibrous stroma. Mucin production is noted as are mitotic figures in this intermediate grade adenocarcinoma (NOS).

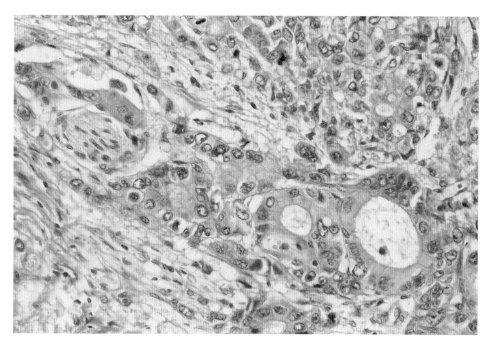

FIGURE 12-4
A higher grade adenocarcinoma (NOS) shows glandular profiles with perineural invasion. Mitotic figures are easily identified.

ANCILLARY STUDIES

IMMUNOHISTOCHEMICAL FEATURES

There are no characteristic immunohistochemical features and immunostaining is carried out merely to exclude other tumor types.

FINE NEEDLE ASPIRATION

The aspirates of AC (NOS) are often diagnosed as "salivary gland neoplasm" which covers a wide variety of benign and malignant tumors. Salivary gland tumors are well known to have variable patterns within the same tumor, making FNA smears difficult to accurately interpret. However, in general, separation into benign and malignant tumors can be accomplished, with low- versus high-grade designation. Obvious cellular features of malignancy, remarkable cytologic variability, vague glandular differentiation, and rare mucin production may help in establishing a high-grade neoplasm, with definitive classification reserved for the surgical specimen (Figs. 12-5, 12-6).

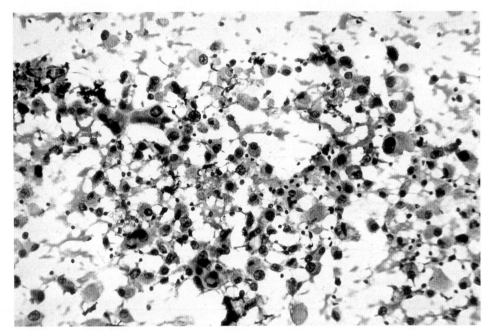

FIGURE 12-5
Highly cellular smear with slight dis-
cohesion of cells with a high nuclear
to cytoplasmic ratio and focal mucin
production (alcohol-fixed, Papanicolaou stain).

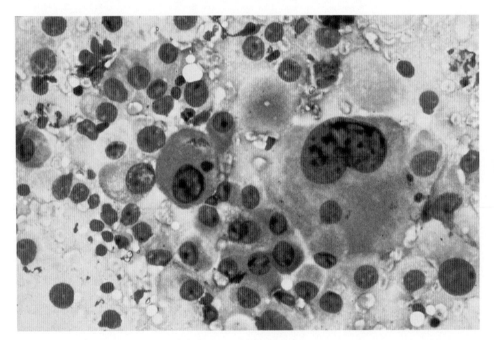

FIGURE 12-6
High power shows profound nuclear
pleomorphism, confirming a high-
grade malignancy, but no specific type
(air-dried, MGG stain).

DIFFERENTIAL DIAGNOSIS

The diagnosis of AC (NOS) is based on the exclusion of
other specific tumor types. The possibility of metastatic
disease, therefore, must always be considered. Evidence
of ductal differentiation aids the distinction from undifferentiated carcinoma.

PROGNOSIS AND THERAPY

The variability of the criteria used to define these
tumors makes the determination of prognostic factors
and assessment of outcome problematic. In addition,
many of the older series will have included tumors that
would now be allocated to more specific categories.

Prognostic factors include tumor grading, clinical stage, and location. Tumors involving minor glands have a better prognosis than those in major glands. In the largest survey of this tumor the 15-year survival rates for low-, intermediate, and high-grade tumors were 54%, 31%, and 3%, respectively. Low-grade and low-stage tumors are treated by complete surgical excision, and in higher grade tumors neck dissection and adjuvant radiotherapy need to be considered.

MUCOEPIDERMOID CARCINOMA

CLINICAL FEATURES

Mucoepidermoid carcinoma (MEC) is the most common malignant salivary gland tumor accounting for 12% to

29%. The major glands account for over half of all cases and most involve the parotid gland. MEC can also involve the mouth, particularly the palate (Fig. 12-7), buccal mucosa, lips and retromolar trigone, and the upper and lower respiratory tracts. Rarely, intrabony tumors form in the mandible and maxilla.

Women are more commonly affected than men (3:2), with a mean age in the 5th decade. MEC is the most common salivary gland malignancy in children. The tumor usually forms a painless, fixed, slow growing swelling of widely varying duration, which sometimes shows an accelerated growth phase immediately before clinical presentation. Symptoms include tenderness, pain, evidence of nerve involvement, otorrhea, dysphagia, and trismus. Intraoral tumors are often bluish-red and fluctuant and may resemble mucoceles or vascular lesions. The tumor occasionally invades the underlying bone.

PATHOLOGIC FEATURES

GROSS FINDINGS

MEC may be circumscribed and variably encapsulated or infiltrative and fixed, particularly in the higher grade

---

**MUCOEPIDERMOID CARCINOMA
DISEASE FACT SHEET**

Definition	A malignant glandular epithelial neoplasm characterized by mucus, intermediate, and epidermoid cells
Incidence and location	Most common malignant salivary gland tumor (12%–29%)
	Nearly 60% occur in major salivary glands (parotid usually)
	Others develop in mouth, upper and lower respiratory tracts
Morbidity and mortality	About 40% of cases recur locally
	Spread to regional lymph nodes and distant sites occurs in about 15% of cases
	5-yr survival rate 80%
Gender, race, and age distribution	Female > Male (3:2)
	Mean, 47 yr (range, 8–92 yr)
	Most common salivary malignancy in children
Clinical features	Usually forms a painless, fixed, slow growing swelling
	Intraoral tumors often bluish red and may mimic mucoceles or vascular tumors
	Symptoms include pain, evidence of nerve involvement, otorrhea, dysphagia, and trismus
Prognosis and treatment	Prognosis depends on clinical stage, site, grading, and adequacy of surgical excision
	Most tumors are low grade with excellent prognosis
	Tumors of submandibular gland have poorer prognosis
	Tumors, particularly high grade, can show spread to regional lymph nodes and distant sites including lungs, bone, and brain
	Surgery, with or without neck dissection, is the treatment of choice; palliative radiotherapy in some cases

---

**MUCOEPIDERMOID CARCINOMA
PATHOLOGIC FEATURES**

Gross findings	May be circumscribed and variably capsulated or infiltrative
	Cysts are often present and contain brownish, viscid fluid
Microscopic findings	Consists of mucus, intermediate, and epidermoid cells
	Other cells include clear cells, columnar cells, and oncocytes
	Tumors show cystic and solid areas in varying proportions along with other patterns
	Inflammation and fibrosis are commonly present
	Tumors separated into low, intermediate, and high grades
Immunohistochemical features	Intermediate and epidermoid cells are immunoreactive for cytokeratin and frequently epithelial membrane antigen
Fine needle aspiration	Cellular smears with background of mucinous material
	Cohesive epithelial clusters with sheets of cells and cells streaming in the mucus
	Mucocytes help to confirm diagnosis in presence of intermediate and epidermoid cells
Pathologic differential diagnosis	Necrotizing sialometaplasia, mucocele, cystadenoma, cystadenocarcinoma, squamous cell carcinoma, clear cell neoplasms, metastasis

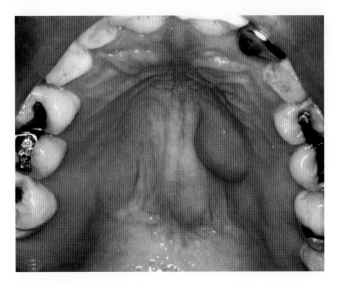

FIGURE 12-7
A mucosal covered slightly bluish mass in the left palate represents a mucoepidermoid carcinoma, although this finding is not specific.

tumors. Areas of scarring are relatively common. Most tumors are less than 4 cm in diameter. Cysts of variable sizes are often present and usually contain brownish, glary fluid.

MICROSCOPIC FINDINGS

The cells of mucoepidermoid carcinomas form sheets, islands, duct-like structures, and cysts of varying sizes (Fig. 12-8). The cysts may be lined by intermediate, mucus, or epidermoid cells, and are filled with mucus. It is common for larger cysts to rupture, spreading tumor cells into the adjacent tissue and evoking an inflammatory reaction with hemorrhage, hemosiderin deposition, cholesterol cleft formation and fibrosis (Fig. 12-9). Papillary processes may extend into the cyst lumina and occasionally this is a conspicuous feature.

The tumor consists predominantly of three cell types in widely varying proportions: epidermoid, mucus, and intermediate. Other less common cell types seen include clear cells, columnar cells, and oncocytes. The intermediate cells frequently predominate and range in size from small, basal cells with scanty basophilic cytoplasm (sometimes referred to as "maternal" cells) to larger and more oval cells with more abundant pale, eosinophilic cytoplasm which appear to merge into epidermoid or mucus cells (Fig. 12-10). The intermediate cells tend to form islands or sheets and may form the basally located cells of intratumoral cysts (Fig. 12-11). Mucus cells (mucocytes) can occur singly or in clusters and have pale and sometimes foamy cytoplasm, a distinct cell boundary, and peripherally placed, small and compressed nuclei. Mucocytes often form the lining of cysts or duct-like structures (Fig. 12-12). Occasionally mucocytes are so scanty they can only be identified with confidence by using stains such as mucicarmine (Fig. 12-13) or Alcian blue. Epidermoid cells may be uncommon and focally distributed. They have abundant eosinophilic cytoplasm but rarely show keratin pearl formation or dyskeratosis unless there has been a biopsy or FNA. Focal areas of clear cells are common and occasionally form the bulk of the tumor. The cells have distinct out-

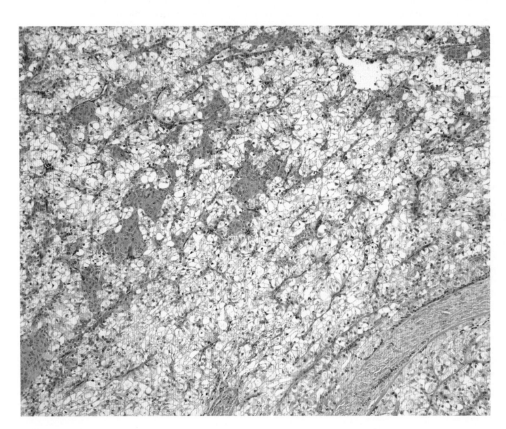

FIGURE 12-8
A sheet like distribution of intermediate and mucus cells in this mucoepidermoid carcinoma.

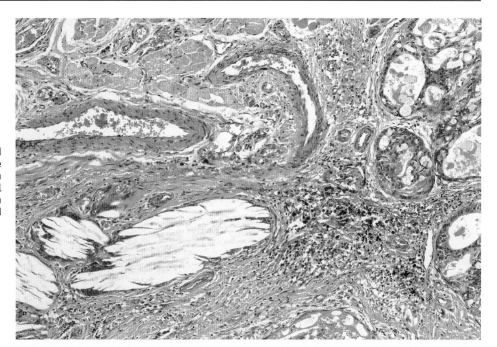

FIGURE 12-9

Small cysts lined by mucocytes and intermediate cells are noted in the right, which have ruptured, eliciting an inflammatory reaction with cholesterol cleft formation and hemosiderin laden macrophages. Skeletal muscle is noted in the upper field.

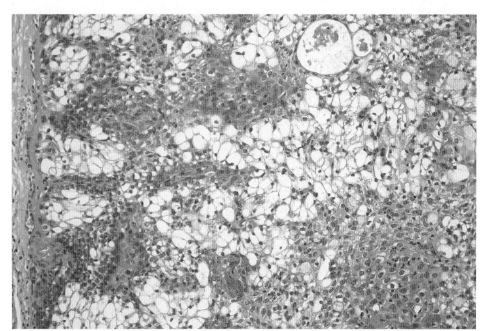

FIGURE 12-10

The intermediate cells are blending imperceptibly with the mucocytes in this mucoepidermoid carcinoma.

lines, water-clear cytoplasm and small, centrally located nuclei. They contain minimal sialomucin but usually have a plentiful glycogen content, as demonstrated with PAS/D staining. Columnar cells are uncommon and typically form the lining of cysts. Focal or generalized oncocytic metaplasia is seen occasionally.

Higher grade tumors have evidence of cytological atypia, a high mitotic frequency, and areas of necrosis, and are more likely to show neural invasion (Fig. 12-14). Rarely, low-grade mucoepidermoid carcinomas undergo de-differentiation. Stromal hyalinization is common and sometimes extensive and there is a scle-

rosing variant with intense central scarring, which may be due to infarction or mucus extravasation. Patchy lymphocytic infiltration is frequently present in MEC, and in some tumors there is extensive lymphocytic proliferation with germinal center formation, resembling lymph node infiltration.

TUMOR GRADING

MEC show remarkable variability in clinical behavior and several microscopic grading systems have been advocated in order to predict outcome. Many systems

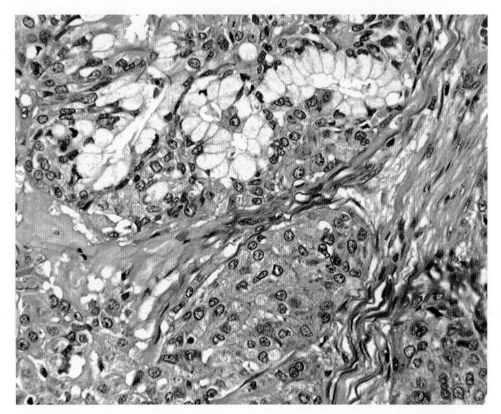

FIGURE 12-11
The intermediate cells are noted in small islands and forming the "basal zone" below the cystic spaces lined by mucocytes.

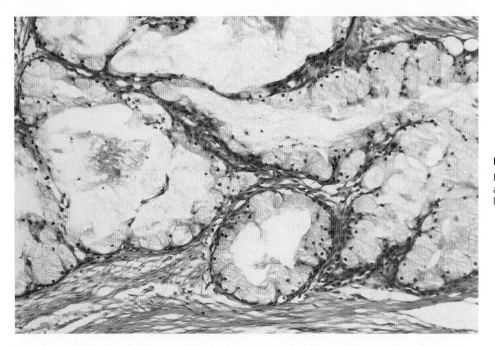

FIGURE 12-12
Mucocytes have fluffy cytoplasm and are seen lining cystic spaces or duct-like structures.

rely on subjective evaluation of the relative proportions of the various cell types, the degree of cellular atypia, mitotic frequency, presence of necrosis, and invasive characteristics. Low-grade tumors tend to be cystic, have abundant mucocytes and show minimal atypia or mitotic activity. They usually show evidence of invasion. Higher grade tumors tend to be more cellular with minimal cyst formation. They have few mucocytes and

consist mainly of cells similar to squamous cell carcinoma and may show necrosis and neural or vascular invasion. A numerical grading system using point scoring of five parameters appears to be very useful in defining the tumors as low-, intermediate, or high-grade and predicting their behavior (Table 12-1). However, the grading of MEC of the submandibular gland using this system was less reliable. A seven point grading

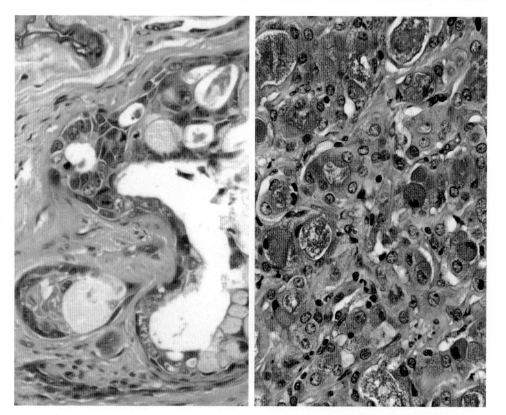

FIGURE 12-13

Left: Mucocytes are identified in a cyst with intermediate cells at the base. *Right:* Mucicarmine highlights intracytoplasmic mucin, especially in cells with eccentric, squashed nuclei.

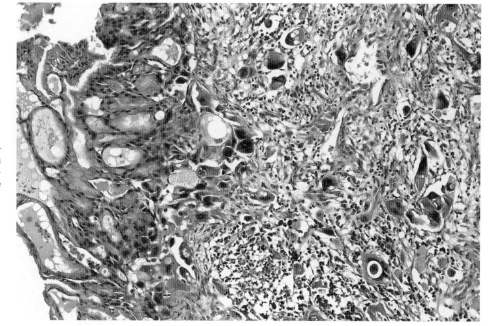

FIGURE 12-14

The left side of the field shows mucocytes within a relatively low-grade area of MEC with areas of much more pleomorphic, high-grade tumor on the right.

TABLE 12-1

Grading and Outcome for Mucoepidermoid Carcinomas

Parameter		Point Value
Intracystic component <20%		+2
Neural invasion		+2
Necrosis		+3
Mitotic figures ≥4/10 HPF		+3
Anaplasia		+4
Grade	Total Score	Death of Disease
Low	0–4	3.3%
Intermediate	5–6	9.7%
High	≥7	46.3%

system, including the additional parameters of the nature of the invasive front and bone invasion, has been recently proposed but requires additional validation.

ANCILLARY STUDIES

IMMUNOHISTOCHEMICAL FEATURES

Intermediate, squamous, and columnar cells are usually positive for cytokeratin but clear cells show inconsistent reactivity and mucocytes are negative. Epithelial membrane antigen is positive in most tumor cells, but staining with this and other immunocytochemical agents does not correlate with histological grading and is rarely of diagnostic value.

FINE NEEDLE ASPIRATION

The smears of a MEC may be difficult to separate from a mucocele or other benign cyst. However, MEC usually have cellular smears with abundant mucinous material and debris in the background (Fig. 12-15). There are cohesive groups of epithelial cells arranged in sheets as well as noted to be streaming within the mucin (Fig. 12-16). The cells are separated into mucocytes, intermediate, and epidermoid cells in variable proportions. Most of the cells have ample cytoplasm surrounding nuclei which are only mildly pleomorphic. Higher grade tumors have less mucin and greater nuclear pleomorphism, which may be difficult to accurately diagnose on FNA. Occasionally, a diagnosis of "mucus-producing lesion" may be the only diagnosis which can be rendered with accuracy.

DIFFERENTIAL DIAGNOSIS

Both MEC and necrotizing sialometaplasia (NSM) can show squamous proliferation with foci of mucocytic differentiation in an inflamed, fibrous stroma. NSM, however, has a lobular distribution and usually shows areas of transition from the ducts to the solid islands

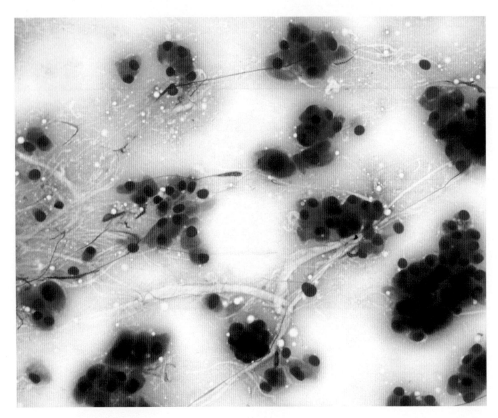

FIGURE 12-15

A cellular smear with a background of mucinous material. Groups of epithelial cells with opaque cytoplasm comprise the intermediate component. Rare mucocytes are present (air-dried, MGG stain).

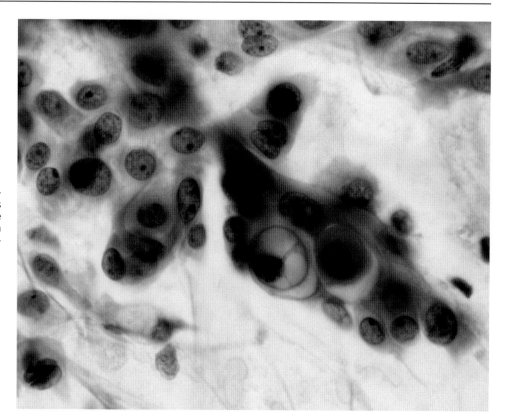

FIGURE 12-16

A cellular smear with intermediate-epidermoid cells arranged in sheets and streaming groups. Note the mucocyte in the center with mucin vacuoles (alcohol-fixed, Papanicolaou stain).

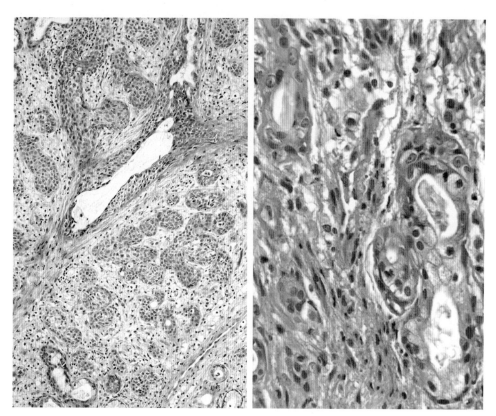

FIGURE 12-17

Left: Necrotizing sialometaplasia has a lobular architecture with squamous metaplasia of the duct/lobular units. *Right:* Residual mucocytes are replaced by metaplastic squamous epithelium. Inflammatory cells are noted in the background.

of squamous cells formed by intraductal regenerative hyperplasia (Fig. 12-17). There are no intermediate cells and cyst formation is not a feature. MEC can usually be distinguished from cystadenoma and cystadenocarcinoma by its much more variable cytological and

morphological characteristics (Fig. 12-18). High-grade tumors may resemble closely squamous cell carcinoma but appropriate stains can demonstrate the presence of scattered mucocytes. In addition, it is very rare for mucoepidermoid carcinomas to show keratinization.

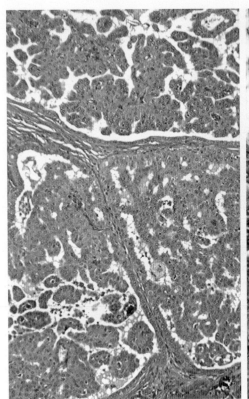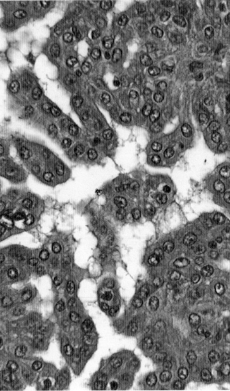

FIGURE 12-18

A papillary cystadenocarcinoma has complex, arborizing papillae (*left*) with nuclear atypia and mitotic figures (*right*).

The sclerosing variant may be confused with chronic sialadenitis. Predominantly clear cell MEC must be distinguished from tumors such as epithelial-myoepithelial carcinoma, clear cell carcinoma (NOS), and metastatic tumors.

PROGNOSIS AND THERAPY

The prognosis is dependent on clinical stage, site, grading, and adequacy of surgery. Most tumors are low grade and the prognosis is generally good. There is a >95% survival for low-grade tumors, with only rare regional metastases. The mortality rate, however, increases to about 45% in the much less common group of high-grade tumors. Tumors that transgress surgical margins have a very high recurrence rate, particularly high-grade tumors. MEC in the submandibular gland, floor of mouth, tongue, and maxillary antrum have a poorer prognosis. Death is usually due to uncontrolled locoregional disease and metastases to lung, bone, and brain. Treatment is by surgical excision with or without neck dissection. Radiotherapy is generally palliative in advanced tumors but has little impact on prognosis.

ACINIC CELL CARCINOMA

CLINICAL FEATURES

Acinic cell carcinoma (AcCC) accounts for about 6% of all salivary gland tumors and between 7% and 17.5% of malignant salivary tumors. About 80% of cases form in the parotid gland, while the minor salivary glands are the second most common site. About 4% arise in the submandibular gland and 1% in the sublingual. Less common locations include the buccal mucosa, lips and palate and, rarely, the lacrimal gland, mandible, and minor glands in the upper and lower respiratory tracts. Women are affected slightly more commonly than men (3:2). The majority of cases are evenly distributed in the 2nd–7th decades, with a mean age of 44 years. It is the second most common malignant salivary gland tumor in children.

AcCC usually presents as a slow growing mass and the reported duration ranges from a few weeks to 40 years. Pain or tenderness is present in up to a half of patients. The tumor may be freely mobile or fixed to the skin or underlying tissues. Facial nerve involvement is seen in up to 10% of cases.

ACINIC CELL ADENOCARCINOMA
DISEASE FACT SHEET

Definition	A malignant epithelial neoplasm demonstrating serous acinar cell differentiation with cytoplasmic zymogen secretory granules
Incidence and location	Accounts for about 6% of salivary gland tumors
	80% involve the parotid gland
	Minor salivary glands second most common site
Morbidity and mortality	About 35% of cases recur locally
	5-yr and 10-yr survival rates 82% and 68%, respectively
Gender, race, and age distribution	Female > Male (3 : 2)
	2nd–7th decades (mean, 44 yr)
	Second most common malignant salivary gland tumor in children
Clinical features	History of slow growing mass which may be mobile or fixed
	Duration varies from weeks to several decades
	Pain or tenderness present in up to a half of patients
	Facial nerve involvement present in 5%–10% of cases
Prognosis and treatment	About 35% develop recurrences
	Behavior does not correlate with patterns of growth
	Poor prognosis associated with large size, involvement of the deep lobe of the parotid, multinodularity and regional and distant metastases, cellular pleomorphism, increased mitotic frequency, areas of necrosis, and neural invasion
	Ki-67 staining may be an independent prognostic factor for survival
	Complete surgical excision treatment of choice

ACINIC CELL ADENOCARCINOMA
PATHOLOGIC FEATURES

Gross findings	Rubbery or firm tumors usually <3 cm in diameter
	Usually circumscribed (occasionally irregular)
	May show hemorrhage or cystic change
Microscopic findings	Characteristic cell is serous acinar with granules in the cytoplasm (usually accentuated at the lumen)
	Other cell types include nonspecific glandular, intercalated ductal, vacuolated, and clear
	Wide variety of histomorphological configurations including solid, microcystic, papillary-cystic, and follicular
	May have lymphoid infiltrate, occasionally prominent
Ancillary studies	PAS positive, diastase resistant zymogen granules
	Acinic cells may stain positively for amylase, transferrin, lactoferrin, CEA, VIP, and others
	About 10% show some positivity for S-100 antigen
Fine needle aspiration	Cellular smears with clean background
	Cohesive, small, tight clusters
	Ample, granular to vacuolated cytoplasm surrounding round and regular nuclei with coarse chromatin (lymphocyte-like nuclei)
Pathologic differential diagnosis	Normal salivary gland, sialadenitis, cystadenocarcinoma (especially papillary variants), mucoepidermoid carcinoma, thyroid carcinoma, clear cell tumors

PATHOLOGIC FEATURES

GROSS FINDINGS

Most tumors are less than 3 cm in diameter and usually form a rubbery or firm, circumscribed, oval or round mass. Some are more irregular with poorly defined margins or multifocal nodules and there may be areas of hemorrhage or cystic change.

MICROSCOPIC FINDINGS

AcCC is characterized by serous acinar cells but several other cell types may be present and include intercalated duct, nonspecific glandular, vacuolated, and clear cells. Individual tumors may show several cell types or one type may predominate. Serous acinar cells are the most common type (Fig. 12-19). They resemble serous cells of the normal salivary gland and have abundant pale, basophilic cytoplasm containing dense, grayish or blue zymogen granules. The granules may be fine or coarse and are variably PAS/D positive (Fig. 12-20). Nuclei are round and basophilic or occasionally more vesicular and are usually located peripherally (Fig. 12-21). Intercalated duct-type cells are smaller as they contain less cytoplasm. The cytoplasm is usually eosinophilic and the nuclei tend to be central. These cells surround luminal spaces of varying sizes. Vacuolated cells are common and may be a conspicuous feature. They have clear, PAS/D negative, cytoplasmic vacuoles, and some cells also contain zymogen granules. Cells with clear cytoplasm and conspicuous cell boundaries are usually only seen focally. They do not contain glycogen and may be a fixation or processing artifact. Nonspecific glandular cells are polygonal or round, and are usually smaller than acinar cells. The cytoplasm is eosinophilic or amphophilic, PAS/D negative, and lacks granules. There is greater variability in the size and staining characteristics of the nuclei. The nonspecific glandular cells often form sheets of cells with indistinct borders.

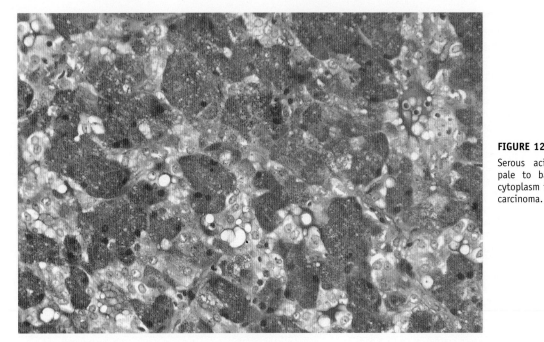

FIGURE 12-19
Serous acinar cells have abundant pale to basophilic, heavily granular cytoplasm in this low-grade acinic cell carcinoma.

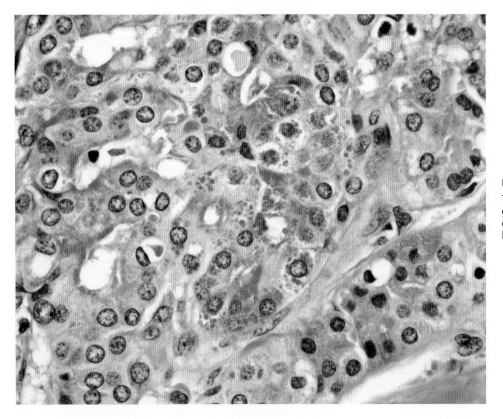

FIGURE 12-20
The granules, representing zymogen granules, are variable in size and often accentuated along the luminal border in acinic cell carcinoma.

The growth patterns of AcCC include solid, microcystic, papillary-cystic and follicular; individual tumors may show several configurations. In the solid type the cells are closely aggregated in sheets or nodules. Cytologically bland acinic cells are the most common form, but nonspecific glandular and clear cells may also be seen. The microcystic pattern is the most common and small spaces develop in the tumor giving it a lattice-like appearance (Fig. 12-22). In addition to the acinic cells, vacuolated and intercalated type cells are common. In the papillary-cystic variant the cysts are usually prominent and show intraluminal papillary projections. The cells on the luminal layer may show a hobnail appearance. Intratumoral and intracystic hemorrhage is

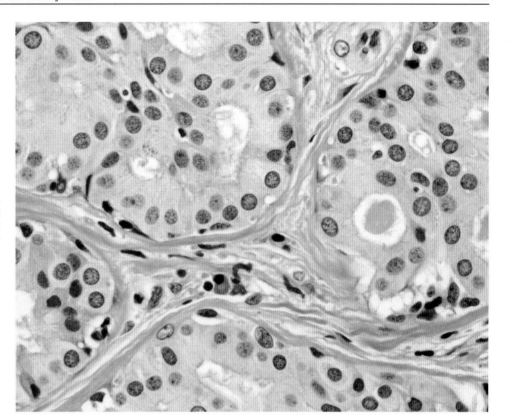

FIGURE 12-21

Small gland-like spaces are lined by cells whose nuclei are peripherally located. Note the small, eosinophilic granules at the luminal border. Fibrosis separates the acinic cells.

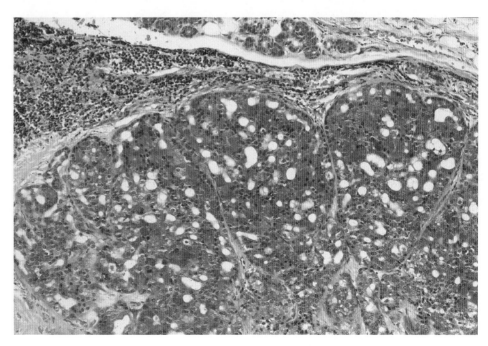

FIGURE 12-22

A microcystic pattern is seen in this acinic cell carcinoma.

common in this variant and sometimes the tumor cells phagocytose hemosiderin (Fig. 12-23). The follicular variant consists of multiple, variably sized cystic spaces. These are lined mostly by intercalated duct-type cells and contain homogeneous, eosinophilic, proteinaceous fluid, and the appearance closely mimics follicular car-

cinoma of the thyroid (Fig. 12-24). Psammoma bodies are sometimes seen in a variety of AcCC types and may be a conspicuous feature (Fig. 12-25).

Many tumors show focal areas of stromal infiltration by lymphocytes but some have a very striking lymphocytic stroma in which germinal centers develop

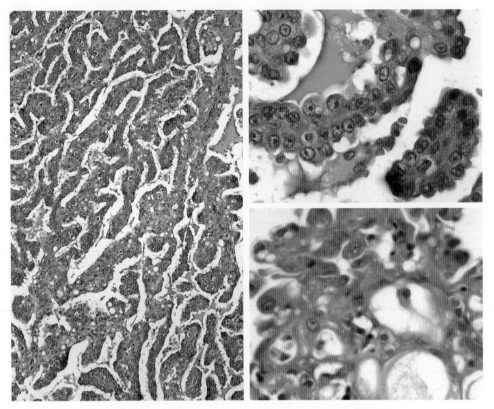

FIGURE 12-23

Left: A papillary-cystic variant has abundant papillary projections. *Right upper:* Acinic cells lining the papillary projections. *Right lower:* Note the hobnail appearance with cystic spaces.

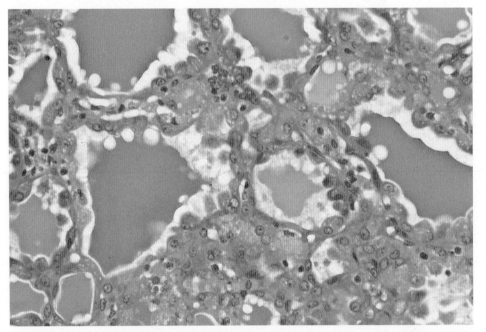

FIGURE 12-24

This follicular variant has cystic spaces lined by intercalated duct-type cells with eosinophilic, scalloped proteinaceous fluid.

(Fig. 12-26). These tumors are well circumscribed or encapsulated and usually of the solid or microcystic type. They may have a better prognosis than conventional types. Stromal fibrosis or sclerosis may be associated with a slightly worse prognosis. Rare dedifferentiated tumors showing high-grade malignant areas in an otherwise conventional AcCC have been described. Bilateral, multifocal, and hybrid tumors have also been reported.

ANCILLARY STUDIES

ULTRASTRUCTURAL FEATURES

While uncommonly used to identify tumors in modern practice, identification of secretory zymogen granules in the cytoplasm can help to confirm the diagnosis (Fig. 12-27).

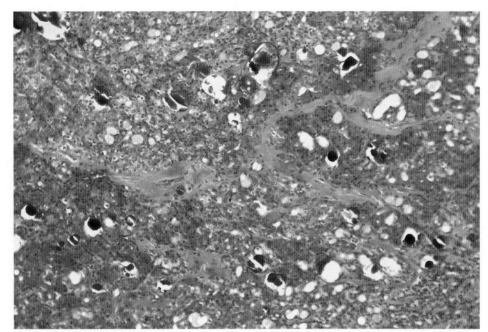

FIGURE 12-25

Psammoma bodies are sometimes a prominent feature in acinic cell carcinoma.

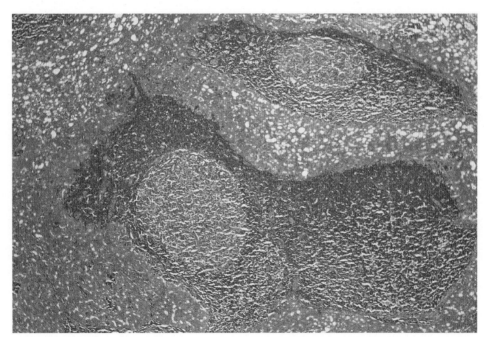

FIGURE 12-26

The stroma is infiltrated by lymphocytes which have formed germinal centers in this acinic cell carcinoma.

IMMUNOHISTOCHEMICAL FEATURES

AcCC show reactivity with a variety of immunoagents but staining tends to be unpredictable and is of little value in diagnosis. The acinic cells may stain positively for amylase, transferrin, lactoferrin, CEA, VIP, and others. However, staining for amylase is frequently weak or absent in routinely processed tissue. About 10 % of tumors show some positivity for S-100 antigen.

FINE NEEDLE ASPIRATION

AcCC tend to yield cellular smears with a clean background. The tumor cells are cohesive, arranged in small, tight clusters, occasionally demonstrating a small central, fibrovascular core (Fig. 12-28). The nuclei are usually round and regular with little pleomorphism surrounded by abundant, eosinophilic, finely granular to vacuolated cytoplasm (Fig. 12-29). Separating other tumors from acinic cell on FNA preparations may be difficult.

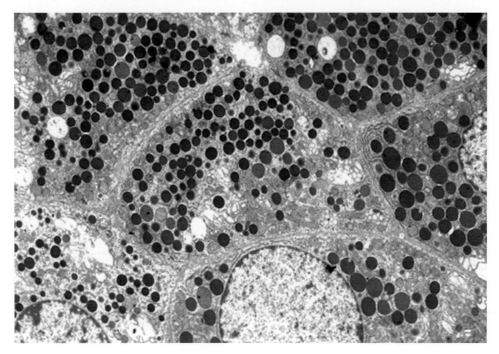

FIGURE 12-27
This ultrastructural examination demonstrates secretory dense zymogen granules. (Courtesy of Dr. I. Dardick.)

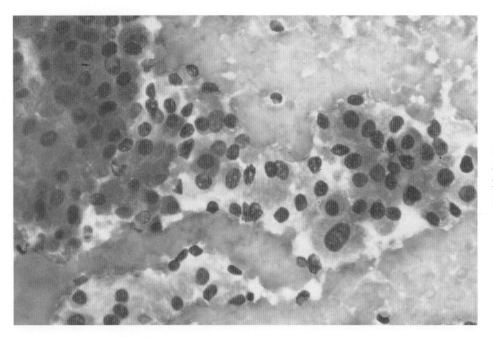

FIGURE 12-28
A sheet and cohesive cluster of cells are noted in a background of blood. There is only slight nuclear variability (alcohol-fixed, H&E stain).

DIFFERENTIAL DIAGNOSIS

The variants of AcCC may cause problems in diagnosis. The neoplasm needs to be separated from normal serous acini or sialadenitis, especially if there is limited material. Microcystic and papillary-cystic tumors need to be differentiated from cystadenocarcinoma, particularly its papillary variant. The presence of zymogen granules, vacuolated cells, and intercalated ductal differentiation supports the diagnosis of AcCC. Microcystic variants may be misdiagnosed as mucoepidermoid carcinomas due to the strong mucicarmine positivity of the cystic spaces and the presence of small spaces being interpreted as mucocytes. Follicular variants can resemble thyroid carcinomas so closely that immunostaining for thyroglobulin is needed to separate the tumors. Although clear cell tumors are included in the differential diagnosis, this is rarely a practical problem as the clear cells in AcCC are usually focal.

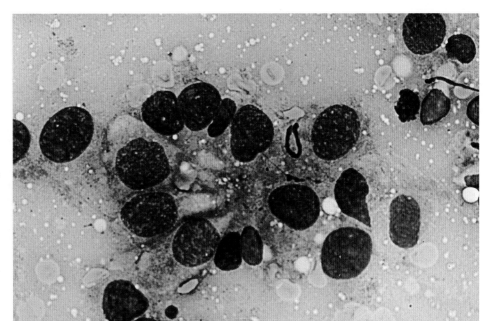

FIGURE 12-29

An acinar arrangement of cells with round, regular nuclei and granular cytoplasm (air-dried, MGG stain).

PROGNOSIS AND THERAPY

Recurrences develop in about 35% of patients. There is an overall 5-year and 10-year survival rate of 82% and 68%, respectively. The tumor may involve regional lymph nodes and the most common sites for distant spread are lung and bones. Grading is not universally accepted and there is no correlation between prognosis and the four main histomorphological patterns. Histological features thought to be associated with poor prognosis include cellular pleomorphism, increased mitotic frequency, areas of necrosis, and neural invasion. Ki-67 staining may be an independent prognostic factor for survival. However, the clinical stage at presentation may be better predictor of behavior than grading. Large size, involvement of the deep lobe of the parotid, multiple recurrences, multinodularity, and regional and distant metastases are indictors of poor prognosis. Tumors involving minor glands have a much better prognosis than those in major glands. Complete surgical excision is the treatment of choice and failure to clear the tumor is associated with a poor outcome.

ADENOID CYSTIC CARCINOMA

CLINICAL FEATURES

Adenoid cystic carcinoma (ACC) accounts for about 10% of all malignant salivary gland tumors. It affects a

ADENOID CYSTIC CARCINOMA DISEASE FACT SHEET

Definition	Adenoid cystic carcinoma is a basaloid tumor consisting of epithelial and myoepithelial cells in variable morphologic configurations, including cribriform, tubular, and solid patterns
Incidence and location	Accounts for about 10% of salivary gland neoplasms
	About 75% arise in minor glands, particularly in palate, with 25% in major glands, mainly the submandibular gland
Morbidity and mortality	5-yr and 10-yr survival rates 62% and 40%, respectively
	Most patients die of, or with, tumor
Gender, race, and age distribution	Female > Male (3 : 2)
	Peak in 5th–7th decades (wide age range)
	Rare in children
Clinical features	Usually forms a slow growing mass which may be painful
	Cranial nerve involvement common, especially facial nerve palsy
	Submucosal tumors may ulcerate
Prognosis and treatment	Main prognostic factors are site, tumor size, clinical stage, histological pattern (solid has a worse prognosis)
	Frequent recurrence, especially in first 5 postoperative yr
	Submandibular gland tumors have a worse prognosis
	Metastasis to lung, bone, brain and liver seen in up to 60%
	Treated with wide local excision and adjuvant radiotherapy

wide age range with a peak incidence in 40–60 year olds. There is a slight female preponderance. Minor glands of the mouth, particularly the palate and the upper aerodigestive tract, account for about half of all cases. Other common sites include the parotid (21%), submandibular gland (13%), and sinonasal tract (11%). Tumors usually present as a slow growing mass of long duration. It may be tender or painful, and cranial nerve lesions, particularly facial nerve palsy, may be the presenting feature. Tumors of minor glands often show ulceration of the overlying mucosa.

PATHOLOGIC FEATURES

GROSS FINDINGS

The tumor is usually firm and may be well circumscribed, particularly when small. Most are unencapsu-

---

ADENOID CYSTIC CARCINOMA PATHOLOGIC FEATURES	
Gross findings	Usually firm, often well circumscribed, but unencapsulated
Microscopic findings	Comprised of duct lining cells and abluminal modified myoepithelial cells
	Main patterns are cribriform, tubular, and solid in that order of frequency, although many tumors show mixture of types
	Pseudocysts are filled with basophilic mucoid ("blue-goo") or hyaline eosinophilic material (reduplicated basement membrane material)
	Perineural invasion common and frequently extensive
	Cells are small with high nuclear to cytoplasmic ratio
	Nuclei are peg shaped ("carrot" shaped) to columnar with heavy nuclear chromatin distribution
	Stroma is hyalinized
Ancillary studies	Pseudocysts positive for PAS, Alcian blue, laminin, and type IV collagen
	Epithelial cells positive for low-molecular weight keratins and EMA
	Myoepithelial cells positive with calponin, SMA, S-100 protein, p63
Fine needle aspiration	Usually cellular smears with cohesive sheets of monotonous, only mildly atypical epithelial cells
	Cells surround spherical, hyaline globules (reduplicated basement membrane material), best seen on air-dried preparations (Romanovsky stains)
	Nuclei are hyperchromatic and peg shaped/cuboidal within cells that have high nuclear to cytoplasmic ratios
Pathologic differential diagnosis	Polymorphous low-grade adenocarcinoma, pleomorphic adenoma, basaloid squamous cell carcinoma, epithelial-myoepithelial carcinoma

---

lated. The gross appearance belies the true extent of the tumor, as neural infiltration is not discernible on macroscopic examination.

MICROSCOPIC FINDINGS

ACC has three main morphological patterns: cribriform or cylindromatous, tubular, and solid, in that order of frequency. A mixture of these patterns may be seen. The cribriform variant consists of islands of modified myoepithelial cells containing rounded, pseudocystic areas forming a characteristic "Swiss cheese" appearance (Fig. 12-30). The pseudocysts are basophilic and mucoid, or consist of hyaline, eosinophilic material. They are composed of glycosaminoglycans and reduplicated basement membrane material (Fig. 12-31). Foci of ductal cells are present within the myoepithelial areas but may require careful examination to detect. The tubular variant is double-layered and has more conspicuous ductal differentiation. There is an inner layer of eosinophilic, duct-lining cells and the abluminal myoepithelial cells often show clear cytoplasm and irregular, angular nuclei (Fig. 12-32). The uncommon solid variant consists of islands or sheets of basaloid cells with larger and less angular nuclei (Fig. 12-33). Duct lining cells may be sparse and inconspicuous and central comedonecrosis is common. Mitoses are sparse in the cribriform and tubular patterns but may be frequent in the solid type.

ACC is composed of luminal ductal cells and abluminal, modified myoepithelial cells. The latter predominate and have indistinct cell borders and frequently sparse, amphophilic or clear cytoplasm. The nuclei are uniform in size, with heavy chromatin and may be round or angular (peg shaped). The ductal cells surround small and sometimes indistinct lumina. They are cuboidal and have more abundant, eosinophilic cytoplasm and round, uniform nuclei that may contain small nucleoli.

The stroma of ACC is usually hyalinized and in some cases is so abundant that tumor cells are attenuated into strands (Fig. 12-34). Perineural or intraneural invasion is a common and frequently conspicuous feature and the tumor can extend along nerves over a wide area (Fig. 12-35). The tumor may invade bone extensively before there is any radiological evidence of bone destruction. Lymph node involvement is often due to contiguous spread rather than lymphatic permeation or embolization.

ANCILLARY STUDIES

HISTOCHEMICAL AND IMMUNOHISTOCHEMICAL FEATURES

The pseudocysts are positive for PAS and Alcian blue and react with antibodies to basement membrane components such as laminin and type IV collagen. The epithelial cells are positive for low-molecular weight keratins and epithelial membrane antigen (EMA), and

FIGURE 12-30

Left: The characteristic cribriform or cylindromatous pattern is seen in this adenoid cystic carcinoma. *Right:* Note a more trabecular appearance.

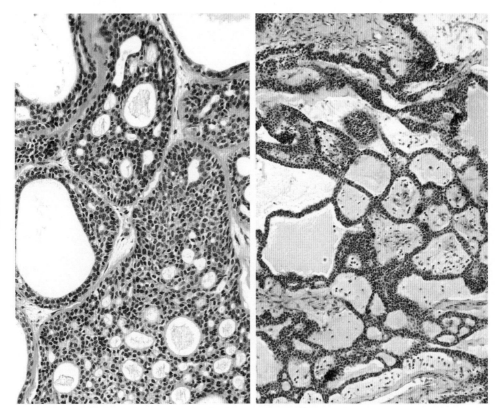

FIGURE 12-31

Left: Pseudocystic spaces with mucoid and eosinophilic material. *Right:* A cylinder appearance with mucoid, basophilic material in the center. Note the "peg-shaped" nuclei surrounding these spaces in an ACC.

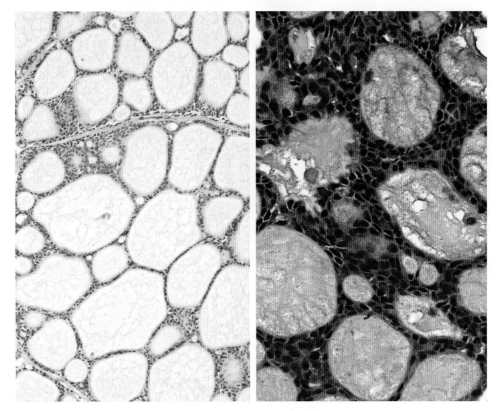

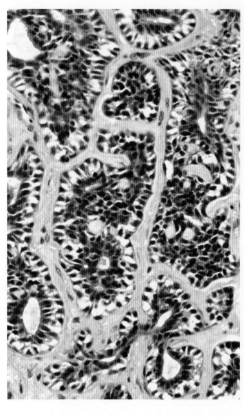

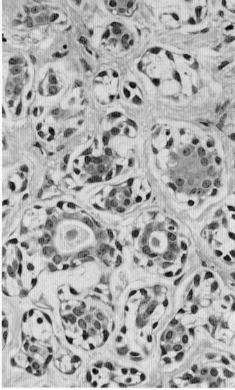

FIGURE 12-32
The tubular variant of ACC has a double-layered appearance with inner ductal cells and outer myoepithelial cells.

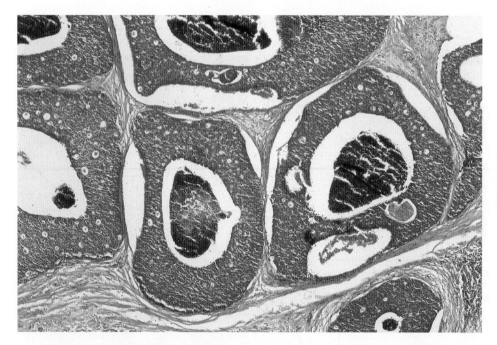

FIGURE 12-33
The solid variant of ACC has large nests of cells with high nuclear to cytoplasmic ratio. Central comedonecrosis is noted.

the myoepithelial cells are positive for markers such as calponin, SMA, p63, and S-100 protein (Fig. 12-36).

FINE NEEDLE ASPIRATION

ACC contain spherical hyaline globules which represent the reduplicated basement membrane material, intimately surrounded by the neoplastic cells (Fig. 12-

37), best seen on air-dried preparations. The globules do not have a fibrillar or feathery edge as seen in pleomorphic adenoma. There are often rounded stromal structures between the nests of tumor cells. The tumor cells are cohesive, often showing high cellularity and cellular overlap of cells that have little pleomorphism (Fig. 12-38). The nuclei are often peg shaped, identified in cells with a high nuclear to cytoplasmic ratio. The chromatin

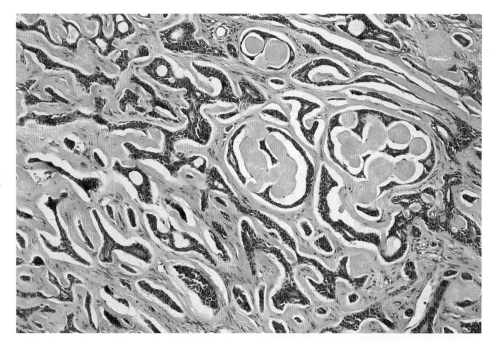

FIGURE 12-34

A heavily hyalinized stroma has compressed the neoplastic cells in this adenoid cystic carcinoma.

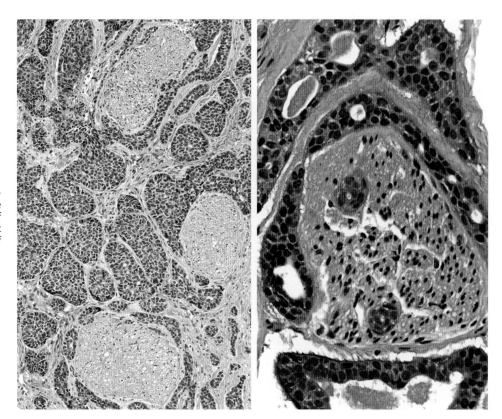

FIGURE 12-35

Left: Nerves are surrounded by neoplastic cells. *Right:* Not only is there perineural invasion by the cells of this adenoid cystic carcinoma, but there are also intraneural nests of tumor.

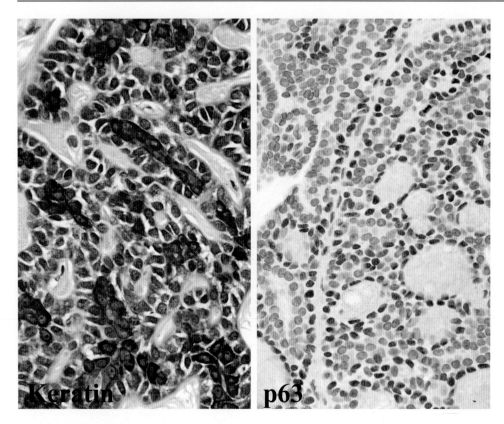

FIGURE 12-36

Left: Keratin immunohistochemistry highlights the lumenal epithelial cells. *Right:* p63 immunohistochemistry highlights the basal/myoepithelial cells.

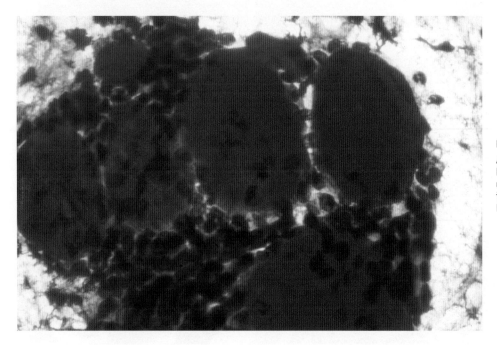

FIGURE 12-37

Air-dried, Romanovsky stained material highlights the spherical hyaline globules with the associated cells containing small, hyperchromatic nuclei in this FNA smear.

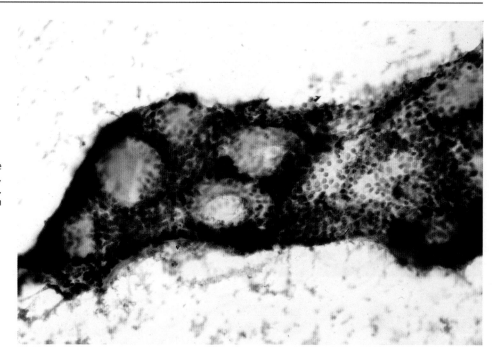

FIGURE 12-38
The epithelial cells form cohesive sheets which show rounded void areas, corresponding to the hyaline globules. These globules do not stain with Papanicolaou-stained preparations.

is heavy and coarse in distribution. Fine needle aspiration of ACC is often difficult to separate from a pleomorphic adenoma.

DIFFERENTIAL DIAGNOSIS

It is important to distinguish ACC from polymorphous low-grade adenocarcinoma (PLGA) in tumors from minor salivary glands. While both neoplasms have similar patterns of growth, PLGA consists of a uniform cell population with cytologically bland, round or oval and vesicular nuclei, and pale eosinophilic cytoplasm. PLGA has infiltrating single cords of cells and also has a striking targeted arrangement, often centered on a nerve. Immunohistochemical separation still requires further validation, with CD117 and galectin-3 showing promise. Occasional foci in pleomorphic adenoma can resemble ACC but the presence of typical myxochondroid matrix and plasmacytoid or spindle-shaped cells helps to avoid confusion. Basaloid squamous cell carcinoma can resemble the solid variant of ACC, but typically involves the hypopharynx and glottic region, shows squamous differentiation, and often involves the overlying mucosa. Both epithelial-myoepithelial carcinoma and the tubular variant of ACC can show double-layered duct-like structures with an abluminal layer of clear cells. However, the other cytologic features allow for separation.

PROGNOSIS AND THERAPY

The 5- and 10-year survival rates are 62% and 40%, respectively, although the majority of patients usually die of or with the tumor. Local recurrence is very common, especially in the first 5 years after surgery. The main prognostic factors are site, tumor size, clinical stage, and histological pattern. Bone involvement and failure of primary surgery are associated with poor prognosis. Correlations between tumor morphology and outcome have yielded conflicting results due to the overall poor long-term prognosis. However, it appears that the tubular and cribriform variants have a better outcome than tumors with a solid component, especially if the solid component exceeds 30% of the tumor volume. Tumors in the submandibular gland have a poorer prognosis than those in the parotid. The relationship between nerve involvement and survival is also contentious but invasion of larger nerves appears to correlate with more aggressive behavior. Lymph node involvement is relatively uncommon but distant metastases to lung, bone, brain, and liver are seen in up to 60% of cases. Wide local excision, together with adjuvant radiotherapy, offers the best hope of local control.

POLYMORPHOUS LOW-GRADE ADENOCARCINOMA

CLINICAL FEATURES

Polymorphous low-grade adenocarcinoma is found almost exclusively in minor glands and accounts for about a quarter of the malignant tumors in these sites. Most tumors present in patients aged 50–70 years, with women affected twice as frequently as men. The most common site is the palate (60% of cases), especially at the junction of the hard and soft palates (Fig. 12-39).

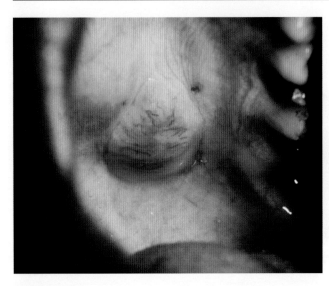

FIGURE 12-39
An intact mucosa overlies a mass at the junction of the hard and soft palate. Note the vascular pattern. No surface ulceration is present.

PATHOLOGIC FEATURES

GROSS FINDINGS

The tumor usually forms a circumscribed, nonencapsulated, pale yellow or tan colored mass. Most measure up to 3 cm in diameter.

MICROSCOPIC FINDINGS

PLGA is an invasive tumor that is often circumscribed but not encapsulated, frequently identified below an intact surface epithelium (Fig. 12-40). There is typically a wide variety of morphological patterns within individual tumors (Fig. 12-41). The most common configurations include lobular, solid nests or theques, cribriform areas, and duct-like structures of varying sizes. Concentric targeting or whorling, often by cells in a single file arrangement, can often be seen around nerves and, less commonly, blood vessels and small ducts (Fig. 12-42). This perineural infiltration is usually present within, or close to, the body of the tumor. Foci of oncocytic, mucus and squamous metaplasia are occasionally present. Normal salivary gland acini are frequently incarcerated within the tumor (Fig. 12-43). A characteristic stromal hyalinization with a slate-gray appearance is common (Fig. 12-44), but chondroid or myxochondroid areas are not seen.

POLYMORPHOUS LOW-GRADE ADENOCARCINOMA DISEASE FACT SHEET	
Definition	A malignant epithelial tumor characterized by an infiltrative growth of cytological uniform cells arranged in architecturally diverse patterns
Incidence and location	Accounts for about 25% of intraoral malignant salivary gland tumors
	60% of cases involve the palate; other sites include lip, buccal mucosa, retromolar areas, and tongue
Morbidity and mortality	Spread to regional lymph nodes 9%–15% of cases
	Death due to disease is uncommon
Gender, race, and age distribution	Female > Male (F : M = 2 : 1)
	Peak in 6th–8th decades (wide age range)
	Rare in children
Clinical features	Usually forms a painless, slow growing mass
	Tumors often present for many years
	Tumors may be mobile or fixed
	Ulceration, pain, and bleeding are uncommon
Prognosis and treatment	Prognosis usually excellent
	Local recurrences 9%–17% of cases
	Questionable aggressive behavior in younger patients
	Conservative surgery is the treatment of choice

POLYMORPHOUS LOW-GRADE ADENOCARCINOMA PATHOLOGIC FEATURES	
Gross findings	Circumscribed, but usually nonencapsulated mass
	Usually 1–3 cm in diameter
Microscopic findings	Cytologically uniform and architecturally diverse
	Wide variety of morphological patterns in individual tumors
	Concentric targeting around nerves and blood vessels
	Encasement of benign residual salivary gland tissue
	Stromal hyalinization or mucinosis (slate-gray)
	Isomorphic, small to medium cells with eosinophilic cytoplasm
	Cytologically bland, pale-staining (vesicular), round or oval nuclei
	Mitoses and necrosis uncommon
Immunohistochemical features	Cytokeratin, vimentin, and S-100 protein positive
	Variable results with immunohistochemistry and rarely of diagnostic value
Pathologic differential diagnosis	Limited biopsy specimens make diagnosis difficult, pleomorphic adenoma, adenoid cystic carcinoma

Other intraoral sites include lip (particularly the upper), buccal mucosa, retromolar areas, and posterior third of tongue. Rarely tumors may arise in the lacrimal gland, sinonasal tract, nasopharynx, and the upper and lower respiratory tracts. Tumors usually form a slow growing mass that may have been present for many years. Ulceration, bleeding, and pain are uncommon presenting features.

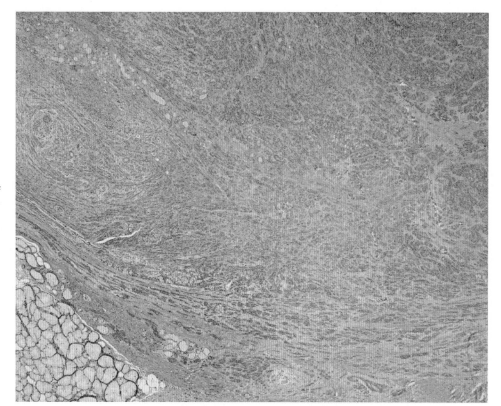

FIGURE 12-40

A low-power magnification of polymorphous low-grade adenocarcinoma showing a well-circumscribed, although unencapsulated, mass with a variety of different growth patterns.

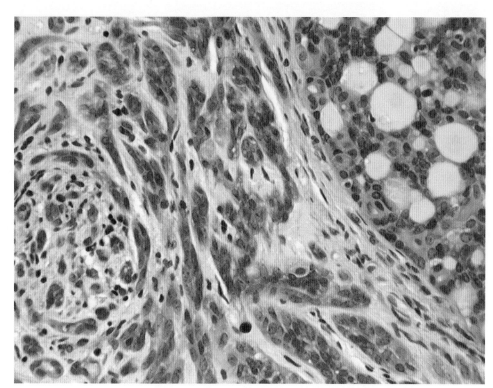

FIGURE 12-41

Variable architectures are seen within a single tumor, including cribriform, tubular, and trabecular. Note the bluish stroma in the background.

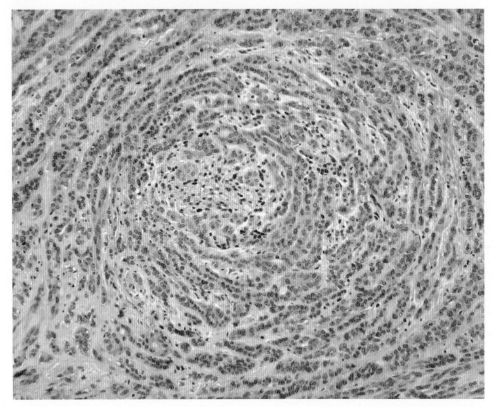

FIGURE 12-42

A targetoid pattern with single-file, concentric arrangement of the cells. Nerves are usually in the center of these targets.

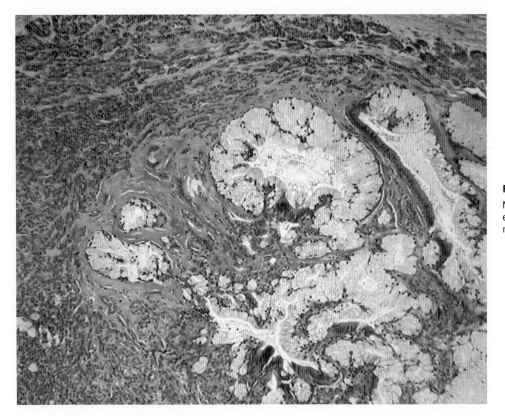

FIGURE 12-43

Non-neoplastic mucinous glands are encased by the neoplasm, although not destroyed.

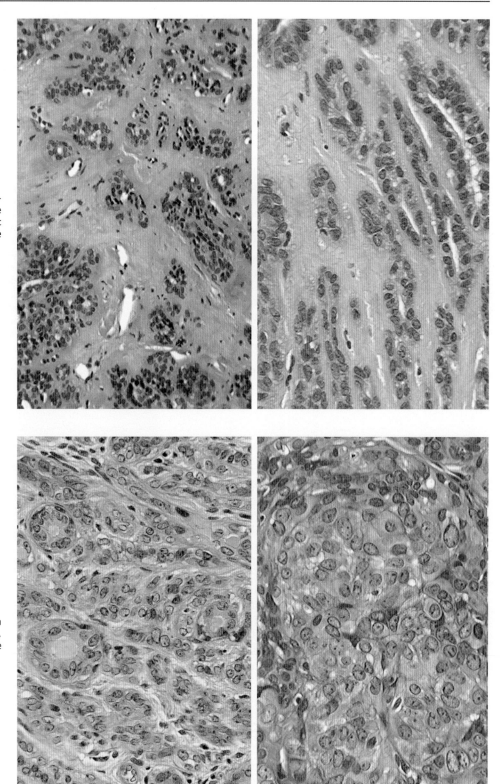

FIGURE 12-44

Stromal hyalinization and a slate-gray to blue mucinous material in the background is quite characteristic for a polymorphous low-grade adenocarcinoma.

FIGURE 12-45

The nuclei are round to oval, with vesicular, pale nuclear chromatin, and small nucleoli. Mitotic figures are inconspicuous.

PLGA is characterized by cytological uniformity even though there is architectural diversity. The cells are isomorphic, small to medium in size, with pale eosinophilic cytoplasm. They have cytologically bland, pale-staining (vesicular), round or oval nuclei (Fig. 12-45). It is uncommon to see mitotic figures or areas of necrosis.

ANCILLARY STUDIES

The immunohistochemical profile can be extremely variable and is rarely of diagnostic value. Cytokeratin, vimentin, and S-100 are the most consistent markers and will decorate some cells in the large majority of tumors, but the intensity and distribution is variable. Most cases of PLGA appear to over-express bcl-2.

DIFFERENTIAL DIAGNOSIS

The differential diagnosis includes pleomorphic adenoma, adenoid cystic carcinoma and papillary variants of cystadenocarcinoma. This separation is hampered if the biopsy is small or limited. Adequate biopsy size is necessary to render a definitive diagnosis. Typically, pleomorphic adenoma is circumscribed and often shows plasmacytoid differentiation in minor glands. In addition, although both tumors can show stromal mucinosis and elastosis, myxochondroid or chondroid matrix is not seen in PLGA. It has been reported that staining for glial fibrillary acidic protein is very strong in pleomorphic adenomas but weak or absent in PLGA. ACC has hyperchromatic nuclei with a much higher nuclear to cytoplasmic ratio and tends to be destructive of the surrounding gland. Cystadenocarcinoma is a tumor which displays papillary architecture and has nuclear pleomorphism with mitotic figures.

PROGNOSIS AND THERAPY

The long-term prognosis is usually excellent. There is local recurrence in 9% to 17% of cases and spread to regional lymph nodes is seen in 9% to 15% of cases. Distant metastases are very rare and death due to disease is uncommon. Cribriform adenocarcinoma of the tongue may be a variant of PLGA with a high frequency of regional lymph node metastases, but this is unsettled. Whether papillary PLGA exists is debated, but papillary tumors have a much more aggressive behavior, suggesting they may not belong in this category. Complete but conservative surgery is the treatment of choice, together with neck dissection in cases with proven regional metastases.

EPITHELIAL-MYOEPITHELIAL CARCINOMA

CLINICAL FEATURES

Epithelial-myoepithelial carcinoma (EMC) is a malignant neoplasm demonstrating a characteristic bi-phasic pattern of inner duct-like lining cells and an outer layer of myoepithelial like-cells. EMC accounts for about 1% of salivary gland tumors. It is usually seen in older age groups (50–60 yr) and is rare in children. Women are affected twice as often as men. Most cases arise in the parotid gland where they typically form a slow growing,

EPITHELIAL-MYOEPITHELIAL CARCINOMA DISEASE FACT SHEET	
Definition	A malignant neoplasm with bi-phasic duct-like structures composed of an inner layer of duct lining, epithelial-type cells and an outer layer of clear, myoepithelial-type cells
Incidence and location	About 1% of salivary gland tumors
	60% of cases involve the parotid gland
	Can also be seen in the mouth, upper and lower respiratory tracts
Morbidity and mortality	About 40% of cases recur locally
	Spread to regional lymph nodes and distant sites occur in about 15% of cases
	5-yr survival rate 80%
Gender, race, and age distribution	Female > Male (F : M = 2 : 1)
	Peak incidence in 50–60 yr
	Rare in children
Clinical features	Usually forms a painless, slow-growing mass
	Tumors are often present for long periods before presentation
	Tumors involving mucosal sites often ulcerate
	Occasionally tumors are rapidly growing and painful and may cause nerve palsies
Prognosis and treatment	Prognosis is usually good (80% 5-yr survival), although recurrences are common (40%)
	Clinical indicators of poor prognosis include incomplete surgical excision, large size, rapid growth, involvement of minor salivary glands
	Microscopic features associated with a poor outcome include cellular atypia, high mitotic frequency, and aneuploidy
	Surgery is the treatment of choice, supplemented by radiotherapy in advanced or recurrent cases

painless mass, often of long duration. It can also arise from minor salivary glands of the mouth and the upper and lower respiratory tracts. In these sites the tumor has a tendency to ulcerate. Higher grade tumors may undergo rapid growth and cause pain or facial nerve palsy.

PATHOLOGIC FEATURES

GROSS FINDINGS

The tumor typically forms a well-defined, but usually nonencapsulated mass, 2–8 cm in diameter. It is often lobulated, with cystic areas common on the cut surface. Tumors in minor glands tend to be less well demarcated.

EPITHELIAL-MYOEPITHELIAL CARCINOMA
PATHOLOGIC FEATURES

Gross findings	Well defined, but usually nonencapsulated mass, 2–8 cm in diameter Often lobulated, and cystic areas are common on cut surface Tumors in minor glands are less well demarcated		Papillary and cystic areas are present in 20% of cases Spindle cell areas and squamous metaplasia occasionally present Mitoses uncommon (2/10 HPF) Perineural and vascular invasion commonly seen
Microscopic findings	Double-layered duct-like structures Inner cuboidal duct-lining cells and outer, single or multiple layers of myoepithelial cells with clear cytoplasm and eccentric, vesicular nuclei Wide variation in the proportions of each cell type The duct-like structures may be widely separated by fibrous tissue or merge into cohesive sheets	Immunohistochemical features Pathologic differential diagnosis	Inner cells positive with keratins Outer myoepithelial cells calponin, smooth muscle actin, p63 and, less reliably, S-100 protein positive Pleomorphic adenoma, adenoid cystic carcinoma (tubular variant), myoepithelioma, clear cell oncocytoma, mucoepidermoid carcinoma, clear cell carcinoma (NOS), and metastases from the kidney and thyroid gland

MICROSCOPIC FINDINGS

The characteristic feature of EMC is the formation of double-layered, duct-like structures (Fig. 12-46). The luminal cells form a single, cuboidal, or columnar layer and have finely granular, eosinophilic cytoplasm, and a central round or oval nucleus. The outer cells may form single or multiple layers and have abundant, clear cytoplasm that is usually rich in glycogen, and typically have eccentric and vesicular nuclei (Fig. 12-47). The proportion of each cell type and their architectural arrange-

ments are extremely variable. The duct-like structures may be surrounded and separated by hyaline material or fibrous tissue (Fig. 12-48). They can also form more cohesive sheets, and the ductal configuration may not be immediately apparent. Tumors may consist predominantly of clear cells with only scattered duct-lining cells that may form solid islands without canalization. Cystic or papillary areas are seen in about 20% of cases. Less commonly, areas show spindle cell or squamous dif-

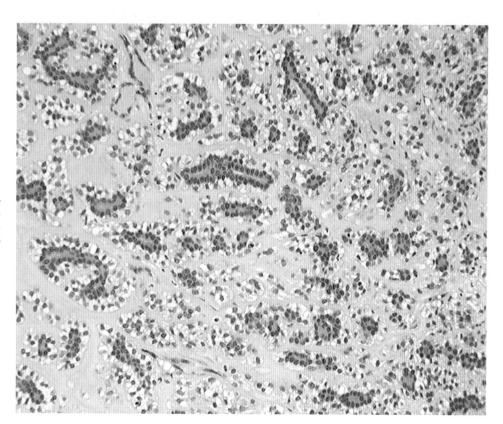

FIGURE 12-46

Duct-like structures separated by fibrous connective tissue. Note the double layer of inner cuboidal cells surrounded by clear, myoepithelial cells.

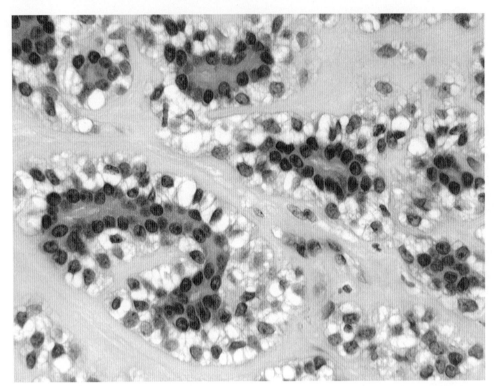

FIGURE 12-47
High power shows eosinophilic cyto-plasm of the inner luminal duct-like cells. The myoepithelial cells have cleared cytoplasm with more vesicu-lar nuclear chromatin.

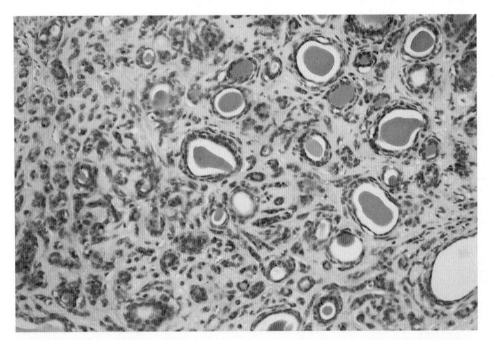

FIGURE 12-48
Hyaline material separates these gland-like structures with secretions in the lumen.

ferentiation, or oncocytic metaplasia, typically of the luminal cells. Mitoses are usually sparse and rarely exceed 2/10 HPF. Perineural and vascular involvement is relatively common and bone invasion is occasionally seen (Fig. 12-49). EMC can arise from a pleomorphic adenoma and a few cases of hybrid tumors have been described. Recently, cases of EMC showing de-differen-tiation have been reported.

ANCILLARY STUDIES

The inner duct lining cells stain with low-molecular weight cytokeratins, CAM5.2, and EMA (Fig. 12-50). The outer clear cells stain with myoepithelial markers such as calponin, α-SMA, p63 and, less reliably, with S-100 protein (Fig. 12-50).

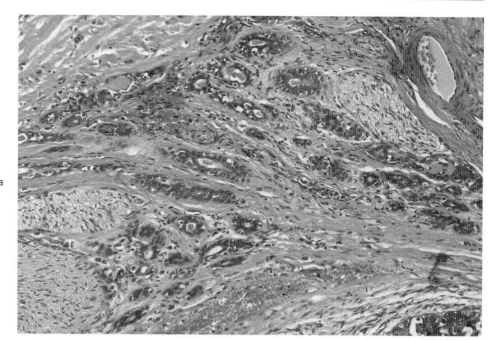

FIGURE 12-49

An epithelial-myoepithelial carcinoma demonstrates perineural invasion.

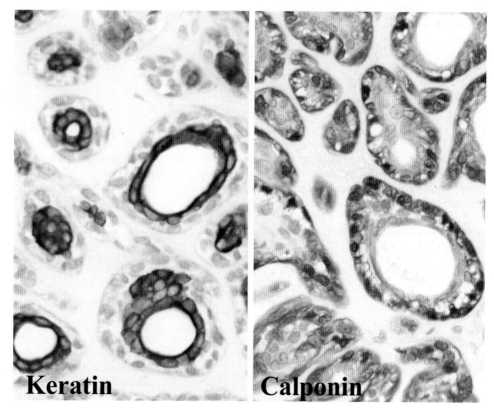

FIGURE 12-50

Left: Keratin highlights the inner ductal type cells. *Right:* A calponin stain accentuates the outer myoepithelial cells.

DIFFERENTIAL DIAGNOSIS

The differential diagnosis of EMC includes tumors showing the formation of double-layered duct-like structures and those consisting predominantly of clear cells. Double-layered duct-like structures can be seen in pleomorphic adenoma and the tubular variant of adenoid cystic carcinoma. The clear cells in these tumors tend to have less abundant cytoplasm and hyperchromatic, angular nuclei. In addition, the clear cells of EMC are typically rich in glycogen. However, these variants usually form focal areas of more typical tumors, and the main problem arises in the interpretation of limited biopsy material. In such circumstances it may not be possible to distinguish between these tumors with confidence. A wide range of benign and malignant salivary tumors can show focal or extensive areas of predominantly clear cells. These include clear cell variants of pleomorphic adenoma, myoepithelioma, oncocytoma, mucoepidermoid carcinoma, and clear cell carcinoma (NOS). In addition, metastases from the kidney and thyroid glands may need to be excluded by staining for CD10, renal cell carcinoma (RCC) marker, thyroglobulin, and TTF-1.

PROGNOSIS AND THERAPY

EMC is a moderately aggressive salivary tumor with a high recurrence rate (40%) and metastasis to regional lymph nodes and distant sites such as lung, liver, and kidney in nearly 15% of cases. The 5-year survival rate is 80% and the 10-year survival is 72%. Clinical features indicating poorer prognosis include incomplete surgical excision, large size, rapid growth, and involvement of minor salivary glands. Microscopic features associated with a poor outcome include cellular atypia, high mitotic frequency, and aneuploidy. Surgery is the treatment of choice and neck dissection should be included in patients with evidence of regional lymph node spread. This can be supplemented by radiotherapy in advanced or recurrent cases.

SALIVARY DUCT CARCINOMA

CLINICAL FEATURES

Salivary duct carcinoma (SDC) can arise ab initio and is also a relatively common malignant element of carcinoma ex pleomorphic adenoma. It accounts for about 9% of malignant salivary gland tumors. The age at presentation ranges from 22–91 years and most patients are over 50 years old. There is a striking male predominance of at least 4:1. The vast majority of cases arise in the

SALIVARY DUCT CARCINOMA DISEASE FACT SHEET	
Definition	Salivary duct carcinoma is an aggressive adenocarcinoma that resembles high-grade breast ductal adenocarcinoma
Incidence and location	Represents about 9% of malignant salivary gland tumors
	Common type of malignancy arising ex pleomorphic adenoma
	Overwhelming majority affect major glands (usually parotid)
Morbidity and mortality	About a third of cases recur locally
	Regional lymph node metastasis in about 60% with distant spread in about 50% of cases
	65% of patients die from disease
Gender, race, and age distribution	Male >> Female (4 : 1)
	Peak incidence in 6th–7th decades
Clinical features	Present with a rapidly growing tumor
	Ulceration and facial nerve palsy common
	If it is in a carcinoma ex pleomorphic adenoma, there is rapid enlargement in a long-standing mass
Prognosis and treatment	Most aggressive salivary gland tumor with regional metastasis in about 60% with distant spread in about 50% of cases
	Features associated with a poor outcome include large tumor size, presence of distant metastases and overexpression of HER-2/neu
	Radical surgery with adjuvant radiotherapy

major glands (96%), predominantly the parotid, and rarely in the sinonasal tract and larynx. They usually present as a rapidly growing mass, with ulceration and facial nerve palsy relatively common. In carcinomas arising ex pleomorphic adenoma, there may be a history of a long-standing mass with recent enlargement.

PATHOLOGIC FEATURES

GROSS FINDINGS

The cut surface is predominantly solid, white, gray or tan, with cysts, necrosis, and hemorrhage common. The tumor usually shows invasion into surrounding tissues but occasional cases appear to be relatively well circumscribed. Macroscopic features typical of a preexisting pleomorphic adenoma may be present.

MICROSCOPIC FINDINGS

SDC resembles in situ and infiltrative ductal adenocarcinoma of breast (Fig. 12-51). The most characteristic feature is the formation of large ducts with cribriform configurations, "Roman-bridging," and

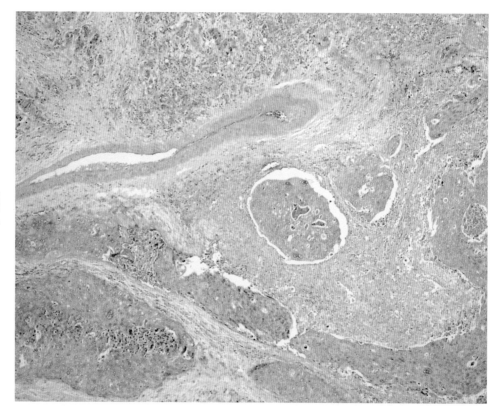

FIGURE 12-51

Large nests of tumor have replaced and expanded the salivary gland ducts. There is vascular invasion, comedonecrosis, and heavy fibrosis.

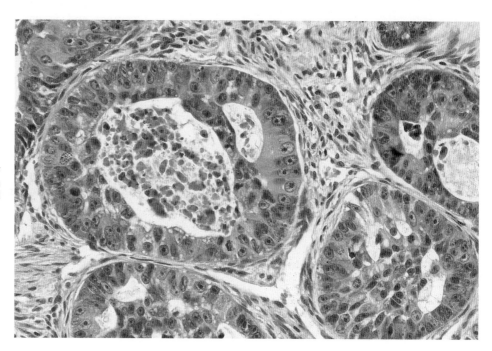

FIGURE 12-52

Cribriform areas with "Roman-bridge" formation and comedonecrosis are seen in this SDC. Note the pleomorphism and mitotic figures.

comedonecrosis (Fig. 12-52). In addition, solid and papillary areas and evidence of squamous differentiation may be present (Fig. 12-53). Stromal fibrosis and inflammatory infiltration is often a conspicuous feature. Vascular and neural invasion are common and frequently extensive. The tumor typically consists of cytologically pleomorphic cells with abundant pink, granular cyto-

plasm (Fig. 12-54). Oncocytic metaplasia is a common and sometimes striking feature. The nuclei are large and hyperchromatic with prominent nucleoli and there is usually a high mitotic frequency. Tumors are occasionally biphasic and have a malignant spindle-cell, sarcomatoid stroma (Fig. 12-55). Several other variants have recently been described. The mucin-rich variant shows

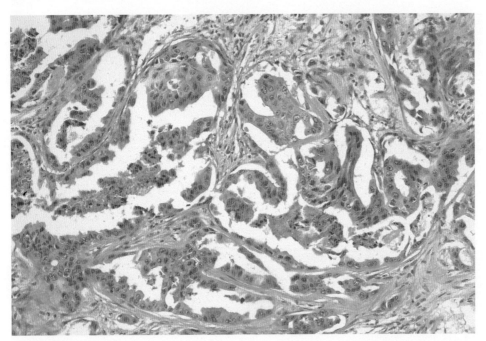

FIGURE 12-53
A papillary pattern of growth is noted in this salivary duct carcinoma.

SALIVARY DUCT CARCINOMA PATHOLOGIC FEATURES	
Gross findings	Predominantly solid white, gray or tan
	Cysts, necrosis, and hemorrhage common
	Usually shows invasion into surrounding tissues
	Macroscopic features typical of a preexisting pleomorphic adenoma may be present
Microscopic findings	Resembles ductal adenocarcinoma of breast, both intraductal and infiltrative
	Vascular and neural invasion
	Large ducts with cribriform configurations, Roman-bridging, and comedonecrosis
	Solid, papillary areas, and squamous differentiation may be present
	Cytologically pleomorphic cells, often with granular or oncocytic cytoplasm
	Large, hyperchromatic nuclei with prominent nucleoli and high mitotic frequency
Immunohistochemical features	Positive for a wide range of cytokeratins, CEA and EMA
	Strongly positive for androgen receptor (negative with estrogen/progesterone receptors)
	Most show overexpression of HER-2/neu protein
Pathologic differential diagnosis	Metastatic breast carcinoma, squamous cell carcinoma, oncocytic carcinoma, may be part of carcinoma ex pleomorphic adenoma

ANCILLARY STUDIES

SDC is usually positive for a wide range of cytokeratins, carcinoembryonic antigen, and epithelial membrane antigen. It shows strong nuclear positivity for androgen receptors and is usually negative for myoepithelial, estrogen, and progesterone markers. There is variable positivity for prostate-specific antigen and prostatic acid phosphatase. Peroxisome proliferator-activated receptor gamma is expressed in 80 % of SDC, often at high levels, and is topographically localized to the cytoplasm. Most tumors show overexpression of HER-2/neu protein with strong membrane staining.

DIFFERENTIAL DIAGNOSIS

SDC must be distinguished from metastatic breast carcinoma. Although areas can resemble poorly differentiated squamous cell carcinoma, more typical cribriform, duct-like structures are typically present. Papillary areas can resemble cystadenocarcinoma but are usually only focally present and there is usually more cellular pleomorphism in SDC. Some tumors are extensively oncocytic but their histomorphologic characteristics should aid differentiation from oncocytic carcinoma.

PROGNOSIS AND THERAPY

SDC is the most aggressive salivary gland tumor, with an overall survival rate of about 35 %, most patients dying within 4 years. About a third of cases show

lakes of epithelial mucin containing malignant cells, in addition to more typical areas. Some tumors have an invasive, micropapillary component and a strong propensity for angiolymphatic and neural spread; these have a particularly poor prognosis.

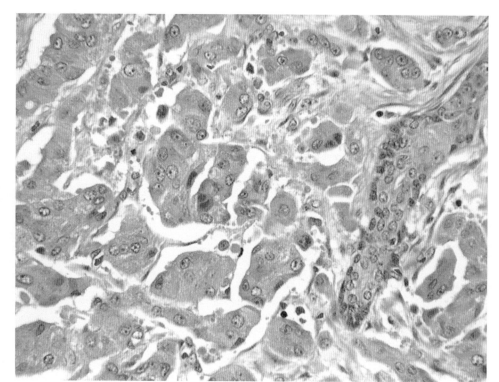

FIGURE 12-54

A benign duct (*right side*) is contrasted with the cytologically pleomorphic cells that have granular, eosinophilic cytoplasm.

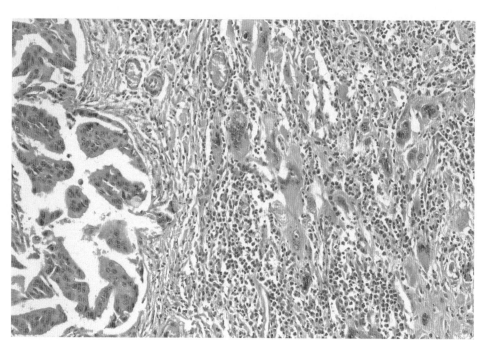

FIGURE 12-55

A papillary architecture blends into an area of spindle cell or "sarcomatoid" transformation in this salivary duct carcinoma.

local recurrence and approximately 60% develop metastasis to regional lymph nodes. Systemic metastases to lung and bone is seen in up to 50% of cases. A large primary tumor, evidence of metastases, and overexpression of HER-2/neu protein appear to be indicators of poorer prognosis. Aneuploidy, proliferation rate, and expression of p53 show no correlation with outcome. The treatment usually includes a total parotidectomy with a neck dissection and adjuvant radiotherapy.

CARCINOMA EX PLEOMORPHIC ADENOMA

CLINICAL FEATURES

Carcinoma ex pleomorphic adenoma (Ca ex PA) accounts for about 4% of all salivary tumors and 12% of salivary malignancies. The sites of origin are usually parotid (67%), followed by minor glands (18%), submandibular (15%), and sublingual gland (<1%). Most cases are seen in 6th and 7th decades; it is rare in children. There is equal gender distribution. The typical history is that of long-standing mass with recent rapid enlargement or previous surgery for a PA. Some tumors, however, appear to have a relatively short duration. They are often painless but some are painful, and about 40% of patients have nerve palsies.

PATHOLOGIC FEATURES

GROSS FINDINGS

Tumors range up to 25 cm. An area of circumscribed PA may be apparent, associated with an extensively infiltrative component, often showing areas of hemorrhage and necrosis. The preexisting PA may be represented by an area of scarring.

MICROSCOPIC FINDINGS

The relative proportions of preexisting PA and Ca ex PA are widely variable. Some tumors show a carcinoma in direct juxtaposition to a typical PA (Fig. 12-56); sometimes the benign remnant may be difficult to find,

particularly in scarred tumors. The malignant component may overgrow the benign element, but the diagnosis can be made on the basis of clinical history. The malignant component is frequently a poorly differentiated carcinoma, high-grade adenocarcinoma (NOS) or salivary duct carcinoma (Fig. 12-57). However, most other types of salivary gland carcinomas have been described in Ca ex PA, and some cases show diverse differentiation with several distinct types within the tumor mass. Adequate sampling of the tumor is required to make an accurate diagnosis. A carcinosarcoma ("true malignant mixed tumor") has been defined by the simultaneous presence of a carcinoma and a sarcoma, and this tumor may be associated with a residual PA; it is vanishingly rare.

Ca ex PA has been subclassified into noninvasive, minimally invasive (≤1.5 mm), and invasive (≥1.5 mm) (Fig. 12-58). Noninvasive carcinomas have also been referred to as intracapsular carcinomas, in situ Ca ex PA, or severely dysplastic PA. They show a PA with focal or diffuse areas of cytologically malignant cells but without evidence of invasion into the surrounding tissues. These areas are commonly associated with increased mitotic activity.

DIFFERENTIAL DIAGNOSIS

FNA or spontaneous infarction of PA can cause secondary degenerative changes that may be confused with Ca ex PA. These include hemorrhage, necrosis, inflammation, reactive cellular atypia, and squamous or

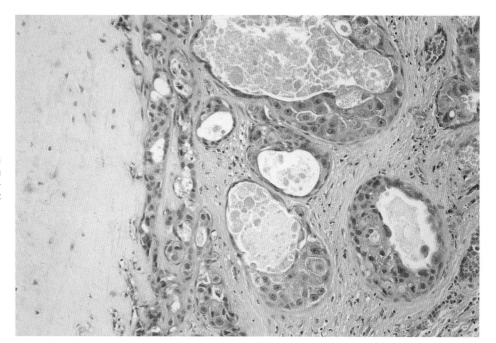

FIGURE 12-56

Benign pleomorphic adenoma (*left*) blends with a high-grade carcinoma with features of a salivary duct carcinoma in this carcinoma ex pleomorphic adenoma.

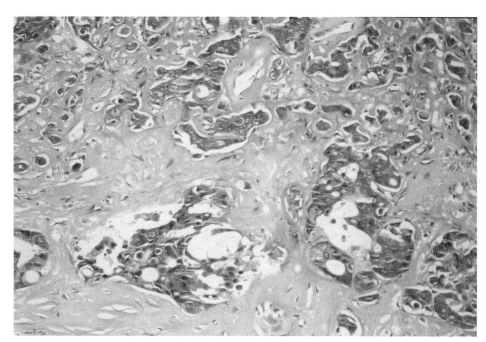

FIGURE 12-57

High-grade carcinoma infiltrating into the surrounding fibrous tissue.

mucus metaplasia. It is important to distinguish between noninvasive, minimally invasive, and invasive tumors, as there are clear prognostic implications. Carcinomas can also arise in other salivary adenomas and, though uncommon, these appear to have a better prognosis. Foci of carcinoma may develop in a hyalinized PA and are easily missed, particularly in large tumors. A *metastasizing PA* may be caused by iatrogenic manipulation of a PA (during surgery), with benign appearing epithelial elements in the sites of metastasis.

PROGNOSIS AND THERAPY

Noninvasive carcinomas have the same prognosis as conventional PA. Invasive carcinomas are usually aggressive but do show a range of behavior. About 25% to 50% of cases undergo one or more local recurrences, usually within 5 years. About 70% show regional or distant metastases, usually to lung, bone liver, brain,

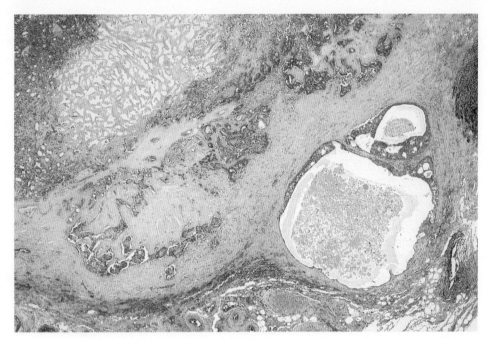

FIGURE 12-58
The benign pleomorphic adenoma (*left upper*) associated with areas of invasion beyond the contour of the tumor in this invasive carcinoma ex pleomorphic adenoma.

and elsewhere. Tumors with invasion of >1.5 mm have a poor prognosis ranging from 26% to 65% at 5 years to 0% to 38% at 20 years. Minimally invasive tumors (<1.5 mm) appear to have a relatively good prognosis. Large and histologically high-grade tumors have a poor prognosis. Wide resection is the treatment of choice.

EXTRANODAL MARGINAL ZONE B CELL LYMPHOMA OF SALIVARY GLANDS

CLINICAL FEATURES

Extranodal marginal zone B cell lymphoma (EMZBCL) of mucosa-associated lymphoid tissue is an uncommon but important low-grade B cell neoplasm of salivary glands. It is usually seen in the context of lympho-epithelial sialadenitis (LESA), previously referred to as either benign lymphoepithelial lesion or myoepithelial sialadenitis (MESA) associated with either primary or secondary Sjögren's syndrome. Most patients are in the 55–65 years range, with a significant female predilection (F:M = 9:1). Over 80% of cases involve the parotid glands, either unilaterally or bilaterally, and they usually cause painless swellings. Despite their neoplastic nature, these swellings may be remarkably episodic and, in some cases, enlargement can be exacerbated by secondary ascending bacterial infection, when pain may also be a feature.

EXTRANODAL MARGINAL ZONE B CELL LYMPHOMA OF SALIVARY GLANDS DISEASE FACT SHEET	
Definition	An extranodal low-grade B cell lymphoma arising in mucosa-associated lymphoid tissue
Incidence and location	Predominantly seen in patients with Sjögren's syndrome
	80% of cases involve the parotid gland
	May be bilateral
Morbidity and mortality	Typically indolent, without significant morbidity or mortality
	Spontaneous regression reported
Gender, race, and age distribution	Female >>> Male (9 : 1)
	Age range 55–65 yr
Clinical features	Patients may have xerostomia and xerophthalmia associated with Sjögren's syndrome
	Chronic and sometimes episodic parotid enlargement
	Occasionally painful due to superimposed ascending infection
Prognosis and treatment	Most patients can be followed up without active treatment
	Infrequent transformation into higher grade lymphomas may require additional therapy

PATHOLOGIC FEATURES

GROSS FINDINGS

The tumor forms a firm mass with a yellowish, tan to pale, "fish-flesh" cut surface. This is usually homogeneous but small cysts are occasionally present.

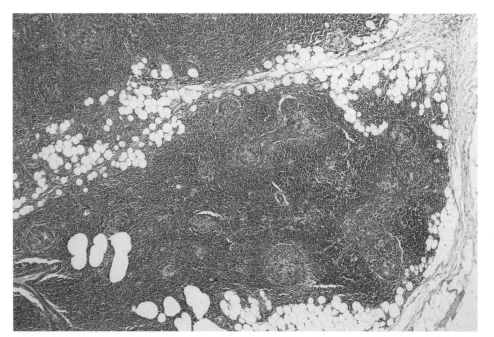

FIGURE 12-59

Lymphoepithelial sialadenitis shows a multifocal inflammatory infiltrate with "epimyoepithelial" islands and reactive germinal centers in a major salivary gland.

MICROSCOPIC FINDINGS

EMZBCL is usually seen in salivary glands involved with MESA. The two components of LESA are lymphoid infiltration and epimyoepithelial islands. The lymphoid infiltrate is initially multifocal and periductal and spreads centrifugally, progressively destroying the acinar tissue (Fig. 12-59). Reactive follicles frequently develop and consist of polytypic B cells and the interfollicular lymphoid tissue consists predominantly of T cells. The epimyoepithelial islands consist of ducts that have undergone hyperplasia and frequently show luminal obliteration (Fig. 12-60). The role, if any, of myoepithelial cells in this process is contentious. The islands frequently contain hyaline material, which is derived from basement membrane. In addition, the islands are infiltrated by both B and T cells. When EMZBCL develops in LESA, halos of monocytoid and centrocyte-like B cells surround and progressively

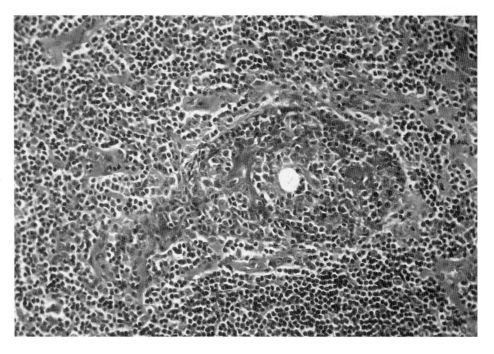

FIGURE 12-60

An "epimyoepithelial" island has small hyperplastic ducts associated with a mixed inflammatory infiltrate.

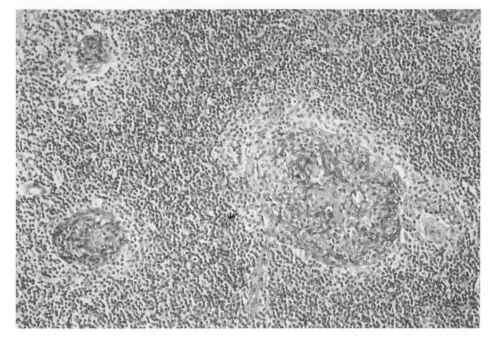

FIGURE 12-61

Halos of monocytoid cells around "epimyoepithelial" islands, a few containing hyaline material in this extranodal marginal zone B cell lymphoma.

invade and destroy the epimyoepithelial islands or "lymphoepithelial islands" (Fig. 12-61). In addition, immunoblasts and lymphoplasmacytic cells are present and plasma cell differentiation may be a striking feature. Colonization of reactive germinal follicles by neoplastic B cells is frequently present. A few large cells are commonly present and infrequently they are more numerous and form focal aggregates (Fig. 12-62). Occasionally, diffuse large B cell lymphoma develops within this setting. The lymphoid cells infiltrate the interlobular septa and gland capsule and extend into the periglandular tissues.

ANCILLARY STUDIES

The predominance of B cells in these tumors can be confirmed by immunostaining for CD20 or CD79a. The neoplastic nature of the infiltrate can be demonstrated by light-chain restriction (kappa or lambda). The significance of clonal rearrangements of immunoglobulin genes in diagnosing malignant transformation of LESA is less clear. Neoplastic B cells colonizing reactive follicles often show bcl-2 positivity. Remnants of the epithelial islands can be readily highlighted with keratin immunohistochemistry (Fig. 12-63).

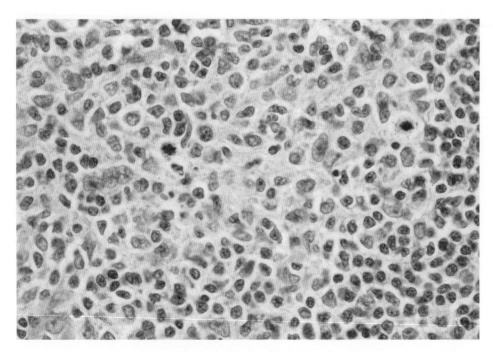

FIGURE 12-62

Immunoblasts, lymphoplasmacytic cells with increased mitotic figures in this area of extranodal marginal zone B cell lymphoma.

EXTRANODAL MARGINAL ZONE B CELL LYMPHOMA OF SALIVARY GLANDS PATHOLOGIC FEATURES	
Gross findings	Firm, with yellowish-tan, "fish-flesh" cut surface
	Usually homogeneous or may show microcysts
Microscopic findings	Background of lymphoepithelial sialadenitis (LESA)
	Epimyoepithelial islands, frequently infiltrated by the lymphoid infiltrate
	Nodular of diffuse heterogeneous B cell infiltrate
	Halos of monocytoid B cells around follicles
	Infiltrate consists of atypical small lymphocytes, centrocyte-like cells, monocytoid B cells, immunoblasts, and plasma cells
	Reactive germinal centers common and may be colonized by neoplastic B cells
Immunohistochemical features	B cell phenotype of CD20 and/or CD79a
	B cells colonizing reactive follicles are often bcl-2 reactive
	Monoclonality demonstrated by light-chain restriction
	Remnants of epimyoepithelial islands highlighted by cytokeratin staining
Pathologic differential diagnosis	LESA, follicular lymphoma, rarely diffuse large B cell lymphoma

DIFFERENTIAL DIAGNOSIS

In some cases it may not be possible to distinguish between EMZBCL and LESA using conventional

microscopy. Effacement of the interlobular septa and infiltration of lymphocytes into periglandular tissue suggest lymphomatous transformation. Both may contain reactive follicles but in EMZBCL colonizing B cells are usually bcl-2 positive. Demonstration of light-chain restriction is typical of a B cell lymphoma. Nodular tumors may be confused with follicular lymphoma but, in addition to more extensive immunoreactivity for bcl-2, the latter is typically also positive for CD10 and bcl-6, although follicular lymphoma is very rare in salivary glands. Rarely there is development of a diffuse large B cell lymphoma.

PROGNOSIS AND THERAPY

EMZBCL usually has an excellent prognosis and most patients can be followed up without active treatment. Some cases appear to show spontaneous regression. Occasionally there is transformation into higher grade tumors and development of extra salivary gland lymphoma. Treatment is usually limited to the procedure performed to obtain the specimen.

UNCOMMON CARCINOMAS

BASAL CELL ADENOCARCINOMA

Basal cell adenocarcinoma consists of basaloid epithelial cells cytologically and histomorphologically similar to those of basal cell adenoma, but in an infiltrative epithelial neoplasm (Fig. 12-64) with a potential for metasta-

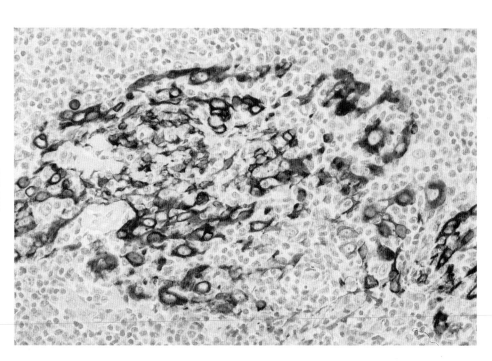

FIGURE 12-63
A keratin immunohistochemistry highlights the epithelial component in the lymphoepithelial lesion which develops in extranodal marginal zone B cell lymphoma.

UNCOMMON CARCINOMAS (BASAL CELL ADENOCARCIOMA, CLEAR CELL CARCINOMA, SEBACEOUS CARCINOMA, ONCOCYTIC CARCINOMA) FACT SHEET

Basal cell adenocarcinoma	*Clinical:*
	Basaloid cell neoplasm with invasive growth
	Represents <2% of salivary gland tumors
	Adults, mean 60 yr
	>90% occur in the parotid gland
	Locally destructive, but good long-term prognosis
	Pathology:
	Infiltrative border
	Basaloid cells which may be small and dark with scant cytoplasm or larger, polygonal cells with eosinophilic/amphophilic cytoplasm
	Solid, membranous, and tubulo-trabecular patterns
	Separated by variable hyalinizing material
	Mitotic figures scant
	Perineural and vascular invasion can be seen
Clear cell carcinoma (NOS)	*Clinical:*
	Malignant epithelial tumor of monotonous optically clear cytoplasm (no other tumor features present)
	Represents <2% of salivary gland tumors
	Adults, peak in 40–70 yr range
	About 60% occur in minor salivary gland (palate)
	Locally infiltrative, but low grade, cured by surgery
	Pathology:
	Unencapsulated with infiltrative growth
	Uniform population of polygonal/round cells with distinct borders, cleared cytoplasm, small nuclei, and fibrosis separating the tumor groups
	Must be separated from metastatic renal cell carcinoma and other clear-cell variants of salivary gland neoplasms
Sebaceous carcinoma	*Clinical:*
	Malignant tumor with sebaceous cells of variable maturity with pleomorphism and invasive growth
	Represent <1% of salivary gland tumors
	Adults, peak in 3rd–7th decades
	>90% occur in the parotid gland
	May be very painful with facial nerve palsy
	Wide excision yields an approximately 70% 5-yr survival
	Pathology:
	Sheets, islands, and trabeculae with duct structures which may become cystic
	Sebaceous differentiation is variable, with occasional tumors showing only rare sebaceous cells
	Cytologic atypia and mitotic figures usually in basaloid and squamous cells
	Necrosis is common, with perineural invasion seen in about 20%
Oncocytic carcinoma	*Clinical:*
	Cytomorphologically malignant oncocytes arranged in an adenocarcinoma pattern with invasion
	Represent <1% of salivary gland tumors
	Adults, mean 65 yr, M > F
	80% occur in the parotid gland
	A mass lesion which may be associated with pain or facial palsy
	A high-grade tumor with frequent recurrences and metastasis
	Pathology:
	Unencapsulated tumors composed of large, round, polygonal cells with abundant, granular, eosinophilic cytoplasm
	Large nuclei with prominent nucleoli
	Variable pleomorphism
	Neural and vascular invasion is common
	Ki67 staining usually positive in malignant tumors
	Must be separated from oncocytic variants of other salivary gland tumors

sis. Rare cases have arisen from a preexisting basal cell adenoma. Basal cell adenocarcinoma accounts for <2% of all salivary gland tumors. It has only been reported in adults, with an average age of 60 years at presentation. Over 90% of cases involve the parotid gland, and tumors in the oral cavity are rare. Most present as painless swellings, sometimes of many years duration.

The tumor consists of basaloid epithelial cells which may be small and dark with scanty cytoplasm, or larger and polygonal, with eosinophilic or amphophilic cytoplasm (Fig. 12-65). As in basal cell adenoma, there are three main histomorphologic patterns: solid, membranous, and tubulo-trabecular. In the solid variant the tumor islands are separated by collagenous septa of vari-

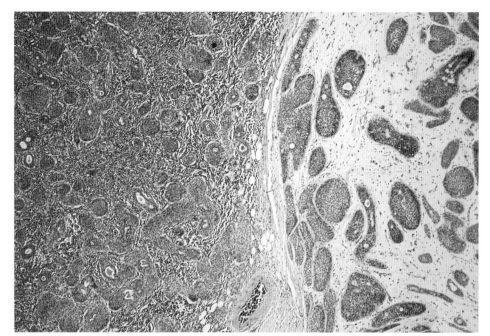

FIGURE 12-64

The basaloid cells of this basal cell adenocarcinoma are seen invading adjacent lymphoid tissue.

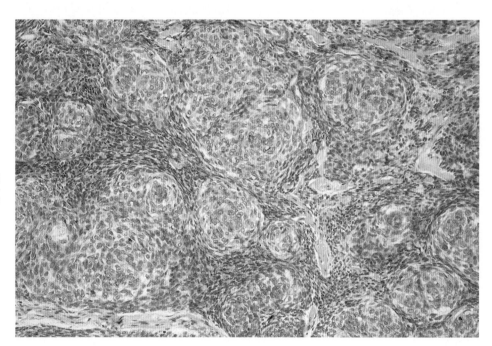

FIGURE 12-65

Small dark cells with scant cytoplasm are noted surrounding larger, polygonal cells with eosinophilic cytoplasm in this basal cell adenocarcinoma.

able thickness. The basement membrane zone of the membranous variant is thick and densely hyalinized and frequently there are hyaline droplets within the tumor islands. Peripheral palisading and cellular whorling, sometimes with squamous differentiation, may be seen in both of these variants. The tubulo-trabecular pattern consists of interconnecting cords of basaloid cells with variable degrees of luminal differentiation. Cellular and nuclear pleomorphism is rarely conspicuous and mitotic activity is often minimal. Ki-67 and PNCA indices are low. However, these tumors show an infiltrative growth pattern and frequently extend widely into the sur-

rounding tissues. Perineural and vascular invasion is present in about a quarter of cases but regional and distant metastases are uncommon. Although basal cell adenocarcinoma is locally destructive, the long-term prognosis is good and the tumor is regarded as low grade.

CLEAR CELL CARCINOMA (NOS)

Clear cell carcinoma (NOS) is a malignant epithelial neoplasm composed of a monomorphous population of cells that have optically clear cytoplasm. It is distinguished from other salivary gland tumors containing clear cells by the absence of the characteristic features of these other neoplasms and its monomorphous population of cells. The peak incidence is in the 40–70 years age range and about 60% involve intraoral minor glands, particularly the palate. Most present as a painless swelling without ulceration with a history ranging from a few weeks to many years.

Clear cell carcinoma is unencapsulated and infiltrates the surrounding tissues. Microscopy shows a uniform population of polygonal or round cells with distinct cell borders. The cytoplasm in most cells is optically clear, although in a few cells it may be faintly eosinophilic (Fig. 12-66). The cytoplasm contains variable amounts of glycogen but has no significant mucin content. Nuclei are round and eccentric and, though occasionally there may be moderate pleomorphism, mitoses are few. The cells are arranged in nests, sheets and cords with no evidence of ductal differentiation. There is a fibrous stroma of variable thickness and cellularity. In the so-called hyalinizing variant, the stroma is densely collagenized and forms thick bands between tumor nests. This tumor must be separated from clear cell variants of other salivary gland neoplasms, and from metastatic renal cell carcinoma. Clear cell carcinoma is locally infiltrative and may invade nerves. The tumor is usually low grade and cured by conservative surgery.

SEBACEOUS CARCINOMA

Sebaceous carcinoma is a malignant tumor composed of sebaceous cells of varying maturity that are arranged in sheets and/or nests with different degrees of pleomorphism, nuclear atypia and invasiveness. It is a rare tumor with peaks of age incidence in the 3rd and 7th decades of life. Over 90% arise in the parotid gland and the tumor usually presents as a variably painful mass, sometimes with facial nerve palsy.

The tumor can form sheets, islands and trabeculae. Ductal structures are common and may become cystic (Fig. 12-67). The degree of sebaceous differentiation is very variable and in some tumors basaloid or squamous cell types predominate and sebaceous cells may be difficult to find. Cytological atypia and mitotic activity are usually seen in these basaloid and squamous cells. Areas of necrosis are common and neural invasion is present in about a fifth of cases. The 5-year survival in the small number of reported cases was about 70%, and wide surgical excision is the treatment of choice.

ONCOCYTIC CARCINOMA

Oncocytic carcinoma is a proliferation of cytomorphologically malignant oncocytes with an adenocarcinomatous architectural phenotype, including infiltrative qualities. It is rare and accounts for less than 1% of all salivary gland tumors. About 80% involve the parotid gland with the remainder arising in the submandibular and minor glands. The age ranges from 29–91 years (mean, 65 yr) and there is a male predominance. Parotid tumors usually form a nondescript mass that is often associated with pain or facial palsy.

Microscopically the tumor is unencapsulated and consists of large, round, or polyhedral cells with abundant, granular, and eosinophilic cytoplasm and large, centrally placed nuclei with prominent nucleoli (Fig. 12-68). The mitochondrial-rich cytoplasm usually shows intensely blue granular positivity with PTAH stain.

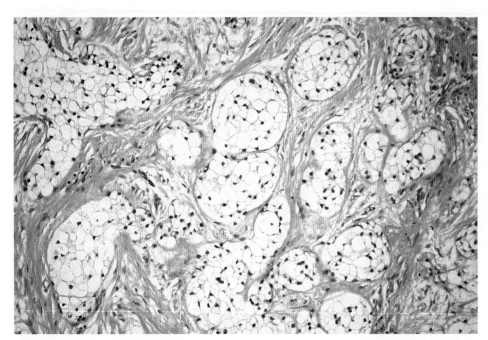

FIGURE 12-66

A monotonous population of cells with clear cytoplasm containing small, hyperchromatic nuclei. Fibrous bands separate the nodules of tumor. There is no ductal differentiation.

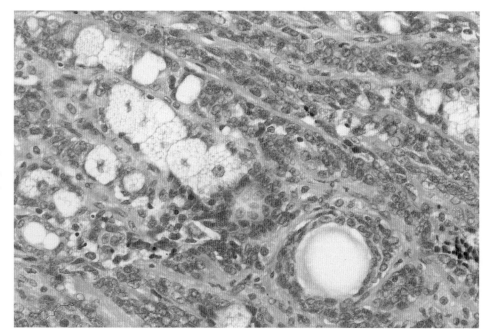

FIGURE 12-67

Basaloid cells arranged in trabeculae with a duct-like structure in this sebaceous carcinoma. Note the areas of sebaceous differentiation in the center of the field.

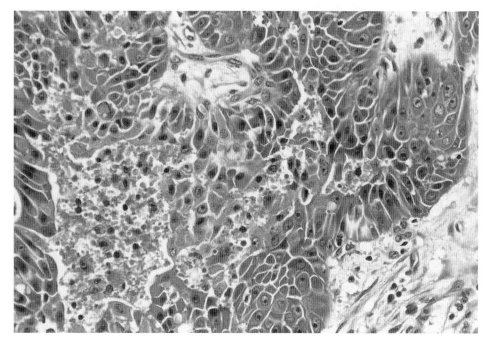

FIGURE 12-68

Large, polygonal cells with ample oncocytic/oxyphilic cytoplasm surround nuclei with prominent nucleoli. Note the areas of necrosis.

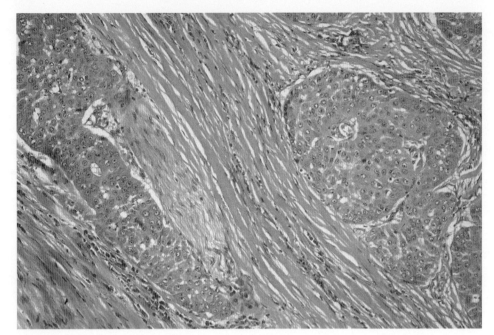

FIGURE 12-69

Oncocytic carcinoma cells are arranged in a gland- or duct-like structure, seen surrounding a nerve in this infiltrative neoplasm.

There is variable pleomorphism and some tumors have cytologically bland areas, suggesting that they have arisen from a preexisting oncocytoma. Ki-67 staining may be of value in differentiating between benign and malignant oncocytic tumors. The cells are arranged in sheets, theques, and cords, and sometimes duct-like structures are present. The tumor shows infiltration into surrounding tissue, and neural and vascular invasion are common (Fig. 12-69). The tumor is often a diagnosis of exclusion after oncocytic variants of other salivary gland malignancies have been excluded. Oncocytic carcinoma is often high grade, showing frequent local recurrence and both regional and distant metastases.

SUGGESTED READING

Adenocarcinoma, Not Otherwise Specified

1. Auclair P, van der Wal JE: Adenocarcinoma, not otherwise specified. In: Barnes EL, Eveson JW, Reichart P, Sidransky D, eds. Pathology and Genetics of Head and Neck Tumours. Kleihues P, Sobin LH, series eds. World Health Organization Classification of Tumours. Lyon, France: IARC Press, 2005:238–239.
2. Ellis GL, Auclair PLL Tumors of the salivary glands, 3rd ed. Washington, DC: Armed Forces Institute of Pathology, 1996.
3. Matsuba HM, Mauney M, Simpson JR, et al.: Adenocarcinomas of major and minor salivary gland origin: a histopathologic review of treatment failure patterns. Laryngoscope 1988;98:784–788.
4. Nagao K, Matsuzaki O, Saiga H, et al.: Histopathologic studies on adenocarcinoma of the parotid gland. Acta Pathol Jpn 1986;36:337–347.
5. Sheahan P, Byrne M, Hafidh M, et al.: Neck dissection findings in primary head and neck high-grade adenocarcinoma. J Laryngol Otol 2004;118:532–536.
6. Spiro RH, Huvos AG, Strong EW: Adenocarcinoma of salivary origin. Clinicopathologic study of 204 patients. Am J Surg 1982;44:423–431.
7. Wahlberg P, Anderson H, Biorklund A, et al.: Carcinoma of the parotid and submandibular glands—a study of survival in 2,465 patients. Oral Oncol 2002;38:706–713.

Mucoepidermoid Carcinoma

1. Auclair PL, Goode RK, Ellis GL: Mucoepidermoid carcinoma of intraoral salivary glands. Evaluation and application of grading criteria in 143 cases. Cancer 1992;69:2021–2030.
2. Boahene DK, Olsen KD, Lewis JE, et al.: Mucoepidermoid carcinoma of the parotid gland: the Mayo clinic experience. Arch Otolaryngol Head Neck Surg 2004;130:849–856.
3. Brandwein MS, Ivanov K, Wallace DI, et al.: Mucoepidermoid carcinoma: a clinicopathologic study of 80 patients with special reference to histological grading. Am J Surg Pathol 2001;25:835–845.
4. Ellis GL: Clear cell neoplasms in salivary glands: clearly a diagnostic challenge. Ann Diagn Pathol 1998;2:61–78.
5. Fadare O, Hileeto D, Gruddin YL, Mariappan MR: Sclerosing mucoepidermoid carcinoma of the parotid gland. Arch Pathol Lab Med 2004;128:1046–1049.
6. Goode RK, Auclair PL, Ellis GL: Mucoepidermoid carcinoma of the major salivary glands: clinical and histopathologic analysis of 234 cases with evaluation of grading criteria. Cancer 1998;82:1217–1224.
7. Goode RK, El-Naggar AK: Mucoepidermoid carcinoma. In: Barnes EL, Eveson JW, Reichart P, Sidransky D, eds. Pathology and Genetics of Head and Neck Tumours. Kleihues P, Sobin LH, series eds. World Health Organization Classification of Tumours. Lyon, France: IARC Press, 2005:219–220.
8. Guzzo M, Andreola S, Sirizzotti G, Cantu G: Mucoepidermoid carcinoma of the salivary glands: clinicopathologic review of 108 patients treated at the National Cancer Institute of Milan. Ann Surg Oncol 2002;9: 688–695.
9. Nagao T, Gaffey TA, Kay PA, et al.: Dedifferentiation in low-grade mucoepidermoid carcinoma of the parotid gland. Hum Pathol 2003;34:1068–1072.

Acinic Cell Adenocarcinoma

1. Colmenero C, Patron M, Sierra I: Acinic cell carcinoma of the salivary glands. A review of 20 new cases. J Craniomaxillofac Surg 1991;19: 260–266.
2. Ellis GL, Corio RL: Acinic cell adenocarcinoma. A clinicopathologic analysis of 294 cases. Cancer 1983;52:542–549.
3. Ellis GL, Auclair PL: Tumors of the salivary glands, 3rd ed. Tumor Fascicle Series. Washington, DC: Armed Forces Institute of Pathology, 1996.

4. Ellis G, Simpson RHW: Acinic cell carcinoma. In: Barnes EL, Eveson JW, Reichart P, Sidransky D, eds. Pathology and Genetics of Head and Neck Tumours. Kleihues P, Sobin LH, series eds. World Health Organization Classification of Tumours. Lyon, France: IARC Press, 2005:216–218.
5. Hellquist HB, Sundelin K, Di Bacco A, et al.: Tumour growth fraction and apoptosis in salivary gland acinic cell carcinomas. Prognostic implications of Ki-67 and bcl-2 expression and of in situ end labelling (TUNEL). J Pathol 1997;181:323–329.
6. Ihrler S, Blasenbreu-Vogt S, Sendelhofert A, et al.: Differential diagnosis of salivary acinic cell carcinoma and adenocarcinoma (NOS). A comparison of (immuno-)histochemical markers. Pathol Res Pract 2002;198:777–783.
7. Michal M, Skalova A, Simpson RH, et al.: Well-differentiated acinic cell carcinoma of salivary glands associated with lymphoid stroma. Hum Pathol 1997;28:595–600.
8. Seifert G: Histopathology of malignant salivary gland tumours. Eur J Cancer B Oral Oncol 1992;28B:49–56.
9. Timon CI, Dardick I, Panzarella T, et al.: Clinico-pathological predictors of recurrence for acinic cell carcinoma. Clin Otolaryngol 1995;20:396–401.

Adenoid Cystic Carcinoma

1. Edwards PC, Bhuiya T, Kelsch RD: C-kit expression in the salivary gland neoplasms adenoid cystic carcinoma, polymorphous low-grade adenocarcinoma, and monomorphic adenoma. Oral Surg Oral Med Oral Pathol Oral Radiol Endod 2003;95:586–593.
2. El-Naggar AK, Huvos AG: Adenoid cystic carcinoma. In: Barnes EL, Eveson JW, Reichart P, Sidransky D, eds. Pathology and Genetics of Head and Neck Tumours. Kleihues P, Sobin LH, series eds. World Health Organization Classification of Tumours. Lyon, France: IARC Press, 2005:221–222.
3. Garden AS, Weber RS, Morrison WH, et al.: The influence of positive margins and nerve invasion in adenoid cystic carcinoma of the head and neck treated with surgery and radiation. Int J Radiat Oncol Biol Phys 1995;32:619–626.
4. Hamper K, Lazar F, Dietel M, et al.: Prognostic factors for adenoid cystic carcinoma of the head and neck: a retrospective evaluation of 96 cases. J Oral Pathol Med 1990;19:101–107.
5. Martins C, Fonseca I, Roque L, et al.: Cytogenetic similarities between two types of salivary gland carcinomas: adenoid cystic carcinoma and polymorphous low-grade adenocarcinoma. Cancer Genet Cytogenet 2001;128:130–136.
6. Spiro RH, Huvos AG: Stage means more than grade in adenoid cystic carcinoma. Am J Surg 1992;164:623–628.
7. Spiro RH: Distant metastasis in adenoid cystic carcinoma of salivary origin. Am J Surg 1997;174:495–498.

Polymorphous Low-Grade Adenocarcinoma

1. Castle JT, Thompson LD, Frommelt RA, et al.: Polymorphous low grade adenocarcinoma: a clinicopathologic study of 164 cases. Cancer 1999;86:207–219.
2. Curran AE, White DK, Damm DD, Murrah VA: Polymorphous low-grade adenocarcinoma versus pleomorphic adenoma of minor salivary glands: resolution of a diagnostic dilemma by immunohistochemical analysis with glial fibrillary acidic protein. Oral Surg Oral Med Oral Pathol Oral Radiol Endod 2001;91:194–199.
3. Darling MR, Schneider JW, Phillips VM: Polymorphous low-grade adenocarcinoma and adenoid cystic carcinoma: a review and comparison of immunohistochemical markers. Oral Oncol 2002;38:641–645.
4. Evans HL, Luna MA: Polymorphous low-grade adenocarcinoma: a study of 40 cases with long-term follow up and an evaluation of the importance of papillary areas. Am J Surg Pathol 2000;24:1319–1328.
5. Kumar M, Stivaros N, Barrett AW, et al.: Polymorphous low-grade adenocarcinoma—a rare and aggressive entity in adolescence. Br J Oral Maxillofac Surg 2004;42:195–199.
6. Luna MA, Wenig BM: Polymorphous low-grade adenocarcinoma. In: Barnes EL, Eveson JW, Reichart P, Sidransky D, eds. Pathology and Genetics of Head and Neck Tumours. Kleihues P, Sobin LH, series eds. World Health Organization Classification of Tumours. Lyon, France: IARC Press, 2005:223–225.
7. Nagao T, Gaffey TA, Kay PA, Minato H, et al.: Polymorphous low-grade adenocarcinoma of the major salivary glands: report of three cases in an unusual location. Histopathology 2004;44:164–171.
8. Penner CR, Folpe AL, Budnick SD: C-kit expression distinguishes salivary gland adenoid cystic carcinoma from polymorphous low-grade adenocarcinoma. Mod Pathol 2002;15:687–691.

Epithelial-Myoepithelial Carcinoma

1. Cho KJ, El Naggar AK, Ordonez NG, et al.: Epithelial-myoepithelial carcinoma of salivary glands. A clinicopathologic, DNA flow cytometric, and immunohistochemical study of Ki-67 and HER-2/neu oncogene. Am J Clin Pathol 1995;103:432–437.
2. Fonseca I, Soares J: Epithelial-myoepithelial carcinoma of the salivary glands. A study of 22 cases. Virchows Arch A Pathol Anat Histopathol 1993;422:389–396.
3. Fonseca I, Felix A, Soares J: Dedifferentiation in salivary gland carcinomas. Am J Surg Pathol 2000;24:469–471.
4. Fonseca I, Soares J: Epithelial-myoepithelial carcinoma. In: Barnes EL, Eveson JW, Reichart P, Sidransky D, eds. Pathology and Genetics of Head and Neck Tumours. Kleihues P, Sobin LH, series eds. World Health Organization Classification of Tumours. Lyon, France: IARC Press, 2005:225–226.
5. Nagao T, Sugano I, Ishida Y, et al.: Hybrid carcinomas of the salivary glands: report of nine cases with a clinicopathologic, immunohistochemical, and p53 gene alteration analysis. Mod Pathol 2002;15:724–733.
6. Tralongo V, Daniele E: Epithelial-myoepithelial carcinoma of the salivary glands: a review of literature. Anticancer Res 1998;18:603–608.
7. Wang B, Brandwein M, Gordon R, et al.: Primary salivary clear cell tumors—a diagnostic approach: a clinicopathologic and immunohistochemical study of 20 patients with clear cell carcinoma, clear cell myoepithelial carcinoma, and epithelial-myoepithelial carcinoma. Arch Pathol Lab Med 2002;126:676–685.

Salivary Duct Carcinoma

1. Barnes L, Rao U, Krause J, et al.: Salivary duct carcinoma. Part I. A clinicopathologic evaluation and DNA image analysis of 13 cases with review of the literature. Oral Surg Oral Med Oral Pathol 1994;78:64–73.
2. Brandwein-Gensler MS, Skálová A, Nagao T: Salivary duct carcinoma. In: Barnes EL, Eveson JW, Reichart P, Sidransky D, eds. Pathology and Genetics of Head and Neck Tumours. Kleihues P, Sobin LH, series eds. World Health Organization Classification of Tumours. Lyon, France: IARC Press, 2005:236–237.
3. Etges A, Pinto DS Jr, Kowalski LP, et al.: Salivary duct carcinoma: immunohistochemical profile of an aggressive salivary gland tumour. J Clin Pathol 2003;56:914–918.
4. Fan CY, Wang J, Barnes EL: Expression of androgen receptor and prostatic specific markers in salivary duct carcinoma: an immunohistochemical analysis of 13 cases and review of the literature. Am J Surg Pathol 2000;24:579–586.
5. Mukunyadzi P, Ai L, Portilla D, et al.: Expression of peroxisome proliferator-activated receptor gamma in salivary duct carcinoma: immunohistochemical analysis of 15 cases. Mod Pathol 2003;16:1218–1223.
6. Nagao T, Gaffey TA, Serizawa H, et al.: Sarcomatoid variant of salivary duct carcinoma: clinicopathologic and immunohistochemical study of eight cases with review of the literature. Am J Clin Pathol 2004;122:222–231.
7. Nagao T, Gaffey TA, Visscher DW, et al.: Invasive micropapillary salivary duct carcinoma: a distinct histologic variant with biologic significance. Am J Surg Pathol 2004;28:319–326.
8. Simpson RH, Prasad AR, Lewis JE, et al.: Mucin-rich variant of salivary duct carcinoma: a clinicopathologic and immunohistochemical study of four cases. Am J Surg Pathol 2003;27:1070–1079.
9. Skalova A, Starek I, Vanecek T, et al.: Expression of HER-2/neu gene and protein in salivary duct carcinomas of parotid gland as revealed by fluorescence in-situ hybridization and immunohistochemistry. Histopathology 2003;42:348–356.

Carcinoma Ex Pleomorphic Adenoma

1. Brandwein M, Huvos AG, Dardick I, et al.: Noninvasive and minimally invasive carcinoma ex mixed tumor: a clinicopathologic and ploidy

study of 12 patients with major salivary tumors of low (or no?) malignant potential. Oral Surg Oral Med Oral Pathol Oral Radiol Endod 1996;81:655–664.

2. Gnepp DR: Carcinosarcoma. In: Barnes EL, Eveson JW, Reichart P, Sidransky D, eds. Pathology and Genetics of Head and Neck Tumours. Kleihues P, Sobin LH, series eds. World Health Organization Classification of Tumours. Lyon, France: IARC Press, 2005:244.

3. Gnepp DR: Metastasizing pleomorphic adenoma. In: Barnes EL, Eveson JW, Reichart P, Sidransky D, eds. Pathology and Genetics of Head and Neck Tumours. Kleihues P, Sobin LH, series eds. World Health Organization Classification of Tumours. Lyon, France: IARC Press, 2005:245.

4. Gnepp DR: Malignant mixed tumors of the salivary glands: a review. Pathol Annu 1993;28 Pt 1:279–328.

5. Gnepp DR, Brandwein-Gensler MS, El-Naggar AK, Nagao T: Carcinoma ex pleomorphic adenoma. In: Barnes EL, Eveson JW, Reichart P, Sidransky D, eds. Pathology and Genetics of Head and Neck Tumours. Kleihues P, Sobin LH, series eds. World Health Organization Classification of Tumours. Lyon, France: IARC Press, 2005:242–243.

6. Li S, Baloch ZW, Tomaszewski JE, LiVolsi VA: Worrisome histologic alterations following fine-needle aspiration of benign parotid lesions. Arch Pathol Lab Med 2000;124:87–91.

7. LiVolsi VA, Perzin KH: Malignant mixed tumors arising in salivary glands. I. Carcinomas arising in benign mixed tumors: a clinicopathologic study. Cancer 1977;39:2209–2230.

8. Olsen KD, Lewis JE: Carcinoma ex pleomorphic adenoma: a clinicopathologic review. Head Neck 2001;23:705–712.

9. Skálová A, Jäkel KT: Myoepithelial carcinoma. In: Barnes EL, Eveson JW, Reichart P, Sidransky D, eds. Pathology and Genetics of Head and Neck Tumours. Kleihues P, Sobin LH, series eds. World Health Organization Classification of Tumours. Lyon, France: IARC Press, 2005:240–241.

10. Tortoledo ME, Luna MA, Batsakis JG: Carcinomas ex pleomorphic adenoma and malignant mixed tumors. Histomorphologic indexes. Arch Otolaryngol 1984;110:172–176.

Extranodal Marginal Zone B Cell Lymphoma of Salivary Glands

1. Anaya JM, McGruff HS, Banks PM, Talal N: Clinicopathological factors relating to malignant lymphoma in Sjögren's syndrome. Semin Arthritis Rheum 1996;25:337–346.

2. Chan ACL, Chan JKC, Abbondanzo SL: Haematolymphoid tumours. In: Barnes EL, Eveson JW, Reichart P, Sidransky D, eds. Pathology and Genetics of Head and Neck Tumours. Kleihues P, Sobin LH, series eds. World Health Organization Classification of Tumours. Lyon, France: IARC Press, 2005:277–280.

3. Isaacson PG, Wright DH: Malignant lymphoma of the salivary gland. In: Isaacson PG, Norton AJ, eds. Extranodal Lymphomas. New York: Churchill Livingstone, 1994.

4. Jaffe ES, Harris NL, Stein H, Vardiman JW: Pathology and Genetics of Tumors of Haemopoietic and Lymphoid Tissues. Lyon, France: IARC Press, 2001.

5. Masaki Y, Sugai S: Lymphoproliferative disorders in Sjögren's syndrome. Autoimmun Rev 2004;3:175–182.

6. Quintana PG, Kapadia SB, Bahler DW, et al.: Salivary gland lymphoid infiltrates associated with Lymphoepithelial lesions: a clinicopathologic, immunophenotypic, and genotypic study. Hum Pathol 1997;28:850–861.

7. Royer B, Cazals-Hatem D, Sibilia J, et al.: Lymphomas in patients with Sjögen's syndrome are marginal zone B-cell neoplasms, arise in diverse extranodal sites, and are not associated with viruses. Blood 1997;90:766–777.

Uncommon Carcinomas (Basal Cell Adenocarcinoma, Clear Cell, Sebaceous Carcinoma, Oncocytic Carcinoma)

1. Brandwein MS, Huvos AG: Oncocytic tumors of salivary glands. A study of 68 cases with follow-up of 48 cases. Am J Surg Pathol 1991;15:514–528.

2. Ellis G: Clear cell carcinoma, not otherwise specified. In: Barnes EL, Eveson JW, Reichart P, Sidransky D, eds. Pathology and Genetics of Head and Neck Tumours. Kleihues P, Sobin LH, series eds. World Health Organization Classification of Tumours. Lyon, France: IARC Press, 2005:227–228.

3. Ellis G: Basal cell adenocarcinoma. In: Barnes EL, Eveson JW, Reichart P, Sidransky D, eds. Pathology and Genetics of Head and Neck Tumours. Kleihues P, Sobin LH, series eds. World Health Organization Classification of Tumours. Lyon, France: IARC Press, 2005:229–230.

4. Ellis GL, Auclair PL, Gnepp DR, Goode RK: Other malignant epithelial neoplasms. In: Ellis GL, Auclair PL, Gnepp DR, eds. Surgical Pathology of Salivary Glands. Philadelphia: WB Saunders, 1991:455–488.

5. Ellis GL, Wiscovitch JG: Basal cell adenocarcinomas of the major salivary glands. Oral Surg Oral Med Oral Pathol 1990;69:461–469.

6. Gnepp DR: Sebaceous neoplasms of salivary gland origin: a review. Pathol Annu 1983;18(Part 1):71–102.

7. Gnepp DR: Malignant sebaceous tumours. In: Barnes EL, Eveson JW, Reichart P, Sidransky D, eds. Pathology and Genetics of Head and Neck Tumours. Kleihues P, Sobin LH, series eds. World Health Organization Classification of Tumours. Lyon, France: IARC Press, 2005:231.

8. Ito K, Tsukuda M, Kawabe R, et al.: Benign and malignant oncocytoma of the salivary glands with an immunohistochemical evaluation of Ki-67. ORL J Otorhinolaryngol Relat Spec 2000;62:338–341.

9. O'Regan E, Shandilya M, Gnepp DR, et al.: Hyalinizing clear cell carcinoma of salivary gland: an aggressive variant. Oral Oncol 2004;40:348–352.

10. Quddus MR, Henley JD, Affify AM, et al.: Basal cell adenocarcinoma of the salivary gland: an ultrastructural and immunohistochemical study. Oral Surg Oral Med Oral Pathol Oral Radiol Endod 1999;87:485–492.

11. Sciubba JJ, Shimono M: Oncocytic carcinoma. In: Barnes EL, Eveson JW, Reichart P, Sidransky D, eds. Pathology and Genetics of Head and Neck Tumours. Kleihues P, Sobin LH, series eds. World Health Organization Classification of Tumours. Lyon, France: IARC Press, 2005:235.

12. Simpson RH, Sarsfield PT, Clarke T, Babajews A: Clear cell carcinoma of minor salivary glands. Histopathology 1990;17:433–438.

13

Non-Neoplastic Lesions of the Ear and Temporal Bone

Carol Adair

FIRST BRANCHIAL CLEFT ANOMALIES

First branchial cleft anomalies include fistulas, sinuses, and cysts, and result from incomplete fusion of the first and second branchial arches, with persistence of the ventral component of the first branchial cleft. The most commonly used classification of the first branchial cleft anomalies is the Work and Proctor type I: ectodermal origin with close proximity to the external auditory canal; and type II: ectodermal elements of the first branchial cleft and mesodermal components of the first and second branchial arches, and is more medially and inferiorly located.

CLINICAL FEATURES

Type I branchial cleft anomalies usually manifest as periauricular cysts rather than sinuses or fistulas. They are usually located posterior, inferior, and medial to the conchal cartilage and pinna; if a sinus tract is present it parallels the external auditory canal. Although most are discovered in childhood, they are sometimes not diagnosed until adulthood, and are often misdiagnosed as abscesses due to secondary infection, or as epidermal inclusion cysts. Females are affected twice as often as males. Incision and drainage results in persistence or recurrence for years.

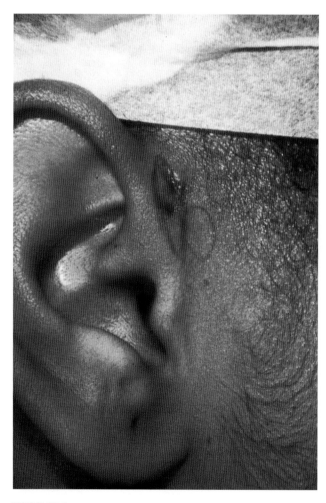

FIGURE 13-1

A pre-auricular fistula is present in a patient with a first branchial cleft anomaly. The lesion was secondarily infected and produced purulent drainage.

FIRST BRANCHIAL CLEFT ANOMALIES
DISEASE FACT SHEET

Definition	A spectrum of cysts, fistulas, and sinuses resulting from incomplete fusion of the first and second brachial arches
Incidence and location	Uncommon (<10% of all branchial cleft anomalies)
	Periauricular with sinuses/fistulas in anteriolateral neck or external auditory canal
Morbidity and mortality	Secondary infection common with potential facial nerve injury
Gender, race, and age distribution	Female > Male (2 : 1)
	Most discovered in early childhood, but type I anomalies may present in adults (range: 13–81 yr)
Clinical features	Painless cyst, draining sinus tract on skin of neck, otorrhea or purulent drainage from ear canal
Prognosis and treatment	Benign
	Complete excision of cyst, sinus, and/or fistula with antibiotic treatment prior to surgery if infected

371

Type II branchial cleft anomalies usually come to medical attention in the first year of life as a result of a draining sinus tract with otorrhea or periauricular drainage; the lesions are frequently infected at the time of diagnosis. They may be represented by a cystic lesion with a sinus, or a fistulous tract between the neck and the ear canal (Fig. 13-1). A sinus may open from a fistulous track, usually anterior to the sternocleidomastoid muscle and superior to the hyoid bone, or in the external auditory canal. The spatial relationship to the facial nerve is variable, requiring a cautious surgical approach.

A careful physical examination with particular attention to the periauricular region and lateral neck is essential, including otologic examination to exclude a tract which communicates with the external auditory canal or rarely, the middle ear space. High-resolution computed tomography (CT) is the preferred radiologic study for accurate delineation of the extent and course of the anomaly prior to surgery.

PATHOLOGIC FEATURES

GROSS FINDINGS

Discrete cysts, sinuses, or fistulas, or a combination of structures may be seen, with the cysts frequently containing viscous cloudy fluid, or, if infected, purulent material and necrotic debris. Cartilaginous components may be noticed on sectioning.

MICROSCOPIC FINDINGS

The cysts, sinuses, and fistulas may be lined by either stratified squamous epithelium or ciliated respiratory epithelium (Fig. 13-2). The cyst wall may contain lymphoid aggregates, sometimes with germinal centers (Figs. 13-3, 13-4), as commonly seen in second branchial cleft anomalies. If the lesion is infected the

FIRST BRANCHIAL CLEFT ANOMALIES PATHOLOGIC FEATURES	
Gross findings	Cyst with viscous cloudy fluid
	Sinus tracts/fistulas extending from neck skin or from external auditory canal
	Abscess with purulent contents if secondarily infected
Microscopic findings	Cyst, sinus or fistula lined by stratified squamous or ciliated respiratory epithelium
	Lymphoid aggregates may be present in cyst wall
	Granulation tissue or purulent material if infected, with denuded epithelium
	Type I: epithelial component only
	Type II: epithelial lining and cutaneous adnexal structures and/or cartilage
Pathologic differential diagnosis	Epidermal inclusion cyst, cholesteatoma, cystic squamous cell carcinoma, abscess, and second branchial cleft anomalies

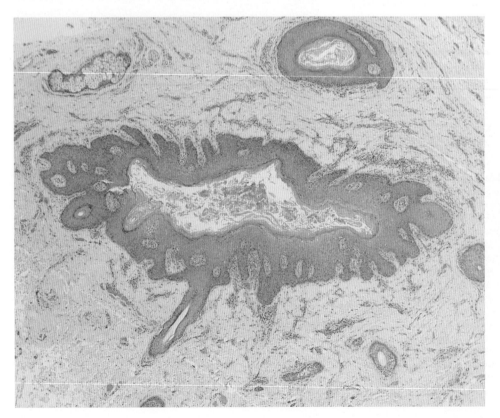

FIGURE 13-2

This series of sections (Figs. 13-2 to 13-5) was taken along the course of a fistulous tract which represented a Work type II anomaly of the first branchial cleft. Near the skin surface, the tract is lined by keratinizing squamous epithelium with cutaneous adnexal structure.

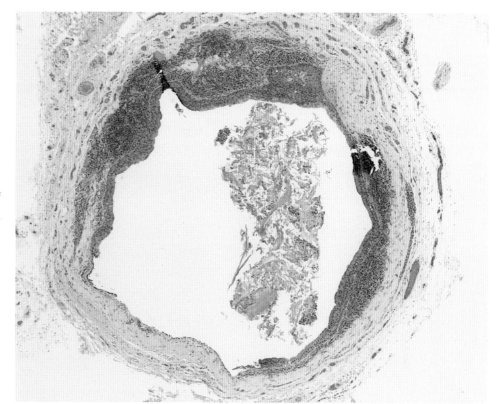

FIGURE 13-3

The lining of the deepest portion of the tract transitions to ciliated respiratory epithelium, surrounded by lymphoid tissue.

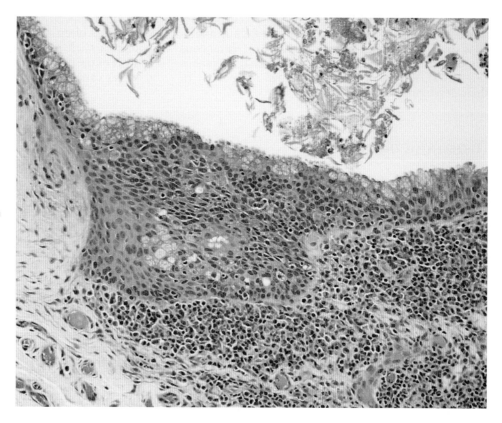

FIGURE 13-4

Ciliated respiratory epithelium with heavy lymphoid component.

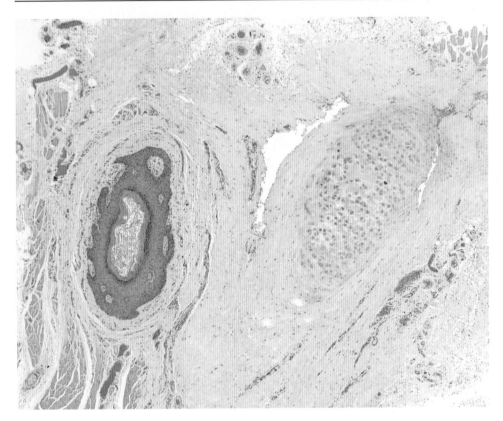

FIGURE 13-5
Cartilage appears adjacent to the tract in deeper sections of this Work Type II anomaly.

epithelium may be largely denuded, replaced by heavily inflamed granulation tissue. Type I and type II anomalies are distinguished by the presence of cutaneous adnexal structures and cartilage in the type II anomalies (Fig. 13-5), the result of a mesodermal component in their development.

DIFFERENTIAL DIAGNOSIS

The pathologic differential diagnosis includes epidermal inclusion cyst, cholesteatoma, and, in adults, cystic metastatic squamous cell carcinoma. Epidermal inclusion cysts and cholesteatomas contain intracystic keratinous debris. The benign cytologic features contrasts with the atypia and loss of polarity encountered in cystic metastatic squamous cell carcinoma.

PROGNOSIS AND THERAPY

First branchial cleft anomalies are congenital benign lesions, commonly given to secondary infection. Treatment consists of complete surgical excision of the malformation, including cysts, and any associated sinus or fistula. Superficial parotidectomy may be required for complete removal. Complications of surgery include recurrence, often with infection, injury of adjacent structures such as the facial nerve, and infection or stenosis of the external auditory canal or middle ear due to an ear canal defect.

CYSTIC CHONDROMALACIA

Idiopathic cystic chondromalacia, also known as pseudocyst of the auricle, is an uncommon degenerative cystic lesion of the auricular cartilaginous plate. Without a well-established etiology, ischemic necrosis (rarely related to trauma), abnormal release of lysosomal enzymes by chondrocytes, and an embryologic fusion defect are considerations.

CLINICAL FEATURES

Cystic chondromalacia tends to be more common in young males, although either gender and all ages may be affected. An increased incidence has been noted in

CYSTIC CHONDROMALACIA
DISEASE FACT SHEET

Definition	A non-neoplastic degenerative change in the auricular cartilage resulting in a cleft-like pseudocyst within the cartilaginous plate
Incidence and location	Rare Usually involves helix or antihelix, with 80% in the scaphoid fossa
Gender, race, and age distribution	Male > Female Higher incidence in Chinese population Any age, but commonly young to middle-aged adults
Clinical features	Usually unilateral, painless, fusiform swelling of helix or antihelix with normal overlying skin Often fluctuant; viscous clear fluid may be aspirated
Prognosis and treatment	Benign Usually treated for cosmetic reasons with aspiration followed by compression sutures; unroofing of anterior wall of pseudocyst followed by application of sclerosing agent

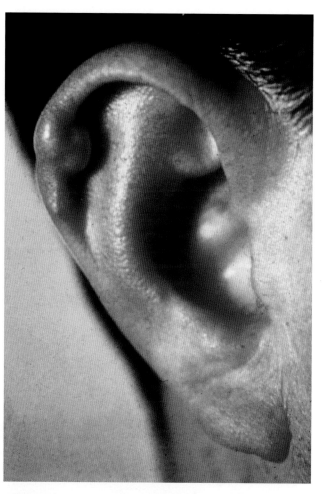

FIGURE 13-6

A young adult male has a fusiform fluctuant mass on the helix which was histologically idiopathic cystic chondromalacia. (Used by permission. Hyams VJ: Pathology of the Ear. Chicago: ASCP Press, 1976.)

Chinese males. The typical presentation is a unilateral, fusiform, slightly fluctuant, swelling of the helix or antihelix (Fig. 13-6). The scaphoid fossa is the most common site. The lesion is painless, and there are no changes in the overlying skin.

PATHOLOGIC FEATURES

GROSS FINDINGS

If the full thickness of the cartilaginous plate has been excised, a central, slit-like cleft can be seen in the cartilage (Fig. 13-7). When incised, the cyst exudes viscous, clear to olive-oil colored fluid, usually <2 mL in volume. The cystic area, especially in long-standing lesions may be lined by a thin brown-tinged layer, representing old hemorrhage and granulation tissue. Often the specimen is fragmented, especially if the cyst is "unroofed," making knowledge of the clinical appearance helpful in diagnosis.

MICROSCOPIC FINDINGS

The cartilaginous plate contains a central cleft with no epithelial lining, hence the term "pseudocyst." The contour of the cleft may be slightly irregular, and a thin inner rim of fibrous tissue or granulation tissue with plump fibroblasts may be seen (Figs. 13-8, 13-9). Hemosiderin deposits may be present. In long-standing cases the fibrous tissue may obliterate the cystic space.

CYSTIC CHONDROMALACIA
PATHOLOGIC FEATURES

Gross findings	Cleft-like space centrally located within cartilaginous plate Cleft filled with viscous clear to olive oil-colored fluid Obliterated by fibrous tissue or granulation tissue in long-standing lesions
Microscopic findings	Central slit-like cleft in cartilage without an epithelial lining Cleft may contain fibrous tissue, granulation tissue with hemosiderin
Pathologic differential diagnosis	Relapsing polychondritis, chondrodermatitis nodularis helicis

DIFFERENTIAL DIAGNOSIS

Cystic chondromalacia is easily distinguished from relapsing polychondritis by its lack of an inflammatory component, and from chondrodermatitis nodularis

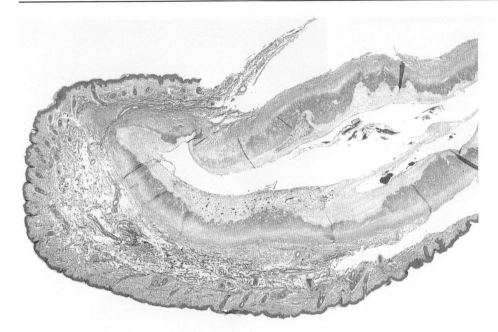

FIGURE 13-7
The cartilaginous plate contains an elongated cleft and has lost some of its normal basophilic staining in this idiopathic cystic chondromalacia.

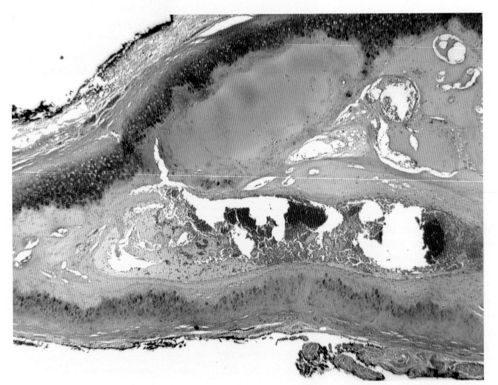

FIGURE 13-8
A blood-filled cyst is associated with granulation-type tissue. The cartilage plate is separated, with fluid in part of the spaces.

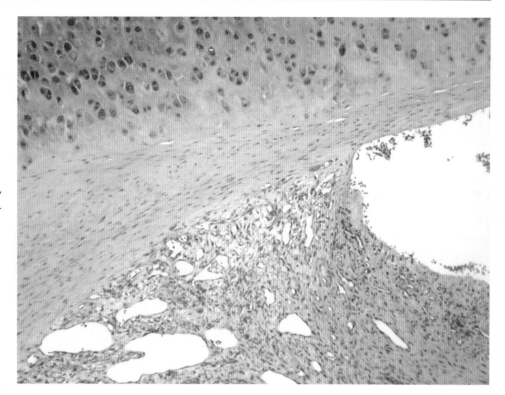

FIGURE 13-9

Granulation tissue forms the "cyst" lining, seen adjacent to the degenerating cartilaginous plate.

helices by the normal skin overlying it. Likewise, both lesions in the differential are associated with pain.

PROGNOSIS AND THERAPY

Cosmetic concerns for this benign lesion often prompt therapeutic intervention. Treatment is usually directed at extirpation of the pseudocyst while preserving the underlying architecture of the cartilaginous plate. Incision and drainage with curettage has had variable success. Needle aspiration alone has limited value, but, when combined with suture compression, is quite effective. Unroofing of the pseudocyst by removal of its anterior wall followed by application of a sclerosing agent, such as tincture of iodine, is also highly effective.

CHONDRODERMATITIS NODULAR HELICIS

Chondrodermatitis nodularis helicis (CDNH) is a nonneoplastic inflammatory and degenerative process of the external ear characterized by necrobiotic changes in the dermis which extend down to the perichondrium, with associated alterations in the cartilaginous plate. The dermal injury is thought to be caused by a combination of factors: local trauma, actinic damage, and the relatively tenuous vascularity of the auricle. The necrobiotic dermal collagen, and sometimes cartilaginous matrix, are extruded through a crater-like defect in the

epidermis; thus, CDNH is considered to be one of the transepidermal elimination disorders.

CLINICAL FEATURES

CDNH presents as an exquisitely painful nodule, usually on the helix or antihelix; however, it may

CHONDROMDERMATITIS NODULAR HELICIS DISEASE FACT SHEET

Definition	Inflammatory transepidermal elimination disorder characterized by necrobiosis of dermal collagen and degenerative changes in the cartilaginous plate
Incidence and location	Relatively common
	Helix most often, followed by antihelix (more common in females)
Gender, race, and age distribution	Male > Female
	Usually 6th decade
Clinical features	Unilateral, painful, circumscribed indurated nodule with central crater filled with brown debris
Prognosis and treatment	Benign disorder, often removed to alleviate pain
	Intralesional steroid injection successful in 50% of cases
	Persistent or recurrent lesions adequately treated by conservative excision or deep shave biopsy

develop on any portion of the auricle. Lesions of the helix are twice as common as those of the antihelix. CDNH begins as a reddish, round, indurated nodule, measuring several millimeters in diameter; over a period of days to a few weeks, the nodule develops a central crater which contains crust-like material (Fig. 13-10). CDNH is more common in males; lesions of the antihelix, however, are more common in females. Most patients are in the 6th decade.

PATHOLOGIC FEATURES

GROSS FINDINGS

CDNH is usually removed by shave biopsy. The nodule is firm, round, circumscribed, and nodular, with a central crater containing yellow to brown necrotic material. Most examples measure between 5 and 15 mm in diameter. Sectioning may demonstrate cartilage at the deep aspect of the biopsy, but the sharp interface between the cartilaginous plate and dermis is obscured.

MICROSCOPIC FINDINGS

There is a central crater filled with acellular necrotic debris, fibrin, and a variable number of inflammatory cells. The epidermis surrounding the crater is acanthotic with hyperkeratosis (Fig. 13-11). The dermal collagen underlying the crater is homogeneous and eosinophilic, admixed with fibrin (Fig. 13-12), with edema in the surrounding viable dermis. The degenerative changes extend to the level of the perichondrium and are associated with loss of the normal basophilia of the underlying cartilage, focal fibrosis with increased cellularity or dropout of chondrocytes. The necrobiotic material and fibrin spew from the crater through a disrupted epi-

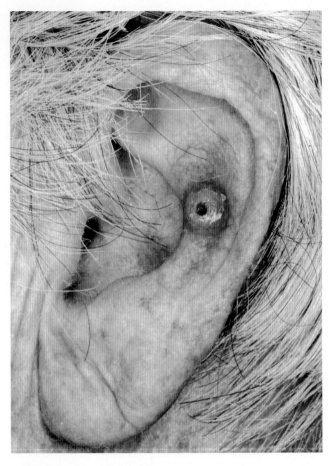

FIGURE 13-10
This firm nodule with a central crater is seen on the antihelix of an elderly female with CDNH; antihelical lesions are more common in women. (Courtesy of Dr. S. A. Norton.)

dermis. In some cases portions of the cartilage are also extruded through the crater.

DIFFERENTIAL DIAGNOSIS

Clinically, CDNH is very commonly confused with squamous cell carcinoma, occasionally leading to over treatment. The histologic findings may be mistaken for squamous cell carcinoma or actinic keratosis because of the prominent squamous epithelial hyperplasia and underlying solar elastosis typically encountered in CDNH.

PROGNOSIS AND THERAPY

Chondrodermatitis nodularis helicis is a benign disorder, which may be treated with intralesional steroid injection, with an up to 50% cure rate. Persistent or recurrent lesions are amenable to conservative excisional biopsy or deep shave excision with excellent

CHONDROMDERMATITIS NODULAR HELICIS PATHOLOGIC FEATURES	
Gross findings	Rounded, circumscribed nodule with central crater filled with necrotic debris
	5–15 mm diameter
	Cartilage may be seen at deep aspect of biopsy
Microscopic findings	Squamous epithelial hyperplasia surrounding central crater
	Crater filled with acellular necrotic debris, fibrin, and inflammatory cells
	Homogenous, eosinophilic dermal collagen may extrude through the crater
	Underlying cartilage looses normal basophilia
	Interface between cartilaginous plate and dermis is blurred
Pathologic differential diagnosis	Squamous cell carcinoma, actinic keratosis

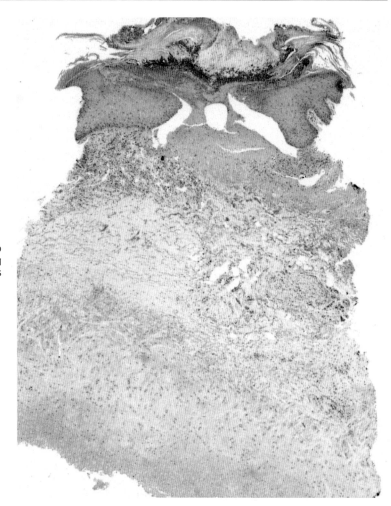

FIGURE 13-11

Eosinophilic degenerative dermal collagen appears ready to extrude from the central crater of this CDNH. The underlying interface between the cartilaginous plate and the dermis is blurred; and the cartilage has lost its normal basophilia.

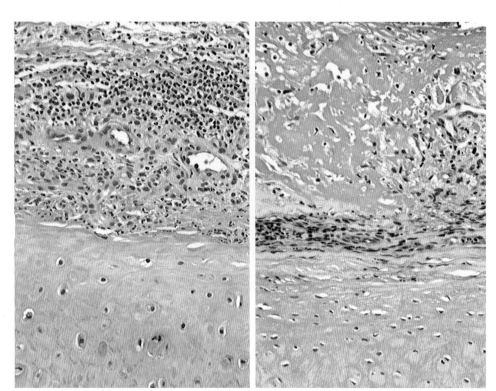

FIGURE 13-12

Deep biopsies of CDNH may show extensive inflammation (*left*) or degenerated collagen and fibrinoid necrosis (*right*), both immediately adjacent to the cartilage.

results. Removal of the lesion often alleviates the associated pain.

RELAPSING POLYCHONDRITIS

Relapsing polychondritis is a rare autoimmune inflammatory disorder with antibodies which target type II collagen usually in cartilage of the ear, nose, joints, and tracheobronchial tree, often resulting in structural damage and deformity. A humoral and cell-mediated immunity seems to play a role in the destructive inflammatory process. There is an increased incidence (up to 35%) of other autoimmune disorders such as rheumatoid arthritis, Hashimoto's thyroiditis, systemic lupus erythematosus, Sjögren's syndrome, inflammatory bowel disease, diabetes mellitus, primary biliary cirrhosis, and myelodysplastic syndromes, to name just a few.

CLINICAL FEATURES

Relapsing polychondritis has an estimated incidence of 3.5 cases per million in the United States. Occurring in a wide age range, the disease is most often in the 5th–6th decades (mean, 47 yr). Females seem to be affected more commonly than men (up to 3 : 1 ratio).

The most common site of involvement is the auricle, with 40% of patients initially affected, although eventually about 85% will have ear involvement. The ears become red to purple, swollen, and painful, except for the noncartilaginous lobule, which is spared. Inflammatory episodes may last a few days or several weeks. After repeated attacks or a prolonged episode, the cartilaginous framework is damaged, feeling flabby and may result in a "cauliflower ear" deformity (Fig. 13-13).

RELAPSING POLYCHONDRITIS DISEASE FACT SHEET	
Definition	Rare, autoimmune inflammatory disorder with antibodies to type II collagen which lead to destruction of cartilaginous or proteoglycan-rich tissues of the auricle, nose, tracheobronchial tree, eye, heart, and blood vessels
Incidence and location	3.5/1,000,000 in United States
	Auricle most common site, affected in up to 85%
Morbidity and mortality	Leading cause of death is airway compromise due to tracheobronchial damage
	10-yr survival of 55%–94%
	Associated with myelodysplasia or leukemia
Gender, race, and age distribution	Female > Male (up to 3 : 1 ratio)
	Perhaps higher incidence in Caucasians
	5th–6th decades
Clinical features	In acute phase the ears become red, edematous, and tender although noncartilaginous lobule is spared
	After repeated bouts, floppy ear, saddle nose deformity
	Other symptoms relate to other anatomic sites, including laryngotracheal disease, nonerosive arthritis, ophthalmologic disease, and cardiovascular disease
	Associated autoimmune disorder in 25%–35%
	Myelodysplastic syndrome or leukemia may be associated
Prognosis and treatment	Depends on severity of disease and number of anatomic sites affected, with airway compromise, secondary infections and cardiovascular disease the most common causes of death
	Corticosteroids, nonsteroidal anti-inflammatory drugs and immunomodulators have variable success
	Advanced age, anemia, and tracheobronchial stricture are poor prognostic factors

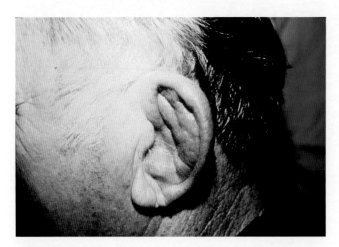

FIGURE 13-13

After multiple acute episode of auricular chondritis this patient's auricle is deformed and floppy as a result of destruction of the cartilaginous plate in this relapsing polychondritis. (Courtesy of Dr. V. J. Hyams.)

When the external auditory canal and Eustachian tube are involved, they may become narrowed, leading to decreased auditory acuity (conductive type) and otitis media. Other anatomic sites may be affected, with nasal chondritis (25%–50%) producing a saddle nose deformity; laryngotracheal disease (50%) yielding obstruction, collapse, and a predisposition to pulmonary infections. Relapsing polychondritis arthropathy is the second most common clinical symptom, typically nonerosive arthritis and most often affecting the knees and the small joints of the hands. Cardiovascular disease (up to 50%) presents with vasculitis.

Biopsy is unnecessary as the diagnosis can be made clinically based on the presence of chondritis in two of three sites (auricle, nose, laryngotracheal tree) or in one of those sites along with two other features (ocular inflammation, audiovestibular damage, or seronegative arthritis).

PATHOLOGIC FEATURES

GROSS FINDINGS

After long-standing or repeated episodes of active inflammation the auricular cartilage becomes "floppy," leading to loss of structural integrity of the pinna.

MICROSCOPIC FINDINGS

The initial histologic finding in relapsing polychondritis is loss of the normal basophilia of the cartilage. The perichondrium is infiltrated by neutrophils, lymphocytes, plasma cells, and eosinophils, blurring the usually sharp interface between the cartilaginous plate and the surrounding soft tissue (Figs. 13-14, 13-15). The

RELAPSING POLYCHONDRITIS PATHOLOGIC FEATURES	
Gross findings	Acute phase: erythematous, edematous pinna, with sparing of lobule
	After multiple episodes: floppy, deformed pinna with loss of cartilaginous structure
Microscopic findings	Loss of basophilia in cartilaginous plate (earliest change)
	Perichondrium infiltrated by mixed inflammation
	Damaged cartilage has moth-eaten appearance and areas are replaced by granulation tissue
Pathologic differential diagnosis	Malignant external otitis, Wegener's granulomatosis and extranodal NK/T cell lymphoma, sinonasal type

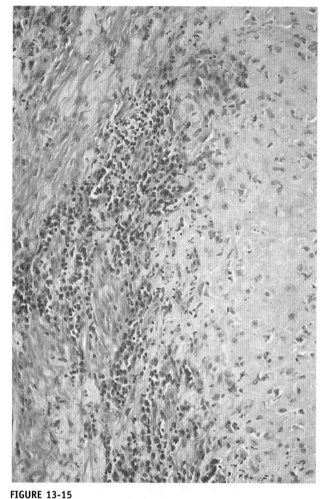

FIGURE 13-15
The inflammatory cells are predominantly small lymphocytes and plasma cells. The normal basophilia of the cartilage has been lost.

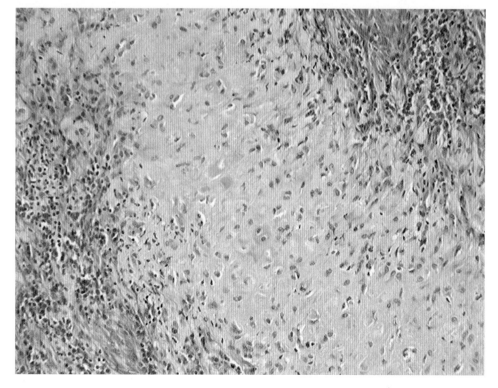

FIGURE 13-14

The interface between the cartilage and perichondrium is blurred by a mixed inflammatory infiltrate in relapsing polychondritis.

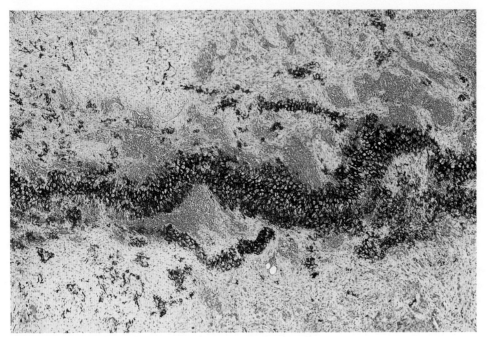

FIGURE 13-16
A Movat stain highlights the extensive damage to the cartilaginous plate, which appears black. The moth-eaten appearance is typical of relapsing polychondritis.

damaged cartilage is gradually replaced by granulation tissue and fibrous tissue, with any residual cartilage demonstrating an irregular moth-eaten border (Fig. 13-16). Immunofluorescence studies may show deposition of immunoglobulins and C3 at the periphery of the cartilage and within the walls of perichondral vessels.

DIFFERENTIAL DIAGNOSIS

The differential diagnosis includes necrotizing (malignant) external otitis (an infection due to *Pseudomonas aeruginosa*), Wegener's granulomatosis and extranodal NK/T cell lymphoma, sinonasal type in upper aerodigestive tract locations. The ears are not usually affected by these latter disorders.

PROGNOSIS AND THERAPY

The disorder is uncommon, making management difficult. Various medical therapies, including corticosteroids, nonsteroidal anti-inflammatory drugs, and immunomodulators (e.g., methotrexate, azathioprine, and cyclosporine A), have all had some degree of success depending on the severity of disease. Autologous stem cell transplantation has induced complete remission of disease in some patients who have failed other treatments. Ear treatments are usually not important, but surgery may be needed for patients with severe airway compromise or aortic grafting and valve replacement for cardiovascular disease. The leading causes of death in patients with relapsing polychondritis

are airway compromise, secondary infections, and cardiovascular disease. Factors which have a negative impact on survival include advanced age at diagnosis, anemia, and tracheobronchial stricture. The 10-year survival rate varies from 55% to 94%, depending on the study.

OTIC POLYP

Otic or aural polyp is a benign proliferation of granulation tissue with chronic inflammatory cells, usually lined by attenuated squamous metaplastic or cuboidal glandular epithelium, in response to a long-standing inflammatory process in the middle ear.

CLINICAL FEATURES

Aural, or otic, inflammatory polyps develop following chronic otitis media; although they form within the middle ear, they may perforate the tympanic membrane, presenting as a mass in the external auditory canal (Fig. 13-17). Aural polyps usually affect young men (mean, 30 yr) more commonly than women (2 : 1). The most common presenting symptom is otorrhea, although conductive hearing loss is almost always present. Other symptoms include otalgia, aural bleeding, and sensation of a mass. Physical examination shows a solitary, polypoid, reddish mass in the middle ear. Radiologic studies are an important adjunct in assessing the likelihood of an underlying cholesteatoma, which makes surgical therapy inevitable.

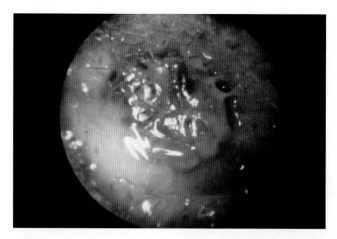

FIGURE 13-17

An otoscopic view of an inflammatory otic, or aural, polyp. Note the erythematous cobblestone appearance of the mucosa in this patient with chronic middle ear disease.

MICROSCOPIC FINDINGS

The polyp contains edematous stroma with a high density of capillaries (granulation tissue) and a chronic inflammatory infiltrate which includes small lymphocytes, plasma cells, histiocytes, and eosinophils (Figs. 13-18, 13-19). In florid cases, plasma cells containing Russell bodies and Mott cells (large eosinophilic globules of immunoglobulin) may be seen. Multinucleated giant cells, cholesterol granulomas, and calcifications may be present. Epithelium may be metaplastic squamous epithelium or cuboidal to columnar glandular epithelium. Glandular inclusions may be seen within the stroma in chronic cases (Fig. 13-20). Stratified squamous epithelium with surface layers of acellular keratinous debris should be noted as evidence of an associated cholesteatoma.

OTIC POLYP DISEASE FACT SHEET	
Definition	Benign polypoid proliferation of granulation tissue with chronic inflammation
Incidence and location	Common companion of chronic middle ear disease
Morbidity and mortality	Associated with other destructive lesions such as cholesteatoma
Gender, race, and age distribution	Male > Female (2 : 1)
	Mean, 30 yr (but wide range, 17–60 yr)
	Socioeconomic status and lack of access to medical care predispose to development of chronic middle ear disease
Clinical features	Chronic otitis media
	Otorrhea most commonly, with otalgia, aural bleeding, sensation of mass in ear canal, and conductive hearing loss
	Red, polypoid mass on otoscopic examination
	Radiographic exams to exclude cholesteatoma
Prognosis and treatment	Prognosis related to presence of other lesions (cholesteatoma) and extent of mastoid disease
	Antibiotics as initial therapy with polypectomy for persistent disease; radical surgery if extensive mastoid disease

PATHOLOGIC FEATURES

GROSS FINDINGS

If the lesion is removed intact, it appears as a reddish friable polypoid soft tissue fragment. All material must be processed to exclude an associated cholesteatoma.

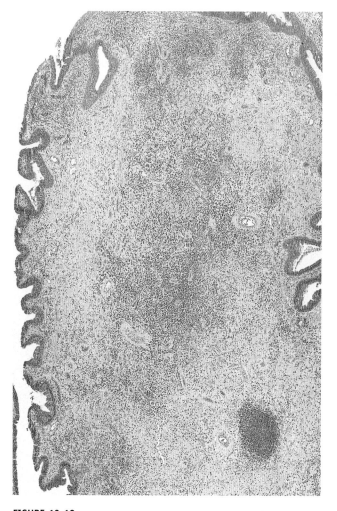

FIGURE 13-18

The polypoid mass of inflamed and edematous stroma is lined by ciliated respiratory mucosa of the middle ear.

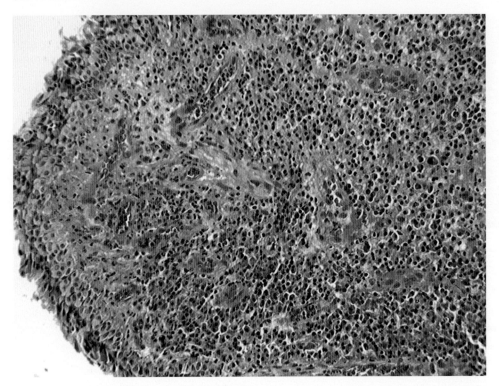

FIGURE 13-19

The inflammatory infiltrate is rich in plasma cells, eosinophils, and "granulation"-type tissue.

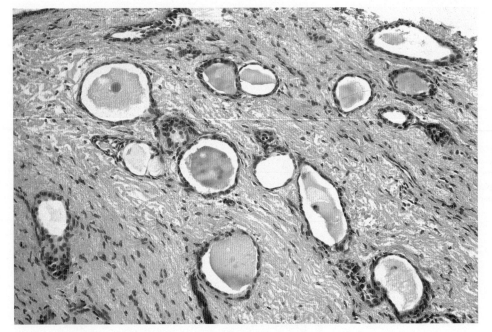

FIGURE 13-20

A more fibrous polypoid mass in the middle ear contains benign glandular inclusions, which may be mistaken for glandular neoplasms of the external auditory canal and middle ear.

OTIC POLYP PATHOLOGIC FEATURES	
Gross findings	Rarely received intact, contents are friable reddish tissue
	All tissue must be processed to exclude cholesteatoma
Microscopic findings	Polypoid mass with edematous stroma, granulation tissue and chronic inflammatory infiltrate
	Plasma cells with Russell bodies or Mott cells
	When present, epithelium may be metaplastic squamous or ciliated cuboidal or columnar glandular type
	Small, glandular cyst-like inclusions in the stroma
	Cholesterol granulomas, calcifications, and giant cells may be present
	Stratified squamous epithelium with acellular keratinous debris must be diagnosed as associated cholesteatoma
Pathologic differential diagnosis	Plasmacytoma, ceruminous adenoma, middle ear adenoma (NAME), rhabdomyosarcoma ("sarcoma botryoides")

DIFFERENTIAL DIAGNOSIS

The differential diagnosis is limited. A lymphoproliferative disorder, such as plasmacytoma, is excluded by a polyclonal immunohistochemistry. Glandular inclusions, suggesting a ceruminous neoplasm, have no myoepithelial cells and the nuclei lack neuroendocrine features.

PROGNOSIS AND THERAPY

Traditionally antibiotic therapy has been the first line of therapy in patients with aural polyps, followed by polypectomy for persistent disease. However, if there is chronic persistent disease, recurrence, unexpected cholesteatoma, and extensive mastoid disease, a more radical surgical approach may be needed. The pathologist's primary concern in examining material submitted as an aural polyp is to carefully evaluate all of the tissue to exclude cholesteatoma.

"MALIGNANT" OTITIS

Necrotizing, or "malignant," external otitis is an infection of the external auditory canal which progresses to a highly aggressive, invasive osteomyelitis of the tempo-

ral bone or skull base, occurring most often in immunocompromised patients.

CLINICAL FEATURES

Malignant external otitis (MEO) is most often encountered in elderly patients who have diabetes mellitus; nearly 90% of cases occur in diabetics, most over 60 years. No definitive gender differences are noted, but immunocompromised patients are at increased risk, particularly those with HIV/AIDS, organ transplantation, hematologic malignancies, and other malignancies treated with chemotherapeutic agents.

"MALIGNANT" OTITIS DISEASE FACT SHEET	
Definition	Aggressive external otitis progressing to temporal bone or skull base osteomyelitis, most often caused by *Pseudomonas aeruginosa*, occurring in immunocompromised patients
Incidence and location	Uncommon due to advanced antibiotic therapy
Morbidity and mortality	Early diagnosis and aggressive antibiotic therapy reduced mortality from 50% to 10%–30%
	Cranial nerve deficits may persist in survivors
Gender, race, and age distribution	Equal gender distribution
	Most patients > 60 yr
Clinical features	Approximately 90% are diabetics
	Any immunocompromised patients are at increased risk, especially HIV/AIDS, organ transplantation, hematologic malignancies, treatment with chemotherapeutic agents
	Initiated by minor trauma to external auditory canal lining
	Initial manifestation is simple external otitis, but with pain out of proportion to clinical findings
	Severe headache, purulent otorrhea
	Hallmark is granulation tissue in the external auditory canal
	Cranial nerve dysfunction (facial nerve especially)
Radiologic features	Earliest finding is positive bone scan
	CT scan defines extent of osteomyelitis, with bone erosion, bony sequestration, and abscess formation
	Gallium scan monitors activity of infection
Prognosis and treatment	Recent mortality rate: 10%–30%, improved by prompt aggressive antibiotic therapy
	Complications include sigmoid sinus thrombosis, meningitis, brain abscess
	Strict diabetes mellitus control, careful debridement of necrotic and granulation tissue, and intravenous multidrug antibiotic therapy

The disease is thought to be initiated by minor trauma, especially in a moist environment, to the external auditory canal mucosa. Minor trauma may be using a cotton-tipped swab to clean the ear canal. This slight breach of the mucosa allows entry of an opportunistic organism, most often *Pseudomonas aeruginosa,* although many other organisms have been documented. It has been postulated that, in diabetics, microangiopathy, combined with the necrotizing vasculitis caused by the *Pseudomonas* organism, interferes with antibiotic and inflammatory cell penetration into the area of active infection, facilitating the rapid spread of the disease through adjacent soft tissue (Fig. 13-21).

Initially, there is an erythematous auricle and ear canal with otalgia; however, the pain is out of proportion to the clinical findings. Patients may also complain of severe headache, purulent otorrhea, or temporomandibular joint pain, but are usually afebrile. If patients fail topical antibiotics and lack good aural hygiene, further examination is warranted; MEO will have granulation tissue on the floor of the external auditory canal at the chondro-osseous junction. Progression to more life-threatening temporal bone or skull base osteomyelitis presents with cranial nerve dysfunction, specifically the facial nerve, although glossopharyngeal, vagal, spinal accessory, and hypoglossal nerves are also often affected. Progressive intracranial disease may develop sigmoid sinus thrombosis, meningitis, or brain abscesses.

RADIOLOGIC FEATURES

Radiologic studies are essential for the assessment of MEO, particularly in the recognition of temporal bone and skull base osteomyelitis. Technetium phosphate radionucleotide scans (bone scans) are especially useful in the initial detection of osteomyelitis before there is CT evidence of bone and/or soft tissue destruction.

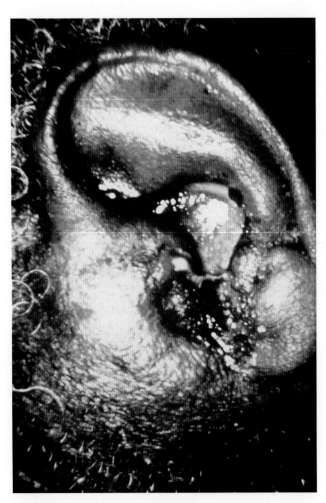

FIGURE 13-21

An elderly diabetic patient with advanced disease has purulent discharge from the ear canal which contains necrotic material and granulation tissue, the hallmark of malignant external otitis. (Used with permission. Hyams VJ: Pathology of the Ear. Chicago: ASCP Press, 1976.)

"MALIGNANT" OTITIS PATHOLOGIC FEATURES	
Gross findings	Necrotic material and granulation tissue
	Must submit cultures from debridement material
Microscopic findings	Necrotic tissue and granulation tissue
	Autopsy findings may include temporal bone and skull base osteomyelitis, purulent meningitis, brain abscess
Pathologic differential diagnosis	Squamous cell carcinoma (may be coexistent)

However, a bone scan cannot be used in follow-up as repair will keep the scan "positive." A gallium scan is a sensitive indicator of active infection, rapidly returning to normal when the infection resolves and is useful for long-term monitoring of treatment response.

PATHOLOGIC FEATURES

The biopsy material shows necrotic material and granulation tissue (Fig. 13-22). Culture of debridement specimens is crucial in the management of MEO. An en block removal of the temporal bone with the entire auditory and vestibular system is helpful at autopsy in demonstrating skull base osteomyelitis, sigmoid sinus thrombosis, brain abscess, and meningitis (Figs. 13-23, 13-24).

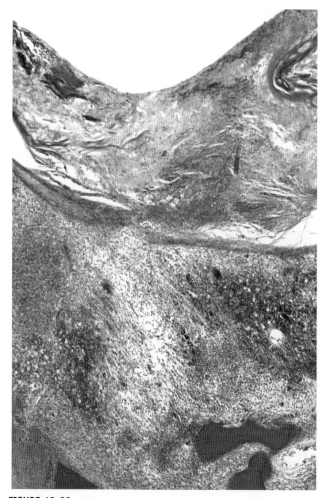

FIGURE 13-22
The external auditory canal is filled with necroinflammatory debris and granulation tissue, which extends into the adjacent bone.

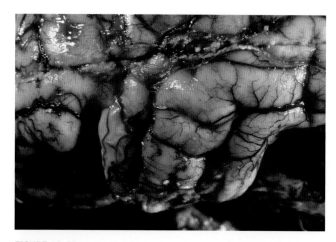

FIGURE 13-23
This patient died of intracranial complications of malignant external otitis. A purulent exudate present on the brain surface indicates suppurative meningitis. (See Fig. 13-24.)

DIFFERENTIAL DIAGNOSIS

Cytologic atypia of the squamous epithelium responding to an infection raises the differential with squamous cell carcinoma. However, the degree of cytologic atypia is well below the threshold of pleomorphism seen in carcinoma. Sometimes the presence of necrosis will make this distinction impossible, requiring further biopsies. Rarely, coexisting MEO and squamous cell carcinoma of the external auditory canal are documented. Most of the separation between uncomplicated otitis externa and MEO is based on the clinical findings listed above.

FIGURE 13-24
The histology demonstrates neutrophils and fibrin in the subarachnoid space as a sequelae of MEO. (See Fig. 13-23.)

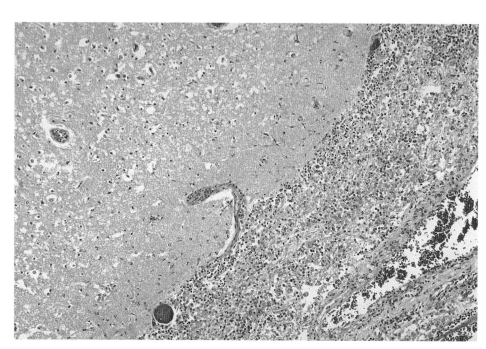

PROGNOSIS AND THERAPY

Treatment of MEO includes strict diabetes control (if applicable), careful debridement until all granulation tissue has resolved, and intravenous, multidrug antibiotic therapy in confirmed osteomyelitis cases. Topical antibiotic therapy is controversial as it may alter or interfere with cultures. With early diagnosis and aggressive antibiotic therapy the mortality rate has been reduced from 50% to between 10% and 30%. Even patients with cranial nerve involvement may now survive.

GOUT

The systemic disease of gout is caused by disordered purine metabolism or abnormal excretion of uric acid, although in most cases the cause is unknown. The symptoms generally relate to the precipitation of monosodium urate crystals in joint spaces or soft tissues, as urates are not soluble in synovial fluid. Arthritis, nephropathy, and soft tissue tophaceous gout are the most common presenting findings. Auricular gouty tophi are seen in chronic tophaceous gout, usually after many years of hyperuricemia and acute episodes of arthritis.

CLINICAL FEATURES

Without an exhaustive discussion of the biochemistry and clinical manifestations of the disease, gout has a number of general predisposing clinical factors including age and duration of hyperuricemia (usually only after 20–30 yr of hyperuricemia), heavy alcohol intake (especially beer), high purine diet, obesity, familial and genetic influences, and drugs. Males are affected twice as often as females. After 20 to 30 years of asymptomatic hyperuricemia, acute attacks of gouty arthritis may begin. After many years of acute gout (average, 12 yr), patients develop chronic tophaceous gout, which in the auricle presents as a firm nodule, which may over time extrude white, chalky material through the skin.

PATHOLOGIC FEATURES

GROSS FINDINGS

Excisional biopsies of tophi may include the overlying skin, or may consist solely of deep dermal or subcutaneous tissue. The cut surface is yellow-white and chalky, often with bands of fibrous tissue separating nodules of amorphous material.

GOUT
DISEASE FACT SHEET

Definition	Gout is a systemic disease of purine metabolism or abnormal uric acid secretion resulting in urate crystal deposition in joints and soft tissues
Incidence and location	Tophaceous gout develops only after multiple episodes of acute gouty arthritis, usually after many years
	Tophaceous gout involves juxta-articular soft tissue, periarticular ligaments, tendons, bursae, and auricle
Morbidity and mortality	Crippling arthritis and renal failure, accounting for 20% of deaths in patients with gout
Gender, race, and age distribution	Male > Female (2 : 1)
	Long history (20–30 yr) of hyperuricemia before clinical gout develops
	5th–6th decades
Clinical features	Predisposing factors include age, duration of hyperuricemia, heavy alcohol intake, obesity, familial and genetic influences, drugs (especially thiazides)
	Acute attacks begin with exquisitely painful joints (feet, knees, hands, elbows)
	Nonpainful tophi develop after several years, firm subcutaneous nodules, which contain white, chalky urate crystals
Prognosis and treatment	While potential fatal (20%) from renal failure, the vast majority of patients have a quality of life issue only
	Crippling arthritis is most severe manifestation in most patients
	Systemic treatment includes antihyperuricemics, colchicine, COX-2 inhibitors, and nonsteroidal anti-inflammatory agents
	Tophi may be excised for cosmetic reasons

GOUT
PATHOLOGIC FEATURES

Gross findings	Subcutaneous nodule with chalky, white cut surface
Microscopic findings	Tophi contain large aggregates of refractile brownish needle shaped crystals in alcohol-fixed material
	In formalin fixed tissue the crystals dissolve, leaving pink hyaline material surrounded by granulomatous inflammation
	Crystals engulfed by multinucleated giant cells, with granulomatous elements palisaded around crystal aggregates
	Polarization demonstrates negative birefringence
Pathologic differential diagnosis	Rheumatoid nodule, amyloidosis

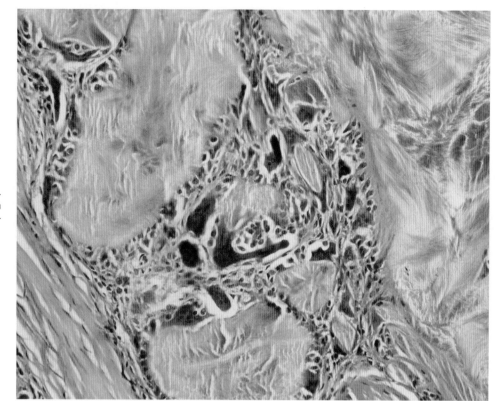

FIGURE 13-25

A gouty tophus of the auricle contains aggregates of gray to brown needle-like crystals with a granulomatous response (alcohol fixed).

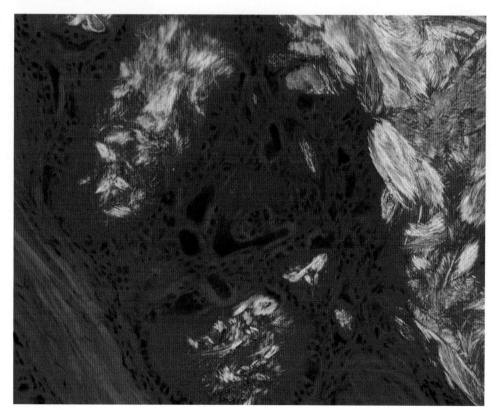

FIGURE 13-26

When polarized with a red compensator, monosodium urate crystals are yellow when parallel to the compensator and blue when perpendicular.

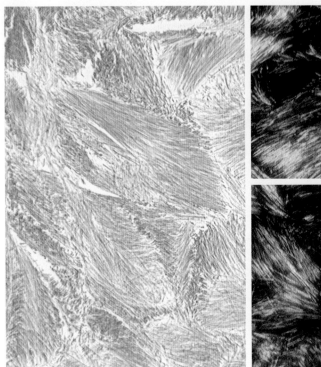
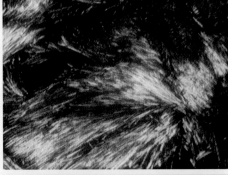
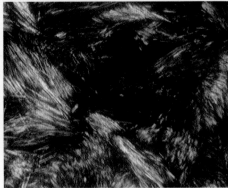

FIGURE 13-27
Left: Unfixed scraped material from a gouty tophus. *Right:* Polarized unfixed sample.

MICROSCOPIC FINDINGS

The pathologic features of gouty tophi are best demonstrated in manually processed tissue, as fixation in an aqueous fixative, such as formalin, dissolves out the urate crystals. Fixation in absolute alcohol followed by hand processing gives the best results. Even in formalin-fixed tissues, the histologic features are usually very characteristic, and, using a nonaqueous alcoholic eosin stain, the polarized appearance is still diagnostic. Sheaves of elongated needle-shaped, refractile crystals are slightly brown in alcohol-processed material (Fig. 13-25). With polarization they are negatively birefringent (Fig. 13-26). The aggregates of crystals are surrounded by mononuclear histiocytes and foreign body giant cells which may engulf individual crystals. The granulomatous elements usually palisade around crystalline masses, mimicking rheumatoid nodules. If alcohol processing is not feasible, it is quite simple to scrape some of the chalky material from the cut surface of a suspected tophus and to prepare an unfixed smear for examination with polarization (Fig. 13-27). This can then be correlated with the histologic findings in routinely processed and stained sections.

DIFFERENTIAL DIAGNOSIS

The differential diagnosis of gouty tophi is a rheumatoid nodule or amyloidosis, but urate crystals clinch the diagnosis.

PROGNOSIS AND THERAPY

Renal failure accounts for death in up to 20% of patients with gout; but for the most part the disorder is largely a quality of life issue in the majority of those affected. The arthritis, in its chronic phase, may be crippling. Many antihyperuricemics, colchicine, COX-2 inhibitors, and nonsteroidal anti-inflammatory agents are used in the treatment armamentarium. Therapy may mitigate the chronic effects of tophaceous deposits in the joint spaces and in soft tissues.

CHOLESTEATOMA

Cholesteatoma is a misnomer as it contains no "cholesterol" and it is not a "neoplasm." A "neoplasm" is simulated clinically by the propensity to destroy surrounding tissues (including bone) and to recur after excision. Collagenase production by the squamous epithelium ("matrix") is thought to result in the bone destruction. The cystic lesion, filled with keratinous debris and lined by keratinizing squamous epithelium, is found within the middle ear or mastoid region. The presence of squamous epithelium in the middle ear, which is normally lined by cuboidal or columnar glandular epithelium, is abnormal, no matter by which mechanism it arrives there. Acquired and congenital forms of cholesteatoma are recognized.

CLINICAL FEATURES

Cholesteatomas are not uncommon and usually unilateral. Older children and young adults (3rd–4th decades) will present with a foul-smelling aural discharge and conductive hearing loss. The tympanic membrane is perforated (usually at the superior margin) in the acquired form, while intact in the congenital form. Both are usually associated with a long history of severe chronic otitis media, giving an otoscopic appearance of a white-gray to yellow irregular mass associated with chronic otitis media (Figs. 13-28, 13-29). Facial nerve dysfunction, vomiting, severe vertigo, and very severe headaches may indicate advanced destructive disease or a suppurative infection, requiring immediate intervention.

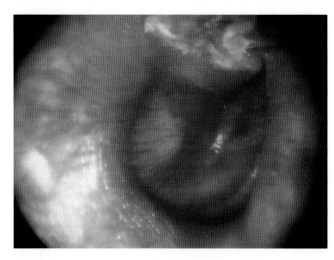

FIGURE 13-28

An otoscopic view demonstrates an irregular yellow to white mass behind the perforated tympanic membrane in this cholesteatoma.

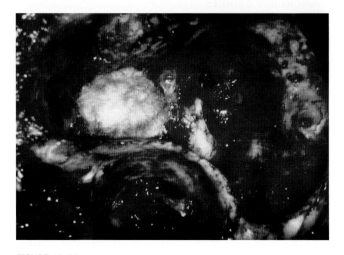

FIGURE 13-29

Surgical exposure reveals the yellow white mass that represents a cholesteatoma. Specimens received in pathology are typically fragmented.

CHOLESTEATOMA DISEASE FACT SHEET	
Definition	Destructive squamous epithelial cyst of middle ear or mastoid region, usually secondary to chronic otitis media, but occasionally congenital
Incidence and location	Common worldwide
	Origin in superior posterior middle ear and/or petrous apex, but may demonstrate locally aggressive growth into adjacent structures
Morbidity and mortality	Chronic middle ear disease and progressive conductive hearing loss
	Intracranial extension may lead to lethal complications such as meningitis, epidural abscess, brain parenchymal abscess, or lateral sinus thrombosis
Gender, race, and age distribution	Equal gender distribution
	Any age, including congenital examples; highest incidence in 3rd–4th decades
Clinical features	Long history of severe, chronic otitis media
	Progressive conductive hearing loss, otalgia, otorrhea (in part due to underlying chronic ear disease); tinnitus and vertigo less common
	Facial nerve palsy, vomiting, severe vertigo, severe headache suggests advanced destructive disease or suppurative infection
	Otoscopic appearance: white-gray to yellow irregular mass associated with chronic otitis media or perforated tympanic membrane
Radiologic features	Bone destruction with medial displacement of the ossicles
	No gadolinium enhancement by CT
	MRI: T1-weighted signal, low intensity; T2-weighted signal, high intensity
Prognosis and treatment	Surgical extirpation of the squamous epithelial lining essential
	Recurrence if incompletely excised (20%)
	Increased incidence of recurrence includes: <20 yr of age, marked ossicular erosion, polypoid mucosal inflammatory disease, extensive disease
	Serious complications include labyrinthine fistula, sigmoid sinus or facial nerve canal erosion, cranial nerve dysfunction, meningitis, epidural or brain parenchymal abscess

RADIOLOGIC FEATURES

CT and magnetic resonance imaging (MRI) show a soft tissue mass displacing the ossicles medially, with a variable degree of bone destruction (Figs. 13-30, 13-31). Associated changes of chronic middle ear infection are common. There is usually prolongation of the signal in both T1 and T2 MRI signals, with T1-weighted signal

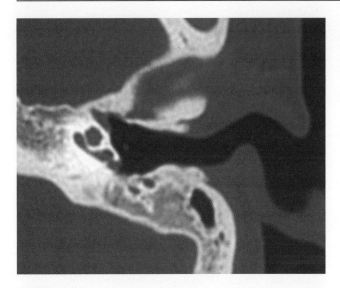

FIGURE 13-30
The CT image of the normal right ear in comparison to a cholesteatoma in Fig. 13-31.

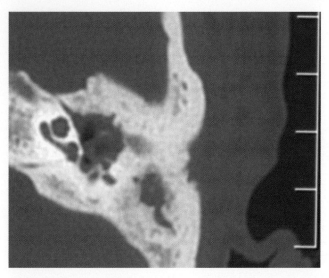

FIGURE 13-31
Contrasted with the previous image, the left ear CT shows a soft tissue mass in the middle ear space. The stapes is present in both views. (See Fig. 13-31).

intensity low, while T2-weighted signal intensity is high by MRI. There may be peripheral enhancement if degenerated.

PATHOLOGIC FEATURES

GROSS FINDINGS

Rarely is a cholesteatoma received intact for pathologic examination. The specimen usually consists of multiple fragments of flakey, white keratinous debris, accompanied by soft tissue fragments. A foul aroma and associated chronic otitis media with bone destruction may be noted at surgery, with bone fragments submitted to pathology.

MICROSCOPIC FINDINGS

Three components are essential for the diagnosis of cholesteatoma: keratinous material, stratified squamous epithelium with a granular layer, and inflamed granulation or fibrous tissue (Figs. 13-32, 13-33). The squamous epithelium is usually bland, atrophic, lacking rete pegs without reactive changes expected in an inflammatory process. A giant cell granulomatous reaction to the keratinous material may be seen. The thin epithelium lines a sac filled with exfoliated anucleate keratin squames. Occasionally, other disorders accompany the cholesteatoma and include, cholesterol granuloma, aural polyps, tympanosclerosis, and acquired encephalocele (herniation of normal brain tissue through a bony defect).

ANCILLARY STUDIES

Fluorescence in situ hybridization studies have demonstrated extra number 7 chromosomes in over half of cholesteatomas, which correlates with proliferative activity; this abnormality may be useful in identifying those cases which will exhibit more aggressive behavior. Other proliferation markers, such as ErbB-2 and Ki-67, may also prove to be helpful in predicting behavior of cholesteatomas.

DIFFERENTIAL DIAGNOSIS

The pathologic differential diagnosis is relatively limited to squamous cell carcinoma and cholesterol granuloma. Carcinoma contains pleomorphic epithelium, not seen in cholesteatoma.

CHOLESTEATOMA PATHOLOGIC FEATURES	
Gross findings	Specimen fragmented, but may contain flecks of white to yellow keratinous (grumous) material
	All tissue should be processed
Microscopic findings	Cystic, sac-like mass
	Acellular, keratinous material
	Thin, stratified squamous epithelium with prominent granular layer
	Inflamed granulation or fibrous tissue
	Giant cell granulomatous reaction to keratinous debris and cholesterol granuloma may coexist
Immunohistochemical features	Strong Ki67 immunoreactivity confirms proliferation
Pathologic differential diagnosis	Cholesterol granuloma, squamous cell carcinoma

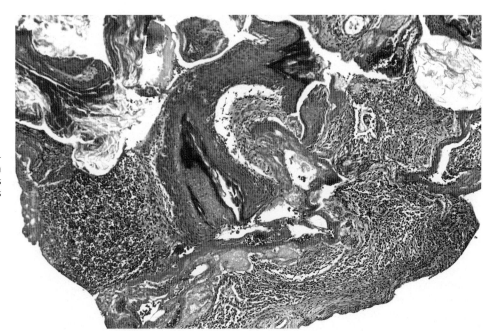

FIGURE 13-32
The essential elements of a cholesteatoma include inflamed granulation or fibrous tissue, keratinizing squamous epithelium, and acellular keratinous material.

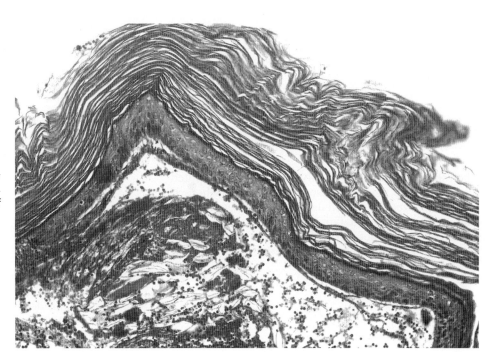

FIGURE 13-33
The squamous epithelium, or "matrix" has a granular layer in a cholesteatoma, associated with flakes of keratin and debris.

PROGNOSIS AND THERAPY

An excision or exteriorization of a cholesteatoma can be achieved by a modified radical (all ossicles left) or radical mastoidectomy (stapes left). Recurrence can occur if incompletely excised, with a rate of about 20%.

Other factors associated with increased incidence of recurrence include age <20 years, marked ossicular erosion, polypoid mucosal inflammatory disease, and extensive disease. Serious complications include a labyrinthitis, labyrinthine fistula, sigmoid sinus or facial nerve canal erosion, cranial nerve dysfunction, meningitis, and epidural or brain parenchymal abscess.

CHOLESTEROL GRANULOMA

Cholesterol granuloma of the mastoid or middle ear is a stromal reaction to hemorrhage and cholesterol crystals associated with breakdown of red blood cells and other necrotic tissues.

CLINICAL FEATURES

Cholesterol granuloma is seen at any age, with no gender preference, usually in patients with a history of chronic ear disease, such as serous otitis media or acute suppurative otitis media. Trauma or surgical procedures that produce obstruction may also predispose to these lesions. Patients present with unilateral conductive hearing loss, tinnitus, disturbances of balance, or episodes of bloody otorrhea. Otoscopic examination often demonstrates a blue to black tympanic membrane secondary to a middle ear bloody effusion. When cholesterol granulomas occur in the petrous apex the clinical course may be more aggressive, with sensorineural hearing loss, deficits of other cranial nerves (V, VI, VII), and, in advanced cases, extension into the middle or posterior cranial fossa.

RADIOLOGIC FEATURES

Cholesterol granuloma is readily identified by computed tomography or magnetic resonance imaging where it is characterized by a well-defined intraosseous cystic lesion with associated bone remodeling. Gadolinium enhancement is not present; cholesterol granuloma demonstrates high-intensity signal with both T1- and T2-weighted images by MRI.

PATHOLOGIC FEATURES

GROSS FINDINGS

The specimen is usually fragmented, consisting of yellow-brown or red friable tissue, sometimes with overlying mucosa. Process all material to exclude associated cholesteatoma or neoplasm.

MICROSCOPIC FINDINGS

The cholesterol granuloma consists of granulation tissue or fibrous tissue, with recent hemorrhage, elon-

CHOLESTEROL GRANULOMA DISEASE FACT SHEET	
Definition	Stromal reaction to hemorrhage and cholesterol crystals from cell breakdown of erythrocytes
Incidence and location	Incidence unknown due to coexistence with other diseases
	Middle ear and petrous apex, but occur in any location
Morbidity and mortality	Conductive hearing loss and chronic middle ear disease
	Petrous apex lesions may be more aggressive, with sensorineural hearing loss, cranial nerve deficits, or intracranial extension
Gender, race, and age distribution	Equal gender distribution
	Any age
Clinical features	History of chronic middle ear disease
	Trauma or surgical procedure predispose in some cases
	Otoscopic appearance: Blue to black tympanic membrane if associated with bloody middle ear effusion, or submucosal brown mass
	Unilateral conductive hearing loss, tinnitus, balance disturbances, bloody otorrhea
Radiologic features	Well-defined intraosseous cystic lesion with bone remodeling
	No gadolinium enhancement by CT
	MRI T1- and T2-weighted high-intensity signal
Prognosis and treatment	Drainage and aeration of middle ear-mastoid compartment
	Aggressive petrous apex lesions may require more aggressive surgery

gated clefts (left by cholesterol crystals dissolved by processing) surrounded by multinucleated giant cells, foamy and hemosiderin-laden histiocytes, and extracellular accumulations of hemosiderin pigment (Fig. 13-34). The overlying mucosa may demonstrate reactive changes, but a pure cholesterol granuloma will not include a proliferation of keratinizing squamous epithelium, which would indicate a coexisting cholesteatoma.

DIFFERENTIAL DIAGNOSIS

The cholesterol granuloma is frequently simultaneously present with other lesions, such as cholesteatoma, neuroendocrine adenoma of the middle ear, and endolymphatic sac tumors. Therefore, it is imperative to search for these other possible lesions.

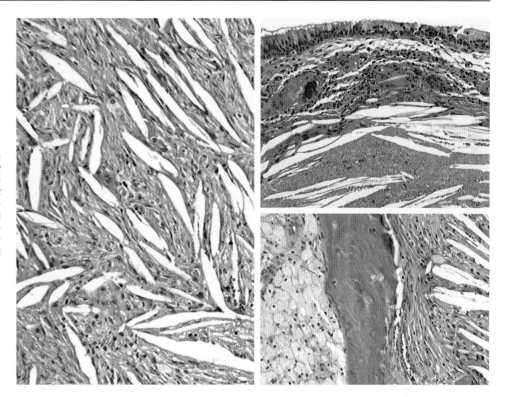

FIGURE 13-34

Right: The submucosal stroma demonstrates fusiform clefts left by cholesterol crystals which have been dissolved during processing. *Right upper:* Many of the cholesterol crystals are engulfed by multinucleated giant cells below an intact respiratory-type epithelium. *Right lower:* Bone with histiocytes (*left side*) and cholesterol clefts (*right side*).

CHOLESTEROL GRANULOMA PATHOLOGIC FEATURES	
Gross findings	Fragmented, friable, yellow-brown to red friable tissue
	Process all material to exclude associated cholesteatoma or neoplasm
Microscopic findings	Granulation or fibrous tissue with recent hemorrhage
	Elongated clefts (left by cholesterol crystals) surrounded by multinucleated giant cells, foamy and hemosiderin-laden macrophages
	Extracellular aggregates of hemosiderin pigment
	Reactive epithelium, but no keratinizing squamous epithelium in pure cholesterol granuloma
Pathologic differential diagnosis	Look for associated lesions: cholesteatoma, neuroendocrine adenoma of middle ear (NAME), endolymphatic sac tumor

PROGNOSIS AND THERAPY

Treatment of a cholesterol granuloma requires drainage and aeration of the middle ear-mastoid compartment, removing the predisposing factors for development of these lesions. Petrous apex lesions may require drainage (through a variety of techniques), depending on the presence or absence of residual hearing; nonaggressive petrous apex lesions, often incidental, may be followed clinically and radiographically.

SUGGESTED READING

First Branchial Cleft Anomalies

1. Barnes L: Surgical Pathology of the Head and Neck, 2nd ed. New York: Marcel Dekker, 2001:1486–1491.
2. Ford GR, Balakrishnan A, Evans JNG, Bailey CM: Branchial cleft and pouch anomalies. J Laryngol Otol 1992;106:137–143.
3. Hickey SA, Scott GA, Traub P: Defects of the first branchial cleft. J Laryngol Otol 1994;108:240–243.
4. Lambert PR, Dodson EE: Congenital malformations of the external auditory canal. Otolaryngol Clin North Am 1996; 29:741–760.
5. Triglia J-M, Nicollas R, Ducroz V, et al.: First branchial cleft anomalies. A study of 39 cases and a review of the literature. Arch Otolaryngol Head Neck Surg 1998;124:291–295.

Cystic Chondromalacia

1. Heffner DK, Hyams VJ: Cystic chondromalacia (endochondral pseudocyst) of the auricle. Arch Pathol Lab Med 1986;110:740–743.
2. Michaels L: Idiopathic pseudocystic chondromalachia. In: Barnes EL, Eveson JW, Reichart P, Sidransky D, eds. Pathology and Genetics of Head and Neck Tumours. Kleihues P, Sobin LH, series eds. World Health Organization Classification of Tumours. Lyon, France: IARC Press, 2005:341.
3. Secor CP, Farrell HA, Haydon RC: Auricular endochondral pseudocysts: diagnosis and management. Plast Reconstr Surg 1999;103:1451–1457.
4. Tan BY, Hsu PP: Auricular pseudocyst in the tropics: a multi-racial Singapore experience. J Laryngol Otol 2004;118:185–188.
5. Zhu L, Wang X: Histological examination of the auricular cartilage and pseudocysts of the auricle. J Laryngol Otol 1992;106:103–104.

Chondrodermatitis Nodular Helicis

1. Elgart ML: Cell phone chondrodermatitis. Arch Dermatol 2000;136:1568.
2. Michaels L: Chondrodermatitis nodularis chronica helicis. In: Barnes EL, Eveson JW, Reichart P, Sidransky D, eds. Pathology and Genetics of Head and Neck Tumours. Kleihues P, Sobin LH, series eds. World Health Organization Classification of Tumours. Lyon, France: IARC Press, 2005:341.
3. Moncrief M, Sassoon EM: Effective treatment of chondrodermatitis nodularis chronica helices using a conservative approach. Br J Dermatol 2004;150:892–894.
4. Munnoch DA, Hernert KJ, Morris AM: Chondrodermatitis nodularis helices et antihelices. Br J Plast Surg 1996;49:473–476.
5. Santa Cruz DJ: Chondrodermatitis nodularis helices: a transepidermal perforating disorder. J Cutan Pathol 1980;7:70–76.
6. Weedon D: Skin Pathology, 2nd ed. Philadelphia: Churchill Livingstone, 2002:363–364.

Relapsing Polychondritis

1. Frances C, el Rassi R, Laporte JL, et al.: Dermatologic manifestations of relapsing polychondritis. A study of 200 cases at a single center. Medicine 2001;80:173–179.
2. Kent PD, Michet CJ, Luthra H: Relapsing polychondritis. Curr Opin Rheumatol 2003;16:56–61.
3. Letko E, Panayotis Z, Baltatzis S, et al.: Relapsing polychondritis: a clinical review. Semin Arthritis Rheum 2002;31:384–395.
4. Myers B, Gould J, Dolan G: Relapsing polychondritis and myelodysplasia: a report of two cases and a review of the current literature. Clin Lab Hematol 2000;22:45–48.
5. O'Connor Reina C, Garcia Iriarte MT, Barron Reyes FJ, et al.: When is a biopsy justified in a case of relapsing polychondritis? J Laryngol Otol 1999;113:663–665.
6. Richez C, Dumoulin C, Coutouly X, Schaeverbeke T: Successful treatment of relapsing polychondritis with infliximab. Clin Exp Rheumatol 2004;22:629–631.
7. Saif MW, Hopkins JL, Gore SD: Autoimmune phenomen in patients with myelodysplastic syndrome and chronic myelomonocytic leukemia. Leuk Lymphoma 2002;43:2083–2092.
8. Trentham DE, Le CH: Relapsing polychondritis. Ann Intern Med 1998;129:114–122.
9. Vroman D, Solomon KD: Images in medicine: relapsing polychondritis. N Engl J Med 2003;17:349.

Otic Polyp

1. Brugler G: Tumors presenting as aural polyps. Pathology 1992;24:315–319.
2. Gliklich RE, Cunningham MJ, Eavey RD: The cause of aural polyps in children. Arch Otolaryngol Head Neck Surg 1993;119:669–671.
3. Hussain SS: Histology of aural polyp as a predictor of middle ear disease activity. J Laryngol Otol 1991;105:268–269.
4. Milroy CM, Slack RWT, Maw AR, et al.: Aural polyps as predictors of underlying cholesteatoma. J Clin Pathol 1989;42:460–465.
5. Prasannaraj T, De N, Narasimhan I: Aural polyps: safe or unsafe disease? Am J Otolaryngol 2003;24:155–158.
6. Tay HL, Hussain SS: The management of aural polyps. J Laryngol Otol 1997;111:212–214.

"Malignant" Otitis

1. Grandis JR, Curtin HD, Yu VL: Necrotizing (malignant) external otitis: prospective comparison of CT and MR imaging in diagnosis and follow-up. Radiology 1995;196:499–504.
2. Handzel O, Halperin D: Necrotizing (malignant) external otitis. Am Fam Phys 2003;68:309–312.
3. Kohut RI, Lindsay JR: Necrotizing ("malignant") external otitis: histopathologic processes. Ann Otol 1979;88:714–720.
4. Rajbhandari SM, Wilson RM: Unusual infections in diabetes. Diabetes Res Clin Pract 1998;39:123–128.
5. Ress BD, Luntz M, Telischi FF, et al.: Necrotizing external otitis in patients with AIDS. Laryngoscope 1997;107:456–460.
6. Slattery WH, Brackmann DE: Skull base osteomyelitis: malignant external otitis. Otolaryngol Clin North Am 1996;29:795–805.

Gout

1. Bieber JD, Terkeltaub RA: Gout: on the brink of novel therapeutic options for an ancient disease. Arthritis Rheum 2004;50:2400–2414.
2. Choi HK, Atkinson K, Karlson EW, et al.: Purine-rich foods, dairy and protein intake, and the risk of gout in men. N Engl J Med 2004;11:1093–1103.
3. Choi HK, Atkinson K, Karlson EW, et al.: Alcohol intake and risk of incident gout in men: a prospective study. Lancet 2004;363:1277–1281.
4. Kim KY, Schumacher H, Hunsche E, et al.: A literature review of the epidemiology and treatment of acute gout. Clin Ther 2003;25:1593–1617.
5. Monu JU, Pope TL: Gout: a clinical and radiologic review. Radiol Clin North Am 2004;42:169–184.
6. Pascual E, Pedraz T: Gout. Curr Opin Rheumatol 2004;16:282–286.
7. Terkeltaub RA: Clinical practice. Gout. N Engl J Med 2003;23:1647–1655.

Cholesteatoma

1. Adamczyk M, Sudhoff H, Jahnke K: Immunohistochemical investigations on external auditory canal cholesteatomas. Otol Neurotol 2003;24:705–708.
2. Ferlito A, Devaney KO, Wenig BM, et al.: Clinicopathological consultation. Ear cholesteatoma versus cholesterol granuloma. Ann Otol Rhinol Laryngol 1997;106:79–85.
3. Goycoolea MV, Hueb MM, Muchow D, Paparella MM: The theory of the trigger, the bridge, and the transmigration in the pathogenesis of acquired cholesteatoma. Acta Otolaryngol 1999;119:244–248.
4. Huisman MA, De Heer E, Grote JJ: Cholesteatoma epithelium is characterized by increased expression of Ki-67, p53, and p21, with minimal apoptosis. Acta Otolaryngol 2003;123:377–382.
5. Michaels L, Soucek S, Beale T: Cholesterol granuloma and cholesteatoma. In: Barnes EL, Eveson JW, Reichart P, Sidransky D, eds. Pathology and Genetics of Head and Neck Tumours. Kleihues P, Sobin LH, series eds. World Health Organization Classification of Tumours. Lyon, France: IARC Press, 2005:342–344.
6. Sie KCY: Cholesteatoma in children. Ped Clin North Am 1996;43:1245–1252.
7. Soldati D, Mudry A: Knowledge about cholesteatoma, from the first description to modern histopathology. Otol Neurotol 2001;22:723–730.
8. Stenfors L-E: Does occurrence of keratinizing stratified squamous epithelium in the middle-ear cavity always indicate a cholesteatoma? J Laryngol Otol 2004;118:757–763.
9. Thompson JW: Cholesteatomas. Ped Review 1999;20:134–136.

Cholesterol Granuloma

1. Brackmann DE, Toh EH: Surgical management of petrous apex cholesterol granulomas. Otol Neurotol 2002;230:529–533.
2. DeGuine C, Pulec JL: Blue ear drum and cholesterol granuloma. Ear Nose Throat J 2000;79:542.
3. Ferlito A, Devaney KO, Wenig BM, et al.: Clinicopathological consultation. Ear cholesteatoma versus cholesterol granuloma. Ann Otol Rhinol Laryngol 1997;106:79–85.
4. Jaisinghani VJ, Paparella MM, Schachern PA, Le CT: Tympanic membrane/middle ear pathologic correlates in chronic otitis media. Laryngoscope 1999;109:712–716.
5. Mosnier I, Cyna-Gorse F, Grayeli AB, et al.: Management of cholesterol granulomas of the petrous apex based on clinical and radiologic evaluation. Otol Neurotol 2002;23:522–528.
6. Schuknecht HF: Pathology of the ear, 2nd ed. Philadelphia: Lea & Febiger, 1993:405–411.

14

Benign Neoplasms of the Ear and Temporal Bone

Lester D. R. Thompson

CERUMINOUS ADENOMA

Variable nomenclature has been used in the past to describe benign tumors of ceruminal gland origin, to include ceruminoma, ceruminal adenoma, syringocystadenoma papilliferum, mixed tumor, apocrine adenoma, and cylindroma. However, due to the remarkable difference in clinical behavior and treatment alternatives, "ceruminous adenoma" conveys the anatomic site of origin and the underlying benign tumor type most succinctly.

CLINICAL FEATURES

There is an equal gender distribution with a wide age at initial presentation, although the 6th decade is the mean age at initial presentation. Patients most frequently present with a mass lesion accompanied by hearing changes and occasionally pain.

CERUMINOUS ADENOMA DISEASE FACT SHEET	
Definition	Benign ceruminal gland neoplasm
Incidence and location	Rare
	Outer half of the external auditory canal
Morbidity and mortality	None
Gender, race, and age distribution	Equal gender distribution
	Wide age range, but usually 6th decade
Clinical features	Mass with hearing changes
Prognosis and treatment	Excellent; successfully treated by surgery alone

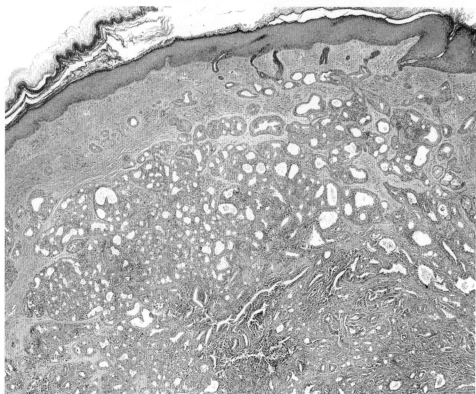

FIGURE 14-1
Keratinized squamous epithelium overlies a circumscribed, although unencapsulated, neoplastic proliferation of ceruminous glands. The glandular and cystic profiles are visible even at low magnification.

PATHOLOGIC FEATURES

GROSS FINDINGS

The tumor is usually a nonulcerating superficial mass found in the outer one-third to one-half of the external auditory canal measuring about 1 cm in greatest dimension, covered by intact skin. As benign tumors, extension into the mastoid bone, middle ear, and base of the skull is not identified.

MICROSCOPIC FINDINGS

Ceruminous adenomas are circumscribed, although not truly encapsulated (Fig. 14-1). Surface involvement (not *origin*) can be seen, while ulceration is absent. They are divided into three major groups based on spe-

CERUMINOUS ADENOMA PATHOLOGIC FEATURES	
Gross findings	Nonulcerated, superficial mass in outer half of external auditory canal about 1 cm
Microscopic findings	Circumscribed mass with glandular and cystic pattern
	Dual cell population, with inner apocrine cells showing decapitation secretion and cerumen granules and outer basal-myoepithelial cells
Immunohistochemical features	CK7 positive secretory cells
	CK5/6 and p63 positive basal-myoepithelial cells
Pathologic differential diagnosis	Paraganglioma, neuroendocrine adenoma of the middle ear (NAME), ceruminal gland adenocarcinoma

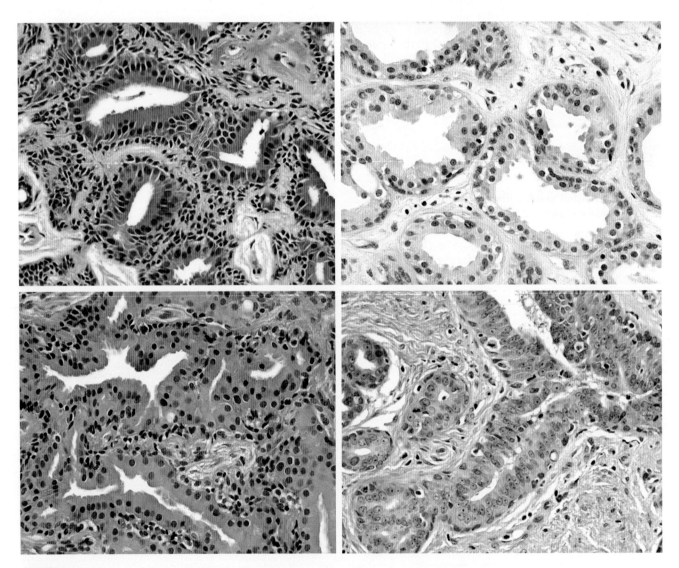

FIGURE 14-2

A variety of different patterns and histologic appearances. *Upper left:* Inner luminal secretory cells subtended by basal myoepithelial cells demonstrate the dual cell population. *Upper right:* Abundant eosinophilic-granular cytoplasm is seen in the luminal cells which show focal decapitation secretion. *Lower left:* Glandular structures are separated by fibrous connective tissue. *Lower right:* Stratification of the nuclei with moderate nuclear pleomorphism and a mitotic figure.

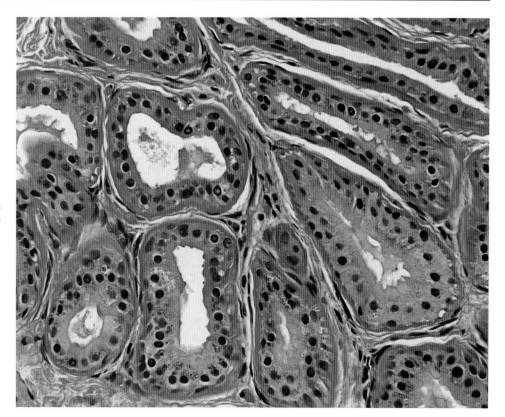

FIGURE 14-3

Yellow-brown "ceroid" lipofuscin-like material is seen in the cytoplasm are the ceruminous cells.

cific histologic findings: ceruminous adenoma, ceruminous pleomorphic adenoma (chondroid syringoma), and syringocystadenoma papilliferum (too rare to be discussed here). Ceruminous adenomas contain neoplastic cells arranged in a variety of different patterns. Whereas a glandular pattern predominates in most lesions, cystic spaces are frequently noted. Ceruminous adenomas demonstrate a dual cell population composed of inner luminal epithelial cells subtended by basal/myoepithelial cells adjacent to the basement membrane (Fig. 14-2). The luminal cells frequently reveal apocrine-type decapitation secretion and/or contain yellow-brown cerumen (wax) granules (acid-fast fluorescent ceroid pigment; Fig. 14-3). The tumors tend to have a low to moderate cellularity composed of cells with mild to moderate nuclear pleomorphism. Nucleoli can be found, rare mitotic figures can be counted, but necrosis is not seen. The presence of a more abundant myoepithelial cell population juxtaposed to areas of myxoid-chondroid matrix material (not native cartilage of the external auditory canal) and the presence of ceruminal apocrine cells within the "duct-like" structures, confirms the diagnosis of a ceruminous pleomorphic adenoma. The apocrine decapitation secretion and cerumen granules are usually identified within the luminal cells of the duct-like structures of the pleomorphic adenomas.

ANCILLARY STUDIES

The lesion cells usually react strongly and diffusely with keratin while only weakly and focally with epithelial membrane antigen (EMA). The dual cell population shows differential immunoreactions with CK7 in the luminal cells and strong and diffuse immunoreactivity with S-100 protein, CK5/6 and p63 in the basal-myoepithelial cells (Fig. 14-4).

DIFFERENTIAL DIAGNOSIS

Paraganglioma, neuroendocrine adenoma of the middle ear, and ceruminal gland adenocarcinoma are the differential diagnostic considerations in the anatomic location of ceruminal gland primaries. The "zellballen" architectural, slightly basophilic cytoplasm, nuclear pleomorphism, and chromogranin, and S-100 immunoreactivity will define a paraganglioma. Neuroendocrine adenoma of the middle ear also has a similar biphasic tumor growth, but arises within the middle ear. The nuclear chromatin distribution is coarse and granular, there are no decapitation apocrine secre-

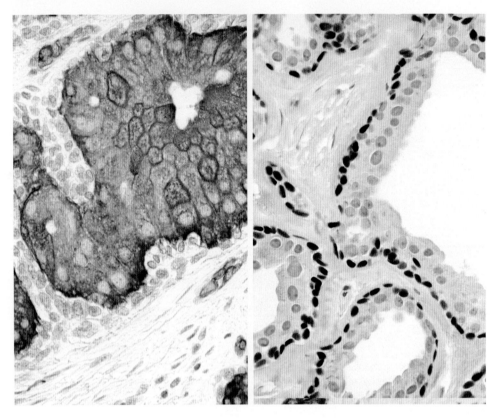

FIGURE 14-4

Differential immunohistochemical staining highlights the luminal cells (CK7) (*left*) while the myoepithelial, basal cell nuclei are accentuated with a p63 immunoreaction (*right*).

tions, a lack of cerumen, and the cells are immunoreactive with chromogranin. The most difficult differential is with ceruminal gland adenocarcinoma. The latter are much more cellular (sometimes difficult to assess on a small biopsy), have a cribriform, solid and infiltrating growth, have increased mitotic figures (including atypical forms), demonstrate moderate to severe nuclear pleomorphism, have prominent nucleoli, develop tumor necrosis, and in general lack cerumen. While these features overlap, it is the aggregate of the findings in either entity that helps with the diagnosis.

PROGNOSIS AND THERAPY

While complete surgical removal of the tumor is ideal, it is frequently impossible due to the complex anatomy of the ear. Therefore, in a small percentage of patients, residual tumor may develop a recurrence. After additional surgery, the patients enjoy a disease-free survival.

PERIPHERAL NERVE SHEATH TUMOR (SCHWANNOMA)

Schwannoma (acoustic neuroma or neurilemmoma) is the most common neoplasm of the temporal bone, many

of which arise at the cerebropontine angle. About 95% of tumors are unilateral and sporadic, but if bilateral or presenting in a young patient, association with neurofibromatosis type 2 (NF2) is high.

CLINICAL FEATURES

The tumors occur equally in the genders with most patients presenting in the 5th or 6th decade, although much younger in patients with NF2. Progressive unilateral sensorineural (not *conductive*) hearing loss and tinnitus are the clinical manifestations, occasionally accompanied by headache, vertigo, facial pain, and facial weakness.

RADIOLOGIC FEATURES

In most schwannomas, the mass is isodense to the cerebellum, with internal auditory canal (IAC) widening. Calcifications and hemorrhage are rare. Magnetic resonance imaging (MRI) scanning shows a mass which is iso- to hypointense on T1-weighted images, and hyperintense with T2-weighted images, with intense enhancement into the porus acousticus (Fig. 14-5).

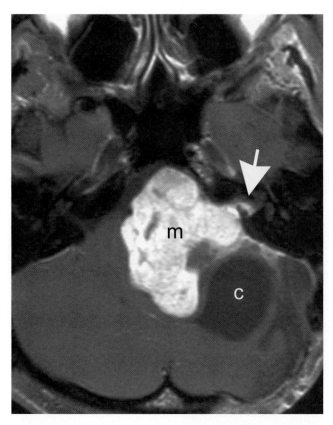

FIGURE 14-5
Contrast-enhanced axial T1-weighted MRI demonstrates large heterogeneously enhancing mass (m) of the left cerebellopontine angle. There is involvement of the left internal auditory canal which is expanded. A peripheral cyst (c) is also present. At surgery, involvement of the posterior margin of the internal auditory canal was confirmed.

PATHOLOGIC FEATURES

GROSS FINDINGS

Schwannomas of the temporal bone usually arise from and are attached to the vestibular division of cranial nerve VIII, growing centrally onto the cerebellopontine angle and peripherally along the IAC. The eccentric, globular, firm to rubbery yellow mass may expand the IAC bone, often creating a mushroom shape (the stalk is within the canal and the "mushroom" is in the CP angle). Cross-section shows a tan-grey, yellowish, solid to myxoid and cystic tumor, commonly with hemorrhage.

MICROSCOPIC FINDINGS

Schwannoma is a neoplasm of the nerve sheath (Schwann) cells. The tumor is composed of cellular Antoni A areas with Verocay bodies (Fig. 14-6) and hypocellular Antoni B areas with a loose reticular pattern and microcystic degeneration. The cells are fusiform with elongated fibrillary cytoplasm, and buckled to spindled nuclei which show little pleomorphism, although scattered large pleomorphic or bizarre cells can be present in some cases. Nuclear palisading is often evident (Fig. 14-7). There are frequently small to medium-sized vessels with ectasia and perivascular hyalinization. Mitotic figures are rare. Extensive degenerative changes can occur (including xanthoma-type histiocytes), and may result in only a thin rim of recognizable tumor.

PERIPHERAL NERVE SHEATH TUMOR DISEASE FACT SHEET

Definition	Benign Schwann cell–derived neoplasm
Incidence and location	Most common cerebellopontine angle tumor
	95% unilateral and sporadic
	If bilateral or young age, NF2 association is high
Morbidity and mortality	Loss of hearing, especially in NF2 associated tumors
	No mortality
Gender, race, and age distribution	Equal gender distribution
	5th to 6th decade for most patients; younger for NF2 patients
Clinical features	Progressive sensorineural hearing loss
Radiologic features	Widening of the internal auditory canal
	MRI: hypointense on T1 versus hyperintense on T2
Prognosis and treatment	Excellent prognosis
	Surgery or serial MRI scans to follow slow growing lesions

PERIPHERAL NERVE SHEATH TUMOR PATHOLOGIC FEATURES

Gross findings	Attached to the vestibular division of the cranial nerve VIII
	Globular, rubbery yellow mass, myxoid, and cystic
Microscopic findings	Cellular Antoni A areas with Verocay bodies
	Hypocellular Antoni B areas with microcystic degeneration
	Fusiform cells with fibrillar cytoplasm
	Spindled, wavy/buckled nuclei
	Medium sized dilated vessels with hyalinization
Immunohistochemical features	Diffuse, strong S-100 protein and vimentin immunoreactivity
	CD34 may stain fibroblasts within Antoni B areas
Ultrastructural features	Thin interdigitating cytoplasmic process with continuous basal lamina and long spacing collagen (Luse body)
Pathologic differential diagnosis	Meningioma and neurofibroma

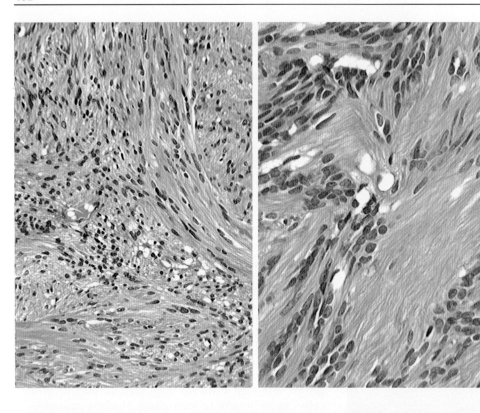

FIGURE 14-6
Hypercellular Antoni A area with fascicular arrangement of cells with fibrillar cytoplasm.

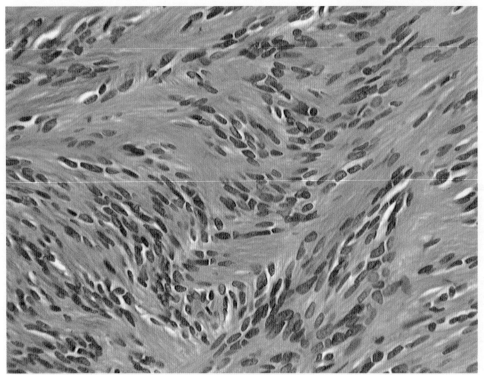

FIGURE 14-7
Fibrillar cytoplasm creates a syncytial arrangement. Nuclear palisading is present.

ANCILLARY STUDIES

ULTRASTRUCTURAL FEATURES

Electron microscopy is not required to make a diagnosis but would show Schwann cells with thin interdigitating cytoplasmic processes covered with a discrete, continuous basal lamina wrapping stromal long spacing collagen with its distinct periodicity (Luse body).

IMMUNOHISTOCHEMICAL FEATURES

The tumor cells and nuclei are strongly and diffusely immunoreactive for S-100 protein, while also expressing vimentin (though not specific). Glial fibrillary acidic protein and neuron-specific enolase may occasionally be positive. CD34 only stains some more slender cells in the Antoni B areas. Neurofilament is absent. The proliferation index (using Ki67 antibody) is higher in schwannomas of NF2 patients than in solitary lesions.

GENETIC STUDIES

NF2 (not the same as NF1 or von Recklinghausen disease) is an autosomal dominant condition characterized by a high incidence of bilateral vestibular schwannomas. The gene for NF2 is a suppressor gene on the long arm of chromosome 22 (22q12). About 90% of the mutations of the protein coded for by the gene (MERLIN or schwannomin) result in a loss of the protein's function.

DIFFERENTIAL DIAGNOSIS

The unique anatomic site raises only meningioma and neurofibroma in the differential diagnosis. The whorled architecture, psammoma bodies, intranuclear cytoplasmic inclusions, and EMA immunoreactivity confirm a meningioma. Neurofibromas are exceptionally rare in the ear and temporal bone.

PROGNOSIS AND THERAPY

Schwannoma is a benign tumor with a very low recurrence potential. Surgical removal by a number of approaches (translabyrinthine, suboccipital, middle cranial fossa, or by stereotactic gamma knife surgery) is standard therapy. However, in small, slowly growing tumors, a "wait-and-see" approach using MRI scanning at intervals to observe growth can be used. It is more difficult to preserve hearing and facial nerve function in schwannomas of NF2 patients, as they tend to infiltrate the nerves to a greater extent and also grow more rapidly.

PARAGANGLIOMA

A neoplasm arising from the paraganglia situated in the vicinity of the jugular bulb (glomus jugulare) or the medial cochlea promontory of the middle ear (glomus tympanicum). Paraganglioma is the preferred term for this most common neoplasm of the middle ear, but jugulotympanic chemodectoma, jugular glomus tumor, and tympanic glomus tumor are frequently used clinically. It is important to note that "glomus" used here is not synonymous with *glomus tumor*, which is a specific tumor arising from perivascular smooth muscle, usually in a subungual location.

CLINICAL FEATURES

Familial and solitary paragangliomas are recognized. Solitary lesions occur predominantly in women (F:M = 5:1), while familial lesions arise more frequently in men. There is a wide age range at initial presentation, although most arise in the 6th decade. Multicentric, bilateral, and coexistent pheochromocytomas are seen in up to 10% of patients. Most patients have conductive hearing loss, while pain, facial paralysis, and pulsatile tinnitus are reported less frequently. Biopsy of the richly vascularized mass behind or protruding through the tympanic membrane can result in profound bleeding. Rarely, catecholamine function may be found.

RADIOLOGIC FEATURES

Modern imaging techniques accurately define the location, size and extent of the paraganglioma. Computed tomography (CT) with contrast shows a homogenous, hypervascular, well-defined mass, sometimes heterogeneous ("moth eaten") if there has been hemorrhage or thrombosis. Bony expansion and erosion of the

PARAGANGLIOMA DISEASE FACT SHEET	
Definition	A benign neoplasm arising from the paraganglia of the jugular bulb or medial cochlea promontory of the middle ear
Incidence and location	Uncommon
	Jugular bulb, middle ear
	Multifocal, bilateral and coexistent pheochromocytomas in about 10%
Morbidity and mortality	About 15% mortality
Gender, race, and age distribution	90% are solitary lesions, more common in women
	10% are familial lesions, more common in men
	Most patients present in the 6th decade
Clinical features	Conductive hearing loss and pulsatile tinnitus
Radiologic features	CT shows a well-defined hypervascular, heterogeneous mass
	MRI shows serpentine signal voids on T1 with hyperintense areas on T2
	Octreotide scintigraphy may find clinically occult tumors
Prognosis and treatment	Slow growing, but invasive with 15% mortality rate
	Embolization, surgery, and radiation therapy

jugular foramen or ossicular chain may be seen. MRI with gadolinium shows a well-defined hypointense mass with areas of serpentine signal void on T1-weighted images, while T2-weighted images amplify areas of high vascularity (slow flow or hemorrhage) (Fig. 14-8). Octreotide or ^{131}I-meta-iodobenzylguanidine scintigraphy confirms the "neuroendocrine" nature of the neoplasm and may help identify clinically occult tumors, especially in familial cases. Preoperative embolization under angiographic guidance is also frequently used.

PATHOLOGIC FEATURES

GROSS FINDINGS

Due to the complex anatomic confines of the region, most surgical specimens are fragmented. However, they are well circumscribed to irregular, reddish, firm masses filling the petrous temporal bone and/or middle ear. The tympanic membrane is usually intact. There is a variegated cut surface, with areas of hemorrhage and degeneration.

MICROSCOPIC FINDINGS

The histological appearances of jugular and tympanic paragangliomas are identical. The tumors are

PARAGANGLIOMA PATHOLOGIC FEATURES	
Gross findings	Fragmented, irregular, reddish firm mass with hemorrhage
Microscopic findings	Poorly encapsulated
	Clusters or Zellballen architecture
	Small, uniform cells with granular basophilic cytoplasm
	Rare pleomorphic or multinucleated cells
	Richly vascularized stroma
Immunohistochemical features	Pheochromocytes are chromogranin and synaptophysin positive
	Sustentacular cells are S-100 protein positive
Pathologic differential diagnosis	Schwannoma, meningioma, neuroendocrine adenoma of the middle ear (NAME)

poorly encapsulated, sometimes giving an "infiltrative" appearance. The tumors are of medium cellularity, demonstrating degenerative changes (cyst formation, hemorrhage, and hemosiderin laden macrophages) especially in embolized tumors. Fibrosis is prominent in a few cases (Fig. 14-9). The tumor cells are arranged in the characteristic clusters or Zellballen architecture with peripherally flattened cells (Fig. 14-10). The cells are small and relatively uniform with finely granular basophilic cytoplasm, separated by an arborizing vascular stroma. Occasionally, there may be nuclear pleomorphism or multinucleate cells (Fig. 14-11). Mitotic figures are inconspicuous or absent in most cases.

ANCILLARY STUDIES

ULTRASTRUCTURAL FEATURES

Paraganglioma cells contain membrane-bound, electron-dense neurosecretory granules in the cytoplasm.

IMMUNOHISTOCHEMICAL FEATURES

The pheochromocytes will be immunoreactive with chromogranin (Fig. 14-12), synaptophysin, NSE and/or CD56 (membrane staining), confirming the neuroendocrine differentiation of the cells. The supporting sustentacular framework cells will react with S-100 protein.

GENETIC STUDIES

Up to 10% of head and neck paragangliomas are familial and inherited as an autosomal dominant trait with genomic imprinting. The most common genetic loci associated with paragangliomas are: paraganglioma 1 (PGL1) on chromosome 11q23, PGL2 on chromosome 11q13.1, and PGL3 on chromosome 1q21–q23, which can be found by genetic analysis to identify early on patients at risk for familial paragangliomas.

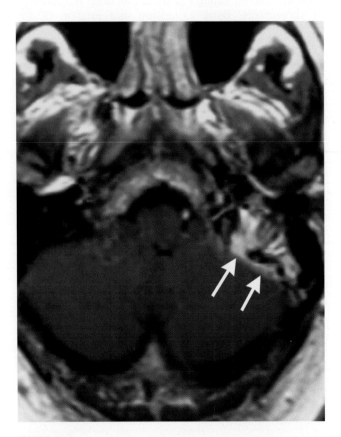

FIGURE 14-8
Contrast-enhanced axial T1-weighted MRI shows heterogeneously enhancing mass (*arrows*) of the left jugular foramen.

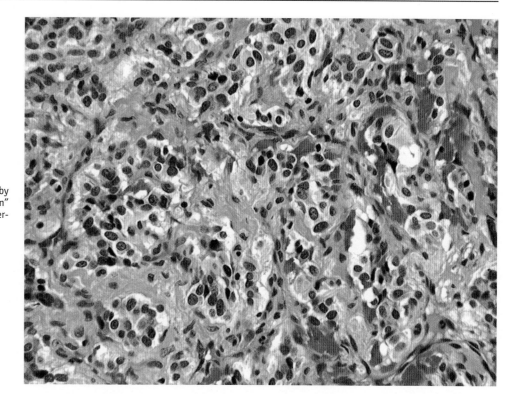

FIGURE 14-9

Nests of tumor cells are separated by a fibrovascular stroma. "Infiltration" into the stroma can be misinterpreted as malignancy.

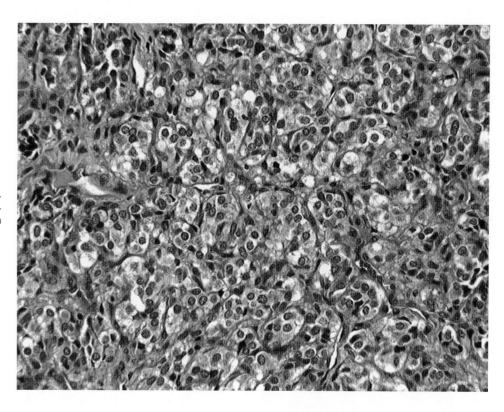

FIGURE 14-10

The characteristic Zellballen architecture with small nests of cells separated by a richly vascularized stroma in this paraganglioma.

DIFFERENTIAL DIAGNOSIS

Based on the anatomic site, nearly 90% of masses in the jugular foramen are paraganglioma, with schwannoma and meningioma accounting for the remaining lesions.

In small biopsies, a neuroendocrine adenoma of the middle ear may cause confusion, but keratin immunoreactivity should make the distinction obvious. Necrosis due to embolization may suggest an underlying malignancy. The presence of embolic material will assist in confirming the correct diagnosis.

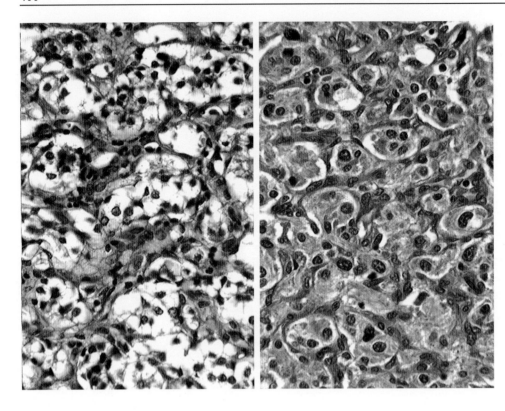

FIGURE 14-11
Left: The cells are small and relatively uniform with basophilic, granular to clear cytoplasm. *Right:* Slight nuclear pleomorphism can be seen, but the nested pattern is still obvious.

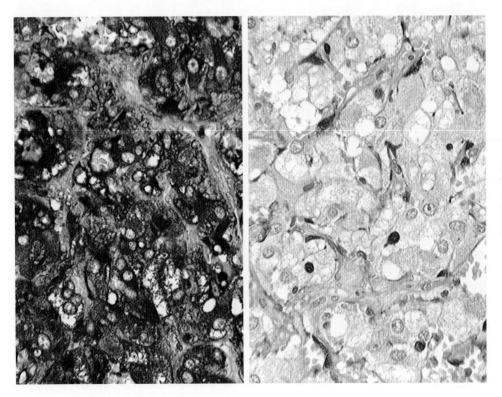

FIGURE 14-12
The paraganglia cells are strongly and diffusely immunoreactive with chromogranin (*left*), while the supporting, sustentacular cells are highlighted by S-100 protein (*right*).

PROGNOSIS AND THERAPY

Jugulotympanic paragangliomas are slow growing, but can be locally invasive. Due to the vital structures in the region, mortality rates of 15% can be expected even though it is a benign neoplasm. Distant metastases have been reported rarely. Radiation therapy plays a role in poor surgical candidates.

MENINGIOMA

Meningioma is a common intracranial neoplasm (15%–18% of all neoplasms) with a variety of histomorphologic growth patterns, which are usually easy to recognize. Clinicopathologically, extraneuraxial (extracranial, ectopic, extracalvarial) meningiomas are usually divided into four groups based on suggested etiologies: (1) Direct extension of a primary intracranial meningioma through pressure necrosis/absorption of the bone, or through an iatrogenic or natural opening. (2) Extracranial metastasis from an intracranial meningioma. (3) Extracranial meningioma originating from pia-arachnoid cell clusters in the sheaths of the cranial nerves (or vessels) as they exit through the foramina or suture lines of the skull. (4) Extracranial meningioma without any apparent demonstrable connection with foramina, cranial nerves, or cranial primaries. Most of the reported cases involving the ear and temporal bone represent secondary extension from an intracranial lesion, a phenomenon in up to 20% of intracranial meningiomas. A true primary meningioma of the ear and temporal bone should only be diagnosed when there is clinical and radiographic support, i.e., a lack of any detectable intracranial mass or "dural enhancement."

CLINICAL FEATURES

Similar to their intracranial counterparts, there is a nearly 2:1 female to male ratio for ear and temporal bone lesions. The patients' ages range from 10 to 90 years, although there is an overall mean age of 50 years. Women tend to present at an older age at initial presentation. Patients present with nonspecific findings, including hearing loss, otitis, pain, headaches, dizziness, and/or vertigo. The mean duration of symptoms is usually between 2 and 3 years, although shorter if more than one anatomic site is simultaneously affected (i.e., external auditory canal and middle ear).

RADIOLOGIC FEATURES

Roentgenographic temporal air cell opacification is often noted, with focal bone erosion, sclerosis or hyperostosis, i.e., a "destructive" lesion. The tumor is usually isointense to gray matter on T1-weighted MRI images, while iso- to hyperintense on T2-weighted images. A direct extension or central nervous system association should be sought and/or excluded. Frequently, the meningiomas' intracranial component will be attenuated or "en plaque."

PATHOLOGIC FEATURES

GROSS FINDINGS

Meningiomas occur at a number of sites in the temporal bone, including the internal auditory meatus, the

---

MENINGIOMA
DISEASE FACT SHEET

Definition	A benign neoplasm of meningothelial cells
Incidence and location	Up to 10% of ear and temporal bone tumors
	Internal auditory meatus, jugular foramen, middle ear (cleft)
Morbidity and mortality	Mastoiditis
	80% 5-yr survival
Gender, race, and age distribution	Female > Male (2:1) (women are usually older at presentation)
	10–90 yr (mean, 50 yr)
Clinical features	Hearing loss, otitis, pain, headaches, dizziness, vertigo
Radiologic features	Focal bone erosion, sclerosis or hyperostosis
	Direct extension from CNS should be sought or excluded
Prognosis and treatment	80% 5-yr survival
	20% recurrence rate
	Complete surgical excision

MENINGIOMA
PATHOLOGIC FEATURES

Gross findings	Infiltrative into bone, sparing mucosa/skin
	Usually <1.5 cm
	Granular mass with gritty consistency and calcifications
Microscopic findings	Meningothelial and whorled architecture
	Epithelioid cells with indistinct borders
	Bland, round nuclei with delicate chromatin and inclusions
	Psammoma bodies
Immunohistochemical features	Epithelial membrane antigen focal and weak
	Vimentin positive
Pathologic differential diagnosis	Neuroendocrine adenoma of the middle ear (NAME), schwannoma, paraganglioma, meningocele

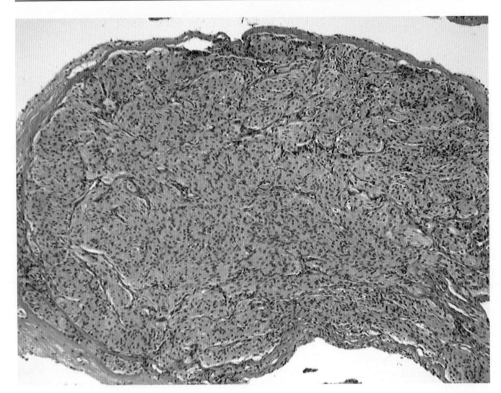

FIGURE 14-13

Typical meningotheliomatous meningioma with a whorled syncytial architecture growing in a polypoid fashion.

jugular foramen, the geniculate ganglion region, roof of the eustachian tube, and middle ear (cleft). Tumors of the ear and temporal bone are on average <1.5 cm in greatest dimension. Macroscopically, the tumors are usually infiltrative into the bone, sparing the mucosal surface (or skin if it involves the external auditory canal) (Fig. 14-13). The cut surface is a grey-white, granular mass with a gritty consistency, with calcifications and fragments of bone frequently macroscopically visible.

MICROSCOPIC FINDINGS

Most meningiomas are typical meningothelial (syncytial) or psammomatous meningiomas. The meningothelial tumors are composed of lobules and whorls of neoplastic epithelioid cells with indistinct borders (Fig. 14-13). The nuclei are generally bland, round to oval with delicate chromatin, and occasional intranuclear cytoplasmic inclusions (Fig. 14-14). Psammoma bodies are typically found (Fig. 14-14). Other ear and temporal bone subtypes of meningiomas include transitional and fibroblastic. Multiple patterns of growth are seen (Fig. 14-15). An infiltrative growth pattern, whether assessed radiographically or histologically (bone or soft tissue invasion), identified in many cases, does not appear to have a bearing on overall patient outcome. Malignant meningiomas, if they exist, must be vanishingly uncommon.

ANCILLARY STUDIES

Nearly all meningiomas react with vimentin and epithelial membrane antigen (EMA), although often only weakly and focally with EMA (Fig. 14-16). It is not uncommon to also exhibit focal immunoreactivity with keratin and S-100 protein. Proliferation markers are not of prognostic value in extraneuraxial meningiomas.

DIFFERENTIAL DIAGNOSIS

The differential diagnosis for meningiomas includes neuroendocrine adenoma of the middle ear, schwannoma, paraganglioma, and meningocele. The general histologic features and immunohistochemical findings can usually separate between these tumors. A neuroendocrine adenoma of the middle ear has a more organoid growth with neuroendocrine nuclear features and strong keratin, chromogranin, and human pancreatic polypeptide immunoreactivity. Schwannoma tends to have alternating cellular and hypocellular areas with areas of cystic degeneration. S-100 protein immunoreactive will be strong and diffuse. Paragangliomas have an organoid growth pattern, with clear to basophilic cytoplasm surrounding hyperchromatic nuclei and a dis-

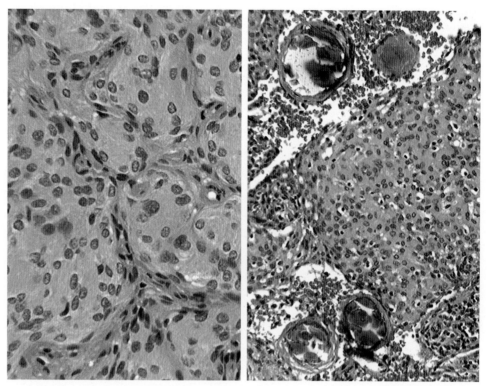

FIGURE 14-14

Whorled architecture is maintained, with the meningothelial cells having indistinct borders and delicate nuclear chromatin. Psammoma bodies are identified in many cases.

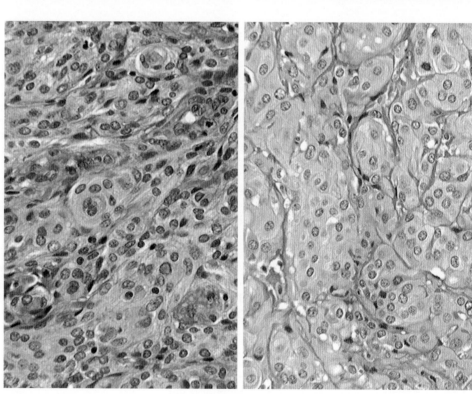

FIGURE 14-15

A variety of different growth patterns can be seen, but the meningothelial nature of the neoplasm is maintained (*left*). A paraganglioma-like growth pattern is occasionally seen (*right*).

tinctive immunoprofile (chromogranin-positive paraganglia cells and S-100 protein-positive supporting sustentacular cells). A meningocele can occur in the middle ear and temporal bone, but histologically they are cystic, have a connection to the central nervous system, and are usually congenital or "acquired" after surgery, infection, or trauma.

PROGNOSIS AND THERAPY

All patients should be treated by complete surgical excision, although complete surgical removal of the tumor is not always possible as a result of the complex anatomy of the ear and temporal bone. Adjuvant radiation

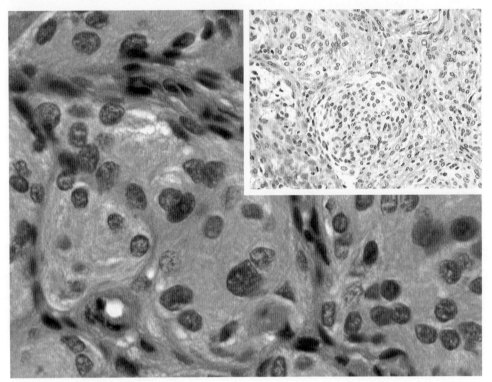

FIGURE 14-16
Nuclear variability is limited, but a whorled architecture is present and may even be highlighted by weak and focal epithelial membrane antigen immunoreactivity (*inset*).

therapy is generally not used. The overall survival rate is usually good (80% 5-yr survival), although patients will not infrequently develop local recurrence (~ 20%). These recurrences may in fact represent incompletely excised residual disease. In spite of additional surgery, occasionally patients will die with disease (although "from" disease is difficult to determine). Involvement of the base of the skull region where complete surgical eradication of the tumor is complicated by the anatomic confines of the region makes the complete resection of recurrences nearly impossible. Mastoiditis is the most frequent complication, occasionally leading to sepsis which results in the patient's death.

NEUROENDOCRINE ADENOMA OF THE MIDDLE EAR (MIDDLE EAR ADENOMA)

"Adenoma" or "carcinoid tumor" of the middle ear are rare neoplasms with indistinguishable morphologies. These benign neuroendocrine lesions of the middle ear have been described by many names (carcinoid tumor, middle ear adenoma, adenomatous tumor of the middle ear, adenocarcinoid, and amphicrine tumor). It is probably best to think of these tumors as a single entity which displays numerous different architectural patterns but similar cytomorphologic and immunohistochemical reactivity patterns. "Neuroendocrine adenoma of the middle ear" (NAME) provides the correct morphologic and behavioral outcome of this rare neoplasm.

CLINICAL FEATURES

Patients, on average, present in the 5th decade of life with an equal gender distribution. Clinical presentation commonly includes decreased hearing acuity, fullness or pressure, and tinnitus. The tympanic membrane is usually intact. Otoscopy shows an intact tympanic membrane in the first stage with a dark brown-reddish colored structure behind it. Tumor may later expand and involve the ossicular chain causing conductive hearing loss and may penetrate the tympanic membrane.

NEUROENDOCRINE ADENOMA OF THE MIDDLE EAR DISEASE FACT SHEET	
Definition	Benign neuroendocrine neoplasm arising in the middle ear
Incidence and location	Uncommon
	Middle ear
Morbidity and mortality	Mastoiditis
	No mortality
Gender, race, and age distribution	Equal gender distribution
	Mean, 5th decade
Clinical features	Decreasing hearing acuity, fullness and tinnitus
Prognosis and treatment	Excellent, although recurrences/re-growth in about 15%
	Complete surgical excision, including ossicular chain

PATHOLOGIC FEATURES

GROSS FINDINGS

Patients present with unilateral disease. Most of the lesions are excised in a piecemeal fashion, with an overall small size (<1 cm) due to the anatomic confines of the middle ear. The tumor by definition occurs within the middle ear and occasionally may extend into the external auditory canal or into the mastoid bone and eustachian tube. There is usually intimate association with the ossicular chain. Tumors are avascular, soft or rubbery, unencapsulated masses with a variegated cut surface. The lesions tended to be gray-tan, brown-red, or pale yellow.

MICROSCOPIC FINDINGS

Tumors are unencapsulated and most are of moderate cellularity. Architectural patterns vary within each tumor and include glandular spaces, trabeculae, festoons, anastomosing cords, and solid sheets, although the glandular pattern predominates (Fig. 14-17). The glandular pattern consists of duct-like structures with focal "back-to-back" gland configuration. The ducts are lined by a dual cell population composed of an inner (luminal), flattened, slightly more intensely eosinophilic cell surrounded by a basally positioned cuboidal to short columnar cell with indistinct cytoplasmic borders. The cytoplasm is eosinophilic and homogenous to finely granular (Fig. 14-18). The nuclei tend to be round to oval, eccentrically placed ("plasmacytoid"), with minimal pleomorphism and "salt-and-pepper" chromatin distribution. Nucleoli are inconspicuous and mitoses are essentially absent. The glandular lumen are occasionally filled with an amorphous secretion. An "infiltrative" pattern is characterized by small irregular groups and strands of cells in a moderately desmoplastic stroma. This pattern gives the illusion of tumor cells dissecting the collagen bundles in an uncontrolled and aggressive fashion. The cells tend to be smaller than those within the other patterns with a higher nuclear-

NEUROENDOCRINE ADENOMA OF THE MIDDLE EAR PATHOLOGIC FEATURES	
Gross findings	<1 cm fragmented mass within the middle ear
	Avascular, rubbery, unencapsulated gray-yellow mass
Microscopic findings	Glandular, ribbon-like, festoon and solid architecture
	"Infiltrative" growth is common
	Dual cell population: inner luminal cells with eosinophilic cytoplasm and outer, cuboidal/columnar cells with indistinct cytoplasm
	Ovoid, eccentrically placed nuclei with "salt-and-pepper" nuclear chromatin distribution and no nucleoli
Immunohistochemical features	Keratin and CK7 (the latter in luminal cells)
	Chromogranin, synaptophysin, and human pancreatic polypeptide
Pathologic differential diagnosis	Ceruminous adenoma, paraganglioma, meningioma, metastatic adenocarcinoma

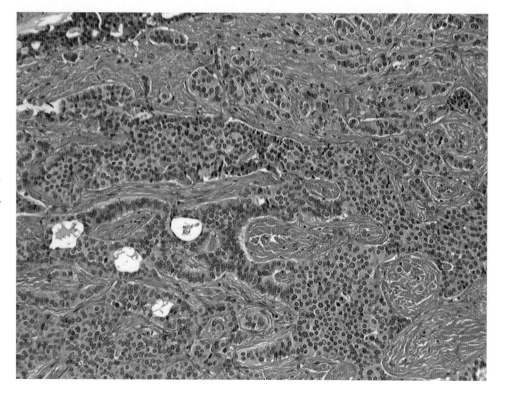

FIGURE 14-17

Neuroendocrine adenoma of the middle ear displaying multiple growth patterns, to include infiltrative (*upper right*), organoid (*upper central*), solid, trabecular, and glandular.

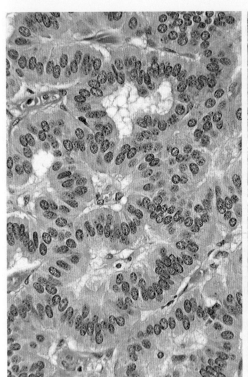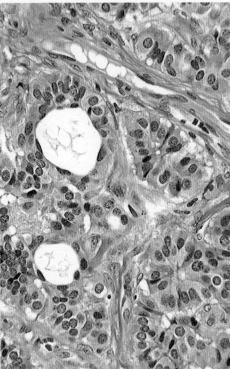

FIGURE 14-18
Left: Columnar cells with oval nuclei demonstrating "salt-and-pepper" nuclear chromatin. *Right:* Glandular pattern with easily identifiable inner, flattened cellular layer and an outer cuboidal-to-columnar layer. Note the lightly basophilic amorphous material within the lumina.

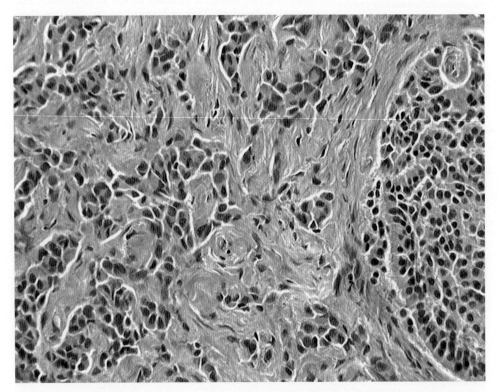

FIGURE 14-19
An "infiltrative" pattern associated with an organoid island in this adenoma. Fibrosis separates the neoplastic cells.

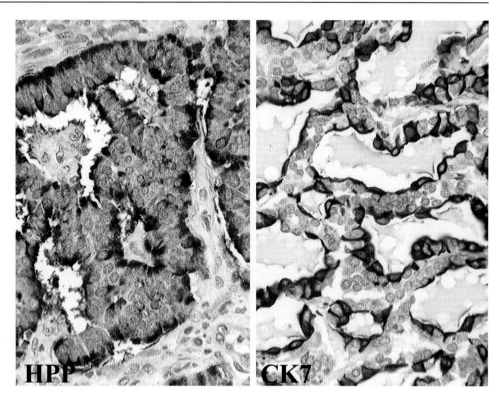

FIGURE 14-20

Left: Human pancreatic polypeptide. *Right:* CK7. Note the predominantly basilar staining pattern of the human pancreatic polypeptide and the inner, luminal pattern of the CK7.

to-cytoplasmic ratio (Fig. 14-19). However, features of malignancy such as mitotic activity, pleomorphism, necrosis, bone, and perineural or lymph-vascular space invasion are not noted. Definitive surface derivation is not seen.

ANCILLARY STUDIES

ULTRASTRUCTURAL FEATURES

Electron microscopy demonstrates two distinct cell types: type A (apical cells with elongated microvilli and secretory mucus granules) and type B (basal cells with cytoplasmic dense-core neurosecretory granules) cells. Transitional forms with features of both cell types have been described.

IMMUNOHISTOCHEMICAL FEATURES

The tumor cells are immunoreactive with a variety of keratin antibodies, including cytokeratin cocktail, CK7, and CAM5.2, although CK7 preferentially highlights the inner (luminal) layer of the glandular cells (Fig. 14-20). Neuroendocrine marker immunoreactivity (although not systemic production) includes chromogranin, NSE, synaptophysin, along with various hormone polypeptides (serotonin, glucagon, leu-7, human pancreatic polypeptide). Neuroendocrine markers are usually in the basal cell layer of the glan-

dular areas while more diffusely reactive in the other architectural patterns. Reactivity, however, is not uniform and varies both between cases and in level of intensity.

DIFFERENTIAL DIAGNOSIS

Histologically, ceruminous adenoma, paraganglioma, meningioma, and metastatic adenocarcinoma can be included in the differential diagnosis. However, the anatomic site of origin makes this a unique tumor, distinctly separable from the other lesions by histology and immunohistochemistry.

PROGNOSIS AND THERAPY

The tumors are usually tightly adherent to the middle ear cavity, commonly encasing the ossicular chain. Complete surgical removal of the neoplasm, including the ossicles, is the treatment of choice. Recurrence (regrowth) is likely to develop in about 15% of patient, especially when the ossicular chain is involved but not removed. Facial nerve paralysis or paresthesias is usually mass-related compression rather than invasion. No well-documented cases of metastatic disease are reported.

ENDOLYMPHATIC SAC TUMOR

This tumor arises from within the endolymphatic sac as a papillary neoplasm with a biologic potential to destroy the temporal bone. Growth into the middle ear is common. This tumor is intermediate, behaving in more than a benign, but not quite malignant fashion as there is no metastatic potential.

CLINICAL FEATURES

There is an equal gender distribution with many patients presenting at a young age (mean, 30 yr), although any age can be affected. Ipsilateral hearing loss (sensorineural > conductive, although can be mixed), tinnitus, facial nerve palsy, and vestibular dysfunction (vertigo, ataxia) are the most common symptoms (similar to Ménière's disease), frequently reported to be present for years, suggesting a slow growing lesion. There is a very strong association with Von Hippel-Lindau syndrome (VHL), sufficient to suggest clinical assessment for the gene mutations [short arm of chromosome 3 (3p25–26)] in patients who present with an endolymphatic sac tumor. Bilateral tumors are associated with VHL.

RADIOLOGIC FEATURES

Bone destruction by a lytic lesion at or near the posterior-medial face of the petrous bone (centered on the endolymphatic sac between the internal auditory canal and the sigmoid sinus) can be seen on CT images, with a hyperintense lesion on T1-weighted MRI images (hypervascular) (Fig. 14-21). The tumor may extend beyond the temporal bone into the cranial fossa and middle ear.

PATHOLOGIC FEATURES

GROSS FINDINGS

The papillary endolymphatic sac neoplasm is centered in the endolymphatic sac and may reach a large

ENDOLYMPHATIC SAC TUMOR PATHOLOGIC FEATURES	
Gross findings	Centered on the endolymphatic sac region, it is often large
Microscopic findings	Unencapsulated with bone invasion
	Coarse, papillary projections into cystic, fluid filled spaces
	Bland, cuboidal cells with little pleomorphism
	Glands with colloid-like material in lumens
Immunohistochemical features	Keratin, EMA and S-100 protein immunoreactive
	Thyroglobulin and TTF-1 negative
Pathologic differential diagnosis	Choroid plexus papilloma, metastatic papillary thyroid carcinoma, neuroendocrine adenoma of the middle ear (NAME), metastatic adenocarcinoma (lung and colon)

ENDOLYMPHATIC SAC TUMOR DISEASE FACT SHEET	
Definition	Papillary epithelial proliferation arising within or near the endolymphatic sac
	Debate about neoplasm versus hamartoma
Incidence and location	Rare, although strong association with Von Hippel-Lindau syndrome
	Temporal bone and occasionally middle ear
Morbidity and mortality	Locally destructive with nerve damage
	Death may result due to large, destructive lesion in vital area
Gender, race, and age distribution	Equal gender distribution
	Wide age range, with mean between 30–40 yr
Clinical features	Ipsilateral hearing loss, vestibular dysfunction and facial nerve palsy
Radiologic features	Bone destruction by a lytic lesion in the petrous bone, sigmoid sinus (specifically endolymphatic sac region)
	Multilocular lesion
	Hyperintense on T1-weighted MRI
Prognosis and treatment	Good, although dependent on extent of tumor
	Recurrent if not completely excised (difficult due to site)
	Surgery

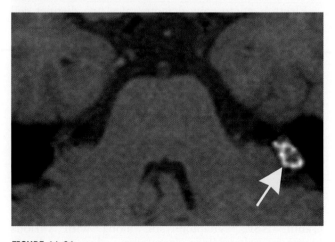

FIGURE 14-21

Axial T1-weighted MRI reveals inherent hyperintensity of mass (*arrow*) located along posterior margin of the left temporal bone.

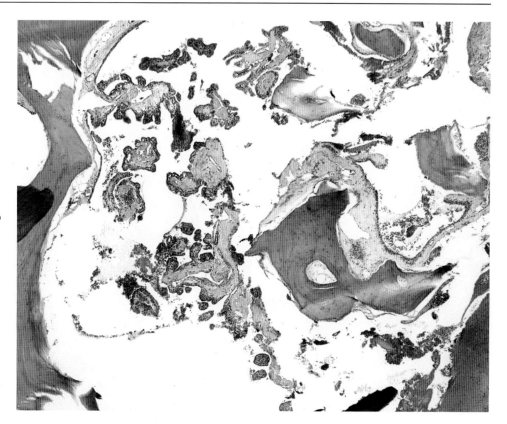

FIGURE 14-22
Complex papillae "invading" into bone.

size (>10 cm), frequently destroying the mastoid air spaces and extending into the middle ear and the cerebellum.

Microscopic Findings

The tumors are unencapsulated with "bone invasion" commonly identified (Fig. 14-22). The coarse pap-

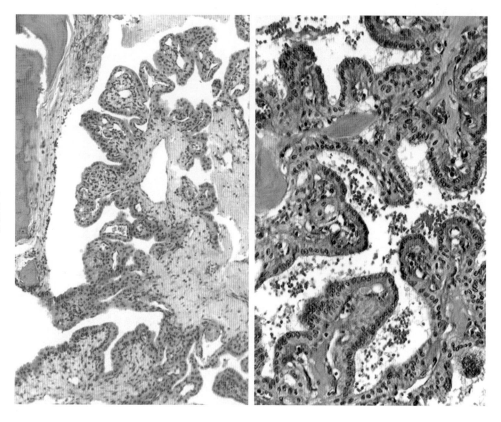

FIGURE 14-23
Left: Complex, although broad papillae within a cystic cavity adjacent to bone. *Right:* Single layer of cuboidal cells with small, hyperchromatic nuclei line the papillary projections.

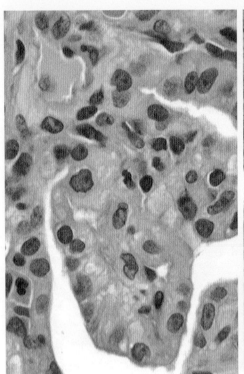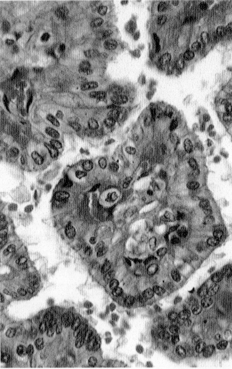

FIGURE 14-24

Left: Papillae are lined by cuboidal to columnar cells which may occasionally have nuclear atypia. Cellular borders are indistinct. *Right:* Cytoplasmic clearing may occasionally be present.

illary projections of the neoplasm are interdigitating, lying within a cystically dilated cavity. The papillae are lined by a single layer of low cuboidal to columnar epithelial cells (Fig. 14-23), similar to the normal endolymphatic sac lining. The cells contain uniformly round to oval nuclei with coarse nuclear chro-

matin deposition. The cell membranes are indistinct and the cytoplasm is eosinophilic and granular (Fig. 14-24). A histologic similarity to thyroid follicles is common (Fig. 14-25), with dilated glands containing secretions. Pleomorphism, mitotic figures, and necrosis are absent.

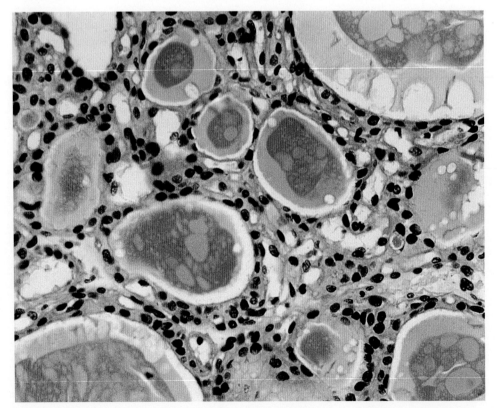

FIGURE 14-25

Thyroid gland-like area of neoplasm of endolymphatic sac: there are acini with eosinophilic secretion resembling thyroid gland follicles with colloid. (Reproduced with permission from Michaels L, Hellquist HB: Ear, Nose, and Throat Histopathology. London: Springer Verlag, 2001.)

ANCILLARY STUDIES

Cytokeratin, EMA, and S-100 protein are immunoreactive, although often focal and weak. Thyroglobulin and TTF-1 are always negative, while glial fibrillary acidic protein may occasionally be weakly positive.

DIFFERENTIAL DIAGNOSIS

A choroid plexus papilloma generally is a mid-line lesion, not destroying the temporal bone. Metastatic carcinomas can be separated by a positive reaction with thyroglobulin and/or TTF-1 in metastatic papillary thyroid carcinoma and TTF-1, CK7, CK20, and carcinoembryonic antigen may be helpful in eliminating metastatic lung and colon carcinoma. A neuroendocrine adenoma of the middle ear does not have a papillary architecture and has neuroendocrine immunoreactivity.

PROGNOSIS AND THERAPY

While surgery is the treatment of choice, it often is radical in order to completely remove the lesion. Since there is a question as to whether the tumor is truly a neoplasm versus a hamartoma, serial radiographic examinations have been suggested if the patients are not symptomatic. The prognosis is dependent on the extent of the disease, with death occasionally reported due to destruction of vital structures as a result of the indolent, but progressive course.

SUGGESTED READING

Ceruminous Adenoma

1. Garin P, Degols JC, Delos M, Marbaix E: Benign ceruminous tumours of the external ear canal. J Otolaryngol 1999;28:99–101.
2. Lynde CW, McLean DI, Wood WS: Tumors of ceruminous glands. J Am Acad Dermatol 1984;11:841–847.
3. Mansour P, George MK, Pahor AL: Ceruminous gland tumours: a reappraisal. J Laryngol Otol 1992;106:727–732.
4. Mills RG, Douglas-Jones T, Williams RG: "Ceruminoma"—a defunct diagnosis. J Laryngol Otol 1995;109:180–188.
5. Thompson LDR, Nelson BL, Barnes EL: Ceruminous adenomas: a clinicopathologic study of 41 cases with a review of the literature. Am J Surg Pathol 2004;28:308–318.
6. Thompson LDR, Michaels L: Ceruminous gland neoplasms of external auditory canals. In: Barnes EL, Eveson JW, Reichart P, Sidransky D, eds. Pathology and Genetics of Head and Neck Tumours. Kleihues P, Sobin LH, series eds. World Health Organization Classification of Tumours. Lyon, France: IARC Press, 2005:331–333.

Peripheral Nerve Sheath Tumor (Schwannoma)

1. Hayashi M, Kubo O, Sato H, et al.: Correlation between MR image characteristics and histological features of acoustic schwannoma. Noshuyo Byori 1996;13:139–144.

2. Irving RM, Moffat DA, Hardy DG, et al.: A molecular, clinical, and immunohistochemical study of vestibular schwannoma. Otolaryngol Head Neck Surg 1997;116:426–430.
3. Kapadia SB: Tumors of the nervous system. In: Barnes EL, ed. Surgical Pathology of the Head and Neck, 2nd ed. New York: Marcel Dekker, Vol 2:787–888.
4. Kasantikul V, Netsky MG, Glasscock ME 3rd, Hays JW: Acoustic neurilemmoma: clinico-anatomical study of 103 patients. J Neurosurg 1980;52:28–35.
5. Michaels L, Beale T, Sandison A, Soucek S: Vestibular schwannoma. In: Barnes EL, Eveson JW, Reichart P, Sidransky D, eds. Pathology and Genetics of Head and Neck Tumours. Kleihues P, Sobin LH, series eds. World Health Organization Classification of Tumours. Lyon, France: IARC Press, 2005:351–352.
6. Samii M, Matthies C: Management of 1000 vestibular schwannomas (acoustic neuromas): surgical management and results with an emphasis on complications and how to avoid them. Neurosurgery 1997;40:11–23.

Paraganglioma

1. Jackson CG, Welling DB, Chironis P, et al.: Glomus tympanicum tumors: contemporary concepts in conservation surgery. Laryngoscope 1989;99:875–884.
2. Kapadia SB: Tumors of the nervous system. In: Barnes EL, ed. Surgical Pathology of the Head and Neck, 2nd ed. New York: Marcel Dekker, Vol 2: 787–888.
3. McCaffrey TV, Meyer FB, Michels VV, et al.: Familial paragangliomas of the head and neck. Arch Otolaryngol Head Neck Surg 1994;120:1211–1216.
4. Mills SE, Gaffey MJ, Frierson HF Jr: Jugulotympanic paraganglioma. In: Mills SE, Gaffey MJ, Frierson HF Jr, eds. Tumors of the upper aerodigestive tract and ear. Atlas of Tumor Pathology, Fascicle 26, Third series. Washington, DC: Armed Forces Institute of Pathology, 2000; 426–431.
5. Rao AB, Koeller KK, Adair CF: From the archives of the AFIP. Paragangliomas of the head and neck: radiologic-pathologic correlation. Armed Forces Institute of Pathology. Radiographics 1999;19:1605–1632.

Meningioma

1. Chang CY, Cheung SW, Jackler RK: Meningiomas presenting in the temporal bone: the pathways of spread from an intracranial site of origin. Otolaryngol Head Neck Surg 1998;119:658–664.
2. Gyure KA, Thompson LD, Morrison AL: A clinicopathological study of 15 patients with neuroglial heterotopias and encephaloceles of the middle ear and mastoid region. Laryngoscope 2001;110:1731–1735.
3. Louis DN, Scheithauer BW, Budka H, et al.: Meningiomas. In: Kleihues P, Cavenee WK, eds. Pathology and Genetics Tumors of the Nervous System. World Health Organization Classification of Tumours. Lyon, France: IARC Press, 2000:176–184.
4. Michaels L, Soucek S: Meningoma of the middle ear. In: Barnes EL, Eveson JW, Reichart P, Sidransky D, eds. Pathology and Genetics of Head and Neck Tumours. Kleihues P, Sobin LH, series eds. World Health Organization Classification of Tumours. Lyon, France: IARC Press, 2005:350.
5. O'Reilly RC, Kapadia SB, Kamerer DB: Primary extracranial meningioma of the temporal bone. Otolaryngol Head Neck Surg 1998;118:690–694.
6. Prayson RA. Middle ear meningiomas. Ann Diagn Pathol 2000;4:149–153.
7. Thompson LDR, Bouffard JP, Sandberg GD, Mena H: Primary ear and temporal bone meningiomas: a clinicopathologic study of 36 cases with a review of the literature. Mod Pathol 2003;16:236–245.

Neuroendocrine Adenoma of the Middle Ear (Middle Ear Adenoma)

1. Batsakis JG: Adenomatous tumors of the middle ear. Ann Otol Rhinol Laryngol 1989;98:749–752.
2. Devaney KO, Ferlito A, Rinaldo A: Epithelial tumors of the middle ear—are middle ear carcinoids really distinct from middle ear adenomas? Acta Otolaryngol 2003;123:678–682.
3. Ketabchi S, Massi D, Franchi A, et al.: Middle ear adenoma is an amphicrine tumor: why call it adenoma? Ultrastruct Pathol 2001;25:73–78.

4. McNutt MA, Bolen JW: Adenomatous tumor of the middle ear. An ultra-structural and immunocytochemical study. Am J Clin Pathol 1985;84: 541–547.

5. Mills SE, Fechner RE: Middle ear adenoma. A cytologically uniform neo-plasm displaying a variety of architectural patterns. Am J Surg Pathol 1984;8:677–685.

6. Torske KR, Thompson LDR: Middle ear adenoma vs. carcinoid tumor: A review of the literature and a unifying concept of 48 cases of neu-roendocrine adenoma of the middle ear (NAME). Mod Pathol 2002;15: 543–555.

Endolymphatic Sac Tumor

1. Devaney KO, Ferlito A, Rinaldo A: Endolymphatic sac tumor (low-grade papillary adenocarcinoma) of the temporal bone. Acta Otolaryngol 2003;123:1022–1026.

2. El-Naggar AK, Pflatz M, Ordonez NG, et al.: Tumors of the middle ear and endolymphatic sac. Pathol Ann 1994;29(Pt 2):199–231.

3. Gaffey MJ, Mills SE, Boyd JC: Aggressive papillary tumor of middle ear/temporal bone and adnexal papillary cystadenoma. Manifestations of von Hippel-Lindau disease. Am J Surg Pathol 1994;18:1254–1260

4. Heffner DK: Low-grade adenocarcinoma of probable endolymphatic sac origin: a clinicopathologic study of 20 cases. Cancer 1989;64: 2292–2302.

5. Kempermann G, Neumann HP, Volk B: Endolymphatic sac tumours. Histopathology 1998;33:2–10.

6. Lonser RR, Kim HJ, Butman JA, et al.: Tumors of the endolymphatic sac in von Hippel-Lindau disease. N Engl J Med 2004;350:2481–2486.

7. Manski TJ, Heffner DK, Glenn GM, et al.: Endolymphatic sac tumors. A source of morbid hearing loss in von Hippel-Lindau disease. JAMA 1997;277:1461–1466.

8. Michaels L, Beale T, Sandison A, Soucek S: Endolymphatic sac tumour. In: Barnes EL, Eveson JW, Reichart P, Sidransky D, eds. Pathology and Genetics of Head and Neck Tumours. Kleihues P, Sobin LH, series eds. World Health Organization Classification of Tumours. Lyon, France: IARC Press, 2005:355–356.

9. Mukherji SK, Albernaz VS, Lo WW, et al.: Papillary endolymphatic sac tumors: CT, MR imaging, and angiographic findings in 20 patients. Radiology 1997;202:801–808.

15 Malignant Neoplasms of the Ear and Temporal Bone

Leslie Michaels • Lester D. R. Thompson

ATYPICAL FIBROXANTHOMA (MFH)

Atypical fibroxanthoma is a low-grade malignant mesenchymal lesion of histiocyte-like cells involving the skin and subcutaneous tissues of the external ear.

CLINICAL FEATURES

The lesion presents in elderly people as a small, raised, sometimes ulcerated nodule on the pinna. In a small number of cases regional node and pulmonary lymph node metastases may be found, but in the majority of cases there is a benign course after surgical excision.

ATYPICAL FIBROXANTHOMA (MFH) DISEASE FACT SHEET	
Definition	Low-grade malignant mesenchymal lesion of histiocyte-like cells
Incidence and location	Uncommon skin tumor
Gender, race, and age distribution	Equal gender distribution
	Elderly patients
Clinical features	Small, raised, sometimes ulcerated nodule on the pinna
Prognosis and treatment	Benign course after complete surgical excision in most cases
	Rare lymph node and pulmonary metastasis

PATHOLOGIC FEATURES

Atypical fibroxanthoma is a cellular neoplasm composed of spindle or oval cells with darkly staining often irregular nuclei with profound pleomorphism occupying the dermis of the skin of the pinna up to the epidermis and frequently extending into the subcutaneous fat (Fig. 15-1). Mitotic figures are frequently found. Multinucleate giant cells are often present. The cytoplasm of the tumor

ATYPICAL FIBROXANTHOMA (MFH) PATHOLOGIC FEATURES	
Microscopic findings	Usually lacks attachment or origin from the surface
	Spindle or oval cells of histiocytic appearance
	Remarkable pleomorphism
	Mitotic figures
	Inflammatory and histiocytic cells
Immunohistochemical features	Vimentin positive and keratin negative
	No characteristic immunohistochemical expression
Pathologic differential diagnosis	Spindle cell squamous cell carcinoma, malignant melanoma

cells is usually abundant and eosinophilic, sometimes foamy (Fig. 15-2).

ANCILLARY STUDIES

ULTRASTRUCTURAL FEATURES

Ultrastructural evidence suggests a transition from fibroblasts to large giant cells, with intermediate forms exhibiting features of both.

IMMUNOHISTOCHEMICAL FEATURES

No diagnostic immunochemical characteristics are recognized. Vimentin is strongly expressed, S-100 protein and muscle specific actin are often so, but keratins are negative.

DIFFERENTIAL DIAGNOSIS

The lesion may be difficult to distinguish from spindle cell squamous cell carcinoma (SCSCC) and melanoma. SCSCC usually shows an in situ or invasive squamous

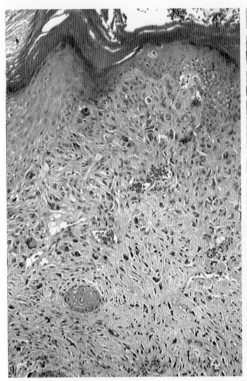

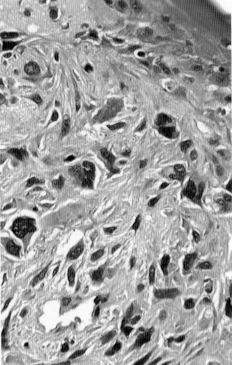

FIGURE 15-1

Left: The overlying epidermis has hyperkeratosis. The stroma contains the atypical spindle cells. *Right:* Remarkable pleomorphism is noted within the spindle and multinucleated cells of this atypical fibroxanthoma.

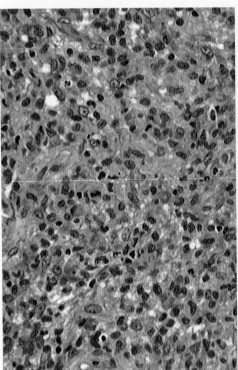

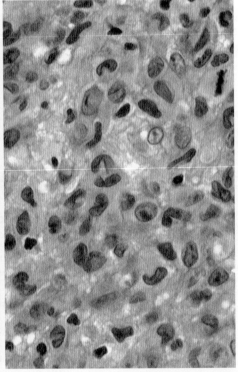

FIGURE 15-2

Left: Inflammatory cells can be part of the reaction to an atypical fibrox-anthoma. *Right:* A histiocytic quality is present with folded and irregular shaped nuclei. Mitotic figures are noted.

cell carcinoma invading into the stroma. Most SCSCCs are keratin reactive, although up to 30% are negative. Amelanotic malignant melanoma may present an appearance similar to that of atypical fibroxanthoma. The use of HMB45, melan A, and S-100 protein will usually help to exclude the diagnosis of malignant melanoma.

PROGNOSIS AND THERAPY

Complete surgical excision (wide) achieves the best result, although Moh's may be considered for cosmetic reasons. Rare cases develop lymph node and/or pulmonary metastasis.

SQUAMOUS CELL CARCINOMA (EXTERNAL AND MIDDLE EAR)

CLINICAL FEATURES

The majority of squamous cell carcinomas (SCC) of the external ear arise in older patients, with men affected more commonly than women. The tumor arises on the pinna most frequently, with a lesser number in the external auditory canal. The pinna lesions, being in a prominent position, are identified early. A serious problem with the canal and middle ear lesions is the delay in diagnosis because of the minimal symptoms that may be present. The pinna SCC display a plaque-like or even polypoid mass (Fig. 15-3). In the later stages ulceration may take place with everted edges (Fig. 15-4).

The canal lesions present as a mass, sometimes warty, occluding the lumen, and often invading deeply into the surrounding tissues. Patients present with an aural discharge and conductive hearing loss. Pain in the ear, bleeding, and facial palsy are also common. In the later stages there is likely to be dissolution of the tympanic membrane with invasion of the middle ear. Entry

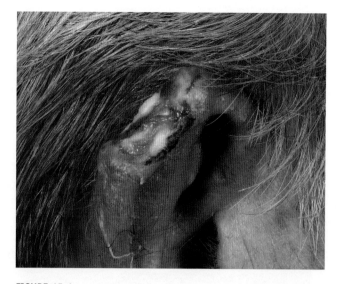

FIGURE 15-4

Marked ulceration of the surface of the squamous cell carcinoma, with everted edges above and below.

SQUAMOUS CELL CARCINOMA (EXTERNAL & MIDDLE EAR) DISEASE FACT SHEET	
Definition	An invasive epithelial tumor with squamous differentiation
Incidence and location	Common tumor (similar frequency to basal call carcinoma)
	Pinna, external canal, and middle ear
Gender, race, and age distribution	Male > Female
	Elderly patients
Clinical features	Mass lesion, often with ulceration
	Pain, hearing loss and drainage of blood or pus
	Tumor plaque, polypoid mass or ulcer with everted edges
	Obstructed external canal
	Conductive hearing loss
Prognosis and treatment	Dependent on stage of disease, but usually good for external ear lesions while less so for external auditory canal tumors
	Recurrences are common
	Death is usually due to intracranial extension
	Surgical excision and/or irradiation

into the middle ear is, however, possible in the presence of an intact tympanic membrane when the tumor passes posteriorly from the canal into the mastoid air spaces and so into the middle ear (Fig. 15-5). In a few cases the neoplasm is confined to the middle ear.

PATHOLOGIC FEATURES

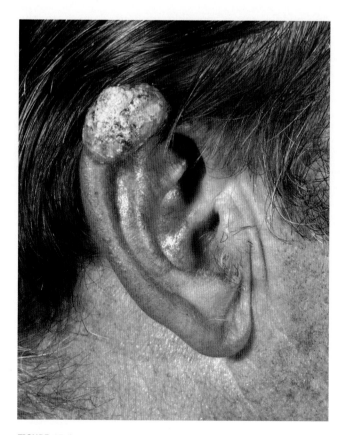

FIGURE 15-3

An oval plaque with early ulceration and exudate on the surface of this squamous cell carcinoma of pinna.

SCC of the external ear usually show origin from the epidermis and demonstrate significant keratinization.

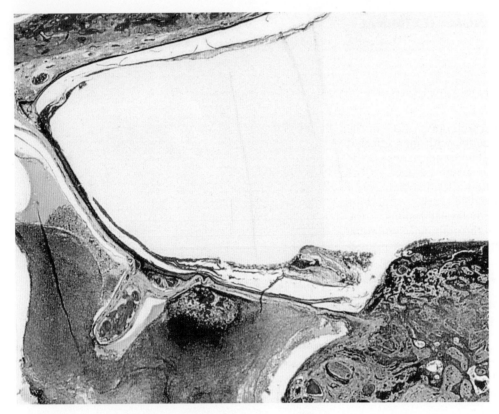

FIGURE 15-5
A low-power temporal bone section shows an intact tympanic membrane with fibrinous and necrotic material resulting from acute inflammation in association with a squamous cell carcinoma at the deep end of the external canal near the eardrum annulus, but not penetrating it.

SQUAMOUS CELL CARCINOMA (EXTERNAL & MIDDLE EAR) PATHOLOGIC FEATURES	
Gross findings	Tumor mass arising from skin
	Invasion of elastic cartilage
Microscopic findings	Squamous cell carcinoma with invasion of atypical cells
	Well, moderately, or poorly differentiated
	Keratinizing or nonkeratinizing
	Multiple patterns of growth
	Stromal response with desmoplasia and inflammation
Immunohistochemical features	Cytokeratin and EGF positive
Pathologic differential diagnosis	Basal cell carcinoma, normal middle ear corpuscles, reactive conditions

The neoplasm may be so well differentiated, with prominent features of eversion, that it can be confused with benign papilloma. The features of squamous cell carcinoma in the ear are no different from those of other sites, displaying keratin pearl formation, atypical keratinization, polarity loss, invasive growth, intercellular bridges, nuclear chromatin condensation, and increased mitotic figures, including atypical forms (Fig. 15-6). In cases arising deeply within the ear canal there is often dissolution of the tympanic membrane and a concomitant origin from middle ear epidermis (metaplastic from the simple cuboidal epithelium), although passage into the middle ear is possible without damage to the eardrum (Fig. 15-5). An origin directly from middle ear epithelium may also be seen. Marked desmoplasia or reactive changes may delay the diagnosis. Verrucous squamous cell carcinoma, spindle cell squamous cell carcinoma, adenosquamous carcinoma, and adenoid squamous carcinoma variants are recognized in this location, displaying similar histologic features to those of upper respiratory tract locations.

While cholesteatoma may be concurrently identified with SCC, SCC does *not* develop from cholesteatoma. Spread of SCC within the middle ear is unique due to the peculiar resistance of the bone of the otic capsule to direct spread of the tumor (Fig. 15-7), but there will be early erosion through the thin bony plate which separates the medial wall of the middle ear at its junction with the eustachian tube from the carotid canal. Only up to 1 mm thick, extension along the carotid canal allows for easy extension to the sympathetic nerves making the tumor impossible to eradicate surgically. Additionally, tumor spreads through the bony walls of the posterior mastoid air cells to the dura of the posterior surface of the temporal bone.

ANCILLARY STUDIES

All SCC of the ear express cytokeratin, epithelial membrane antigen, and epidermal growth factor, although not usually necessary for diagnosis.

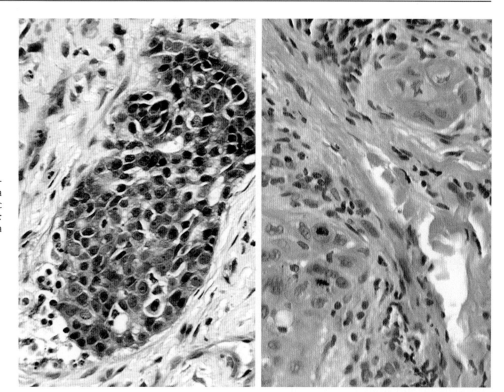

FIGURE 15-6

Left: Moderately differentiated infiltrating squamous cell carcinoma with high nuclear to cytoplasmic ratio, but intercellular bridges. *Right:* Islands of squamous cell carcinoma separated by desmoplastic fibrosis.

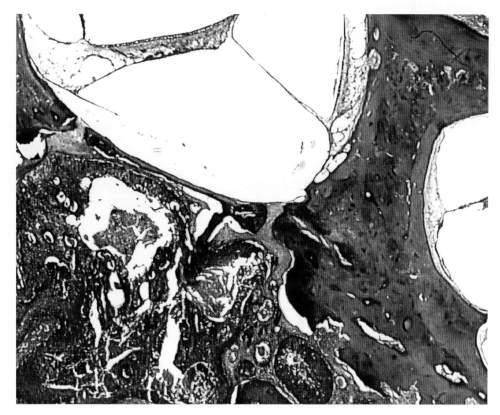

FIGURE 15-7

Low-power view of squamous carcinoma in middle ear showing sparing of otic capsule bone. The vestibule with saccule and utricle lies above. The footplate of the stapes is seen bordering the vestibule below. This thin bony plate is not invaded by the neoplasm. To the right is seen the cochlea, surrounded also by otic capsule bone. There is a little erosion of this bone by adjacent tumor.

DIFFERENTIAL DIAGNOSIS

On the pinna there may sometimes be difficulty in distinguishing poorly differentiated squamous cell carcinoma from basal cell carcinoma. Invocation of the usual histological criteria for the diagnosis of the latter should enable definite diagnosis. Middle ear corpuscles, concentrically laminated balls of collagen formed on bone-free mastoid air cell partitions in the elderly, may be difficult to separate from SCC, particularly in frozen sections. However, there is an absence of cells in the laminated corpuscles.

PROGNOSIS AND THERAPY

Squamous carcinoma of the external canal and middle ear is an aggressive disease with a high propensity for local recurrence. Squamous carcinoma of the pinna is less so. In both the outlook depends on the presenting stage of the disease. Death is usually due to direct intracranial extension. Lymph node metastasis is unusual and spread by the bloodstream even more so.

Both types are treated by surgical excision often with the addition of radiotherapy. If the middle ear is involved the neoplasm it is surgically incurable if either or both (a) the thin plate of bone between the internal carotid artery and the tympanic end of the eustachian tube and (b) the bone in the posterior wall of the mastoid, bordering the posterior cranial fossa, are breached by tumor. In the absence of these features middle ear squamous carcinoma is often treated by "petrosectomy," which is by no means a resection of the whole petrous bone, but extirpation mainly of middle ear components with the neoplasm.

CERUMINOUS ADENOCARCINOMA

Malignant neoplasms derived from the apocrine (ceruminous glands) of the external auditory canal are rare. These neoplasms take the form of adenoid cystic carcinoma, mucoepidermoid carcinoma, and adenocarcinoma, not otherwise specified.

CLINICAL FEATURES

These rare tumors arising from the ceruminal glands of the outer one-third to one-half of the external auditory canal seem to occur in men more frequently than women. Patients tend to be middle to older aged at presentation. Patients present with a mass, hearing changes (conductive hearing loss), drainage, pain, and/or neurologic deficits, most commonly facial nerve paralysis.

CERUMINOUS ADENOCARCINOMA DISEASE FACT SHEET	
Definition	Malignant tumor derived from apocrine glands in the cartilaginous part of the external auditory canal
Incidence	Rare neoplasm
Morbidity and mortality	Hearing loss
	Mortality is variable, but about 50% dead of disease
Gender, race, and age distribution	Male > Female (~2:1)
	Usually 6th–7th decades
Clinical features	Hearing changes (conductive hearing loss)
	Mass lesion
	Drainage
	Paralysis or neurologic deficits
Radiographic features	While nonspecific, CT especially defines the extent of the tumor and excludes a salivary gland primary directly invading into the auditory canal
Prognosis and treatment	Frequent recurrences, direct invasion of the brain, and metastasis (lung) will often result in death
	Some patients survive > 10 yr with radical surgery
	Surgery and/or radiation

Symptoms are frequently present for on average 8–12 months.

RADIOLOGIC FEATURES

Imaging will often demonstrate invasion of middle ear by penetration of the tympanic membrane or of the bony

CERUMINOUS ADENOCARCINOMA PATHOLOGIC FEATURES	
Microscopic findings	Tumors are often polypoid, ranging up to 3 cm
	Tumors are infiltrative
	Range from solid to cystic, glandular or cribriform
	Increased cellularity, nuclear pleomorphism, prominent nucleoli, mitotic figures
	Necrosis is uncommon, but diagnostic of carcinoma
	Adenoid cystic type usually displays the characteristic cribriform pattern with a tendency to perineural infiltration
	Uncommon to identify dual cell population or cerumen
Immunohistochemical features	Keratin, CK7 and CD117 highlights luminal cells
	p63 and S-100 protein highlights basal cells if present
Pathologic differential diagnosis	Metastatic adenocarcinoma, direct extension from salivary gland carcinoma, benign ceruminous adenomas

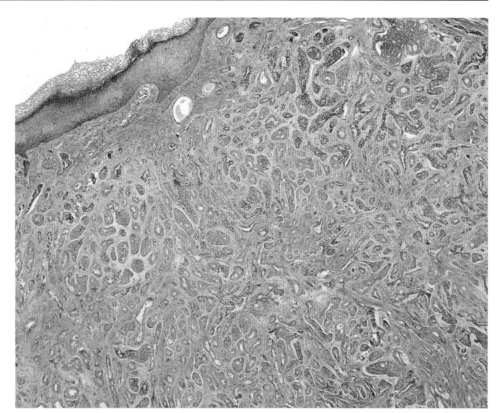

FIGURE 15-8
An invasive ceruminous adenocarcinoma is seen in association with dense fibrosis in the external auditory canal.

wall of the deep external canal. It is most important to exclude involvement of the parotid gland, as adenoid cystic carcinomas may grow into the ear canal by direct extension. Evidence of metastasis to the ipsilateral preauricular lymph node can also be demonstrated by imaging.

PATHOLOGIC FEATURES

Tumors are often polypoid, ranging up to 3 cm. Histologically, all forms of this tumor are invasive (Fig. 15-8). Tumors are solid to cystic, composed of infiltrating glandular to cribriform arrangement of epithelial cells. Uncommonly a dual cell population is noted, but is not the dominant histology. Ceruminous adenocarcinomas may be recognized by the eosinophilic character of the tumor cells, but apocrine-type secretion and a myoepithelial layer are, unlike benign ceruminous adenomas, not usually present in the malignant form (Fig. 15-9). Surface involvement is common. Tumors are cellular, with moderate to severe nuclear pleomorphism and irregular nucleoli. Increased mitotic figures, including atypical forms are present. The adenoid cystic type shows identical features to the same lesion growing from major and minor salivary glands, comprised of masses of small cells with hyperchromatic, carrot-shaped nuclei, surrounding punched-out round spaces containing a basophilic secretion (Figs. 15-10, 15-11). Nerve fiber invasion is frequent. Tumor necrosis, while

uncommon, confirms a malignant diagnosis (Fig. 15-12). Immunohistochemistry may highlight the basal cells if they are present (p63, S-100 protein), but the tumor cells are usually CK7 positive.

DIFFERENTIAL DIAGNOSIS

The most important aspect of the differential diagnosis is to exclude direct invasion from a parotid gland primary, best achieved through careful imaging. Metastatic adenocarcinomas (discussed below) may also be raised in the differential diagnosis, but a clinical history and unique histology should make the distinction. Separation from ceruminous adenoma is difficult on small biopsy. However, carcinomas are invasive, have pleomorphism, mitotic figures and lack ceroid.

PROGNOSIS AND THERAPY

The prognosis is variable, depending on the extent of the disease. The histologic subtype does not seem to influence patient outcome. Multiple recurrences and often metastasis (lung rather than lymph nodes) may be seen. Interestingly, patients may survive > 10 years with wide surgical excision (radical surgery) and radiation.

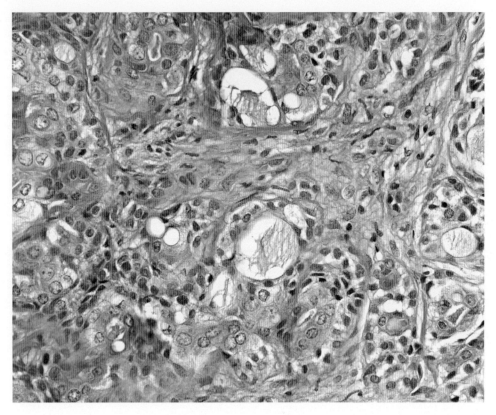

FIGURE 15-9
Atypical epithelial cells arranged in a glandular distribution with mucin present. Note the eosinophilic cytoplasm in this mucoepidermoid carcinoma of ceruminous origin.

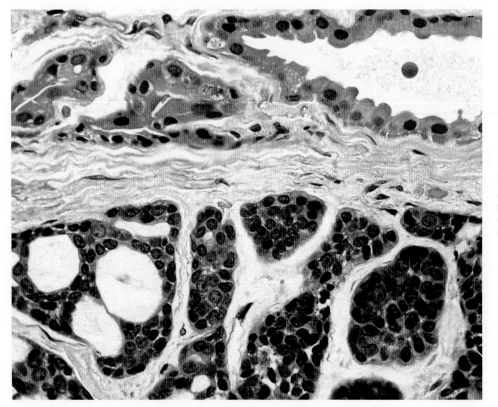

FIGURE 15-10
Adenoid cystic carcinoma is composed of small cells arranged in a cribriform pattern. Note the normal apocrine ceruminous glands above.

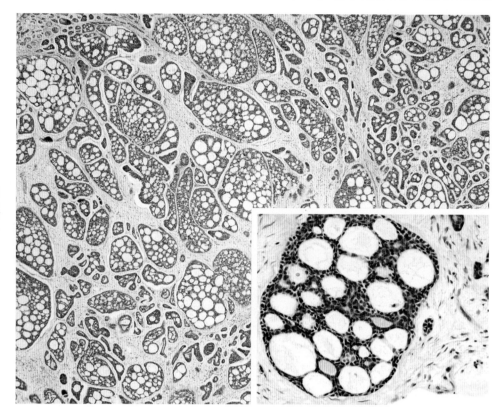

FIGURE 15-11

Multiple patterns are seen in adenoid cystic carcinoma, including the cribriform pattern (*inset*), composed of punched out spaces filled with blue-pink amorphous material.

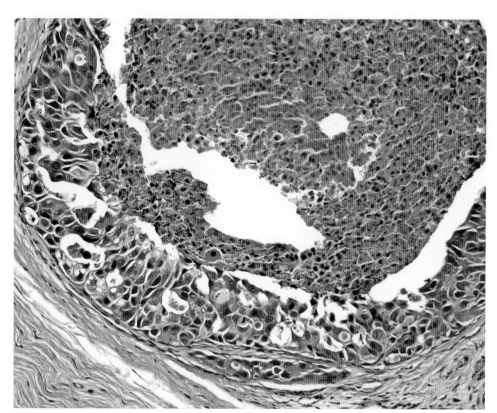

FIGURE 15-12

A high-grade ceruminous adenocarcinoma with central comedo-type necrosis. Severe nuclear pleomorphism is noted.

RHABDOMYOSARCOMA

Rhabdomyosarcoma (RMS) is the most common soft tissue malignancy in the pediatric population. RMS of the ear and mastoid is the most common malignant aural neoplasm in the pediatric population, although it represents <10 % of all head and neck RMS. RMS is generally classified into embryonal, alveolar, pleomorphic, and mixed histologic subtypes. Embryonal RMS is the most common histologic variant seen in the ear and temporal bone.

CLINICAL FEATURES

Almost all the rhabdomyosarcomas of the ear occur in children (2–3 yr) who present with nonspecific symptoms. Symptoms include unilateral refractory otitis media, serosanguinous discharge, otalgia, hearing loss, and neurologic symptoms. These nonspecific symptoms frequently result in clinically misdiagnosed infection or aural polyp. By the time they are diagnosed, there is usually extensive destruction of the bone at the base of the skull, especially the petrous bone, with associated meningeal involvement.

PATHOLOGIC FEATURES

The tumors may present as a polypoid mass (Fig. 15-13). Microscopically, the surface epithelium is usually intact and separated from the neoplastic proliferation (Fig. 15-14). Embryonal RMS is composed of primitive round to spindled mesenchymal cells, called rhabdomyoblasts. The round cells appear similar to lymphocytes, with hyperchromatic, irregular nuclei surrounded by scant, eosinophilic cytoplasm (Fig. 15-15). These cells imperceptibly blend with spindled cells characterized by eosinophilic cytoplasm and an elongated, central, hyperchromatic nucleus. Cross-striations are difficult to identify and are rarely present. Tumor cells are surrounded by a loose myxoid to dense collagenous stroma. Clear spaces in the tumor cell cytoplasm, which may be confirmed as glycogen by the use of the periodic acid Schiff stain with diastase, may be seen in some cases (Fig. 15-16).

ANCILLARY STUDIES

IMMUNOHISTOCHEMICAL FEATURES

Immunohistochemical markers for desmin (Fig. 15-15), myo D1, myogenin and actins confirm the diagnosis of rhabdomyosarcoma, while other "small blue round cell tumor" markers are negative.

RHABDOMYOSARCOMA
DISEASE FACT SHEET

Definition	A malignant neoplasm derived from skeletal muscle
Incidence and location	Rare, although it is the most common sarcoma in children
	Head and neck is most common location of rhabdomyosarcoma (orbit, nasopharynx, ear/temporal bone)
Morbidity and mortality	Loss of hearing
	Dependent on stage, age, and histologic subtype
Gender, race, and age distribution	Equal gender distribution
	Nearly all cases are pediatric (<5 yr old)
Clinical features	Refractory, unilateral, otitis media
	Serosanguinous aural discharge
	Otalgia
	Hearing loss
	Neurologic symptoms, including facial weakness
	Extensive destruction of the bone at the base of the skull
Prognosis and treatment	Good prognosis (~70% 5-year survival) dependent on age, stage, and histologic type
	Multimodality treatment including surgery, chemotherapy, and radiation

---

RHABDOMYOSARCOMA
PATHOLOGIC FEATURES

Gross findings	Polypoid to invasive neoplasm with necrosis
Microscopic findings	Separated into embryonal, alveolar, and pleomorphic types, although embryonal is most common identified
	Intact surface epithelium, separated from neoplastic cells
	Round to spindle-shaped pleomorphic cells
	Hyperchromatic, irregular nuclei with scant, elongated eosinophilic cytoplasm
	Spindle cell morphology with rare cross-striations
	Myxoid to dense collagenous stroma
Ancillary studies	Glycogen in the cytoplasm confirmed with PAS/diastase
	Immunohistochemistry positive for desmin, myo D1, myogenin, and actins
	Mutations of chromosome 11p15 are common
Pathologic differential diagnosis	Inflammatory aural polyp, lymphoma, PNET/Ewing sarcoma, carcinoma, melanoma

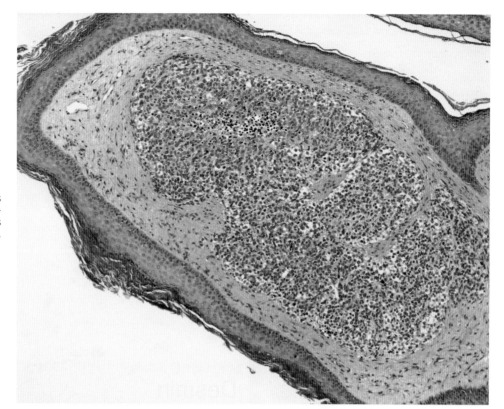

FIGURE 15-13

An intact metaplastic squamous mucosa overlies a compact neoplastic proliferation of rhabdomyoblasts with a small area of central necrosis.

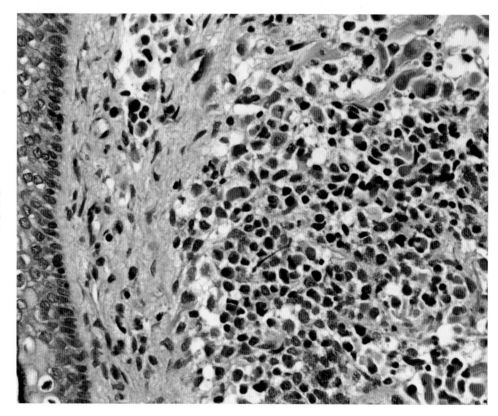

FIGURE 15-14

Atypical-appearing round and spindle cells with eosinophilic cytoplasm pushing the nucleus to the side. Note the covering of an intact epithelium (*left*).

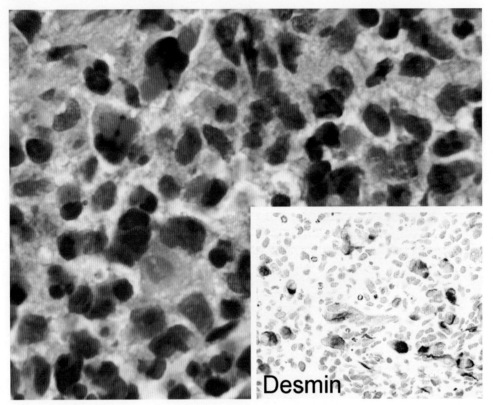

FIGURE 15-15
The cells of embryonal-type rhab-domyosarcoma (RMS) are round to spindle shaped with eccentrically placed eosinophilic cytoplasm. The nuclei are pleomorphic. The inset demonstrates cytoplasmic immunore-activity with desmin, confirming the diagnosis of RMS.

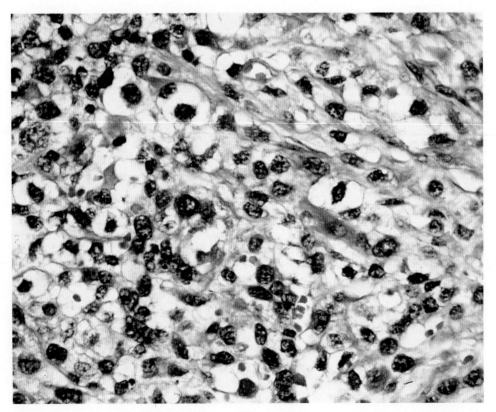

FIGURE 15-16
The tumor cells of this embryonal rhabdomyosarcoma show clear ex-panded cytoplasm, proven to be glycogen with PAS/diastase.

MOLECULAR STUDIES

Mutations in a region mapped to the short arm of chromosome 11 (11p15) have been associated with most rhabdomyosarcomas. Several genes have been mapped to this site. Complex structural and numerical chromosomal rearrangements have also been associated with embryonal rhabdomyosarcoma.

DIFFERENTIAL DIAGNOSIS

The "small blue round cell" appearance makes separation from an aural polyp, lymphoma, melanoma, and other primitive neuroectodermal tumors difficult on routine histologic preparations alone. However, the young age, history of refractory otitis, separation from the epithelium, and pertinent immunohistochemistry studies will aid in the separation of these distinct neoplasms.

PROGNOSIS AND THERAPY

Prognosis for ear RMS is good (70% 5-yr survival) and is related to the age, stage, and histologic subtype. The clinical grouping of rhabdomyosarcomas, according to the Intergroup Rhabdomyosarcoma Study (IRS), is used for "staging" of head and neck rhabdomyosarcomas. Group I is local disease; group II is residual disease or local spread; group III is incomplete resection or biopsy with gross residual disease; and group IV is metastatic disease at onset. It must not be forgotten that RMS of the ear and temporal bone is a highly malignant neoplasm and if left untreated, rapidly spreads into the pharyngeal area or cranial cavity. RMS is usually considered a "systemic" disease for treatment purposes, with treatment based on staging criteria developed by the IRS and consisting of a multimodal approach, including wide local excision, radiation therapy, and multiagent chemotherapy.

METASTATIC NEOPLASMS

Excluding neoplasms which directly invade from a contiguous site into the ear, metastatic tumors spread by blood or lymphatic channels from a noncontiguous site. Metastases to the ear and temporal bone generally occur late in the course of the cancer producing the metastases. While unusual in surgical pathology material during life, autopsy studies show temporal bone involvement in about 20% of patients, virtually all of whom also had disseminated malignant disease.

METASTATIC NEOPLASMS
DISEASE FACT SHEET

Definition	Metastatic tumors spread by blood or lymphatic channels from noncontiguous sites (not direct invasion from adjacent neoplasms)
Incidence and location	About 20% of patients with disseminated malignant tumors will have ear/temporal bone metastasis
	Any part of the region may be affected, including tympanic membrane
Gender, race, and age distribution	Gender differences based on primary site
	Usually older patients with widely disseminated disease
Clinical features	Hearing loss and tinnitus
	Vertigo and nystagmus
	Facial palsy
	Otalgia
	Otorrhea
	External auditory canal mass
Prognosis and treatment	Generally poor outcome reflecting underlying stage of primary tumor
	Surgery may be used in selected case
	Adjuvant therapy may be palliative

METASTATIC NEOPLASMS
PATHOLOGIC FEATURES

Microscopic	Primary adenocarcinoma is vanishingly rare, so metastasis should be excluded first
	Main sources are carcinomas of breast, lung, kidney, stomach, prostate, thyroid, larynx, and cutaneous malignant melanoma
	Histology mimics primary tumor
Immunohistochemical features	Estrogen and progesterone receptors, HER-2/neu for breast primary
	PSA and PAP for prostate primary
	CK7, CK20, TTF-1 may help separate lung and gastrointestinal primary sites
Pathologic differential diagnosis	Ceruminous adenocarcinoma, direct invasion from adjacent sites/organs, primary ear adenocarcinoma

CLINICAL FEATURES

Older patients tend to be affected, with slight differences in gender distribution based on the anatomic site of the primary. Most lesions which metastasize to the ear and temporal bone are carcinomas and melanomas, with few lymphomas or sarcomas identified. Symptoms and signs of metastatic neoplasms in the ear are those of hearing loss, tinnitus, vertigo, nystagmus, facial palsy, otalgia, otorrhea, and external canal mass.

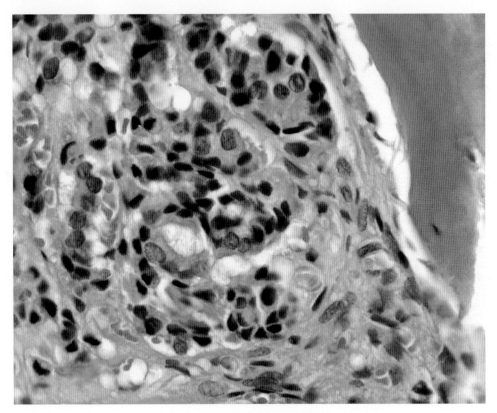

FIGURE 15-17
A metastatic breast carcinoma within the temporal bone. Gland formation is prominent.

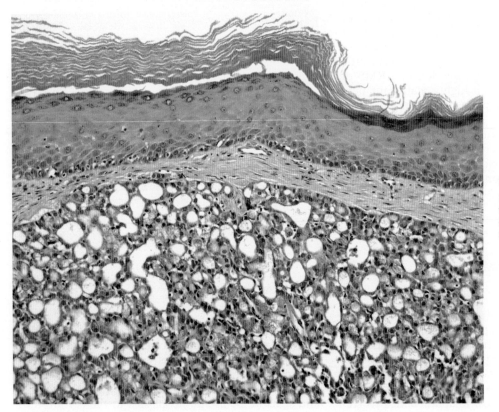

FIGURE 15-18
Direct infiltration into the ear canal from an acinic cell adenocarcinoma of the parotid gland. Note the intact surface epithelium.

FIGURE 15-19

Immunohistochemical studies may sometimes aid in the diagnosis, as this metastatic breast carcinoma is both estrogen receptor (*left*) and HER-2/neu (*right*) immunoreactive.

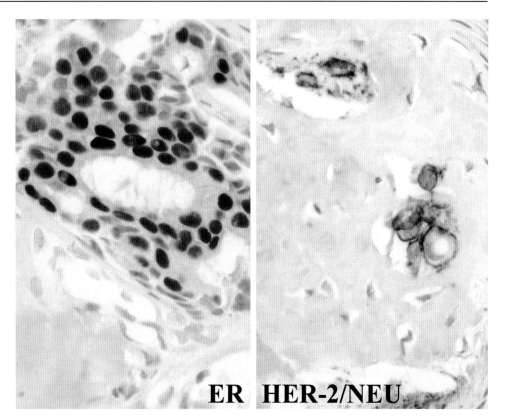

ER HER-2/NEU

PATHOLOGIC FEATURES

Tumors which metastasize to the temporal bone may not yield readily identifiable pathology, but if they extend into more clinically amenable regions, such as the tympanic membrane, they may be more easily diagnosed. Breast carcinomas are the most common primary source (Fig. 15-17), followed by lung, kidney, stomach, prostate, thyroid and larynx; cutaneous malignant melanoma sometimes metastasizes to the ear. In general, metastatic deposits maintain the phenotype of the primary. Rarely are the ear and temporal bone metastases the initial presentation of the disease, and consequently an extensive clinical or histologic workup is seldom necessary. Occasionally, carcinomas may directly extend into the ear and temporal bone via the eustachian tube and from the posterior fossa of the skull through the internal auditory canal. Likewise, parotid malignancies can invade the ear (Fig. 15-18).

ANCILLARY STUDIES

Since primary adenocarcinoma of the ear and temporal bone is vanishingly rare, adenocarcinomas should be presumed to be metastatic. Estrogen and progesterone receptors and HER-2/neu may help with breast carcinoma (Fig. 15-19), while PSA or PAP may identify a prostate carcinoma. TTF-1, CK7, and CK20 are all of value in separating lung and gastrointestinal primaries.

DIFFERENTIAL DIAGNOSIS

Primary carcinoma would be the only real differential diagnosis, but ceruminous adenocarcinomas and primary adenocarcinoma, not otherwise specified, are both vanishingly rare. Immunohistochemical separation helps.

PROGNOSIS AND THERAPY

The prognosis of tumors which have metastasized to the ear and temporal bone is generally dismal, a reflection of the underlying stage of the primary tumor. Surgery may be of value in selected cases, while adjuvant therapy can occasionally have a palliative effect.

SUGGESTED READING

Atypical Fibroxanthoma (MFH)

1. Chilukuri S, Alam M, Goldberg LH: Two atypical fibroxanthomas of the ear. Dermatol Surg 2003;29:408–410.
2. Helwig EB, May D. Atypical fibroxanthoma of the skin with metastases. Cancer 1986;57:368–376.

3. Jones WE. Some special skin tumours in the elderly. Br J Dermatol 1990;122(Suppl 35):71–75.
4. Kamino H, Salcedo E. Histopathologic and immunohistochemical diagnosis of benign and malignant fibrous and fibrohistiocytic tumors of the skin. Dermatol Clin 1999;17:487–505.
5. Starink TH, Hausman R, Van Delden L, Neering H. Atypical fibroxanthoma of the skin. Presentation of 5 cases and a review of the literature. Br J Dermatol 1977;97:167–177.

Squamous Cell Carcinoma (External and Middle Ear)

1. Cooper JR, Hellquist HB, Michaels L: Image analysis in the discrimination of verrucous carcinoma and squamous papilloma. J Pathol 1992;166:383–387.
2. Liang J, Michaels L, Wright A: Immunohistochemical characterization of the epidermoid formation in the middle ear. Laryngoscope 2003;113:1007–1014
3. Michaels L, Soucek S: Squamous cell carcinoma of the external ear. In: Barnes EL, Eveson JW, Reichart P, Sidransky D, eds. Pathology and Genetics of Head and Neck Tumours. Kleihues P, Sobin LH, series eds. World Health Organization Classification of Tumours. Lyon, France: IARC Press, 2005:334.
4. Michaels L: The ear. Chapter 48. In: Sternberg S, ed. Histology for Pathologists, 2nd ed. New York: Raven Press, 1998.
5. Michaels L, Liang J: Origin of middle ear corpuscles. Clin Otolaryngol 1993;18:257–262.
6. Michaels L, Wells M: Squamous cell carcinoma of the middle ear. Clin Otolaryngol 1980;5:235–248.
7. Nyrop M, Grantved A: Cancer of the external auditory canal. Arch Otolaryngol Head Neck Surg 2002;128:834–837.
8. Shockley WW, Stucker FJ Jr: Squamous cell carcinoma of the external ear: a review of 75 cases. Otolaryngol Head Neck Surg 1987;97:308–312.
9. Stafford ND, Frootko NJ: Verrucous carcinoma in the external auditory canal. Am J Otol 1986;7:443–445.

Ceruminous Adenocarcinoma

1. Aikawa H, Tomonari K, Okino Y, et al.: Adenoid cystic carcinoma of the external auditory canal: correlation between histological features and MRI appearances. Br J Radiol 1997;70:530–532.
2. Dehner LP, Chen KT: Primary tumors of the external and middle ear. Benign and malignant glandular neoplasms. Arch Otolaryngol 1980;106:13–19.
3. Mansour P, George MK, Pahor AL: Ceruminous gland tumours: a reappraisal. J Laryngol Otol 1992;106:727–732.
4. Michel RG, Woodard BH, Shelburne JD, et al.: Ceruminous gland adenocarcinoma: a light and electron microscopic study. Cancer 1978;41:545–553.
5. Perzin KH, Gullane P, Conley J: Adenoid cystic carcinoma involving the external auditory canal. A clinicopathologic study of 16 cases. Cancer 1982;50:2873–2883.
6. Pulec JL: Glandular tumors of the external auditory canal. Laryngoscope 1977;87:1601–1612.

7. Thompson LDR, Michaels L: Ceruminous gland neoplasms of external auditory canal. In: Barnes EL, Eveson JW, Reichart P, Sidransky D, eds. Pathology and Genetics of Head and Neck Tumours. Kleihues P, Sobin LH, series eds. World Health Organization Classification of Tumours. Lyon, France: IARC Press, 2005:331–333.

Rhabdomyosarcoma

1. Hawkins DS, Anderson JR, Paidas CN, et al.: Improved outcome for patients with middle ear rhabdomyosarcoma: a children's oncology group study. J Clin Oncol 2001;19:3073–3079.
2. Hicks J, Flaitz C: Rhabdomyosarcoma of the head and neck in children. Oral Oncol 2002;38:450–459.
3. Maroldi R, Farina D, Palvarini L, et al.: Computed tomography and magnetic resonance imaging of pathologic conditions of the middle ear. Eur J Radiol 2001;40:78–93.
4. Pappo AS, Meza JL, Donaldson SS, et al.: Treatment of localized nonorbital, nonparameningeal head and neck rhabdomyosarcoma: lessons learned from intergroup rhabdomyosarcoma studies III and IV. J Clin Oncol 2003;21:638–645.
5. Raney RB, Asmar L, Vassilopoulou-Sellin R, et al.: Late complications of therapy in 213 children with localized, nonorbital soft-tissue sarcoma of the head and neck: a descriptive report from the Intergroup Rhabdomyosarcoma Studies (IRS)-II and -III. IRS Group of the Children's Cancer Group and the Pediatric Oncology Group. Med Pediatr Oncol 1999;33:362–371.
6. Sandison A: Embryonal rhabdomyosarcoma. In: Barnes EL, Eveson JW, Reichart P, Sidransky D, eds. Pathology and Genetics of Head and Neck Tumours. Kleihues P, Sobin LH, series eds. World Health Organization Classification of Tumours. Lyon, France: IARC Press, 2005:335.
7. Simon JH, Paulino AC, Smith RB, Buatti JM: Prognostic factors in head and neck rhabdomyosarcoma. Head Neck 2002;24:468–473.
8. Wiener ES: Head and neck rhabdomyosarcoma. Semin Pediatr Surg 1994;3:203–206.
9. Yang WT, Kwan WH, Li CK, Metreweli C: Imaging of pediatric head and neck rhabdomyosarcomas with emphasis on magnetic resonance imaging and a review of the literature. Pediatr Hematol Oncol 1997;14:243–257.

Metastatic Neoplasms

1. Cumberworth VL, Friedmann I, Glover GW: Late metastasis of breast carcinoma to the external auditory canal. J Laryngol Otol 1994;108:808–810.
2. Davis GL: Secondary tumours. In: Barnes EL, Eveson JW, Reichart P, Sidransky D, eds. Pathology and Genetics of Head and Neck Tumours. Kleihues P, Sobin LH, series eds. World Health Organization Classification of Tumours. Lyon, France: IARC Press, 2005:360.
3. Gloria-Cruz TI, Schachern PA, Paparella MM, et al.: Metastases to temporal bones from primary nonsystemic malignant neoplasms. Arch Otolaryngol Head Neck Surg 2000;126:209–214.
4. Sahin AA, Ro JY, Ordonez NG, et al.: Temporal bone involvement by prostatic adenocarcinoma: report of two cases and review of the literature. Head Neck 1991;13:349–354.

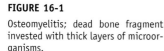

16 Non-Neoplastic Lesions of the Gnathic Bones

Pieter J. Slootweg

OSTEOMYELITIS

Osteomyelitis is an inflammatory process in the marrow cavities of the bone. It may be acute or chronic.

CLINICAL FEATURES

Osteomyelitis is not uncommon, although less common in the gnathic bones than at other anatomic sites. The disease may occur at any age and affects the genders equally. All types of osteomyelitis predominantly affect the mandible. Patients with acute osteomyelitis show all the signs and symptoms of an acute inflammatory disease. In chronic osteomyelitis, signs and symptoms usually are less prominent and may fluctuate in severity; they include swelling, pain, sinus formation, sequestration and, in case of bone loss, pathologic fractures.

Sclerosing osteomyelitis and proliferative periostitis are specific subtypes of chronic osteomyelitis. Sclerosing osteomyelitis causes recurrent pain, swelling of the cheek and restricted jaw movement. The affliction may be either diffuse or focal. Proliferative periostitis represents a hyperplastic periosteal reaction to inflammatory changes in the underlying jaw bone. Facial swelling and bony enlargement of the mandible are the presenting sings. Pain is not a prominent feature. Cortical duplicating or onion-skinning is the radiologic hallmark of this type of osteomyelitis.

RADIOLOGIC FEATURES

Radiographs show an irregular pattern of bone loss and increased density of bone. Periosteal bone apposition may create an onion-skin pattern.

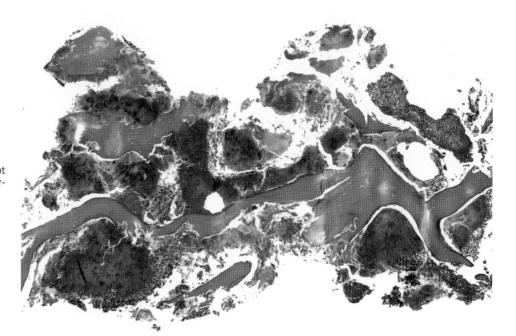

FIGURE 16-1

Osteomyelitis; dead bone fragment invested with thick layers of microorganisms.

OSTEOMYELITIS DISEASE FACT SHEET	
Definition	Osteomyelitis is an inflammatory process of the bone which may be acute or chronic
Incidence and location	Frequent, although not as common in jaw bones
	Mandible more commonly affected
Gender, race, and age distribution	Equal gender distribution
	Mandible most often affected in adults, maxilla in children
Clinical features	Acute osteomyelitis has fever, chills, pain, regional lymphadenopathy
	Chronic osteomyelitis has swelling, pain, and draining fistulae
	Proliferative periostitis has localized bony swelling
Radiologic features	Irregular pattern of mixed radiodense and radiolucent
Prognosis and treatment	Good prognosis with appropriate therapy
	Requires appropriate antibiotics and depends on thorough eradication of causative organisms and necrotic bone

PATHOLOGIC FEATURES

GROSS FINDINGS

Gross findings are nonspecific. Material submitted for analysis mostly consists of irregular bone fragments of

OSTEOMYELITIS PATHOLOGIC FEATURES	
Gross findings	Non-specific soft, granular, hemorrhagic tissues, rarely with bone sequesters
Microscopic findings	Necrotic bone that may be invested with microorganisms
	Infiltrate of polymorphonuclear granulocytes
	Granulation tissue
	Sclerotic bone
	Sinuses lined by squamous epithelium
Pathologic differential diagnosis	Paget's disease, fibrous dysplasia, osseous dysplasia

varying size with attached soft, granular, and hemorrhagic tissue. Sometimes, large bone sequesters are removed that can be recognized as parts of the mandible.

MICROSCOPIC FINDINGS

Acute osteomyelitis shows necrotic bone fragments that are invested with thick layers of microorganisms (Fig. 16-1). At the periphery of the bone and in the haversian canals, an infiltrate of polymorphonuclear granulocytes is present (Fig. 16-2).

In chronic osteomyelitis, dense sclerotic bone masses are seen together with a bone marrow exhibiting edema and small foci of lymphocytes and plasma

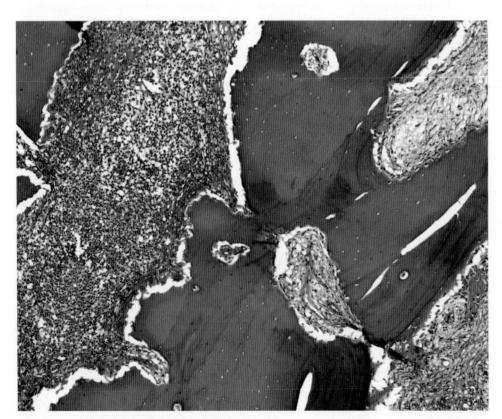

FIGURE 16-2

Osteomyelitis; bone recognizable as dead due to empty osteocyte lacunae. The marrow cavities are partly filled with an infiltrate of polymorphonuclear granulocytes, partly with fibrous tissue. The surface of the bone is irregular and multinuclear osteoclasts form a covering rim in an attempt to resorb the dead bony tissue.

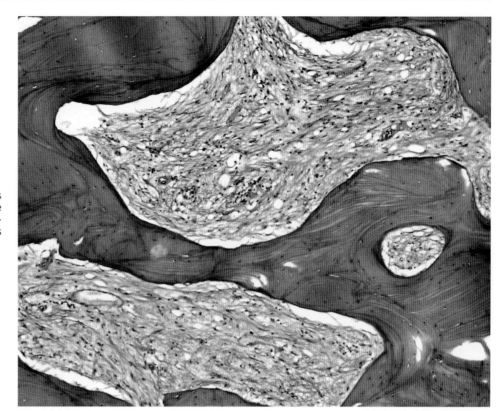

FIGURE 16-3

Chronic sclerosing osteomyelitis is characterized by coarse trabeculae composed of lamellar bone. The intervening marrow cavities contain fibrous tissue with sparse lymphocytes.

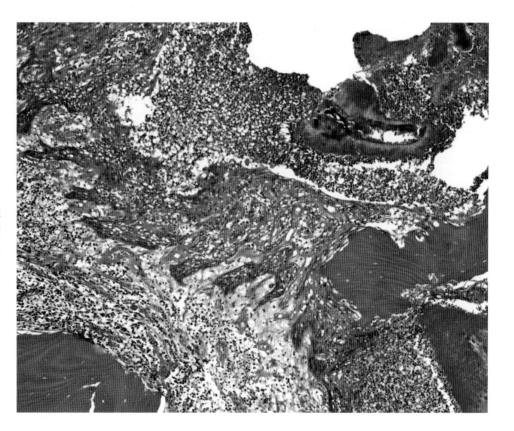

FIGURE 16-4

Fragments of dead bone may lie in contact with sinuses lined by squamous epithelium. This should not be mistaken for invasive squamous cell carcinoma. See also Figs. 16-19 and 16-20 under heading Osteoradionecrosis.

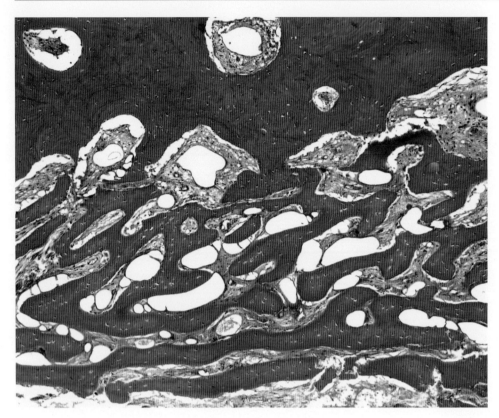

FIGURE 16-5
In case of chronic periostitis, reactive bone formation occurs parallel to the outer surface of the adjacent cortical bone.

cells as well as formation of granulation tissue and fibrosis (Fig. 16-3). Focally abscess formation may be seen. Moreover, sinuses may form, partly lined by squamous epithelium extending from the oral mucosa (Fig. 16-4).

In case of proliferative periostitis, one sees bony trabeculae that lie in a linear parallel pattern. The intervening stroma is composed of fibrous connective tissue sparsely infiltrated with lymphocytes and plasma cells (Fig. 16-5).

DIFFERENTIAL DIAGNOSIS

Acute osteomyelitis does not pose any differential diagnostic problems. Cases of chronic osteomyelitis in which formation of sclerotic bone predominates may be confused with fibrous and osseous dysplasia or Paget's disease. The latter shows highly vascular bone marrow with abundant osteoclasts, features not present in chronic osteomyelitis. A mosaic pattern of reversal lines in the bone is not reliable as it can be seen in both. Fibrous dysplasia has slender trabeculae of woven bone that are sufficiently different from the sclerotic lamellar

bone masses seen in osteomyelitis. Osseous dysplasia is composed of large masses of sclerotic lamellar bone which may occasionally result in diagnostic difficulty.

PROGNOSIS AND THERAPY

Treatment of acute osteomyelitis consists of antibiotics and debridement/removal of dead bone. Chronic osteomyelitis is more difficult to manage, unless all necrotic bone and organisms are removed. Occasionally, resection of large parts of the mandible is needed to obtain this goal.

DENTIGEROUS CYST

A dentigerous cyst is a fluid-filled sac that surrounds the crown of an unerupted tooth, mostly the maxillary canine or the mandibular third molar tooth. They are common.

DENTIGEROUS CYST DISEASE FACT SHEET	
Definition	A cyst arising from fluid accumulation between enamel organ and enamel surface in an unerupted tooth
Incidence and location	Common odontogenic cyst
	Associated with lower 3rd molar or upper canine tooth
Gender, race, and age distribution	Male > Female (2:1)
	Black >> White (5:1)
	2nd–4th decades
Clinical features	Most are incidental discoveries on radiographic studies
	May produce swelling and pain if large or associated with infection/inflammation
Radiologic features	Circumscribed radiolucency surrounding the crown of an unerupted tooth
Prognosis and treatment	Cured by simple enucleation (including involved tooth)

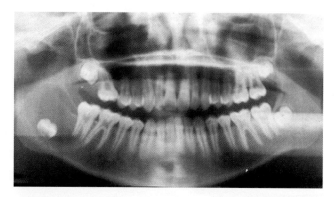

FIGURE 16-6
Panoramic radiograph showing dentigerous cyst in the dorsal area of the right mandible. The tooth crown can be seen to protrude into a well-circumscribed radiolucent bone lesion.

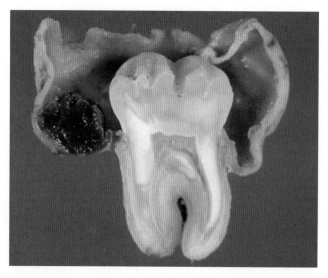

FIGURE 16-7
Gross specimen of a dentigerous cyst. The cyst wall surrounds the tooth crown and is attached at the neck of the tooth at the cemento-enamel junction.

CLINICAL FEATURES

Dentigerous cysts occur twice as often in males as in females and has the highest incidence between 10 and 40 years of age. Blacks are affected much more commonly than whites (5:1). Only when excessively large will dentigerous cysts cause swelling of the involved part of the jaw. Pain is not a conspicuous feature unless there is concomitant infection or inflammation.

RADIOLOGIC FEATURES

Radiologically, dentigerous cysts are radiolucent lesions of varying size in which the crown of an unerupted tooth protrudes (Fig. 16-6). In most instances, they are an incidental finding on oral radiographs.

PATHOLOGIC FEATURES

GROSS FINDINGS

There is a fluid-filled sac from which the roots of the involved tooth protrude. The crown of the tooth is within the cystic cavity. The cyst wall is attached to the tooth at the cemento-enamel junction and forms a collar (Fig. 16-7), a feature difficult to appreciate if the specimen is not carefully dissected.

MICROSCOPIC FINDINGS

The cyst wall has a thin epithelial lining two to three cuboidal cells thick (Fig. 16-8). If there is inflammation,

DENTIGEROUS CYST PATHOLOGIC FEATURES	
Gross findings	A tooth partly covered by a soft tissue sac
Microscopic findings	Epithelial lining of the cyst by a bi- or trilayer of cuboidal cells
	Occasionally, mucus cells and ciliated columnar cells are present
	Spongiotic squamous epithelium in cases with inflammation
	Myxoid change in the fibrous wall and nests and strands of odontogenic epithelium
Pathologic differential diagnosis	Eruption cyst, unicystic ameloblastoma, odontogenic keratocyst, myxoma

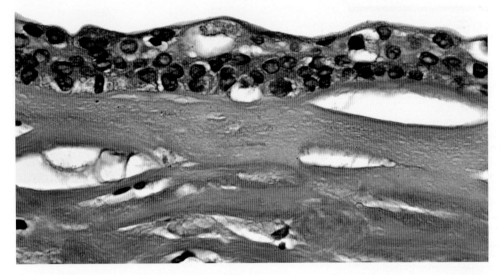

FIGURE 16-8

In its most simple form, the epithelial lining of a dentigerous cyst consists of a few layers of cuboidal epithelial cells.

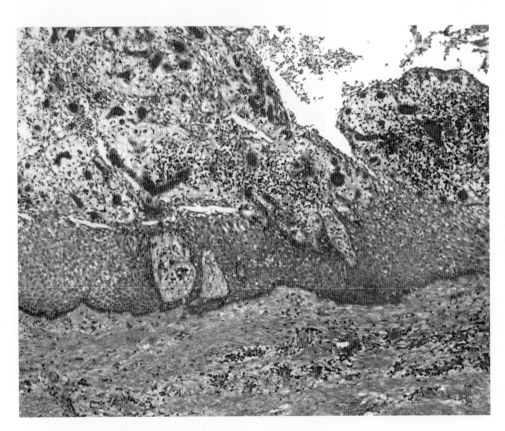

FIGURE 16-9

In case of inflammatory changes, the epithelial lining of a dentigerous cyst transforms into a multilayered squamous epithelium with reactive spongiosis.

the epithelium becomes thicker and will transform into a multilayered squamous epithelium exhibiting spongiosis and elongated rete pegs (Fig. 16-9). Occasionally, mucus-producing cells and ciliated cells may be observed (Fig. 16-10). The connective tissue component of the cyst wall may be fibrous or fibromyxomatous. The cyst wall may contain epithelial nests representing remnants of the dental lamina. The point of attachment in preserved specimens is at the level of the cemento-enamel junction on the root surface (Fig. 16-11).

DIFFERENTIAL DIAGNOSIS

The *eruption cyst* is a specific type of dentigerous cyst located in the gingival soft tissues overlying the crown of an erupting tooth. These cysts burst with progressive eruption of the associated tooth. They are lined by squamous epithelium that is thickened due to inflammatory changes in the underlying connective tissue. While there is radiographic overlap, histologic examination will sep-

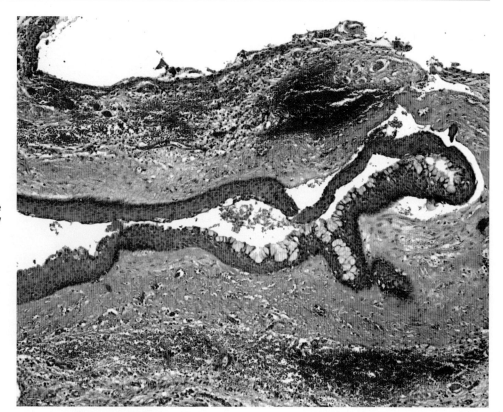

FIGURE 16-10

Goblet cells sometimes occur in the lining of a dentigerous cyst. They may be quite numerous.

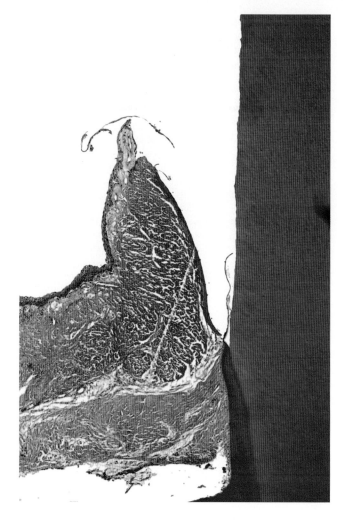

arate keratocyst and unicystic ameloblastoma from dentigerous cyst. Keratocysts are lined by a basal palisade of epithelial cells also demonstrating superficial corrugated parakeratosis. Unicystic ameloblastoma shows a basal layer of cylindrical cells with hyperchromatic nuclei, occasional reverse polarity, with a spindle cell stroma and intervening edema. Fibromyxomatous areas in the connective tissue wall of the dentigerous cyst may be confused with an odontogenic myxoma. However, myxomas are not cystic and lack an epithelial lining.

PROGNOSIS AND THERAPY

Removal of the cyst wall and the involved tooth will yield a permanent cure.

FIGURE 16-11

Wall of dentigerous cyst connected with the tooth at the cemento-enamel junction.

FIBROUS DYSPLASIA

Fibrous dysplasia is a genetically based sporadic disease that occurs in three clinical subtypes: monostotic (one bone), polyostotic (multiple bones), and McCune-Albright syndrome (multiple bones involved with skin hyperpigmentation and endocrine disturbances). Activating missense mutations in the *GNAS1* gene coding for the subunit of the stimulatory G protein are a consistent finding in the various forms of fibrous dysplasia. Also clonal chromosomal aberrations have been described, which suggest that fibrous dysplasia is a neoplastic process.

CLINICAL FEATURES

Fibrous dysplasia occurs in children and adolescents but occasionally it may be seen in older patients. The genders are equally affected. Painless swelling leading to facial asymmetry is the usual clinical presentation. The maxilla is more often involved than the mandible. In the maxilla, the swelling of the involved bones may lead to nasal obstruction and chronic sinusitis. In the skull base, compression of the cranial nerves at their foramina may cause visual impairment or hearing loss.

RADIOLOGIC FEATURES

The classical appearance is described as "orange-skin" or "ground-glass" radiopacity without defined borders (Fig. 16-12). In less typical cases, the afflicted bone may be mainly radiolucent, predominantly sclerotic or show

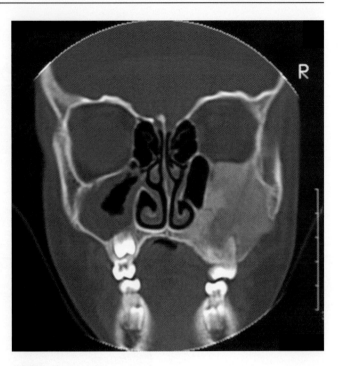

FIGURE 16-13
CT scan showing fibrous dysplasia causing obliteration of right maxillary sinus.

a cotton-wool appearance. There is a gradual merging of the radiologically abnormal bone with its surroundings. In the maxilla, there may be extension across suture lines to involve adjacent bones (Fig. 16-13).

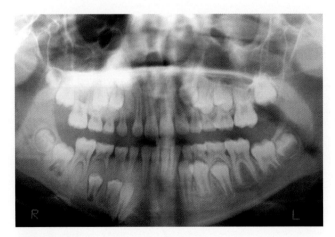

FIGURE 16-12
Panoramic radiograph showing slight increase in size of the right mandibular body. In this area, the ground-glass appearance of the bone, typical of fibrous dysplasia, is clearly visible. This picture also serves to illustrate the radiographic appearance of immature teeth in various stages of development.

FIBROUS DYSPLASIA DISEASE FACT SHEET	
Definition	Thought to be a genetic disorder of bone resulting in bone expansion
Incidence and location	Rare lesion
	Maxilla > mandible
Gender, race, and age distribution	Equal gender distribution
	Adolescents to young adults most often
	Infants may be affected when part of McCune Albright syndrome
Clinical features	Painless swelling with facial asymmetry
	Nasal obstruction and chronic sinusitis (maxilla affected)
	Cranial nerve dysfunction, visual impairment, or hearing loss in cases affecting the skull base
	Pigmented skin spots and endocrine dysfunction in polyostotic cases
Radiologic features	Ground-glass appearance blending with adjacent bone
	Radiolucencies or radiopacities, sometimes coalescing to give a cotton-wool appearance
Prognosis and treatment	Usually a self-limited disease
	Surgery for functional or cosmetic reasons
	Rarely, osteosarcoma may develop

PATHOLOGIC FEATURES

GROSS FINDINGS

Material submitted for examination mostly consists of gritty fragments of bone without further noteworthy features.

MICROSCOPIC FINDINGS

Fibrous dysplasia shows replacement of the normal bone by moderately cellular fibrous tissue containing irregularly shaped ("alphabet letters") trabeculae consisting of woven bone without rimming osteoblasts that fuse with adjacent bone (Figs. 16-14, 16-15, 16-16). Jaw lesions may also show lamellar bone (Fig. 16-17). Sometimes, tiny calcified spherules may be present.

DIFFERENTIAL DIAGNOSIS

Fibrous dysplasia must be distinguished from ossifying fibroma, osseous dysplasia, low-grade osteosarcoma, and sclerosing osteomyelitis. None of these lesions has woven bone trabeculae fusing with adjacent uninvolved bone. Ossifying fibroma and osseous dysplasia have a

FIBROUS DYSPLASIA PATHOLOGIC FEATURES	
Microscopic findings	Fusion of lesional bone with adjacent uninvolved bone
	Moderately cellular fibrous stroma
	Intermingled, immature woven bone with irregular contours/shapes
	Osteoblastic rimming is absent
Pathologic differential diagnosis	Ossifying fibroma, osseous dysplasia, low-grade osteosarcoma, chronic sclerosing osteomyelitis

variety of appearances of mineralized material and stromal cellularity. Low-grade osteosarcoma invades through the cortical bone into soft tissues. Sclerosing osteomyelitis shows coarse trabeculae of lamellar bone with edematous stroma containing lymphocytes.

PROGNOSIS AND THERAPY

In most cases fibrous dysplasia is a self-limiting disease, requiring treatment for cosmetic or functional reasons only. Rarely, an osteosarcoma may arise in fibrous dysplasia.

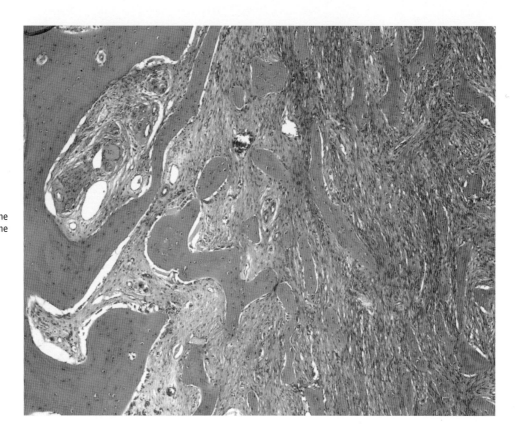

FIGURE 16-14

Continuity between the lesional bone (*right*) and the adjacent cortical bone (*left*) is clearly visible.

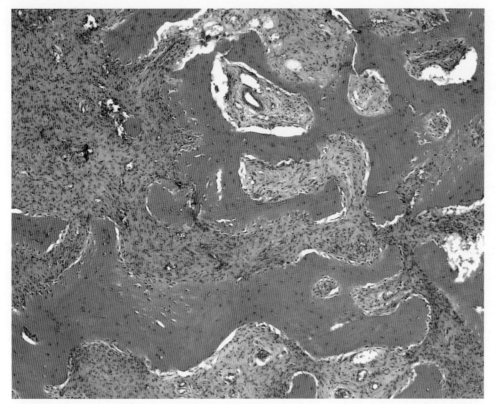

FIGURE 16-15

Irregular, plexiform trabeculae of woven bone with coarse osteocyte lacunae lying in a fibrocellular background are the histologic hallmark of fibrous dysplasia.

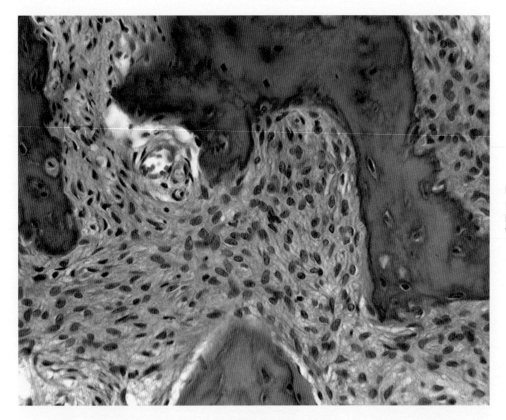

FIGURE 16-16

Fibrous, cellular stroma borders trabeculae of bone that lack osteoblastic rimming.

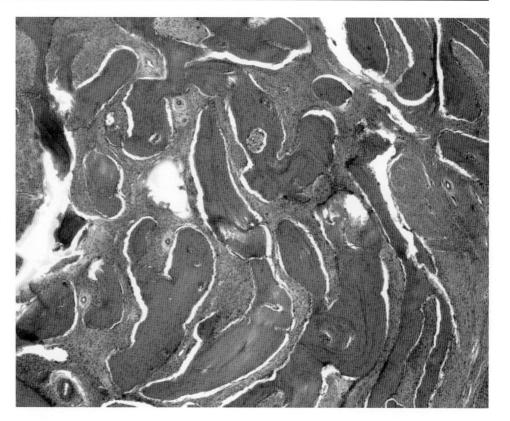

FIGURE 16-17
Bony trabeculae in fibrous dysplasia may show a parallel arrangement. This pattern sometimes is related with the presence of some lamellar bone.

OSTEORADIONECROSIS

Osteoradionecrosis is a complication of irradiation to the head and neck, developing in about 5 % of patients.

Due to a compromised microvasculature, the bone becomes hypoxic. Dead bone that does not heal is the result. Infection may ensue, but is not necessarily present.

CLINICAL FEATURES

Any patient who has received head and neck radiation is a potential candidate for the development of osteoradionecrosis. While usually in older aged male patients, all ages and both genders can be affected. Patients with osteoradionecrosis suffer from severe pain. Sinus tracts and areas of mucosal ulceration will reveal dead bone in the base. Pathologic fractures may result. Most cases involve the mandible.

RADIOLOGIC FEATURES

Ill-defined areas of radiolucency alternate with areas of increased radiopacity.

OSTEORADIONECROSIS DISEASE FACT SHEET	
Definition	Avascular bone necrosis due to irradiation
Incidence and location	A complication of radiation therapy in about 5% of patients
	Mandible is most commonly affected
Gender, race and age distribution	Male > Female (but dependent on reason for radiation)
	Tends to be older patients
Clinical features	Pain
	Sinuses and fistulas may develop
	Pathologic fracture may be presenting symptom
Radiologic features	Non-specific with ill-defined radiolucencies and opacities
Prognosis and treatment	Difficult to cure, in spite of aggressive therapy
	Hyperbaric oxygen and removal of dead bone

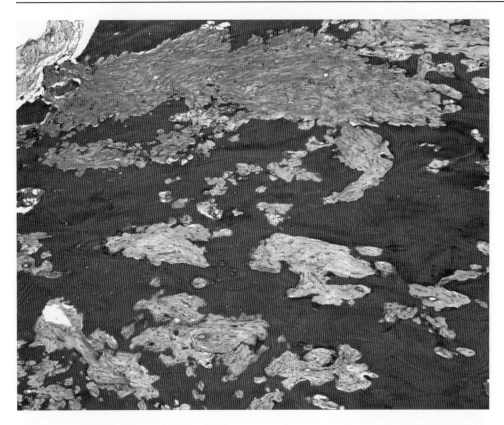

FIGURE 16-18
Large areas of dead sclerotic bone with ragged outlines indicating past resorption are surrounded by cell-poor fibrous tissue in this example of osteoradionecrosis.

PATHOLOGIC FEATURES

The submitted material mostly consists of irregular bone fragments of varying size. Histologically, there is a large overlap with osteomyelitis. Cases with only minor inflammatory changes mimic chronic sclerosing osteomyelitis (Figs. 16-18, 16-19). Cases in which concomitant infection develops, closely resembles acute osteomyelitis. In this setting, clinical history is required for the distinction.

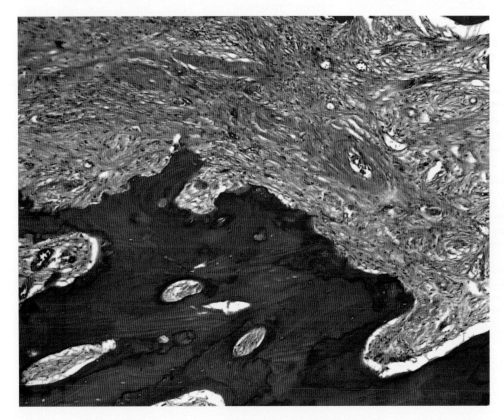

FIGURE 16-19
Prominent reversal lines indicate active bone remodeling. The adjacent stroma contains lymphocytes. The features are virtually identical to chronic sclerosing osteomyelitis.

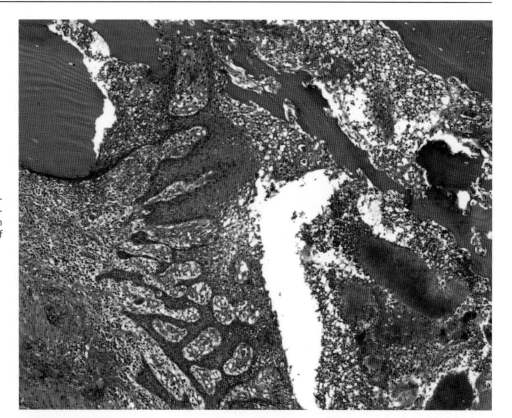

FIGURE 16-20
In case of infection, osteoradionecrosis shows abundant acute inflammatory cells with squamous epithelium lining a fistula tract. Colonies of microorganisms are apparent.

OSTEORADIONECROSIS PATHOLOGIC FEATURES	
Microscopic findings	Fragments of bone that overlap with osteomyelitis
	Sclerotic bone with empty osteocyte lacunae
	Fistula may be lined by reactive metaplastic squamous mucosa
Pathologic differential diagnosis	Osteomyelitis, recurrent squamous cell carcinoma

PROGNOSIS AND THERAPY

In some cases, treatment with hyperbaric oxygen may ameliorate the symptoms. Quite often, cure needs removal of large areas of diseased bone, and even then patients may not be symptom free.

SIMPLE BONE CYST

The solitary bone cyst, also known as *traumatic bone cyst* or *simple bone cyst* is a lesion with a poorly understood pathogenesis, although a remnant of intraosseous hemorrhage is the favored hypothesis.

DIFFERENTIAL DIAGNOSIS

While osteoradionecrosis generally does not pose any diagnostic difficulty per se, the reason for radiation is often a squamous cell carcinoma (or other head and neck malignancy). Therefore, in patients who have a concomitant infection and fistula formation (Fig. 16-20), the separation of recurrent tumor from reactive changes in the fistula epithelium may be a challenge. Frequently, the granulation tissue and squamous epithelium will be in contact with necrotic bone. Careful inspection shows reactive epithelial alterations rather than malignant cytology. In most cases, awareness of the potential pitfall is sufficient to avoid the error.

SIMPLE BONE CYST DISEASE FACT SHEET	
Definition	Fluid-filled bone cavity lacking a definable wall
Incidence and location	Uncommon
	Mandible >>> Maxilla (9:1)
Gender, race, and age distribution	Slight male predominance
	Usually 2nd decade
Clinical features	Incidental finding on radiographs performed for a different reason
Radiologic features	Circumscribed radiolucency
Prognosis and treatment	Excellent without any treatment required

CLINICAL FEATURES

There are seldom clinical findings, as they are discovered incidentally on oral radiographs taken for a different reason. Patients are usually young (2nd decade), with a slight male predominance. The mandible is affected much more commonly than the maxilla (9:1), with lesions usually identified in the molar region.

RADIOLOGIC FEATURES

Radiographs show a well-circumscribed radiolucent cavity of variable size. Mandibular cases may occupy the entire body and ramus.

PATHOLOGIC FEATURES

At surgical exploration, one encounters a fluid-filled cavity. Material for histologic examination may be difficult to obtain, as a soft tissue lining of the bony cavity may be entirely absent or very thin. If present, it usually consists only of loose fibrovascular tissue; it may also contain granulation tissue with signs of previous hemorrhage, such as cholesterol clefts and hemosiderin-laden macrophages. Dystrophic calcification may also

SIMPLE BONE CYST PATHOLOGIC FEATURES	
Microscopic findings	Bony trabeculae with some fibrin and a thin fibrous layer
	May have dystrophic calcification
Pathologic differential diagnosis	Must confirm adequate histologic sample of any gnathic cyst before diagnosing a simple cyst

occur (Figs. 16-21, 16-22, 16-23). Sometimes, this cyst is associated with osseous dysplasia.

DIFFERENTIAL DIAGNOSIS

There are no differential diagnostic considerations, although it is important to realize that insufficiently sampled gnathic cysts may have histologic overlap with a simple bone cyst. Therefore, adequate sampling is imperative to avoid misdiagnosis.

PROGNOSIS AND THERAPY

No therapy is required once the diagnosis has been made.

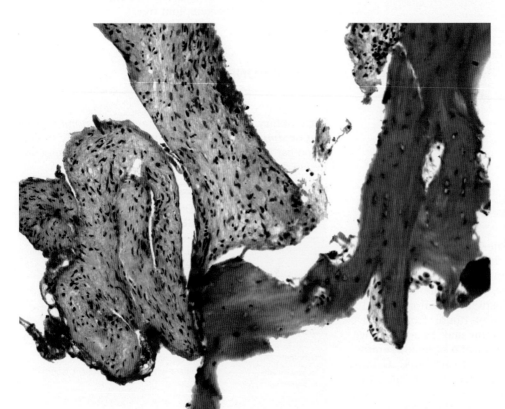

FIGURE 16-21
Biopsies of a simple bone cyst contain thin pieces of lamellar bone and some fibrous tissue.

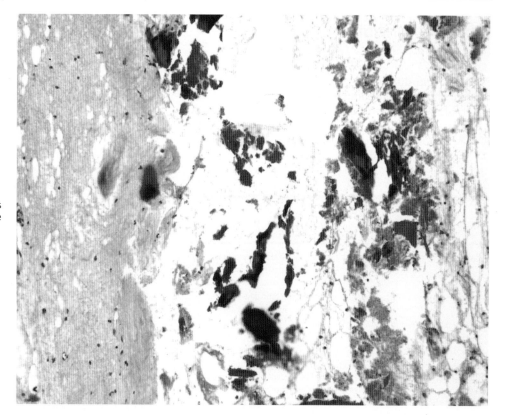

FIGURE 16-22

Fibrin and dystrophic calcifications sometimes are also found in simple bone cysts.

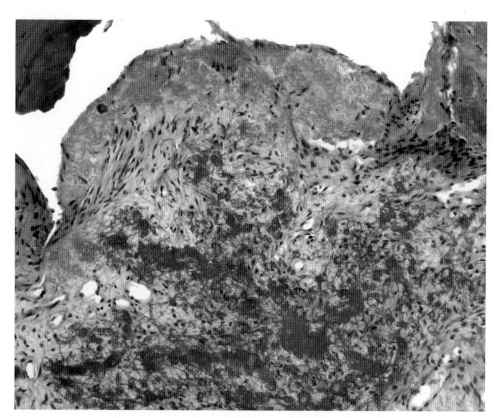

FIGURE 16-23

Rarely, more conspicuous fibrous tissue is present in the wall of a simple bone cyst, usually together with fibrin and threadlike calcifications. These calcifications may also occur in juvenile psammomatoid ossifying fibroma.

NASOPALATINE DUCT CYST

Nasopalatine duct cysts arise within the nasopalatine canal from epithelial remnants of the nasopalatine duct. They are uncommon, accounting for <3% of gnathic cyst-like tumors.

NASOPALATINE DUCT CYST DISEASE FACT SHEET	
Definition	A cyst in the nasopalatine canal and derived from the nasopalatine duct remnants
Incidence and location	One of the more common jaw cysts, confined to the anterior maxilla
Gender and age distribution	Male > Female 4th–6th decades
Clinical features	Swelling of the anterior palate, pain in case of concomitant inflammation
Radiologic features	Pear-shaped radiolucency between roots of left and right central incisor tooth Roots diverging to give way to the expanding cyst
Prognosis and treatment	Excision is curative

CLINICAL FEATURES

Nasopalatine duct cysts are seen most commonly in the 4th–6th decades of life with a male predilection. They manifest as a palatal swelling in the anterior part of the palate, just dorsal to both central incisor teeth. In case of concomitant inflammation, pain may also be present.

RADIOLOGIC FEATURES

Radiologically, they present as radiolucent lesions situated between the roots of both maxillary central incisor teeth.

PATHOLOGIC FEATURES

The cyst lining may be pseudostratified columnar ciliated epithelium, stratified squamous epithelium, columnar or cuboidal epithelium, and combinations of these. As surgical treatment involves emptying the nasopalatine canal, the specimen includes the artery and nerve that run through it (Fig. 16-24). The artery and nerve may be the most diagnostic feature, as the specific epithelial histomorphology may be obscured by inflammatory changes.

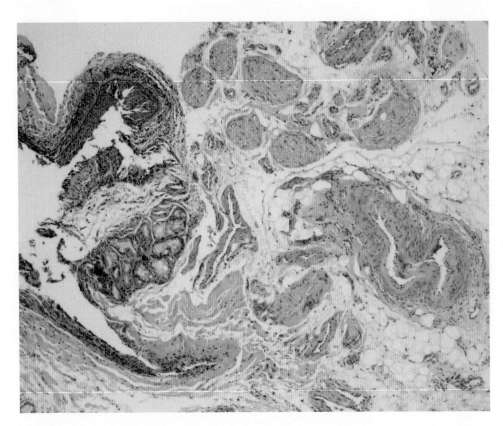

FIGURE 16-24

Note the nerve bundles and vessels in the nasopalatine duct cyst wall. The epithelium may be either squamous or columnar.

NASOPALATINE DUCT CYST PATHOLOGIC FEATURES	
Gross findings	As with any other cyst
Microscopic findings	A fibrous cyst wall lined by columnar, ciliated and mucus cells and containing large vessels and nerve bundles
Pathologic differential diagnosis	Radicular cyst arising from one of the anterior maxillary teeth

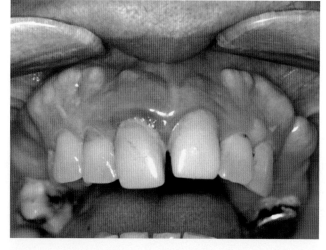

FIGURE 16-25
Photograph showing tori as bony outgrowths on the buccal side of the maxillary alveolar process.

DIFFERENTIAL DIAGNOSIS

Nasopalatine duct cyst may be mimicked by a radicular cyst that has arisen in association with one or both central incisor teeth. When one of these teeth is nonvital and the cyst wall shows inflammatory alterations with its inherent squamous metaplasia of the epithelial lining, distinction between both cyst types may be impossible. When adjacent teeth are vital, radicular cyst can be ruled out as these only arise in association with nonvital teeth.

PROGNOSIS AND THERAPY

Recurrences may develop in up to 11 % of patients. Excision of the cyst and nasopalatine canal is the appropriate treatment.

TORI

Tori are common bony outgrowths on the alveolar process of the jaw.

CLINICAL FEATURES

Women are affected slightly more frequently than men. Blacks are also affected more commonly than whites. The lesion can present at any age. Tori present as irregular, smooth bony outgrowths at the buccal surface of the lower as well as the upper jaw. They may also occur on the lingual side of the mandible and in the midline of the hard palate. The covering mucosa is not involved (Figs. 16-25, 16-26).

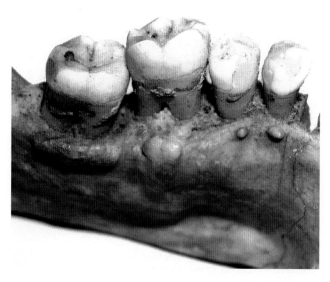

FIGURE 16-26
Dried specimen of mandible showing tori as bony thickenings at its lingual surface.

TORI DISEASE FACT SHEET	
Definition	Benign bony protuberances
Incidence and location	Common intraoral lesion
	Alveolar process or hard palate
Gender, race and age distribution	Females only slightly more common than males
	Black > White
	Any age affected
Clinical features	Bony swellings covered with intact mucosa
Radiologic features	Cloudy radiopacities superimposed on the teeth contour
Prognosis and treatment	Only corrective jaw contouring needed in some cases

TORI
PATHOLOGIC FEATURES

Microscopic findings	Lamellar bone with fibrous or fatty tissue in marrow cavities

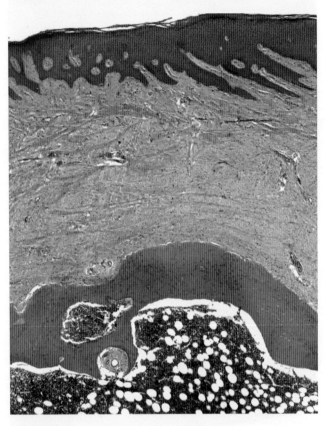

FIGURE 16-27
Tori consists of lamellar bone, with hematopoietic marrow in this case. Periosteum and mucosa do not show any abnormalities.

RADIOLOGIC FEATURES

Tori present themselves as ill-defined cloudy radiopacities.

PATHOLOGIC FEATURES

Tori consist of lamellar bone. The marrow cavities may contain fatty or fibrous tissue. Sometimes hematopoietic marrow is observed (Fig. 16-27).

DIFFERENTIAL DIAGNOSIS

Characteristic clinical appearance precludes any differential diagnostic problem.

PROGNOSIS AND THERAPY

Treatment is not necessary, unless in case of mechanical problems when wearing dentures. In those cases, some recontouring of the jaw may be required.

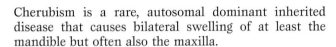

CHERUBISM

Cherubism is a rare, autosomal dominant inherited disease that causes bilateral swelling of at least the mandible but often also the maxilla.

CLINICAL FEATURES

Males are affected more commonly than females and most patients present in early childhood. There is often a history of other afflicted family members. The resulting painless, symmetrical, facial deformity mimics the angelic faces of the cherubs portrayed in Renaissance and Baroque paintings, hence its name (Fig. 16-28). Sometimes there is upward displacement of both eyes. The disease progression is self-limited, stabilizing at

CHERUBISM
DISEASE FACT SHEET

Definition	Rare autosomal dominant inherited disease resulting in bilateral, symmetrical jaw swelling due to proliferation of fibrous tissue with giant cells
Incidence and location	Rare
	Bilateral lower jaws and commonly in upper jaws too
Gender, race, and age distribution	Male > Female
	Young children
Clinical features	Painless, symmetrical facial deformity
	Jaw swelling gives "angelic" facial appearance
	Upward displacement of the eyes uncommon
	Other family members affected
Radiologic features	Bilateral symmetric involvement
	Cortical expansion and attenuation
	Multilocular, soap bubble–like radiolucencies and displaced tooth germs
Prognosis and treatment	Disease burns out with puberty
	Remediation of facial deformity with surgery

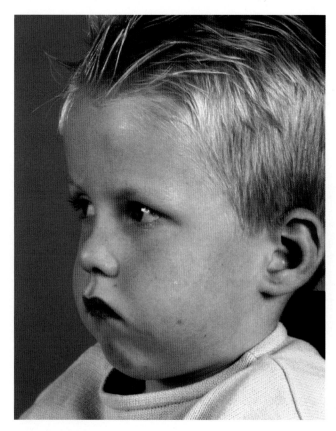

FIGURE 16-28
Young boy showing the maxillary swelling typical for cherubism (shown with permission).

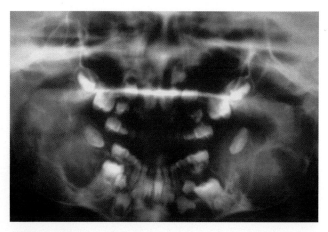

FIGURE 16-29
Cherubism. Panoramic radiograph showing bilateral soap bubble-like radiolucencies with displaced teeth and tooth germs

CHERUBISM PATHOLOGIC FEATURES	
Gross findings	Brown soft tissue fragments, sometimes including teeth or tooth germs
Microscopic findings	Multinucleated, osteoclast-like giant cells, clustered around blood
	Fibrocellular tissue of variable cellularity
	Bone formation is absent, but remodeled bone may be seen at the periphery
Pathologic differential diagnosis	Aneurysmal bone cyst, giant cell granuloma, ameloblastic fibroma, odontogenic myxoma

the end of puberty. Complications developing from the jaw disorder can result in poor or delayed dentition, impacted teeth, and malaligned teeth.

RADIOLOGIC FEATURES

Radiographic findings are not pathognomonic, but the presence of bilateral, usually symmetrical involvement of the maxilla and mandible is certainly most suggested. The affected jaw areas show cortical expansion and attenuation (thinning) as well as a soap bubble-like multilocular radiolucency. Teeth and tooth germs may be displaced (Fig. 16-29).

PATHOLOGIC FEATURES

GROSS FINDINGS

The submitted material mostly consists of brown soft tissue fragments. Teeth or tooth germs may also be recognized if removed as part of the treatment.

MICROSCOPIC FINDINGS

Cherubism shows multinucleated, osteoclast-like giant cells lying in a fibroblastic background tissue (Fig. 16-30). The fibroblastic tissue may vary in cellularity from very dense to cell-poor. Mitotic figures may be encountered but are usually not numerous and not atypical. The giant cells mostly cluster in areas of hemorrhage, but they also may lie more dispersed among the lesion. Bone formation is usually confined to the periphery of the lesion, as a reactive remodeling (Fig. 16-31). There may also be a component consisting of immature odontogenic tissue due to developing tooth germs lying within the lesional tissue.

ANCILLARY STUDIES

Cherubism is an autosomal dominant inherited condition, which has a number of mutations, including mutations in the c-Abl-binding protein SH3BP2 and FGF-RIII (fibroblast growth factor receptor III) gene. Further studies are elucidating the genetic nature of this rare disease.

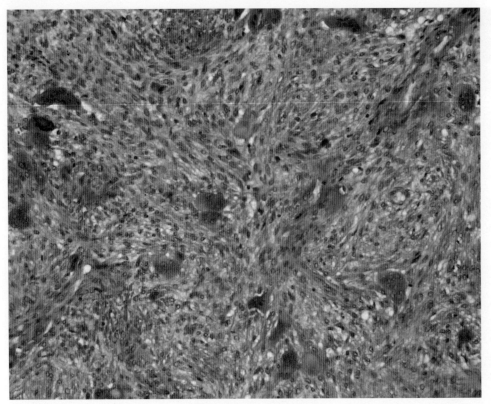

FIGURE 16-30
Histologically cherubism shows moderately cellular fibroblastic tissue with dispersed osteoclast-like giant cells and some extravasation of erythrocytes.

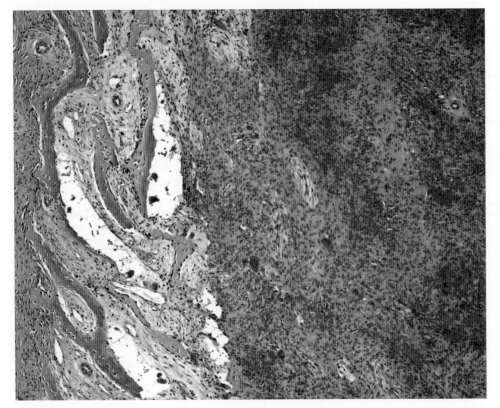

FIGURE 16-31
Cherubism does not show bone formation, but instead, reactive remodeled bone is seen at the border or periphery of the lesion.

DIFFERENTIAL DIAGNOSIS

Cherubism needs to be distinguished from giant cell granuloma and aneurysmal bone cyst. Both are histologically identical but do not show the symmetric involvement of multiple jaw quadrants. Concomitant presence of immature odontogenic tissues should not be interpreted as evidence for an odontogenic tumor, such as an ameloblastic fibroma or immature odontoma.

PROGNOSIS AND THERAPY

With the onset of puberty, the lesions loose their activity and may mature to fibrous tissue and bone. Facial deformity may necessitate cosmetic surgery.

OSSEOUS DYSPLASIA

Osseous dysplasia, formerly called cemento-osseous dysplasia, is a pathologic process of unknown etiology affecting the tooth-bearing jaw areas in the vicinity of the tooth apices and thought to arise from proliferation of periodontal ligament fibroblasts that may deposit bone and cementum.

CLINICAL FEATURES

Osseous dysplasia occurs in various histologically identical but clinically and radiographically different types. Therefore, radiographic studies are imperative before rending a diagnosis. *Periapical osseous dysplasia* occurs in the anterior mandible and involves only a few adjacent teeth. A similar limited lesion in a posterior jaw quadrant is known as *focal osseous dysplasia*. Both types are mostly incidental findings on radiographs taken for some other reason. *Florid osseous dysplasia* is also nonexpansile but involves more than one jaw quadrant, and is typically seen in middle-aged black females. *Familial gigantiform cementoma* is expansile, involves multiple quadrants, and occurs at a young age.

RADIOLOGIC FEATURES

Lesions are either predominantly radiolucent, predominantly radiodense or mixed, depending on the ratio of hard tissue to soft tissue in an individual case. They are characteristically located in the tooth-bearing part of the

OSSEOUS DYSPLASIA DISEASE FACT SHEET	
Definition	Tooth-associated lesions consisting of fibrous tissue and bone separated into several clinical subtypes
Incidence and location	Rare
	Periapical osseous dysplasia: anterior mandible
	Focal osseous dysplasia: posterior mandible
	Florid osseous dysplasia: multifocal simultaneously
	Familial gigantiform cementoma: all jaw quadrants simultaneously
Gender, race, and age distribution	Periapical osseous dysplasia: women, black, rare before 25
	Focal osseous dysplasia: women, white, 4th–5th decades
	Florid osseous dysplasia: women, black, middle aged
	Familial gigantiform cementoma: young children
Clinical features	Periapical and focal osseous dysplasia are incidental findings
	Florid osseous dysplasia: pain and swelling, frequent concomitant infection
	Familial gigantiform cementoma: swelling
Radiologic findings	Mixed radiodense radiolucent lesions adjacent to the roots of teeth, findings dependent on the ratio of hard to soft tissue
Prognosis and treatment	Benign lesion
	Treatment for infection, sclerotic bone masses, and facial deformities

jaw from which they may spread to adjacent areas (Fig. 16-32).

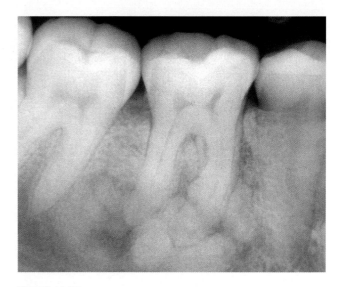

FIGURE 16-32

Radiograph of focal osseous dysplasia showing partly radiolucent, partly radiopaque lesion in the region of the tooth apices.

PATHOLOGIC FEATURES

Osseous dysplasia consists of cellular fibrous tissue, trabeculae of woven and/or lamellar bone and spherules of cementum-like material (Fig. 16-33). Moreover, deeply basophilic amorphous particles may be present (Fig. 16-34). The ratio of fibrous tissue to mineralized material varies, with increased calcification identified in cases of long duration. Osseous dysplasia lacks demarcation and will merge with adjacent cortical or medullary bone, but the mineralized tissue does not connect with the root surface (Fig. 16-35).

DIFFERENTIAL DIAGNOSIS

The differential diagnosis includes ossifying fibroma, fibrous dysplasia, and sclerosing osteomyelitis. Ossifying fibroma usually is a single, localized lesion, predominantly radiolucent with radiodense areas that expand the jaw. Separation on histology alone may be impossible, requiring radiographic and clinical features. Sclerotic lamellar bone trabeculae and well-vascularized fibrous tissue with lymphocytes and plasma cells define sclerosing osteomyelitis, which lacks cementum-like areas and fibrocellular soft tissue. Fibrous dysplasia is composed of irregular trabeculae of woven bone without osteoblastic rimming, whereas osseous dysplasia shows woven as well as lamellar bone, acellular mineralized particles resembling cementum, and amorphous basophilic particles.

PROGNOSIS AND THERAPY

Treatment for all forms of osseous dysplasia is necessitated when there is infection or sclerotic bone masses which result in cosmetic deformities.

OSSEOUS DYSPLASIA PATHOLOGIC FEATURES	
Microscopic findings	Fibrous tissue of varying cellularity
	Woven bone, lamellar bone, amorphous basophilic calcifications and smoothly contoured acellular particles resembling cementum
	May merge with bone, but never touches tooth
Pathologic differential diagnosis	Ossifying fibroma, chronic sclerosing osteomyelitis, fibrous dysplasia

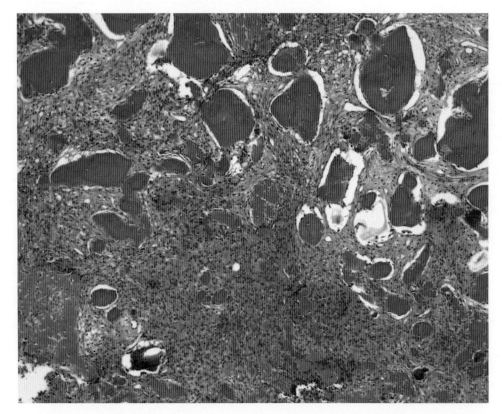

FIGURE 16-33

Focal osseous dysplasia consists of fibroblastic tissue with bony particles of varying size that are lamellar and plexiform.

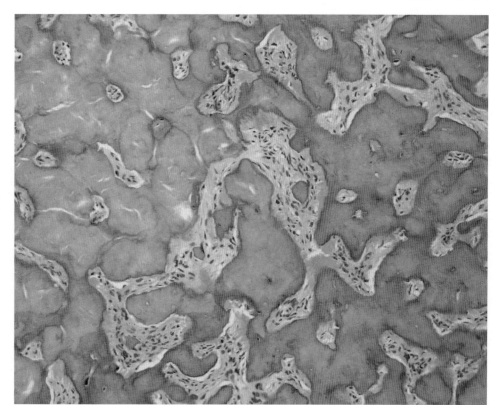

FIGURE 16-34

The bony component in this case of osseous dysplasia consists of slightly basophilic material with a smooth outline and prominent reversal lines.

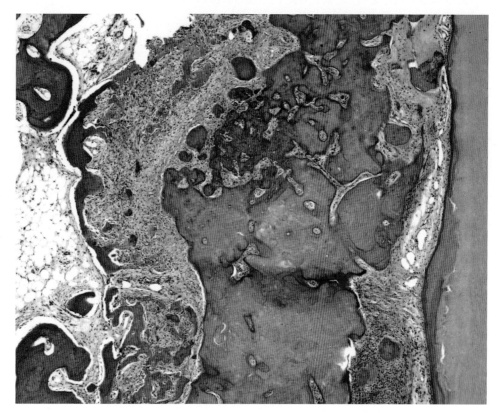

FIGURE 16-35

Osseous dysplasia is interposed between bone (*left side*) and tooth surface (*right side*). The lesional tissue may fuse with surrounding bone but the tooth surface is not touched. The variation in size, outline, and tinctorial qualities of bone in osseous dysplasia is also illustrated in this case.

SUGGESTED READING

Osteomyelitis

1. Hudson JW: Osteomyelitis of the jaws: a 50-year perspective. J Oral Maxillofac Surg 1993;51:1294–1301.
2. Schneider LC, Mesa LM: Differences between florid osseous dysplasia and chronic diffuse sclerosing osteomyelitis. Oral Surg Oral Med Oral Pathol 1990;70:308–312.
3. Suei Y, Tanimoto K, Taguchi A, et al.: Chronic recurrent multifocal osteomyelitis involving the mandible. Oral Surg Oral Med Oral Pathol 1994;78:156–162.

Dentigerous Cyst

1. Dunsche A, Babendererde O, Luttges J, Springer IN: Dentigerous cyst versus unicystic ameloblastoma—differential diagnosis in routine histology. J Oral Pathol Med 2003;32:486–491.
2. Regezi JA: Odontogenic cysts, odontogenic tumors, fibroosseous, and giant cell lesions of the jaws. Mod Pathol. 2002;15:331–341.
3. Shear M: Cysts of the Oral Regions, 3rd ed. Oxford: Wright, 1992.

Fibrous Dysplasia

1. Alawi F: Benign fibro-osseous diseases of the maxillofacial bones. A review and differential diagnosis. Am J Clin Pathol 2002;118(Suppl): S50–S70.
2. Brannon RB, Fowler CB: Benign fibro-osseous lesions: a review of current concepts. Adv Anat Pathol 2001;8:126–143.
3. Ebata K, Takeshi U, Tohnai I, Kaneda T: Chondrosarcoma and osteosarcoma arising in polyostotic fibrous dysplasia. J Oral Maxillofac Surg 1992;50:761–764.
4. Eversole LR, Sabes WR, Rovin S: Fibrous dysplasia: a nosologic problem in the diagnosis of fibro-osseous lesions of the jaws. J Oral Pathol 1972;1:189–220.
5. Jundt G: Fibrous dysplasia. In: Barnes EL, Eveson JW, Reichart P, Sidransky D, eds. Pathology and Genetics of Head and Neck Tumours. Kleihues P, Sobin LH, series eds. World Health Organization Classification of Tumours. Lyon, France: IARC Press, 2005:321–322.
6. Riminucci M, Liu B, Corsi A, et al.: The histopathology of fibrous dysplasia of bone in patients with activating mutations of the Gs a gene: Site-specific patterns and recurrent histological hallmarks. J Pathol 1999;187:249–258.
7. Slootweg PJ: Maxillofacial fibro-osseous lesions: classification and differential diagnosis. Semin Diagn Pathol 1996;13:104–112.

Osteoradionecrosis

1. Marx RE, Johnson RP: Studies in the radiobiology of osteoradionecrosis and their clinical significance. Oral Surg Oral Med Oral Pathol 1987;64:379–390.
2. Nemeth Z, Somogyi A, Takacsi-Nagy Z, et al.: Possibilities of preventing osteoradionecrosis during complex therapy of tumors of the oral cavity. Pathol Oncol Res 2000;6:53–58.
3. Pasquier D, Hoelscher T, Schmutz J, et al.: Hyperbaric oxygen therapy in the treatment of radio-induced lesions in normal tissues: a literature review. Radiother Oncol 2004;72:1–13.
4. Reuther T, Schuster T, Mende U, Kubler A: Osteoradionecrosis of the jaws as a side effect of radiotherapy of head and neck tumour patients—a report of a thirty year retrospective review. Int J Oral Maxillofac Surg 2003;32:289–295.
5. Toljanic JA, Ali M, Haraf DJ, et al.: Osteoradionecrosis of the jaws as a risk factor in radiotherapy: a report of an eight-year retrospective review. Oncol Rep 1998;5:345–349.
6. Vissink A, Burlage FR, Spijkervet FK, et al.: Prevention and treatment of the consequences of head and neck radiotherapy. Crit Rev Oral Biol Med 2003;14:213–225.

Simple Bone Cyst

1. Saito Y, Hoshina Y, Nagamine T, et al.: Simple bone cyst. A clinical and histopathologic study of fifteen cases. Oral Surg Oral Med Oral Pathol 1992;74:487–491.
2. Tong AC, Ng IO, Yan BS: Variations in clinical presentations of the simple bone cyst: report of cases. J Oral Maxillofac Surg 2003;61: 1487–1491.

Nasopalatine Duct Cyst

1. Allard RH, van der Kwast WA, van der Waal I: Nasopalatine duct cyst. Review of the literature and report of 22 cases. Int J Oral Surg 1981;10: 447–461.
2. Choi JH, Cho JH, Kang HJ, et al.: Nasolabial cyst: a retrospective analysis of 18 cases. Ear Nose Throat J 2002;81:94–96.
3. Elliott KA, Franzese CB, Pitman KT: Diagnosis and surgical management of nasopalatine duct cysts. Laryngoscope 2004;114:1336–1340.
4. Swanson KS, Kaugars GE, Gunsolley JC: Nasopalatine duct cyst: an analysis of 334 cases. J Oral Maxillofac Surg 1991;49:268–271.
5. Vasconcelos R, de Aguiar MF, Castro W, et al.: Retrospective analysis of 31 cases of nasopalatine duct cyst. Oral Dis 1999;5:325–328.

Tori

1. Antoniades DZ, Belazi M, Papanayiotou P: Concurrence of torus palatinus with palatal and buccal exostoses: case report and review of the literature. Oral Surg Oral Med Oral Pathol Oral Radiol Endod 1998;85: 552–557.
2. Eckles RL, Miller RI: Tori: a common but neglected entity. Gen Dent 1988;36:417–420.
3. Jainkittivong A, Langlais RP. Buccal and palatal exostoses: prevalence and concurrence with tori. Oral Surg Oral Med Oral Pathol Oral Radiol Endod 2000;90:48–53.
4. Seah YH. Torus palatinus and torus mandibularis: a review of the literature. Aust Dent J 1995;40:318–321.

Cherubism

1. Beaman FD, Bancroft LW, Peterson JJ, et al.: Imaging characteristics of cherubism. AJR Am J Roentgenol 2004;182:1051–1054.
2. Jundt G: Cherubism. In: Barnes EL, Eveson JW, Reichart P, Sidransky D, eds. Pathology and Genetics of Head and Neck Tumours. Kleihues P, Sobin LH, series eds. World Health Organization Classification of Tumours. Lyon, France: IARC Press, 2005:325.
3. Ozkan Y, Varol A, Turker N, et al.: Clinical and radiological evaluation of cherubism: a sporadic case report and review of the literature. Int J Pediatr Otorhinolaryngol 2003;67:1005–1012.
4. Schultze-Mosgau S, Holbach LM, Wiltfang J: Cherubism: clinical evidence and therapy. J Craniofac Surg 2003;14:201–208.
5. Tiziani V, Reichenberger E, Buzzo CL, et al.: The gene for cherubism maps to chromosome 4p16. Am J Hum Genet 1999;65:158–166.
6. von Wowern N: Cherubism: a 36-year long-term follow-up of 2 generations in different families and review of the literature. Oral Surg Oral Med Oral Pathol Oral Radiol Endod 2000;90:765–772.

Osseous Dysplasia

1. Brannon RB, Fowler CB: Benign fibro-osseous lesions: a review of current concepts. Adv Anat Pathol 2001;8:126–143.
2. Schneider LC, Mesa LM: Differences between florid osseous dysplasia and chronic diffuse sclerosing osteomyelitis. Oral Surg Oral Med Oral Pathol 1990;70:308–312.
3. Slootweg PJ: Maxillofacial fibro-osseous lesions: classification and differential diagnosis. Semin Diagn Pathol 1996;13:104–112.
4. Slootweg PJ: Osseous dysplasias. In: Barnes EL, Eveson JW, Reichart P, Sidransky D, eds. Pathology and Genetics of Head and Neck Tumours. Kleihues P, Sobin LH, series eds. World Health Organization Classification of Tumours. Lyon, France: IARC Press, 2005:323.
5. Su L, Weathers DR, Waldron CA: Distinguishing features of focal cemento-osseous dysplasias and cemento-ossifying fibromas. II. A clinical and radiologic spectrum of 316 cases. Oral Surg Oral Med Oral Pathol Oral Radiol Endod 1997;84:540–549.
6. Summerlin DJ, Tomich CE: Focal cemento-osseous dysplasia: A clinicopathologic study of 221 cases. Oral Surg Oral Med Oral Pathol 1994;78: 611–620.

17 Benign Neoplasms of the Gnathic Bones

Brenda Nelson

OSSIFYING FIBROMA

Benign fibro-osseous lesions are characterized by the replacement of native bone by fibrous and mineralized tissues. The ossifying fibroma is unique among these lesions as it is categorized as a neoplasm and requires more extensive treatment. The other benign fibro-osseous lesions, fibrous dysplasia and cemento-osseous dysplasia, can be difficult to differentiate, requiring radiographic and clinical correlation to make an accurate diagnosis. Bone and/or cementum may be present, and so *cementifying fibroma* and *cemento-ossifying fibroma* are also used to describe these lesions.

CLINICAL FEATURES

Ossifying fibromas are found much more commonly in the mandible (90%) than the maxilla, specifically affecting the molar-premolar area. Patients in the 3rd–4th decades are most affected, with a high female to male ratio (5 : 1). Small lesions are usually asymptomatic, often incidental findings on routine dental radiographs, while larger lesions can result in significant cosmetic and functional morbidity, especially with resection and reconstruction.

RADIOLOGIC FEATURES

Radiographic images are essential to the diagnosis, and a diagnosis should not be rendered without radiographs or their reliable interpretation. Ossifying fibromas are characteristically well-demarcated unilocular or multilocular radiolucent lesions with varying degrees of radiopacity (Fig. 17-1). The radiopacities correlate with the mineralized component of the tumor. Large lesions may cause displacement of teeth, root divergence, or alterations of associated structures. Furthermore, a characteristic downward bowing of the mandible may be helpful in developing a radiographic differential diagnosis.

PATHOLOGIC FEATURES

GROSS FINDINGS

Lesions are well demarcated, frequently described as "shelling out" of the bone. The intact tumor is a smooth, glistening, white, firm-elastic mass.

OSSIFYING FIBROMA DISEASE FACT SHEET	
Definition	A well-demarcated neoplasm of gnathic bones composed of fibrocellular tissue and mineralized material of varying appearances
Incidence and location	Mandible >> maxilla (90%), premolar-molar area specifically
Morbidity and mortality	Aggressive behavior is reported with functional morbidity and cosmetic disruption
Gender, race, and age distribution	Female >> Male (5 : 1) Wide age range with a predilection for 3rd–4th decade
Clinical features	Small lesions are asymptomatic, incidentally discovered Larger lesions may cause facial deformity, malocclusion and pain
Prognosis and treatment	Clinical follow-up for recurrences Surgical curettage or enucleation

OSSIFYING FIBROMA PATHOLOGIC FEATURES	
Gross findings	Lesions are well circumscribed, usually with a smooth surface Easily separated from bone ("shell out")
Microscopic findings	Variably cellular fibrous stroma with calcified tissue Mineralized material may be cementum-like basophilic deposits or trabeculae of lamellar or woven bone Osteoblastic rimming is noted along with mitotic figures
Pathologic differential diagnosis	Fibrous dysplasia, cemento-osseous dysplasia, active ossifying fibroma

459

MICROSCOPIC FINDINGS

Microscopically, lesions are composed of varying amounts of fibrous stroma with varying amounts and types of mineralized material. The fibrous tissue can be closely packed (Fig. 17-2) to nearly acellular. The mineralized tissue may present as cementum-like basophillic deposits, trabeculae of lamellar bone, or trabeculae of woven bone (Fig. 17-3). Characteristically, plump osteoblasts are seen to rim the bony trabeculae. Mitotic figures may be seen, in addition to areas of pseudocystic areas of degeneration and hemorrhage.

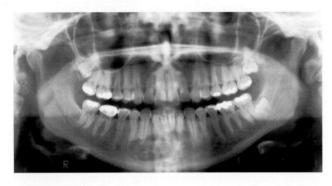

FIGURE 17-1

Panoramic radiograph. The lesion is a well-defined, unilocular, radiolucent defect in the anterior mandible. There is variable radiopacity and a sclerotic border.

DIFFERENTIAL DIAGNOSIS

Quality radiographs and a complete clinical history are *required*, as other benign fibro-osseous lesions may be indistinguishable histologically. Fibrous dysplasia classically appears with an "orange peel" texture in radiographs, while cemento-osseous dysplasia usually has a sclerotic radiodensity. Ossifying fibroma is usually radiolucent. Grossly, both cemento-osseous dysplasia and fibrous dysplasia are submitted as small mineralized fragments, while ossifying fibroma is generally an intact tumor mass or large fragments. Microscopically, osteoblastic rimming is seen less frequently in these other entities. If no radiographic or clinical information is available, only a preliminary diagnosis of benign fibro-osseous lesion should be rendered until more information can be obtained. Definitive diagnosis is important, as the treatment and prognosis of these lesions is different.

PROGNOSIS AND THERAPY

Close clinical follow-up is indicated to monitor the patient for recurrences. Should recurrences be detected, a more aggressive surgical resection may be indicated, with possible reconstruction. Surgical enucleation and curettage is usually the treatment of choice.

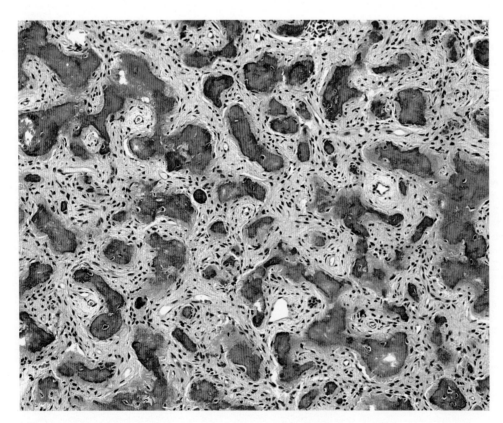

FIGURE 17-2

A cellular fibroblastic stroma with osteoid formation.

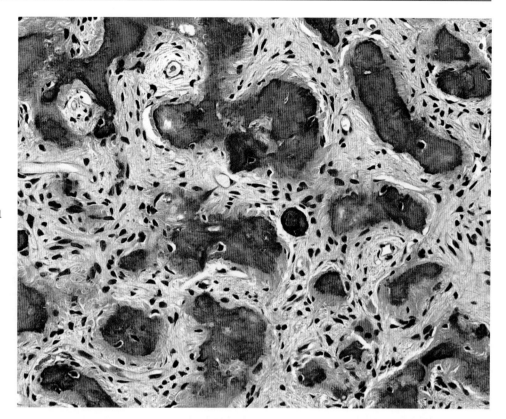

FIGURE 17-3
Osteoid and cementum-like material in a cellular stroma.

JUVENILE/ACTIVE OSSIFYING FIBROMA

Juvenile ossifying fibroma is an ossifying fibroma variant characterized by rapid and destructive growth. The term *active ossifying fibroma* is also used because the tumor does not occur exclusively in young individuals.

CLINICAL FEATURES

Juvenile ossifying fibroma is an uncommon entity, and is considerably more rare than its conventional counterpart. While found most commonly in children <15 years old, older patients can be affected. The maxilla and paranasal sinuses are most often affected, in contrast to ossifying fibroma. Patients present with rapid, disfiguring growth (Fig. 17-4). Radical surgery may be associated with increased morbidity.

RADIOLOGIC FEATURES

Radiographically the lesion presents as a well-delineated, expansile radiolucent lesion with variable focal calcifications. Rarely lesions may demonstrate invasive growth and affect adjacent structures.

JUVENILE/ACTIVE OSSIFYING FIBROMA DISEASE FACT SHEET	
Definition	Ossifying fibroma variant characterized by rapid and destructive growth and an increased cellularity
Incidence and location	Uncommon
	Maxilla and paranasal sinuses more common than mandible
Morbidity and mortality	Radical surgery may be associated with an increased morbidity
Gender, race, and age distribution	Equal gender distribution
	Usually seen in patients <15 yr
Clinical features	Rapid, disfiguring growth
Radiographic features	Well-delineated, expansile radiolucent lesion with variable, focal calcifications
Prognosis and treatment	Recurrences reported up to 58%, requiring potentially disfiguring surgery
	Complete (radical) surgery

PATHOLOGIC FEATURES

GROSS FINDINGS

Lesions are well circumscribed and usually demonstrate a smooth surface. Intraoperative findings may include the tumor "shelling out." Some lesions, however, will grossly have a more infiltrate relationship to the surrounding bone.

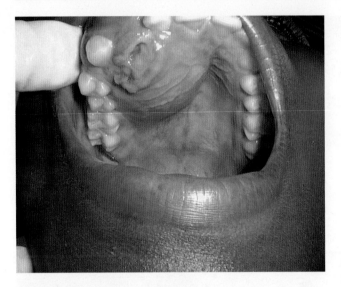

FIGURE 17-4

A young man from a third world nation with a large and distorting juvenile ossifying fibroma of the anterior maxilla. (Courtesy of Dr. S. R. Clarke.)

lagenous rim. Sometimes the ossicles fuse. Concentrically laminated particles may occasionally simulate a genuine psammoma body. Trabeculae of women bone may also be noted. Additionally, multinucleated giant cells and scattered mitotic figures are commonly seen.

DIFFERENTIAL DIAGNOSIS

The differential diagnosis includes ossifying fibroma and extracranial meningioma. Clinical and radiograph history is helpful. The true psammoma bodies of a

MICROSCOPIC FINDINGS

The tumor is characterized by a more cellular proliferation of fibroblast-like spindle cells. Immature osteoid and small spherical ossicles with distinct osteoblastic rimming are seen (Figs. 17-5, 17-6). Cementum-like psammomatous structures are a classic feature of this lesion, although sometimes scant. These particles are spherical or curved, often with a thick, irregular col-

JUVENILE/ACTIVE OSSIFYING FIBROMA PATHOLOGIC FEATURES	
Gross findings	Lesions are well circumscribed, usually with a smooth surface
Microscopic findings	Cellular proliferation of spindle cells
	Immature osteoid and small spherical ossicles with distinct osteoblastic rimming
	Cementum-like psammomatous structures are variably present
	Thick, irregular collagenous rim
	Osteoclastic giant cells are commonly found
	Mitotic figures are noted
Pathologic differential diagnosis	Ossifying fibroma, extracranial meningioma

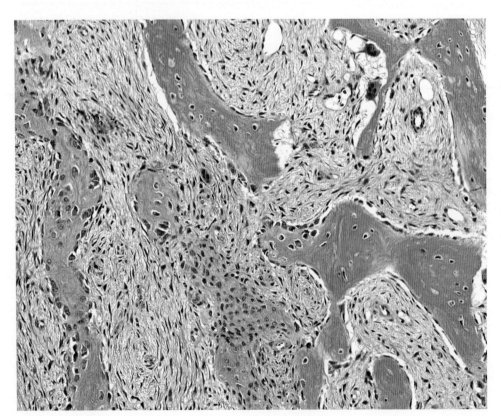

FIGURE 17-5

A network of osteoid rimmed by osteoblasts in a cellular fibrous stroma.

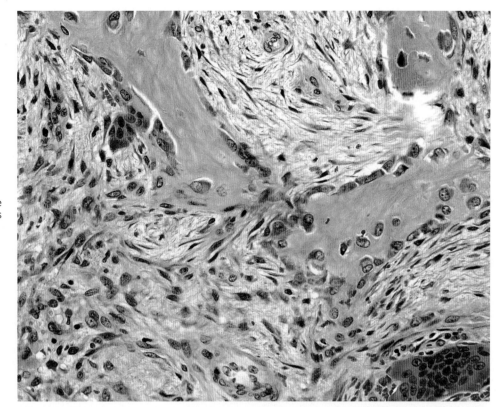

FIGURE 17-6
Plump active osteoblasts lining the osteoid. Multinucleated giant cells are present.

meningioma are different, as is the pattern of growth (whorled, meningothelial architecture).

PROGNOSIS AND THERAPY

Tumors continue to enlarge if left untreated, therefore necessitating complete surgical excision. Recurrences are common (up to 58%), resulting in potentially disfiguring surgery, requiring reconstruction.

OSTEOMA

Osteomas are a benign neoplasm of mature compact or cancellous bone. Surface osteomas are called "periosteal osteomas," while central lesions are called "endosteal osteomas." There is controversy as to whether osteoma is a neoplasm or as a result of trauma or infection.

CLINICAL FEATURES

Osteomas are rare, found almost exclusively in craniofacial bones, and most commonly in the frontal and ethmoid sinuses. Of the gnathic bones, the mandible is affected more than the maxilla. Young adults (2nd–5th

OSTEOMA DISEASE FACT SHEET	
Definition	A benign neoplasm of mature compact or cancellous bone
Incidence and location	Rare
Gender, race, and age distribution	Equal gender distribution Young adults (2nd–5th decades)
Clinical features	Usually solitary lesions, except when associated with Gardner syndrome Usually slow growing painless mass May cause facial deformity, headache, and/or sinusitis Frontal and ethmoid sinuses most commonly, but mandible > maxilla in gnathic bones
Radiographic features	Dense, well-circumscribed sclerotic radiopaque masses Surface tumors called "periosteal" while central tumors are called "endosteal" Central lesions are difficult to identify
Prognosis and treatment	Large lesions may require cosmetic treatment Workup for Gardner syndrome if multiple No treatment is required

decades) are affected without a gender bias. Lesions are usually solitary, except when associated with Gardner syndrome. Gardner syndrome is a rare autosomal dominant disorder characterized by colonic adenomatous polyps, epidermal inclusion cysts, fibromas, and osteomas of the gnathic bones. Osteomas may be an important early sign of the syndrome. Diagnosis is vital as malignant transformation of the colon polyps approaches 100 % in older patients. Osteomas usually present as a slowly growing painless mass which may cause facial deformity, headaches, and/or sinusitis.

RADIOLOGIC FEATURES

Radiographically lesions present as dense, well-circumscribed sclerotic radiopaque masses (Fig. 17-7).

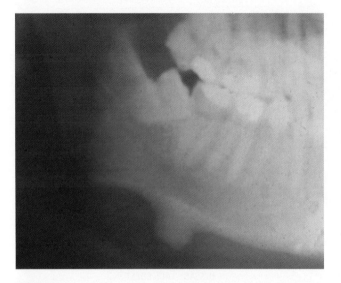

FIGURE 17-7
Radiograph of a periosteal pedunculated osteoma arising from the lower border of the mandible.

Endosteal osteomas are more difficult to separate from reactive jaw lesions.

PATHOLOGIC FEATURES

GROSS FINDINGS

Periosteal lesions may appear as a polypoid bony mass, and may be intact after surgical removal. Conversely, endosteal lesions are usually fragmented during removal and appear as fragments of normal bone.

MICROSCOPIC FINDINGS

Microscopically, osteomas are identical to normal compact or cancellous bone (Fig. 17-8) with variable

OSTEOMA PATHOLOGIC FEATURES	
Gross findings	Periosteal lesions may appear as a polypoid bony mass
	Endosteal lesions are usually fragmented during removal
Microscopic findings	Identical to normal compact or cancellous bone
	Variable fibro-fatty marrow
Pathologic differential diagnosis	Exostoses and tori

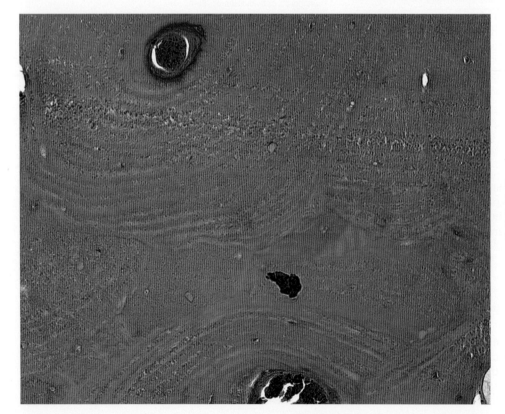

FIGURE 17-8
Compact bone with few marrow spaces, in the correct clinical and radiographic setting is diagnostic of an osteoma.

amounts of fibro-fatty bone marrow, requiring clinical-radiographic correlation for accurate diagnosis.

DIFFERENTIAL DIAGNOSIS

Osteomas should be differentiated from exostoses and tori. Tori are hereditary and developmental bony excrescences covered by normal oral mucosa, commonly found on the hard palate and lingual aspect of the mandible. Exostoses are thought to be related to occlusal stress, but are histologically identical, requiring clinical correlation.

PROGNOSIS AND THERAPY

No treatment is required, but lesions are often removed or sampled to ensure a proper histological diagnosis. Rarely, larger lesions may cause a cosmetic defect requiring treatment. If multiple osteomas are diagnosed, evaluation for Gardner syndrome is recommended.

CEMENTOBLASTOMA

Cementoblastoma is a rare benign neoplasm which forms cementum-like material attached to the tooth root.

CLINICAL FEATURES

Cementoblastomas are rare, accounting for only about 4% of cementum-containing lesions. There is no significant gender predilection and lesions are discovered in the 2nd–3rd decades. Lesions present with varied levels of pain and a swelling of the buccal or lingual aspect of the alveolar ridges as a result of bone expansion. The involved tooth usually remains vital. There is a predilection for the mandibular alveolus, particularly the mandibular permanent first molar.

RADIOLOGIC FEATURES

The tumors are a well-defined, radiopaque or mixed density, rounded mass, intimately associated with the tooth root (Fig. 17-9). Additionally, a thin radiolucent rim surrounds the tumor, representing the periodontal ligament. Root resorption is common. Irregular soft tissue may surround the lesion.

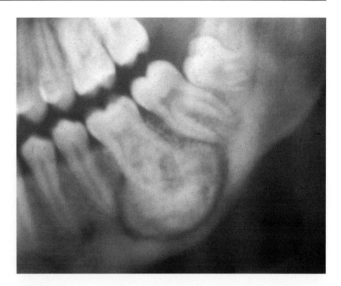

FIGURE 17-9
Radiograph of a radiodense calcified mass attached to the root of the mandibular first molar is characteristic for a cementoblastoma.

CEMENTOBLASTOMA DISEASE FACT SHEET	
Definition	A benign neoplasm of cementum-like material connected with the tooth root
Incidence and location	About 4% of cementum-containing lesions
	Predilection for the posterior mandible, first molar specifically
Gender, race, and age distribution	Equal gender distribution
	Peak in the 2nd–3rd decades
Clinical features	Local expansion of bone causes buccal swelling of the alveolar ridges
	Variable pain
Radiographic findings	Well-defined, radiopaque or mixed density, rounded mass
	Intimately associated with the tooth root
	A narrow radiolucent rim surrounds the tumor, representing the periodontal ligament
Prognosis and treatment	Recurrences only occur if incompletely excised
	Excision of mass and associated tooth

PATHOLOGIC FEATURES

GROSS FINDINGS

The lesion appears as a mass of yellow-white cementum fused to the roots of a tooth.

MICROSCOPIC FINDINGS

A cementoblastoma is composed of a dense mass of cementum in a loose fibrovascular stroma. Lesions usually show prominent cementoblastic rimming and may demonstrate a characteristic basophilic appearance

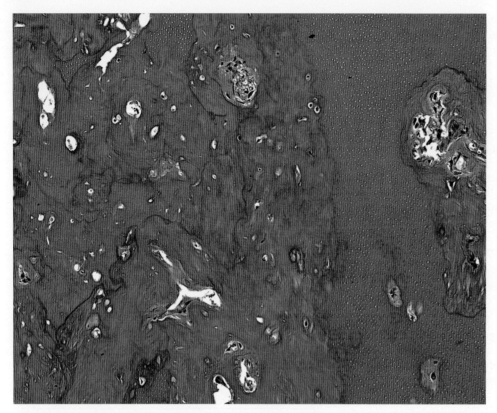

FIGURE 17-10
The relationship between the tooth root (*right*) and the cemental mass (*left*) is demonstrated in this cementoblastoma.

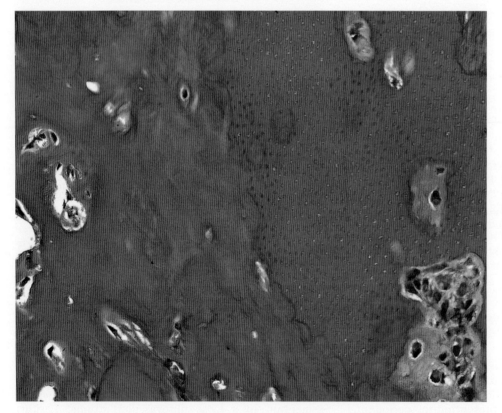

FIGURE 17-11
The dentinal tubules are seen in the root structure adjacent to the nodular mass of cementum, which is lined by plump cementoblasts.

CEMENTOBLASTOMA
PATHOLOGIC FEATURES

Gross findings	A mass of yellow-white cementum fused to the tooth root
Microscopic findings	A dense mass of cementum-like tissue with prominent basophilic reversal lines
	Variably cellular fibrovascular background stroma
	Cementoblasts, cementoclasts, and multinucleated giant cells are found
Pathologic differential diagnosis	Osteoblastoma, osteosarcoma

and reversal lines of the cementum (Fig. 17-10). Multinucleated osteoclastic giant cells are usually present. The periphery may have radiating columns of unmineralized tissue (Fig. 17-11).

DIFFERENTIAL DIAGNOSIS

Cementoblastomas are essentially identical to osteoblastoma microscopically, although the former has a connection to the tooth root. Osteosarcoma must also be excluded. Both lesions need radiographic and clinical correlation.

PROGNOSIS AND THERAPY

Treatment requires removal of the mass and associated tooth, usually a surgical extraction. Recurrences do not occur, unless the lesion is incompletely removed.

OSTEOBLASTOMA

An osteoblastoma is a benign bone-forming tumor within bone, which is sometimes separated into osteoid osteoma and osteoblastoma based on location, size, and symptoms.

CLINICAL FEATURES

Osteoblastoma as a group is a relatively rare bone lesion with approximately 15% occurring in the gnathic bones. The mandible is affected more frequently than the maxilla, particularly the ramus, coronoid process, and condyle. The majority of cases present before 30 years of age and there is a definite male predilection. Pain, particularly nocturnal, is a common symptom in both conventional osteoblastomas and osteoid osteomas, with only the latter being relieved by aspirin.

RADIOLOGIC FEATURES

Osteoid osteomas typically are well-circumscribed lesions with a distinct rim of sclerosis. This is in contrast to conventional osteoblastomas that usually lack surrounding sclerosis and may be more poorly defined. Osteoid osteomas may have an identifiable radiopaque nidus, again a feature not seen in a conventional osteoblastoma. Patchy scattered calcifications may be seen.

PATHOLOGIC FEATURES

GROSS FINDINGS

By definition, conventional osteoblastomas are usually larger than 2 cm, while osteoid osteomas are less than 2 cm. Lesions may cause bone expansion, and are usually sharply circumscribed. They have red to brown gritty bone fragments.

MICROSCOPIC FINDINGS

Although there may be subtle histological differences between conventional osteoblastoma and osteoid osteoma, they are essentially identical. They consist of anastomosing trabeculae of osteoid in a loose fibrovas-

OSTEOBLASTOMA
DISEASE FACT SHEET

Definition	A benign bone forming tumor of bone composed of anastomosing trabeculae of osteoid
Incidence and location	Uncommon
	15% arise in the jaws, involving mandible > maxilla
Morbidity and mortality	May cause functional problems with increased size
Gender, race, and age distribution	Males > Females (2 : 1)
	Peak incidence in 2nd decade; most present <30 yr
Clinical features	Bone expansion may cause pain
	Pain not relieved by aspirin in conventional lesions (as it is in osteoid osteoma)
Radiographic features	Well-circumscribed, radiolucent lesion with a distinct rim of sclerosis
	Small radiopaque nidus may be identified
	Conventional osteoblastomas may be well-defined or ill-defined, lack surrounding sclerosis
	Osteoid osteomas may have an identifiable radiopaque nidus, typically have a distinct rim of sclerosis
Prognosis and treatment	Recurrence is rare, especially for jaw lesions
	Conservative surgery

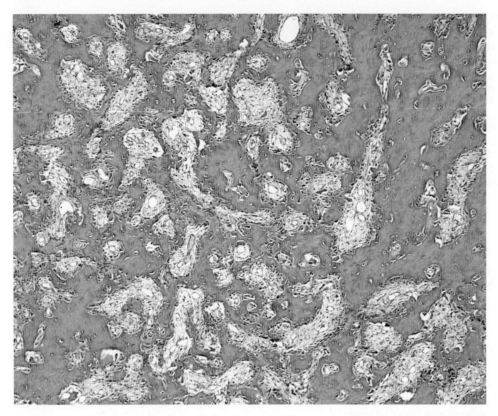

FIGURE 17-12
Anastomosing trabeculae of osteoid with prominent osteoblastic rimming in this osteoblastoma.

cular stroma (Fig. 17-12). The mineralized component usually shows noticeable osteoblastic rimming along with a characteristic basophilic appearance (Fig. 17-13). Osteoclastic giant cells are usually present and may even be a predominate feature. Extravasated erythrocytes are common.

DIFFERENTIAL DIAGNOSIS

Differentiating between an osteoblastoma and a low-grade osteosarcoma is most important. Osteosarcoma

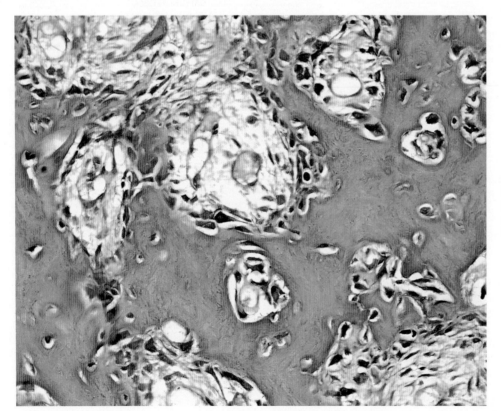

FIGURE 17-13
High power showing characteristic osteoblastic rimming in an osteoblastoma.

OSTEOBLASTOMA PATHOLOGIC FEATURES	
Gross findings	Conventional osteoblastomas larger than 2 cm, osteoid osteoma usually less than 2 cm
	Removed as fragments of red-brown gritty bone
Microscopic findings	Anastomosing trabeculae of osteoid in a loose fibrovascular stroma
	The basophilic mineralized component shows prominent osteoblastic rimming
	Osteoclasts are often present
	Extravasated erythrocytes common
Pathologic differential diagnosis	Osteosarcoma, cementoblastoma, ossifying fibroma

ODONTOMA (COMPLEX AND COMPOUND) DISEASE FACT SHEET	
Definition	A tumor-like malformation (hamartoma) composed of enamel, dentin, pulpal tissue, and cementum separated into compound and complex types
Incidence and location	Most common odontogenic tumor
	Compound odontomas predilect to anterior maxilla
	Complex odontoma predilect to posterior mandible
Gender, race, and age distribution	Equal gender distribution
	Prevalence in the first two decades
Clinical features	Usually asymptomatic
	Unusually large lesions may expand the jaws, preventing normal tooth eruption
Radiographic features	Radiodense calcified mass surrounded by thin radiolucent rim
	Appearance of small, malformed teeth
Prognosis and treatment	Prognosis is good
	Conservative enucleation of odontoma and associated dental follicle or cyst

has atypical features which include pleomorphism, infiltrative growth, and atypical mitosis. The clinical presentation of an osteosarcoma includes pain, loosening of the teeth, and paresthesia. Benign fibro-osseous lesions are also a consideration, although these lesions generally have a distinct clinical and radiographic appearance. Cementoblastoma, which histologically may be essentially identical to osteoblastoma, is distinguished by direct association with the tooth root.

PROGNOSIS AND THERAPY

Usually conservative excision is adequate. Some large lesions may require larger resections resulting in the need for subsequent reconstruction. On rare occasions lesions have been reported to be locally aggressive.

ODONTOMA (COMPLEX AND COMPOUND)

Odontoma is the most common odontogenic tumor, although it may best be classified as a hamartoma composed of enamel, dentin, pulpal tissue, and cementum. Academically, odontomas are subclassified into two types, although management is identical: *compound* when composed of rudimentary teeth-like structures and *complex* when composed of haphazardly arranged tooth structure.

CLINICAL FEATURES

Odontoma occurs more frequently than all other odontogenic tumors combined. Odontomas show no gender predilection. Odontomas develop most commonly in the first two decades, the time normal teeth are developing

and erupting. Most odontomas are asymptomatic, found incidentally on routine dental radiographs, while larger lesions may interfere with eruption of normal adjacent teeth, prompting radiographic investigation.

RADIOLOGIC FEATURES

Odontomas present as a radiodense calcified mass surrounded by a thin radiolucent rim (Fig. 17-14). Compound odontomas will appear like small, malformed teeth while complex odontomas present as radiodense masses of calcified tooth material, slightly more difficult to diagnose.

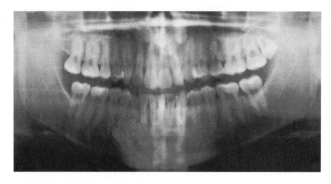

FIGURE 17-14

Panoramic radiograph. A radiopaque mass in the anterior mandible is preventing the eruption of the canine.

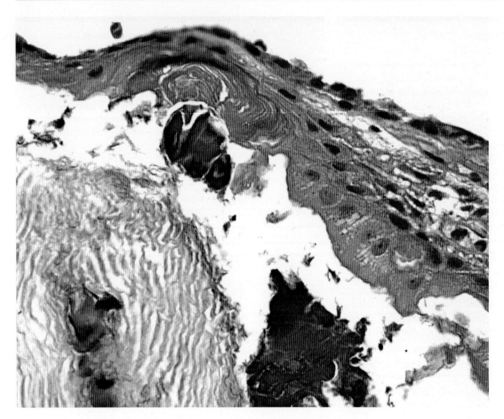

FIGURE 17-15
Enamel matrix and odontogenic epithelium in an odontoma.

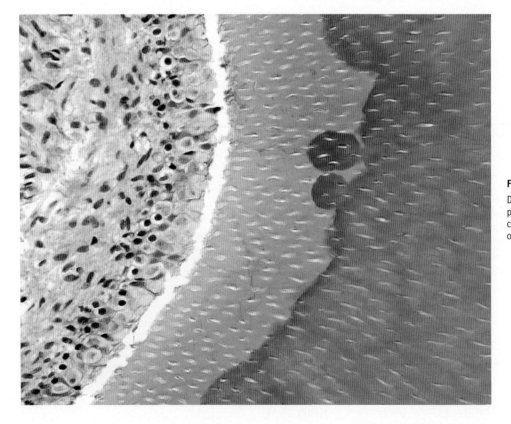

FIGURE 17-16
Distinctive pulpal tissue adjacent to predentin and mature dentin helps to confirm the diagnosis of compound odontoma.

ODONTOMA (COMPLEX AND COMPOUND) PATHOLOGIC FEATURES	
Gross findings	Compound odontomas may appear as a collection of small, malformed teeth
	Complex odontomas may appear as a collection of mineralized material, usually yellow-white
Microscopic findings	Compound odontomas have enamel, dentin, cementum, and pulp tissue recapitulating normal teeth (odontoids)
	Complex odontomas have enamel, dentin, cementum, and pulp tissue arranged in a disorganized, haphazard manner
Pathologic differential diagnosis	Normal teeth

PATHOLOGIC FEATURES

GROSS FINDINGS

Compound odontomas have a predilection for the anterior maxilla, while complex odontomas favor the posterior mandible. Compound odontomas appear as a collection of small malformed teeth. Complex odontomas may appear as a collection of mineralized material, usually yellow-white in color. Both subtypes may be associated with soft fibrous connective tissue. They are frequently described as "shelling out" of the bone.

MICROSCOPIC FINDINGS

Microscopically, odontomas are composed of the normal elements of tooth structure: dentin, enamel, cementum, and pupal tissue (Fig. 17-15). These tissues are histologically characteristic and are usually readily identified. In compound odontomas the normal organized relationship of enamel matrix, dentin, and pulpal elements is intact (Fig. 17-16). By contrast, complex odontoma has a haphazardly arranged enamel matrix, tubular dentin, and pulpal tissue. Dental follicular tissue or a dentigerous cyst may be seen in relation to these tissues.

DIFFERENTIAL DIAGNOSIS

The only real differential diagnosis is normal teeth, which are removed from consideration by clinical and radiographic correlation.

PROGNOSIS AND THERAPY

Treatment is conservative enucleation, including associated dental follicle or cyst. There is no recurrence and prognosis is good. If the eruption of normal teeth was affected, orthodontic procedures may be necessary to correct the resulting malocclusion.

ADENOMATOID ODONTOGENIC TUMOR

The adenomatoid odontogenic tumor (AOT) is a rare benign tumor of odontogenic epithelium with a distinctive duct-like appearance embedded in a mature connective tissue stroma which occurs in the jaws.

CLINICAL FEATURES

AOT accounts for about 4%–5% of odontogenic tumors. Females are affected twice as frequently as males, with >90% of patients diagnosed before age 30 years; nearly 50% as teenagers. Asians and blacks are more commonly affected. The maxilla is affected twice as often as the mandible, particularly at the unerupted canine teeth. The rule of "two-thirds" can be used for this lesion: two-thirds <20 years old, two-thirds females, two-thirds in the maxilla, and two-thirds involve the canines. Peripheral types appear as a nondescript mass of the gingival tissue. Most are asymptomatic, but a bony-hard, palpable mass with or without pain may be the presenting findings. Tooth displacement is also reported. Previously, AOT was considered a variant of ameloblastoma, termed "adenoameloblastoma," but histology and biologic behavior differences warrant separation.

ADENOMATOID ODONTOGENIC TUMOR DISEASE FACT SHEET	
Definition	A benign tumor of odontogenic duct-like epithelium embedded in a mature connective tissue stroma
Incidence and location	About 5% of odontogenic tumors
	Predilection for the anterior maxilla
Gender, race, and age distribution	Female > Male (2 : 1)
	>90% present before 30 yr (peak, 2nd decade)
	Asians and blacks more commonly affected
Clinical features	Usually asymptomatic
	May be bony-hard, palpable mass with or without pain
	Associated with unerupted tooth, most commonly canines
	Tooth displacement is reported
	Rare peripheral type is a nondescript gingival mass
Radiographic features	Intraosseous, well-circumscribed, unilocular radiolucent mass
	Associated with crown or part of the root of an unerupted permanent tooth
	Occasionally, opaque flecks representing calcifications noted
	May cause divergence of adjacent roots
Prognosis and treatment	Recurrence is extremely rare
	Conservative, local excision

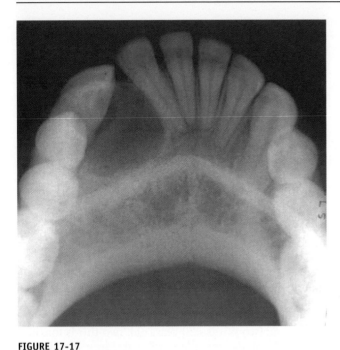

FIGURE 17-17
Occlusal radiograph. Radiolucent lesion of the anterior mandible between the incisor and canine.

RADIOLOGIC FEATURES

Most AOTs present as an intraosseous, well-circumscribed, unilocular radiolucent lesion, often around the crown and part of the root of an unerupted permanent tooth (Fig. 17-17). Some may have opaque flecks that represent small calcifications. Larger lesions may cause divergence of adjacent roots. Peripheral tumors may cause saucerization (erosion) of the alveolar bone.

PATHOLOGIC FEATURES

GROSS FINDINGS

Lesions are well circumscribed, may have a fibrous capsule, and are often associated with the crown of a tooth. Lesions are usually <3 cm. Focal cystic areas and calcifications may be seen on cross-section.

MICROSCOPIC FINDINGS

Nodules of odontogenic epithelium separated by minimal stromal connective tissue are seen on low power. Two cell types comprise the tumor. The duct-like, tubular or cord-like areas are lined by cuboidal to columnar epithelial cells (Fig. 17-18), with nuclei polarized away from the central duct-like space, imparting an appearance reminiscent of ameloblastoma. The duct-like spaces are pseudolumina containing secretions of the columnar cells. The second component is a spindled to polyhedral eosinophilic cell component which creates a nodular, nested, and swirling pattern, often containing collections of eosinophilic, amorphous amyloid-like material (Fig. 17-19). These globular masses may show varying degrees of mineralization, and in its most advanced form may show distinct laminations (Fig. 17-20). Minimal, loose stroma with thin-walled vessels is present, usually accentuated at the periphery.

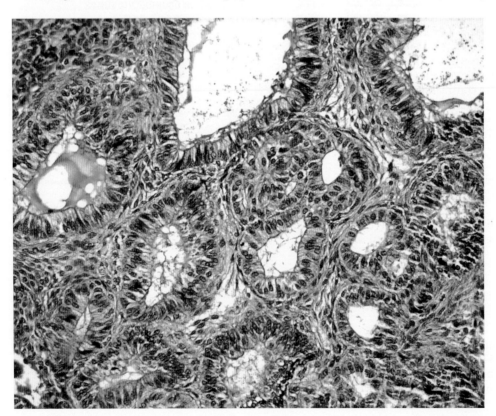

FIGURE 17-18
Nodular duct-like structures set in a spindle cell background in an adenomatoid odontogenic tumor.

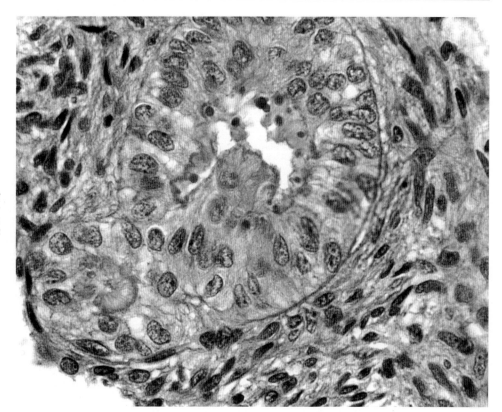

FIGURE 17-19

Gland-like spaces surrounded by cuboidal to columnar cells, surrounded by a spindle cell population is seen in adenomatoid odontogenic tumor.

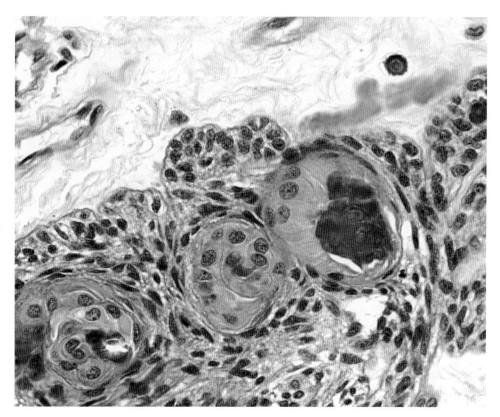

FIGURE 17-20

Calcifications adjacent to the spindle and columnar epithelial cells. Note the area of lamination, a feature helpful in confirming a diagnosis of adenomatoid odontogenic tumor.

ADENOMATOID ODONTOGENIC TUMOR PATHOLOGIC FEATURES	
Gross findings	Well-circumscribed by a fibrous capsule
	Often associated with the crown of an extracted tooth
	Focal cystic areas and calcification may be seen
Microscopic findings	A distinctive fibrous capsule is usually noted
	Nodules of odontogenic epithelium
	Duct-like, tubular or cord-like areas lined by cuboidal to columnar cells with reverse polarized nuclei
	Spindled to polyhedral eosinophilic cells in nodular, nested swirling patterns
	Collections of eosinophilic, amorphous amyloid-like material
	Areas of calcification with lamination may be seen
Ancillary studies	Ultrastructurally appears like enamel matrix
	Histochemical stains support amyloid
Pathologic differential diagnosis	Ameloblastoma

ANCILLARY STUDIES

Ultrastructural findings reveal a fibrillar to granular quality to the eosinophilic deposits, suggesting they may represent enamel matrix or perhaps amyloid.

DIFFERENTIAL DIAGNOSIS

Although AOT histology is characteristic, an ameloblastoma must be ruled out.

PROGNOSIS AND THERAPY

Recurrences are extremely rare. Conservative, local excision is curative, made easy by a thick capsule.

AMELOBLASTOMA

Ameloblastoma is the most common clinically significant odontogenic tumor of the gnathic arches characterized as a benign but persistent and locally aggressive neoplasm. The majority of ameloblastomas occur in the posterior mandible with a wide variety of radiographic and clinical presentations, each carrying treatment and

prognostic implications. The tumor arises from the enamel organ or its progenitor cell lines, resulting in the development of the soft tissue components of the odontogenic tumor without production of any calcified products.

CLINICAL FEATURES

Ameloblastomas clinically presents in three forms: unicystic, multicystic, and peripheral (within soft tissue). Multicystic ameloblastomas are also referred to as conventional or infiltrating because their invasive nature requires more aggressive therapy. Multicystic ameloblastomas occur in the 4th–5th decades, representing 86 % of all ameloblastomas. Sinonasal tumors are unique, as they have a propensity to occur in males, develop in much older patients (6th–7th decades), and present with sinusitis and epitaxis. The majority of ameloblastomas develop at the site of an impacted tooth with 80 % in the posterior mandible; bony expansion is seen, usually at a latter stage of development. Unicystic ameloblastomas occur in a younger population, approximately two decades earlier than multicystic tumors

AMELOBLASTOMA DISEASE FACT SHEET	
Definition	Most common benign epithelial odontogenic tumor which is slow growing, but locally aggressive, persistent, and frequently recurrent
Incidence and location	Most common odontogenic tumor
	80% in mandible and 20% in maxilla
	2/3 located in the posterior mandible (ramus area)
Gender, race, and age distribution	Equal gender and race distribution
	Wide age range, 2nd–6th decade
	Mean age: multicystic (44 yr) while unicystic (22 yr)
Clinical features	Most small tumors are asymptomatic
	Variably sized jaw swellings
	Pain or paraesthesia are rare
Radiographic features	Unilocular or multilocular radiolucencies, resembling cysts with scalloped borders
	An unerupted/impacted tooth is frequently associated
	Resorption of the roots of adjacent teeth is common
	Cortical bony expansion in longstanding tumors
Prognosis and treatment	Prognosis and treatment varies with clinical type of tumor
	Unicystic tumors: enucleation with 5% recurrence
	Multicystic tumors: en bloc resection with 25%–55% recurrence
	Ameloblastic carcinoma: wide resection with 50% mortality

and require the least aggressive treatment. Unicystic ameloblastomas are confined to the lumen or within the wall of the cyst and represent approximately 13% of ameloblastomas. Peripheral ameloblastomas represent only 1% of ameloblastomas and are limited exclusively to the soft tissue. Peripheral tumors are elevated smooth surfaced nodules on the gingiva and appear similar to an irritation fibroma. The superficial nature of peripheral ameloblastomas without bone involvement translates into simple excision, which is curative. All forms of ameloblastomas are asymptomatic until late stages when significant cosmetic deformity and pathologic fracture may occur.

RADIOLOGIC FEATURES

Multicystic lesions form large radiolucent loculations within the cortex of the bone with numerous distinct

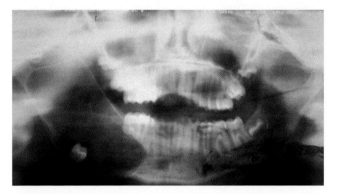

FIGURE 17-21
Radiologic features of an expansive, multiloculated cystic ameloblastoma of right posterior mandible, inferiorly displacing molar and forming fine bony septa in the ramus.

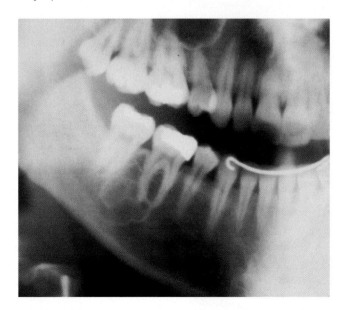

FIGURE 17-22
Radiographic features of an intraosseous ameloblastoma with well-corticated multiloculated mass creating splaying of molar and bicuspid roots.

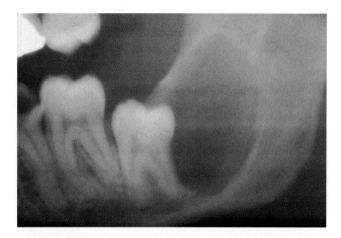

FIGURE 17-23
Radiographic features of a solitary, unilocular radiolucent cystic ameloblastoma of right mandible with distinct sclerotic peripheral margin.

bony septa forming the walls of the compartments (Figs. 17-21, 17-22). Multicystic tumors progress anterior and posterior through the central medullary bone through the path of least resistance. The involved impacted tooth may be significantly displaced, with tooth resorption seen only in later stages of development. Large, long-standing lesions may perforate cortical bone; however, more frequently thinning and expansion of the cortical plate is seen. Unicystic lesions are large solitary radiolucent cysts, associated with an impacted tooth (Fig. 17-23). The cortical plate may be expanded and a dense sclerotic border is seen at the leading edge of the slowing expanding tumor. Maxillary tumors may show less distinct radiographic borders, often filling the maxillary sinus and appearing as a diffuse solid semi-radiopaque mass within the sinus.

PATHOLOGIC FEATURES

GROSS FINDINGS

Early multicystic and unicystic ameloblastomas are typically cysts which have thick walls with rough luminal surface elevations. The cyst wall in early unicystic tumors is thin, uniform, and often filled by gray-brown gelatinous material representing tumor (Fig. 17-24). Unicystic tumor with mural involvement shows mild thickening of the wall with corresponding variegated coloration of the luminal surface. Late stage multicystic tumors are removed as en bloc resections of bone with tumor filling medullary spaces and appearing as dense fibrous tissue with cystic spaces.

MICROSCOPIC FINDINGS

The classic histologic (follicular) features as described by Vickers and Gorlin are seen in conventional tumors and characterized by islands of proliferating odontogenic epithelium reminiscent of the enamel organ. Epithelial tumor islands are enmeshed

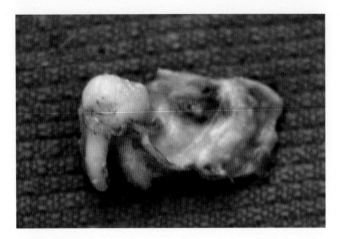

FIGURE 17-24

Gross specimen with attached bisected cyst, showing intact cyst wall with hemorrhagic appearing area representing plexiform unicystic ameloblastoma.

AMELOBLASTOMA PATHOLOGIC FEATURES	
Gross findings	**Unicystic:** Simple cyst with irregular wall filled with gray-brown-yellow gelatinous material
	Multicystic: Compartmentalized bone filled with fibrous stroma containing gray cystic or necrotic foci
Microscopic findings	**Unicystic:** Cyst with lining forming reticulated plexiform, stranded, meshwork of cuboidal cells lacking characteristic ameloblastic features
	Multicystic: Follicular pattern with peripheral columnar cells, reverse polarization, central stellate reticulum, and hyalinized connective tissue epithelial interface
	Desmoplastic: Dense fibrous proliferation with widely placed odontogenic cords without characteristic ameloblastic features
Pathologic differential diagnosis	Dentigerous cyst, odontogenic keratocyst, ameloblastic fibroma, odontogenic myxoma, benign fibro-ossseous lesion, ameloblastic carcinoma

in hyperplastic fibrous connective tissue, displaying pale hyalinized areas at the epithelial connective tissue interface (Fig. 17-25). The odontogenic elements are composed of basophilic columnar cells at the periphery, exhibiting reverse polarization of nuclei away from the connective tissue with vacuolization. The central portions of the epithelial islands are less cellular, edematous, and mimic the stellate reticulum of the enamel organ (Fig. 17-26). Follicular histologic features are seen in most ameloblastomas, however, other patterns are also seen featuring acanthomatous (Fig. 17-27), basaloid, granular cell, desmoplastic, and plexiform variations.

Unicystic tumors and sinonasal tumors seldom show the classic Vickers and Gorlin features, but

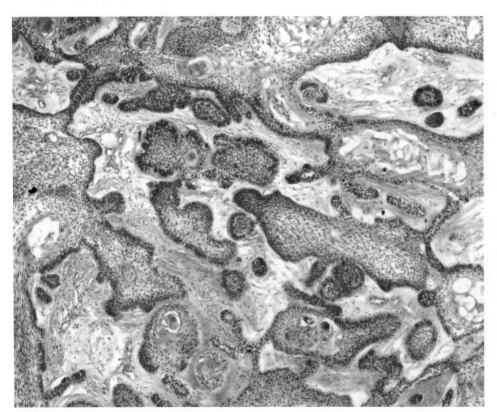

FIGURE 17-25

Low power of follicular pattern ameloblastoma with anastamosing islands of basophilic epithelium set in loose connective tissue stroma with eosinophilic inductive hyalinized change at connective tissue/epithelial interface.

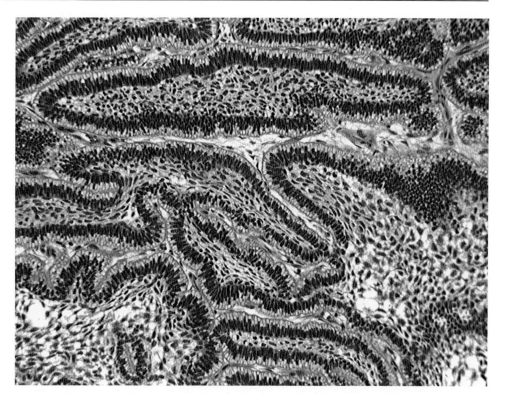

FIGURE 17-26

Hyperchromatic nuclei within columnar basal cells are seen showing vacuolization, reverse polarization, and less cellular central areas reminiscent of stellate reticulum of the enamel organ.

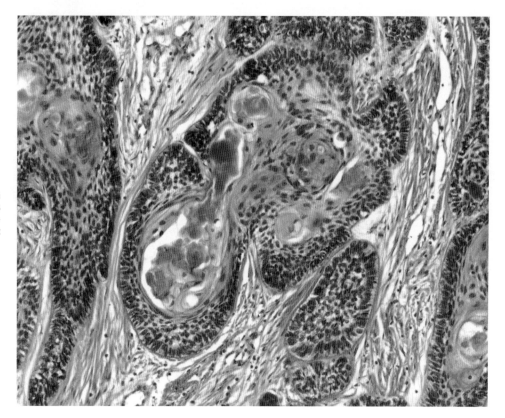

FIGURE 17-27

Medium power of ameloblastoma with follicular and acanthomatous patterns showing cystic acanthomatous central areas with dyskeratotic cells.

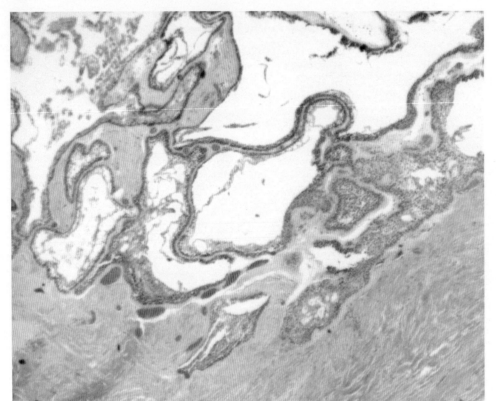

FIGURE 17-28

Low-power view of plexiform amelo-blastoma with reticulated strands of epithelium proliferating into the cystic lumen and focal extension of follicular pattern ameloblastoma in fibrous wall.

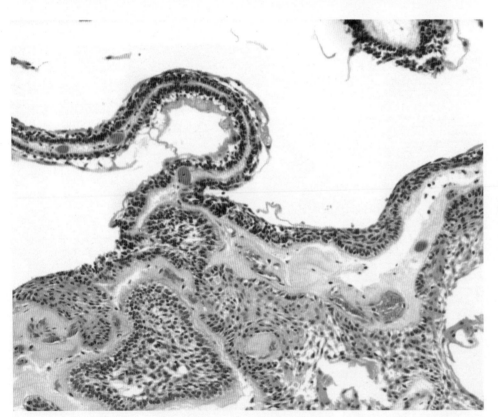

FIGURE 17-29

High power shows strands of plexi-form ameloblastoma free floating in cyst with little reverse polarization and "basket-weave" surface typical of unicystic ameloblastomas.

rather a loose "basket weave" luminal lining with inter-luminal proliferation of plexiform tumor. Unicystic tumors are filled with interlacing strands and cords, forming a reticulated plexiform pattern of cells with little evidence of a follicular character and reverse polarization (Figs. 17-28, 17-29). The desmoplastic variant also shows no evidence of the classic ameloblas-tic features, but rather widely scattered small islands and cords of bland odontogenic epithelium set in a dense collagenous stroma (Fig. 17-30). Peripheral

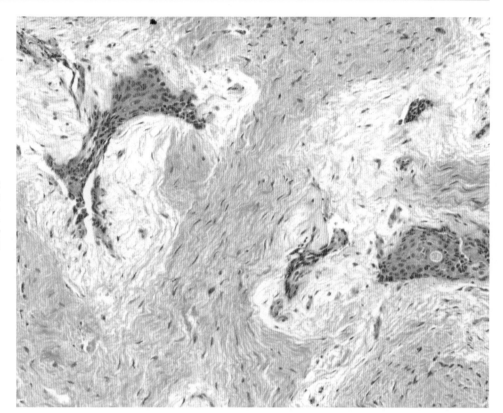

FIGURE 17-30

Medium power of desmoplastic ameloblastoma showing no evidence of Vickers and Gorlin changes, presenting as irregular islands of squamous epithelium circumscribed by edematous halos consistent with inductive effect.

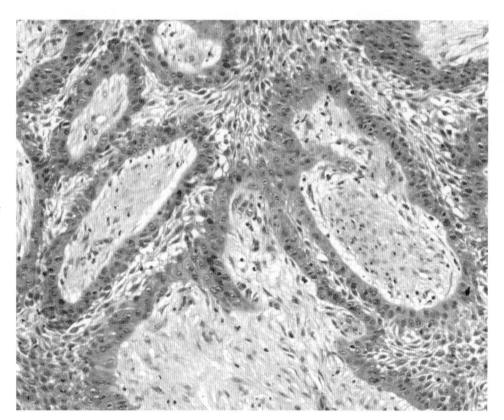

FIGURE 17-31

Medium power of ameloblastic carcinoma shows a condensed layer of atypical peripheral basal cells lacking columnar cells, vacuolar changes, and reverse polarization.

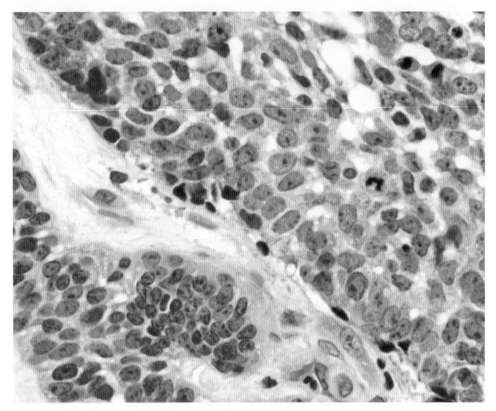

FIGURE 17-32
At high power, ameloblastic carcinoma displays a distinct connective tissue epithelial interface with unorganized basal cell layer, marked pleomorphism, and numerous mitotic figures.

ameloblastomas typically are follicular pattern and circumscribed by dense fibrous connective tissue. All histologic variants of ameloblastomas are cytologically bland with little pleomorphism or mitotic activity. When pleomorphism, hypercellularity, or mitotic activity is encountered, ameloblastic carcinoma should be considered.

DIFFERENTIAL DIAGNOSIS

The clinical differential diagnostic considerations for unicystic lesions includes benign odontogenic cysts and neoplasms. The histologic differential considerations are limited due to the distinctive histology of ameloblastomas. Other histologic considerations include ameloblastic fibroma, ameloblastic fibro-odontoma, and ameloblastic odontoma. Ameloblastic fibroma and ameloblastic fibro-odontoma have a unique character, as the epithelial elements, although ameloblastic appearing are smaller, fail to open into a large follicular island, and are set in a background of primitive mesencyhme containing widely scattered stellate fibroblasts in a myxoid matrix. Ameloblastic odontomas display similar histology in the epithelial elements, however, are associated with hard tissue forming an odontoma.

PROGNOSIS AND THERAPY

Historically ameloblastomas have been treated with wide local surgical resection, margins being 1 cm. Surgical resection continues to be the favored treatment for those tumors which are of the multiloculated conventional type. Multicystic tumors treated with a 1-cm surgical margin have recurrence rates of between 25%–55%. Patients should be placed on long-term periodic follow-up, as tumors frequently recur many years after the initial surgical procedure. Unicystic ameloblastomas require less aggressive therapy, necessitating only enucleation of the cystic tumor with curettage and possible "bone burring" deemed adequate. Recurrence of unicystic lesions treated less aggressively have recurrence rates of approximately 5%. Multicystic conventional ameloblastomas, though locally persistent with high recurrence rates, are subsequently easily treated with surgical en bloc resection.

On rare occasions, an ameloblastoma will metastasize as a benign solitary lesion which has unfortunately been termed "malignant ameloblastoma" in spite of its benignity. The "true malignant" counterpart of ameloblastomas is an ameloblastic carcinoma which is a high-grade tumor, widely metastatic with a 50% mortality rate in some series. The character of ameloblastic carcinomas are reminiscent of the benign counterpart, however, show less polarization at the connective tissue interface, a more solid cellular central area, considerable cytologic pleomorphism, and significant mitotic activity (Fig. 17-31). Ameloblastic carcinoma are often solid basaloid tumors (Fig. 17-32), which clinically are not slowly progressive, but rather locally aggressive, erode bony margins early, and are potentially metastatic.

CENTRAL ODONTOGENIC FIBROMA

Central odontogenic fibroma is a rare benign mesenchymal neoplasm of dental origin which is fraught with some controversy. Early publications separated the lesion into two types but this distinction is only important in ensuring an accurate diagnosis and differential.

CLINICAL FEATURES

Central odontogenic fibromas show a predilection for women (3 : 1), and an increased incidence in the 2nd–4th decades. Lesions may be asymptomatic, although larger lesions may cause jaw expansion and occasional perforation of the cortical plate. It is usually a painless mass. The tumor occurs more frequently in the anterior maxilla, resulting in a distinctive palatal cleft or depression, most suggestive of this tumor.

RADIOLOGIC FEATURES

Radiographically, most central odontogenic fibromas are unilocular, although multilocular lesions are seen. There is often a well-defined sclerotic border. Rarely central odontogenic fibromas may appear as mixed radiolucent-radiopaque lesions. Lesions may be associated with the crown of an unerupted tooth. Additionally, large lesions may affect adjacent structures, move teeth, or even cause root resorption.

PATHOLOGIC FEATURES

GROSS FINDINGS

Specimens are usually encapsulated, firm smooth masses. Surgeons occasionally state that they "shell out."

MICROSCOPIC FINDINGS

There is a wide variation of histological appearances, ranging from densely hyalinized and cellular to loose myxomatous to nearly acellular (Fig. 17-33). Delicate collagen fibers are occasionally identified along with fibromyxoid stroma. It is this variation that has resulted in the controversial separation into two types: WHO (World Health Organization) type and simple type. Inactive-looking odontogenic epithelium is usually identified, although sometimes it can appear proliferative (Fig. 17-34) and occasionally is absent. They form irregular islands or cords. Additionally, calcifications may or may not be present, simulating cementum, osteoid, or dentin. A granular cell odontogenic fibroma variant also exists.

DIFFERENTIAL DIAGNOSIS

The microscopic appearance is similar to a dental follicle and differentiation is based on radiographic and clinical

CENTRAL ODONTOGENIC FIBROMA DISEASE FACT SHEET	
Definition	A benign mesenchymal neoplasm of odontogenic origin
Incidence and location	Rare
	Predilection for the anterior maxilla
Gender, race, and age distribution	Female > Male (3 : 1)
	Peak incidence in 2nd–4th decades
Clinical features	Usually asymptomatic
	Larger lesions may cause painless jaw expansion
	Anterior maxillary lesions result in a distinctive palatal cleft
Radiographic features	Most present as well-defined unilocular radiolucencies
	Well-defined sclerotic border
	Rarely, they may be a mixed radiolucent-radiopaque multilocular lesion
	Occasionally associated with crown of unerupted tooth
Prognosis and treatment	Recurrence is rare
	Enucleation and curettage

CENTRAL ODONTOGENIC FIBROMA PATHOLOGIC FEATURES	
Gross findings	Encapsulated, firm, smooth yellow-white mass
Microscopic findings	Wide variation of histological appearances, ranging from loose myxomatous to densely hyalinized stroma
	Odontogenic epithelium usually inactive, although proliferative type may be present
	Calcifications may or may not be present
Pathologic differential diagnosis	Hyperplastic dental follicle, desmoplastic fibroma

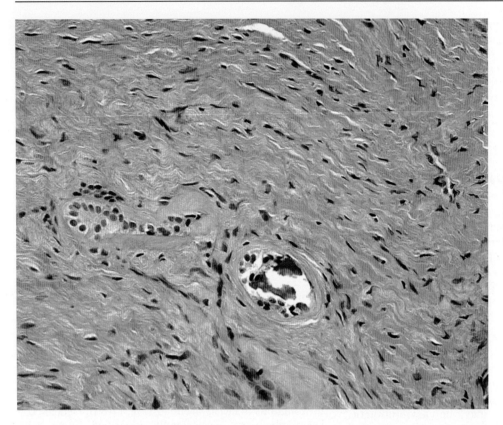

FIGURE 17-33

Loosely arranged fibroblasts and collagen fibrils with a deposit of cementum-like material. Note the small nest of odontogenic epithelium.

appearance including size and location. Usually this is not a difficult distinction, and one should remember that a hyperplastic dental follicle is a very common entity, while the central odontogenic fibroma is exceedingly rare. A cellular central odontogenic fibroma may appear similar to a desmoplastic fibroma. A desmoplastic fibroma does not, however, have an epithelial component nor are they found in association with teeth. Additionally, they will demonstrate a locally infiltrative quality.

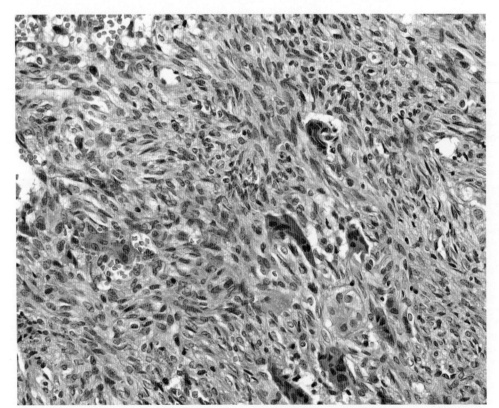

FIGURE 17-34

This more cellular fibrous lesion with focal nest of odontogenic epithelium is characteristic of the World Health Organization (WHO) type central odontogenic fibroma.

PROGNOSIS AND THERAPY

Surgical enucleation and curettage is usually the treatment of choice. Recurrences are rare.

CALCIFYING EPITHELIAL ODONTOGENIC TUMOR

The calcifying epithelial odontogenic tumor (CEOT), also referred to as Pindborg tumor, is a rare, distinctive locally invasive jaw tumor characterized by amyloid-like material that may become calcified.

CLINICAL FEATURES

Accounting for <1% of odontogenic tumors, the tumor occurs without a gender predilection in patients 20–60 years old. Tumors present as slowly, enlarging, and painless masses of the jaw, although rarely the gingiva may be affected. The mandible is affected twice as often as the maxilla, with a distinct predilection for the premolar/molar region.

RADIOLOGIC FEATURES

Tumors are well-circumscribed unilocular or multilocular, mixed radiolucent-radiopaque lesions with variable opaque flecks (Fig. 17-35). The calcifications are described as "driven snow." Up to 60% of lesions are associated with the crown of an unerupted tooth.

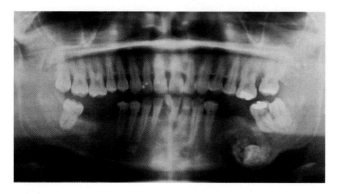

FIGURE 17-35
Panoramic radiograph. A multilocular radiolucent lesion containing larger calcifications in the left posterior mandible.

CALCIFYING EPITHELIAL ODONTOGENIC TUMOR DISEASE FACT SHEET	
Definition	A rare, locally invasive, epithelial odontogenic neoplasm characterized by the presence of amyloid material which may become calcified (also called Pindborg tumor)
Incidence and location	<1% of odontogenic tumors
	Mandible > maxilla (2 : 1), specifically premolar/molar region
Gender, race, and age distribution	Equal gender distribution
	Usually between 20–60 yr
Clinical features	Slowly, enlarging, painless mass of the jaw
	Peripheral (extraosseous) type appears as nondescript gum bumps (6% of cases)
Radiographic features	Well-circumscribed uni- or multilocular radiolucencies with variable opaque flecks
	Calcifications described as "driven snow"
	Up to 60% associated with crown of unerupted tooth
Prognosis and treatment	Long-term follow-up for recurrences (especially if incompletely excised or in clear cell variant)
	Conservative surgery

PATHOLOGIC FEATURES

GROSS FINDINGS

Grossly, lesions appear solid, well circumscribed, with varying amounts of calcification.

MICROSCOPIC FINDINGS

The tumor is composed of sheets and islands of polyhedral epithelial cells with abundant eosinophilic cytoplasm and distinct intercellular bridges. Nuclei show considerable pleomorphism (Fig. 17-36). Mitotic figures are rare. Characteristically, there is abundant, eosinophilic, homogenous, hyaline matrix material, proven to be amyloid (Fig. 17-37). Concentric, basophilic ring calcification of this material results in Liesegang rings. Clear cell and noncalcifying variants are described.

ANCILLARY STUDIES

The amyloid-like material, when stained with Congo red, demonstrates the classic apple-green birefringence when viewed with polarized light. Crystal violet and fluorescence with thioflavin T may also prove the presence of amyloid. Additionally, the tumor cells react with cytokeratins and epithelial membrane antigen.

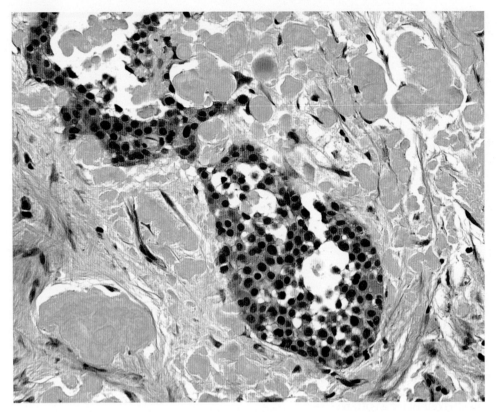

FIGURE 17-36

Sheets of polyhedral epithelial cells. Note the nuclear hyperchromatism and pleomorphism. Focal areas of pink amyloid-like material are readily identified in a CEOT.

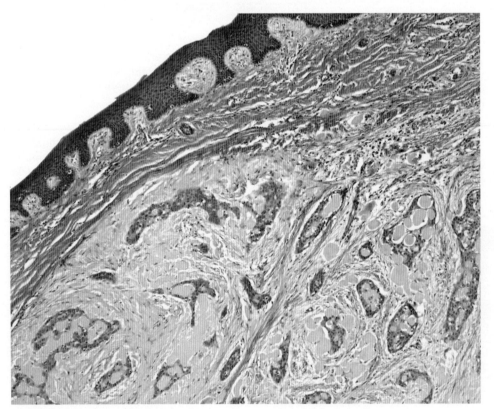

FIGURE 17-37

A rare peripheral variant of CEOT shows islands of epithelial cells and focal areas of acellular amyloid-type material in a fibrous connective tissue stroma surfaced by normal intact oral mucosa.

CALCIFYING EPITHELIAL ODONTOGENIC TUMOR PATHOLOGIC FEATURES

Gross findings	Solid, well-circumscribed mass with calcifications
Microscopic findings	Sheets and strands of polyhedral epithelial cells with abundant eosinophilic cytoplasm with distinct intercellular bridges
	Nuclear pleomorphism may be remarkable
	Mitotic figures are rare
	Abundant, eosinophilic, homogenous, hyaline matrix material (amyloid)
	Concentric, basophilic ring calcification (Liesegang rings)
	"Clear cell" and "noncalcifying" variants described
Ancillary studies	Amyloid material has Congo red apple-green birefringence with polarized light (Crystal violet and thioflavin T may be used)
	Reactivity with cytokeratins and epithelial membrane antigen
Pathologic differential diagnosis	Squamous cell carcinoma, clear cell odontogenic carcinoma, metastatic renal cell carcinoma

DIFFERENTIAL DIAGNOSIS

Squamous cell carcinoma, either primary or metastatic, is sometimes raised in the differential diagnosis. However, a lack of amyloid and the presence calcification will help with the separation. A clear cell odontogenic carcinoma and metastatic renal cell carcinoma may also need to be excluded in the clear cell variant.

PROGNOSIS AND THERAPY

Long-term follow-up is suggested as there is a known recurrence risk, especially if incompletely excised and/or in the clear cell variant. Treatment is usually conservative surgery (enucleation or local resection).

ODONTOGENIC KERATOCYST

The odontogenic keratocyst (OKC) is a distinctive developmental odontogenic cyst, believed to arise from the dental lamina. This cyst is unique in that it demonstrates a neoplastic-like growth potential, making accurate diagnosis essential to manage the high recurrence rate adequately.

CLINICAL FEATURES

Representing between 4%–12% of all odontogenic cysts, OKC is a distinctive developmental cyst of the mandible and maxilla, arising most commonly in the posterior mandible in the region of the 3rd molar specifically. OKCs may develop at any age, although most commonly in the 2nd–3rd decades, with a predilection for males. Many lesions are discovered incidentally during routine dental radiographs. Some patients, however, present with pain, swelling, and drainage, frequently related to a secondary infection of the cyst. Of clinical significance is the presence of OKC as one of the most consistent features of nevoid basal cell carcinoma syndrome (NBCCS), or Gorlin syndrome. Nevoid basal cell carcinoma syndrome is an autosomal dominant disorder (chromosome 9q22; patched [PTCH] tumor suppressor gene). The syndrome has many signs and symptoms including, but not limited to, numerous basal cell carcinomas of the skin, skeletal abnormalities (rib and vertebra), calcification of the falx cerebri, an increased frequency of certain neoplasms, and multiple OKCs.

RADIOLOGIC FEATURES

OKC usually presents as radiolucent, unilocular, well-defined lesion (Fig. 17-38). However, as lesions increase

ODONTOGENIC KERATOCYST DISEASE FACT SHEET

Definition	A developmental odontogenic cyst of the jaw that may exhibit aggressive clinical behavior, characterized by a uni- or multicystic intraosseous tumor with a distinct lining of parakeratinized stratified squamous epithelium
Incidence and location	Represents 4%–12% of odontogenic cysts
Morbidity and mortality	Morbidity is low, although high recurrence may require disfiguring surgery
Gender, race, and age distribution	Male > Female
	Incidence is higher among whites
	Any age, with peak in 2nd–3rd decades
Clinical features	Most lesions are incident and asymptomatic
	If symptomatic, pain, swelling, and drainage are most common
	Lesions of children, as well as multiple lesions, may be associated with nevoid basal cell carcinoma syndrome (NBCCS)
Radiographic findings	Well-defined, radiolucent, unilocular lesion
	Larger lesions may become multilocular
	Smooth corticated borders
	Unerupted tooth present (40%)
Prognosis and treatment	Frequent recurrences require close follow-up
	Association with the NBCCS
	Surgery

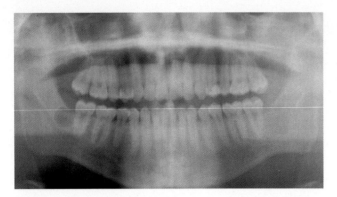

FIGURE 17-38

Panoramic radiograph. A small unilocular cyst of the right posterior mandible; microscopic evaluation revealed the lesion was an odontogenic keratocyst.

ODONTOGENIC KERATOCYST PATHOLOGIC FEATURES	
Gross findings	A thin friable cyst wall filled with either clear fluid or yellow-white keratin
	Unerupted tooth may be seen
Microscopic findings	Uniformly thin epithelium, usually 6 to 8 cells thick, with minimal rete ridges
	Artifactual clefting below epithelium
	Luminal epithelial cells show corrugated parakeratotic surface
	Palisaded cuboidal or columnar basal-cell layer
	Lumen contains keratinaceous debris
	Inflammation may alter the histologic features
Pathologic differential diagnosis	Orthokeratinized odontogenic cyst, dentigerous cyst, calcifying odontogenic cyst, ameloblastoma

in size they may become multilocular. Lesions usually have a smooth margin, without bone expansion, often associated with unerupted teeth (40%).

PATHOLOGIC FEATURES

GROSS FINDINGS

OKC has a fibrous cyst wall with a lumen which may be filled with either clear fluid or yellow-white keratin. The lesion may contain an unerupted tooth.

MICROSCOPIC FINDINGS

The histopathologic features of OKC are distinctive. The epithelial lining is uniformly thin, usually 6 to 8 cells thick (Fig. 17-39). Lesions show a distinct lack of rete ridges, resulting in a characteristic, although artifactual, separation of the epithelial lining from the underlying fibrous connective tissue. The luminal surface shows corrugated parakeratotic epithelial cells, with an underlying basal cell layer composed of pal-

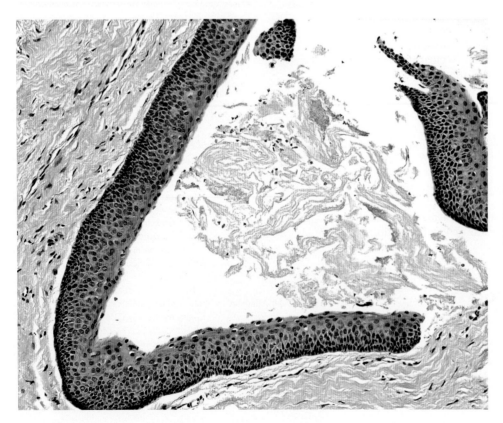

FIGURE 17-39

Note the thin parakeratotic epithelial lining with a focal area of keratinaceous debris in an odontogenic keratocyst.

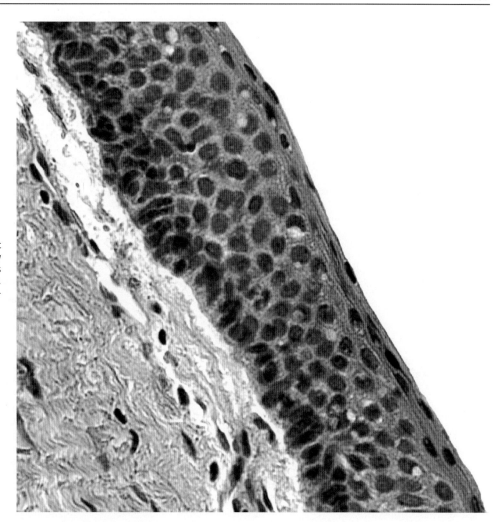

FIGURE 17-40
The epithelial layer is six to eight cells thick and demonstrates darkly stained columnar and cuboidal cells making up the distinct basal layer. The luminal surface shows a characteristic corrugated appearance.

isaded and hyperchromatic cuboidal or columnar epithelial cells (Fig. 17-40). The lumen may contain varying amounts of keratinacious material. OKCs may also show satellite cysts and islands of odontogenic epithelium; the latter features are more common in those patients who have NBCCS. It is important to note that inflammation may alter the features, making definitive diagnosis difficult.

DIFFERENTIAL DIAGNOSIS

Other odontogenic cysts must be considered in the differential diagnosis. A dentigerous cyst, the most common odontogenic cyst, lacks the basal palisading, corrugated parakeratized surface, and usually has numerous rete ridges with thicker epithelium. The orthokeratinized odontogenic cyst may share histologic features with OKC, but is orthokeratinized (not parakeratinized) and lacks the palisaded basal cell layer. A calcified odontogenic cyst has basal palisading, but has very distinctive ghost cells. An ameloblastoma, while in the differential diagnosis radiographically, shows a loosely arranged stellate reticulum, a feature which recapitulates the developing tooth.

PROGNOSIS AND THERAPY

Close patient follow-up is required to monitor for recurrences. Young patients and patients with multiple lesions should be evaluated for NBCCS. Complete removal is essential if recurrences are to be avoided. Controversy about how to achieve complete removal exists, with treatments including peripheral osseous curettage, ostectomy, en bloc resection, and marsupialization followed by surgery.

CENTRAL GIANT CELL LESION

The central giant cell lesion is a localized lytic lesion of the jawbones associated with fibrosis, hemorrhage, hemosiderin laden macrophages, reactive bone, and osteoclastic giant cells. To say this entity is fraught with controversy is an understatement. Suffice it to say that *giant cell reparative granuloma*, *giant cell granuloma*, *aneurysmal bone cyst*, and *giant cell tumor*, all may describe the same entity. Lack of agreement about the

CENTRAL GIANT CELL LESION DISEASE FACT SHEET	
Definition	A localized osteolytic lesion of the jaw bones associated with fibrosis, hemorrhage, hemosiderin laden macrophages, reactive bone and osteoclastic giant cells
Incidence and location	Uncommon
	Mandible > maxilla (2 : 1)
Gender, race, and age distribution	Female > Male (1.5–2 : 1)
	Average 20 yr (>90% before 30 yr)
Clinical features	Separated by radiographic and clinical features into nonaggressive and aggressive
	Usually asymptomatic
	Painless expansion of the jaw, paresthesias, and tooth resorption
Radiographic features	Range from unilocular, well-circumscribed radiolucent lesions to large, expansile multilocular lytic lesions
	Root resorption and displacement of teeth may be seen
	Intralesional bony ("wavy") septae may be seen
Prognosis and treatment	Long-term prognosis is good, although histology doesn't predict behavior
	Complete enucleation, although steroid injection, alpha-interferon injections and calcitonin treatments are effective

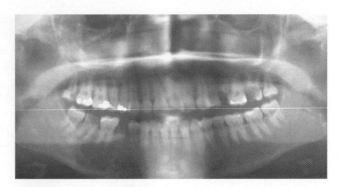

FIGURE 17-41
Panoramic radiograph. A large expanding radiolucent lesion of the posterior mandible.

CENTRAL GIANT CELL LESION PATHOLOGIC FEATURES	
Gross findings	Red to brown hemorrhagic tissue with associated bone
Microscopic findings	Multinucleated, osteoclastic giant cells in a background of ovoid to spindle-shaped fibroblastic cells
	Richly vascularized associated with extravagated erythrocytes, and hemosiderin laden macrophages
	Metaplastic bone and osteoid traverse the lesion
	Mitotic figures are common (although not atypical)
Pathologic differential diagnosis	Brown tumor of hyperparathyroidism, cherubism

true nature of the lesion has led to acceptance of the more neutral "giant cell lesion" until further study resolves these questions.

CLINICAL FEATURES

Central giant cell lesions are found in a wide age range, although the average is 20 years. Women are affected more than men (1.5–2 : 1), and there is a definitive predilection for the mandible. Giant cell lesions of the jaw have traditionally been divided, based on clinical and radiologic features, into two categories: nonaggressive and aggressive. Nonaggressive lesions are usually asymptomatic, incidental findings. Aggressive lesions may present with pain, paresthesias, and resorption of teeth.

RADIOLOGIC FEATURES

Central giant cell lesions present as expansile uni- or multilocular radiolucent defects with scalloped and usually well-defined borders (Fig. 17-41). Tooth displacement can be seen. Intralesional bony septa are helpful, although radiographic findings are not diagnostic.

PATHOLOGIC FEATURES

The lesion consists of oval to spindle-shaped fibroblastic cells; some lesions are highly cellular, others are loose and myxoid (Fig. 17-42). A richly vascularized stroma is associated with extravasated erythrocytes (hemorrhage), hemosiderin laden macrophages, and giant cells (Fig. 17-43). The osteoclastic giant cell population is variable, without an absolute number required for the diagnosis. While multinucleated, the number of nuclei is quite variable. Lobules of collagen and metaplastic bone traverse the lesion, although accentuated at the periphery. Mitoses are common, but are not atypical. Aggressiveness is clinically and radiographically determined.

DIFFERENTIAL DIAGNOSIS

The central giant cell lesion is histologically identical to a brown tumor of hyperparathyroidism. Therefore, the

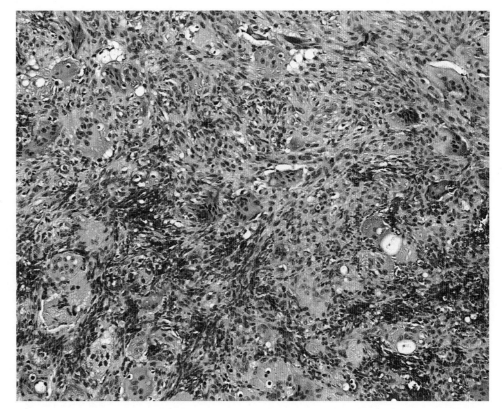

FIGURE 17-42
Large giant cells within a cellular mesenchymal tissue in the bone in a central giant cell lesion.

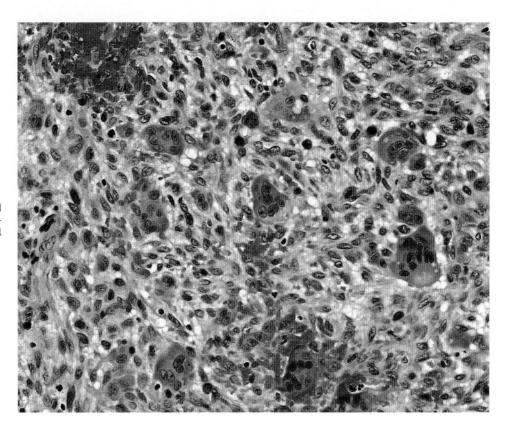

FIGURE 17-43
Large giant cells in a stroma of ovoid to spindle-shaped cells. Note the erythrocyte extravasation in this central giant cell lesion.

diagnosis of this entity as *central giant cell lesion, rule out hyperparathyroidism* may be most prudent, and patient's serum calcium and parathyroid hormone levels should be checked. Histologic separation from cherubism may be difficult; eosinophilic ring-like deposits surrounding vessels and the clinical and radiographic information will allow for proper separation.

PROGNOSIS AND THERAPY

Histology does not predict behavior. Recurrences are rare if there is unaffected bone at the margins of the resection. Complete enucleation has traditionally been the treatment of choice, but steroid injection, alpha-interferon injections, and calcitonin treatments have proven effective. The nonsurgical techniques require months before regression is seen.

SUGGESTED READING

Ossifying Fibroma

1. Eversole LR, Leider AS, Nelson K: Ossifying fibroma: a clinicopathologic study of sixty-four cases. Oral Surg Oral Med Oral Pathol 1985;60: 505–511.
2. Su L, Weathers DR, Waldron CA: Distinguishing features of focal cemento-osseous dysplasia and cemento-ossifying fibromas I. A pathologic spectrum of 316 cases. Oral Surg Oral Med Oral Pathol 1997;84: 301–309.
3. Su L, Weathers DR, Waldron CA: Distinguishing features of focal cemento-osseous dysplasia and cemento-ossifying fibromas II. A clinical and radiologic spectrum of 316 cases. Oral Surg Oral Med Oral Pathol 1997;84:540–549.
4. Sciubba JJ, Fantasia JE, Kahn LB: Fibro-osseous lesions. In: Sciubba JJ, Fantasia JE, Kahn LB, eds. Atlas of Tumor Pathology, Tumors and Cysts of the Jaw. Washington, DC: Armed Forces Institute of Pathology, 1999:145–151.
5. Slootweg PJ, El Mofty SK: Ossifying fibroma. In: Barnes EL, Eveson JW, Reichart P, Sidransky D, eds. Pathology and Genetics of Head and Neck Tumours. Kleihues P, Sobin LH, series eds. World Health Organization Classification of Tumours. Lyon, France: IARC Press, 2005:319–320.
6. Slootweg PJ, Muller H: Differential diagnosis of fibro-osseous jaw lesions. A histologic investigation of 30 cases. J Craniomaxillofac Surg 1990;18:210–214.

Juvenile/Active Ossifying Fibroma

1. Bendet E, Bakon M, Tadmor R, et al.: Juvenile cemento-ossifying fibroma of the maxilla. Ann Otol Rhinol Laryngol 1997;106:75–78.
2. Sciubba JJ, Fantasia JE, Kahn LB: Fibro-osseous lesions. In: Sciubba JJ, Fantasia JE, Kahn LB. Atlas of Tumor Pathology, Tumors and Cysts of the Jaw. Washington, DC: Armed Forces Institute of Pathology, 1999:147–151.
3. Slootweg PJ, Panders AK, Koopmans R, Nikkels PGJ: Juvenile ossifying fibroma. An analysis of 33 cases with emphasis on histopathological aspects. J Oral Pathol Med 1994;23:285–288.
4. Wiendenfeld KR, Neville BW, Hutchins AR, et al.: Juvenile ossifying fibroma of the maxilla in a 6-year-old male: case report. Ped Dentistry 1995;17:365–367.

Osteoma

1. Kaplan I, Calderon S, Buchner A: Peripheral osteoma of the mandible: a study of 10 new cases and analysis of the literature. J Oral Maxillofac Surg 1994;52:467–470.

2. Schneider LC, Dolinsky HB, Grodjesk JE: Solitary peripheral osteoma of the jaws: a report of case and review of literature. J Oral Surg 1980;38:452–455.
3. Sciubba JJ, Fantasia JE, Kahn LB: Nonodontogenic esions. In: Sciubba JJ, Fantasia JE, Kahn LB. Atlas of Tumor Pathology, Tumors and Cysts of the Jaw. Washington, DC: Armed Forces Institute of Pathology, 1999:173–175.

Cementoblastoma

1. Ackermann GL, Altini M: The cementomas—a clinicopathological reappraisal. J Dent Assoc S Afr 1992;47:187–194.
2. Sciubba JJ, Fantasia JE, Kahn LB: Odontogenic cysts. In: Sciubba JJ, Fantasia JE, Kahn LB. Atlas of Tumor Pathology, Tumors and Cysts of the Jaw. Washington, DC: Armed Forces Institute of Pathology, 1999:109–110.
3. Slootweg PJ: Cementoblastoma and osteoblastoma: A comparison of histologic features. J Oral Pathol Med 1996;13:104–112.
4. van der Waal I: Cementoblastoma. In: Barnes EL, Eveson JW, Reichart P, Sidransky D, eds. Pathology and Genetics of Head and Neck Tumours. Kleihues P, Sobin LH, series eds. World Health Organization Classification of Tumours. Lyon, France: IARC Press, 2005:318.
5. Zachariades N, Skordalaki A, Papanicolaou S, et al.: Cementoblastoma: review of the literature and report of a case in a seven-year-old girl. Br J Oral Maxillofac Surg 1985;23:453–461.

Osteoblastoma

1. Ataoglu O, Oygur T, Yamalik K, Yucel E: Recurrent osteoblastoma of the mandible. A case report. J Oral Maxillofac Surg 1994;52:86–90.
2. Lucas DR, Unni KK, McLeod RA, et al.: Osteolastoma: clinicopathologic study of 306 cases. Hum Pathol 1994;25:117–134.
3. Malcolm A, Schiller A, Schneider-Stock R: Osteoblastoma. In: Fletcher DM, Unni KK, Mertens F. Pathology and Genetics, Tumours of Soft Tissue and Bone. Lyon, France: World Health Organization Classification of Tumours, 2002;262–263.
4. Sciubba JJ, Fantasia JE, Kahn LB: Nonodontogenic Lesions. In: Sciubba JJ, Fantasia JE, Kahn LB. Atlas of Tumor Pathology, Tumors and Cysts of the Jaw. Washington, DC: Armed Forces Institute of Pathology, 1999:175–181.
5. van der Waal I, Greebe RB, Elias EA: Benign osteoblastoma or osteoid osteoma of the maxilla. Report of a case. Int J Oral Surg 1983;12:355–358.
6. Weinberg S, Katsikeris N, Pharoah M: Osteoblastoma of the mandibular condyle: review of the literature and report of a case. J Oral Maxillofac Surg 1987;45:350–355.

Odontoma (Complex and Compound)

1. Budnick SD: Compound and complex odontomas. Oral Surg 1976;42:501–506.
2. Kaugars GE, Miller ME, Abbey LM: Odontomas. Oral Surg Oral Med Oral Pathol 1989;67:172–176.
3. Prætorius F, Piattelli A: Odontoma, complex type. In: Barnes EL, Eveson JW, Reichart P, Sidransky D, eds. Pathology and Genetics of Head and Neck Tumours. Kleihues P, Sobin LH, series eds. World Health Organization Classification of Tumours. Lyon, France: IARC Press, 2005:310.
4. Prætorius F, Piattelli A: Odontoma, compound type. In: Barnes EL, Eveson JW, Reichart P, Sidransky D, eds. Pathology and Genetics of Head and Neck Tumours. Kleihues P, Sobin LH, series eds. World Health Organization Classification of Tumours. Lyon, France: IARC Press, 2005:311.
5. Sciubba JJ, Fantasia JE, Kahn LB: Benign odontogenic tumors. In: Sciubba JJ, Fantasia JE, Kahn LB. Atlas of Tumor Pathology, Tumors and Cysts of the Jaw. Washington, DC: Armed Forces Institute of Pathology, 1999:117–120.

Adenomatoid Odontogenic Tumor

1. Aldred MJ, Gray AR: A pigmented adenomatoid odontogenic tumor. Oral Surg Oral Med Oral Pathol 1990;70:86–89.
2. Philipsen HP, Nikai H: Adenomatoid odontogenic tumour. In: Barnes EL, Eveson JW, Reichart P, Sidransky D, eds. Pathology and Genetics of Head and Neck Tumours. Kleihues P, Sobin LH, series eds. World Health

Organization Classification of Tumours. Lyon, France: IARC Press, 2005:304–305.

3. Philipsen HP, Reichart PA, Zhang KH, et al.: Adenomatoid odontogenic tumor: biologic profile on 499 cases. J Oral Pathol Med 1991;20: 149–158.

4. Philipsen HP, Reichart PA: Adenomatoid odontogenic tumour: fact and figures. Oral Oncol 1999;35:125–131.

5. Saku T, Okabe H, Shimokawa H: Immunohistochemical demonstration of enamel proteins in odontogenic tumors. J Oral Pathol Med 1992;21:113–119.

6. Sciubba JJ, Fantasia JE, Kahn LB: Benign odontogenic tumors. In: Sciubba JJ, Fantasia JE, Kahn LB. Atlas of Tumor Pathology, Tumors and Cysts of the Jaw. Washington, DC: Armed Forces Institute of Pathology, 1999:90–95.

Ameloblastoma

1. Corio RL, Goldblatt LI, Edwards PA, Hartman KS: Ameloblastic carcinoma: a clinicopathologic study and assessment of eight cases. Oral Surg Oral Med Oral Pathol 1987;64:570–576.

2. Gardner DG, Corio RL: Plexiform unicystic ameloblastoma. A variant of ameloblastoma with a low recurrence rate after enucleation. Cancer 1984;53:1730–1735.

3. Gardner DG, Heikinheimo K, Shear M, Philipsen HP, Coleman H: Ameloblastomas. In: Barnes EL, Eveson JW, Reichart P, Sidransky D, eds. Pathology and Genetics of Head and Neck Tumours. Kleihues P, Sobin LH, series eds. World Health Organization Classification of Tumours. Lyon, France: IARC Press, 2005:296–300.

4. Leider AS, Eversole LR, Barkin ME: Cystic ameloblastoma: A clinicopathologic analysis. Oral Surg Oral Med Oral Pathol 1985;60:624–630.

5. Mosqueda-Taylor A: Odontoameloblstoma. In: Barnes EL, Eveson JW, Reichart P, Sidransky D, eds. Pathology and Genetics of Head and Neck Tumours. Kleihues P, Sobin LH, series eds. World Health Organization Classification of Tumours. Lyon, France: IARC Press, 2005:312.

6. Philipsen HP, Orminston IW, Reichart PA: The desmo- and osteoblastic ameloblastoma: Histologic variant or clinicopathologic entity? Int J Oral Maxillofac Surg 1992;21:352–357.

7. Schafer DG, Thompson LDR, Smith BC, Wenig BM: Primary ameloblastoma of the Sinonasal tract: a clinicopathologic study of 24 cases. Cancer 1998;82:667–674.

8. Sciubba JJ, Fantasia JE, Kahn LB: Benign odontogenic tumors. In: Rosai J. Tumors and Cyst of the Jaw. Washington, DC: Armed Forces Institute of Pathology, 2001:77–127.

9. Slootweg PJ: Ameloblastic fibroma/fibrodentinoma. In: Barnes EL, Eveson JW, Reichart P, Sidransky D, eds. Pathology and Genetics of Head and Neck Tumours. Kleihues P, Sobin LH, series eds. World Health Organization Classification of Tumours. Lyon, France: IARC Press, 2005:308.

10. Takeda Y, Tomich CE: Ameloblastic fibro-odontoma. In: Barnes EL, Eveson JW, Reichart P, Sidransky D, eds. Pathology and Genetics of Head and Neck Tumours. Kleihues P, Sobin LH, series eds. World Health Organization Classification of Tumours. Lyon, France: IARC Press, 2005:309.

11. Vickers RA, Gorlin RJ: Ameloblastoma: delineation of early histopathologic features of neoplasia. Cancer 1970;26:699–710.

Central Odontogenic Fibroma

1. Dahl EC, Wolfson SH, Haugen JC: Central odontogenic fibroma: review of literature and report of cases. J Oral Surg 1981;39:120–124.

2. Gardner DG: Central odontogenic fibroma current concepts. J Oral Pathol Med 1996;25:556–561.

3. Gardner DG: The central odontogenic fibroma: an attempt at clarification. Oral Surg 1980;5:425–432.

4. Philipsen HP, Reichart PA, Sciubba JJ, van der Waal I: Odontogenic fibroma. In: Barnes EL, Eveson JW, Reichart P, Sidransky D, eds. Pathology and Genetics of Head and Neck Tumours. Kleihues P, Sobin LH, series eds. World Health Organization Classification of Tumours. Lyon, France: IARC Press, 2005:315.

5. Ramer M, Buonocore P, Krost B: Central odontogenic fibroma—report of a case and review of the literature. Periodontal Clin Investig 2002;24:27–30.

Calcifying Epithelial Odontogenic Tumor

1. Hicks MJ, Flaitz CM, Wong ME, et al.: Clear cell variant of calcifying epithelial odontogenic tumor: case report and review of the literature. Head Neck 1994;16:272–277.

2. Philipsen HP, Reichart PA: Calcifying epithelial odontogenic tumour: biological profile based on 181 cases from the literature. Oral Oncol 2000;36:17–26.

3. Pindborg JJ: A calcifying epithelial odontogenic tumor. Cancer 1958;11: 838–843

4. Pindborg JJ, Vedtofte P, Reibel J, Praetoruis F: The calcifying epithelial odontogenic tumor. A review of recent literature and report of a case. APMIS 1991;23(Suppl):152–157.

5. Sciubba JJ, Fantasia JE, Kahn LB: Benign odontogenic tumors. In: Sciubba JJ, Fantasia JE, Kahn LB. Atlas of Tumor Pathology, Tumors and Cysts of the Jaw. Washington, DC: Armed Forces Institute of Pathology, 1999:85–90.

6. Takata T, Slootweg PJ: Calcifying epithelial odontogenic tumour. In: Barnes EL, Eveson JW, Reichart P, Sidransky D, eds. Pathology and Genetics of Head and Neck Tumours. Kleihues P, Sobin LH, series eds. World Health Organization Classification of Tumours. Lyon, France: IARC Press, 2005:302–303.

Odontogenic Keratocyst

1. Brannon RB: The odontogenic keratocyst—a clinicopathologic study of 312 cases. Part I: clinical features. Oral Surg Oral Med Oral Pathol 1976;42:54–72.

2. Brannon RB: The odontogenic keratocyst—a clinicopathologic study of 312 cases. Part II: histologic features. Oral Surg Oral Med Oral Pathol 1977;43:233–255.

3. Daley TD, Wysocki GP, Pringle GA: Relative incidence of odontogenic tumors and jaw cysts in a Canadian population. Oral Surg Oral Med Oral Pathol 1994;77:276–280.

4. Gorlin RJ, Goltz RW: Multiple nevoid basal-cell epithelioma, jaw and bifid rib syndrome. N Engl J Med 1960;262:908–914.

5. Sciubba JJ, Fantasia JE, Kahn LB: Odontogenic cysts. In: Sciubba JJ, Fantasia JE, Kahn LB. Atlas of Tumor Pathology, Tumors and Cysts of the Jaw. Washington, DC: Armed Forces Institute of Pathology, 1999:34–43.

6. Wicking C, Bale AE: Molecular basis of the nevoid basal cell carcinoma syndrome. Curr Opin Pediatr 1997;9:630–635.

Central Giant Cell Lesion

1. Chuong R, Kaban LB, Kozakewich H, Perez-Atayde A: Central giant cell lesions of the jaws: a clinocopathologic study. J Oral Maxillofac Surg 1986;44:708–713.

2. Ficcarra G, Kaban LB, Hansen LS: Giant cell lesions of the jaw: a clinicopathologic and cytometric study. Oral Surg Oral Med Oral Pathol 1987;64:44–49.

3. Jundt G: Central giant cell lesions. In: Barnes EL, Eveson JW, Reichart P, Sidransky D, eds. Pathology and Genetics of Head and Neck Tumours. Kleihues P, Sobin LH, series eds. World Health Organization Classification of Tumours. Lyon, France: IARC Press, 2005: 324.

4. Kaffe I, Ardekian L, Taicher S, et al.: Radiologic features of central giant cell granuloma of the jaws. Oral Surg Oral Med Oral Pathol Radiol Endod 1996;81:720–726.

5. Pogrel MA: Calcitonin therapy for central giant cell granuloma. J Oral Maxillofac Surg 2003;61:649–653.

6. Sciubba JJ, Fantasia JE, Kahn LB: Nonodontogenic lesions. In: Sciubba JJ, Fantasia JE, Kahn LB. Atlas of Tumor Pathology, Tumors and Cysts of the Jaw. Washington, DC: Armed Forces Institute of Pathology, 1999:161–167.

7. Waldrom CA, Shafer WG: The central giant cell reparative granuloma of the jaw. An analysis of 38 cases. Am J Clin Pathol 1966;45:437–447.

8. Whitaker SB, Waldron CA: Central giant cell lesions of the jaws. A clinical, radiologic, and histopathologic study. Oral Surg Oral Med Oral Pathol 1993;75:199–208.

Malignant Neoplasms of the Gnathic Bones

Gary Warnock

OSTEOSARCOMA

CLINICAL FEATURES

Osteosarcoma is the most common primary malignant bone tumor; however, jaw tumors make up only about 7% of all osteosarcomas. While most tumors arise de novo, many arise postradiation therapy, in Paget's disease, osteomyelitis, and in preexisting benign osseous tumors. Extragnathic tumors are most frequently seen in the second decade, whereas jaw tumors occur a full decade later, with a mean age at presentation of 33 years. Males are affected more frequently than females. The maxilla and mandible are equally affected; series suggest maxillary tumors are more common in females, while mandibular tumors are more common in males. Patients present with localized bone expansion and pain, malocclusion (Fig. 18-1), loose teeth, and paresthesia. Conventional intramedullary osteosarcoma comprises the bulk of tumors in the jaws, while paraosteal type are the most common surface bone tumor.

RADIOLOGIC FEATURES

The radiographic picture of osteosarcoma varies widely from lytic to mottled to densely sclerotic (Fig. 18-2). Tumors have poorly defined borders with varying degrees of radiolucency and radiopacity, often with enclaved spicules of residual bone. The irregularity of the sclerotic areas often complicates determining the extent of the tumor (Fig. 18-3). Tumors involving teeth may cause significant tooth resorption along with widening of the periodontal ligament, dissolution of the lamina dura and heightened interdental reactive or malignant bone deposition at the alveolar crest. In mature lesions the radiographic picture is that of "moth-eaten" bone with ragged lytic areas (Fig. 18-4). Radiographic findings in the maxillary osteosarcomas frequently cause opacification of the antrum, mimicking a soft tissue tumor or sinusitis. Approximately a quarter of the tumors will erode through the cortical plate into soft tissue, laying down bone spicules at right angles to

OSTEOSARCOMA DISEASE FACT SHEET	
Definition	The most common primary malignant bone tumor defined by the production of malignant osteoid (bone) from sarcomatous stroma
Incidence and location	Gnathic tumors accounts for about 7% of all osteosarcomas
Gender, race, and age distribution	Male > Female (2 : 1) Mean age, 33 yr
Clinical features	Localized bone expansion with pain Malocclusion with loosening of teeth and paresthesias Maxillary lesions: exophthalmia, diplopia, and nasal stuffiness Associated with Paget's disease, postirradiation, and preexisting benign osseous tumors
Radiographic features	Irregular "moth-eaten" lytic lesions Tooth root resorption Loss of lamina dura and widened periodontal ligament Interdental cortical alveolar bone expansion
Prognosis and treatment	75%–85% overall survival rate Better prognosis in jaws than extragnathic Frequent local recurrence with tumor invading vital structures Preadjunctive chemotherapy with radical tumor resection

the cortical bone and creating a "sun burst" pattern (Fig. 18-5). Defining radiographic margins is accomplished by computed tomography (CT) or magnetic resonance imaging (MRI) scans which best delineates the tumor from the medullary bone.

PATHOLOGIC FEATURES

GROSS FINDINGS

Osteosarcoma at grossing is typically an irregular poorly defined firm yellow-white tumor with focally

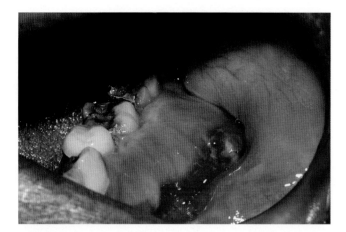

FIGURE 18-1

Clinical presentation of an osteosarcoma of posterior mandible exhibiting significant alveolar expansion, tooth movement, and tumor ulceration in vestibule.

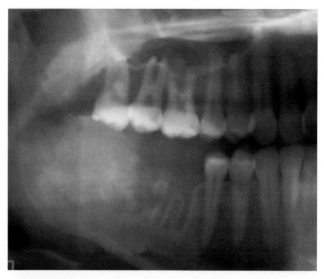

FIGURE 18-2

Osteosarcoma with mixed radiolucent/radiopaque presentation in posterior mandible with expansive sclerotic alveolar lesion in ascending ramus and lytic radiolucency in area of molar tooth loss.

OSTEOSARCOMA PATHOLOGIC FEATURES	
Gross findings	Firm, yellow-white tumor with gritty areas
	Tumor resembles bone marrow
	Reticulated interface with cortical bone
	Opalescent foci of chondroid nodules seen in chondroblastic variant
Microscopic findings	Malignant, irregular osteoid/bone production
	Malignant oval to spindled tumor cells with nuclear atypia, chromatin clumping, and atypical large nucleoli
	Lace-like trabeculae of malignant osteoid
	Increased pleomorphism and mitoses with increased tumor grade
	Chondroid and mucohyalinized ground substance matrix
Immunohistochemical features	CD99 positive; rare cytokeratin and smooth muscle actin reaction
Pathologic differential diagnosis	Osteoblastoma, dedifferentiated chondrosarcoma, malignant fibrous histiocytoma, fibrosarcoma, benign giant cell tumors

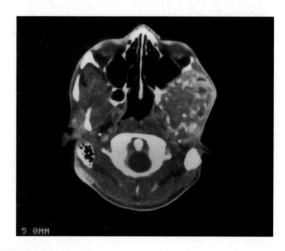

FIGURE 18-3

CT scan showing marked expansion of maxilla with tumor filling maxillary sinus.

gritty areas. Scattered foci of opalescent chondroid appearing lobules are seen in chondroblastic osteosarcoma. Advanced tumors may contain areas of hemorrhage and necrosis intermixed with residual bone marrow.

MICROSCOPIC FINDINGS

The hallmark of osteosarcoma is the production of malignant bone or osteoid from malignant mesenchymal stroma (Fig. 18-6). The sarcomatous stroma varies in degree of aberrancy and cytologic character with tumor grade. Low-grade tumors are only moderately cellular

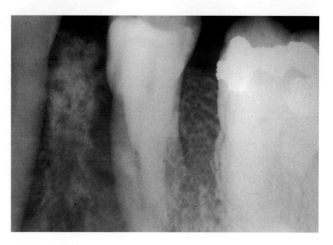

FIGURE 18-4

A maxillary osteosarcoma creating diastemas, widening of periodontal ligament, "moth-eaten" bone, and increased alveolar height.

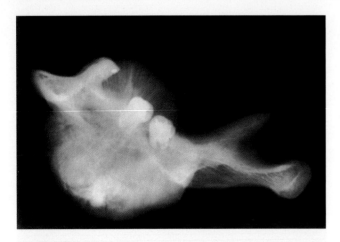

FIGURE 18-5
Mandibular resection specimen displaying significant tumor expansion with "sun-burst" pattern on lingual surface of mandible.

with minimal pleomorphism, few mitotic figures, and produce osteoid and bone that is irregular, lacks lamellae, and has an atypical mineralization pattern. Paraosteal osteosarcomas are well differentiated low-grade tumors, displaying almost no atypia and frequently show focal trabecular rimming, which is not considered a typical feature of conventional osteosarcomas. High-grade tumors are very cellular with closely packed oval, spindled, or polygonal cells with nuclear pleomorphism, chromatin clumping, large nucleoli, and numerous mitotic figures (Fig. 18-7). Malignant osteoid may be difficult to appreciate, because it is minimal and deposited as thin eosinophilic strands interposed between sheets of malignant osteoblasts. Tumors with heavy osteoid and bone production form broad trabecu-

lae with isolated single osteoblasts encompassed in osteoid undergoing normalization through loss of their previous cytologic atypia (Fig. 18-8). Conventional osteosarcomas are histologically subclassified by their most prominent characteristic: fibroblastic (Fig. 18-9), chondroblastic (Fig. 18-10), or osteoblastic. Regardless of the subclassification, deposition of malignant bone or osteoid must be demonstrated to meet the criteria of an osteosarcoma. Telangiectatic and small cell osteosarcoma variants are exceedingly rare in the jaws.

ANCILLARY STUDIES

The difficulty with fine needle aspiration (FNA) of osteosarcoma is the actual sampling technique. However, once the sample is obtained, the smears are cellular, composed of pleomorphic spindle, and rounded tumor cells, occasionally resembling osteoblasts and osteoclasts. Multinucleated tumor cells are often present (Fig. 18-11). Mitotic figures may be appreciated, and amorphous background "osteoid" material may be present, staining eosinophilic with alcohol fixation and magenta with air-dried preparations. There are differing findings for other types of osteosarcoma.

DIFFERENTIAL DIAGNOSIS

Distinguishing osteoblastoma from osteosarcoma both radiographically and histologically is difficult; however, usually osteoblastoma is better circumscribed with a sclerotic margin. Osteoblastoma forms thick trabeculae

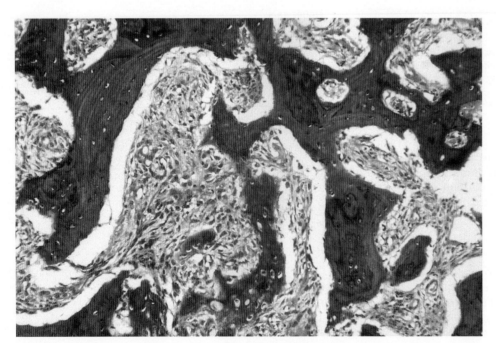

FIGURE 18-6

Medium-power view of osteosarcoma with irregular trabeculae of malignant bone and osteoid arising from sarcomatous stroma characterized by pleomorphic cells with oval and spindled nuclei.

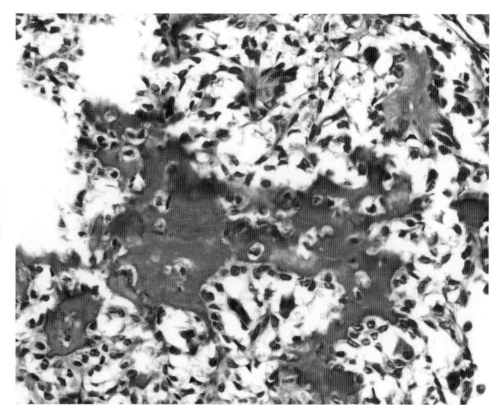

FIGURE 18-7

High-power view of moderately differentiated osteosarcoma with irregular sheeted trabeculae and enclaved pleomorphic osteocytes with oval hyperchromatic nuclei surrounded by edematous stroma.

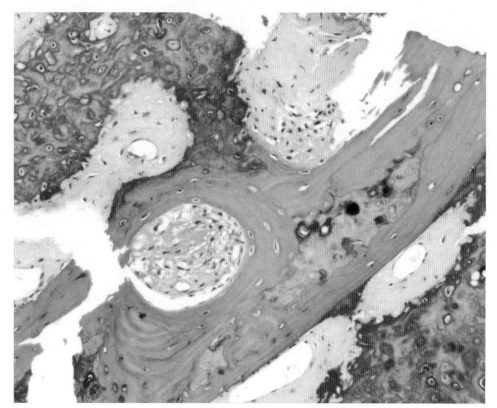

FIGURE 18-8

Aggressive osteosarcoma resorbing residual bone trabeculae with subsequent replacement by malignant tumor bone.

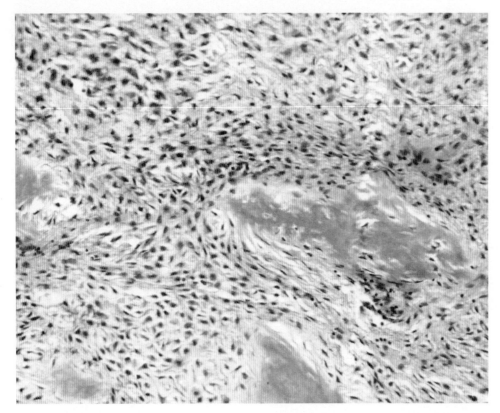

FIGURE 18-9
A fibroblastic osteosarcoma shows a vague fasciculated pattern of spindled and oval cells intertwined in fine collagen fibrils with osteoid arising from the stroma.

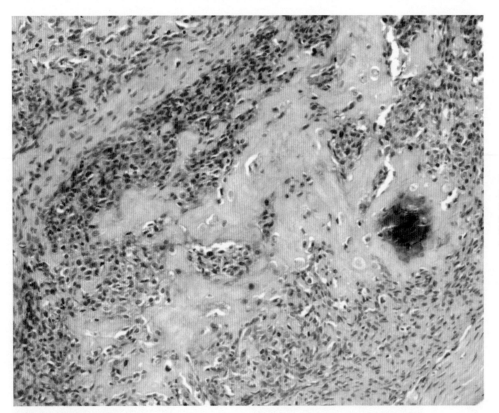

FIGURE 18-10
Chondroblastic osteosarcoma with sheets of small pleomorphic tumor cells circumscribing chondroid appearing osteoid containing chondrocytic cells.

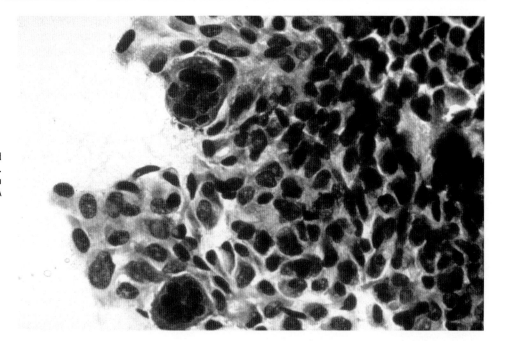

FIGURE 18-11
Malignant oval to spindle-shaped cells are arranged in a dense cluster. Multinucleated giant cells are seen in this osteosarcoma (air-dried FNA preparation).

from broad sheets of epithelioid osteoblasts with trabeculae riming, a feature not seen in osteosarcoma. Osteosarcoma may produce cartilage, whereas osteoblastoma produces cartilage only in areas of previous biopsy. Osteosarcoma is cytologically more pleomorphic and while both are mitotically active, aberrant mitotic figures are not seen in osteoblastoma.

Osteosarcoma on occasion contain large numbers of reactive multinucleated giant cells, resembling benign giant cell tumor. Osteosarcoma with minimal osteoid and giant cells is strikingly similar to benign giant cell tumor and is separated by evaluation of the mononuclear cells which exhibit more pleomorphism with aberrant mitotic figures.

Separation of dedifferentiated chondrosarcoma and chondroblastic osteosarcoma is challenging as each produces chondroid and osteoid. The distinguishing factors are areas of low-grade chondrosarcoma in dedifferentiated chondrosarcoma while chondroblastic osteosarcoma consists of a mixture of high-grade chondrosarcoma intermixed with osteosarcoma. Fibroblastic osteosarcoma producing limited osteoid and malignant bone raises the differential consideration of fibrosarcoma and malignant fibrous histiocytoma (MFH). The production of malignant osteoid favors a diagnosis of osteosarcoma over fibrosarcoma and MFH. As some pathologists accept osteoid in MFH, separation from MFH may be based on the more fasciculated pattern in a MFH.

PROGNOSIS AND THERAPY

Treatment of osteosarcoma is wide surgical resection with neoadjunctive or postsurgical chemotherapy with a variety of agents. Gnathic osteosarcoma survival rates approximate those of extragnathic tumors at about 80 % in patients receiving adequate initial surgical resection. Lesions in the jaws tend to have slightly better prognosis than skeletal lesions and a lower rate of metastasis. Local recurrence and inaccessibility of the tumor frequently causes the demise of patients with jaw lesions, particularly in the maxilla. The lungs are the most frequent site of metastasis and can be treated with resection of solitary metastatic lesions, resulting in a 40 % salvage rate.

CHONDROSARCOMA

CLINICAL FEATURES

Chondrosarcoma is the second most common primary malignant tumor of bone. As in chondrosarcomas of long bones, the most common presenting symptoms in craniofacial bones are cortical expansion and pain. Maxillary tumors may cause nasal obstruction, sinusitis, and secondary ophthalmic aberrations. While chondrosarcomas of long bones favor females 2 : 1, jaw tumors have an equal gender distribution, and equal occurrence in the mandible and maxilla. Tumors present over a broad age range, the bulk seen in the 3rd–6th decades with the mesenchymal variant occurring earlier in the 2nd and 3rd decades. Mandibular tumors occur predominately in the posterior angle and ramus. Maxillary tumors involve primarily the maxillary sinuses and nasal cavity and are less confined as they quickly erode the thin maxillary bone walls. Early jaw symptoms frequently include malocclusion with developing diastemas, loose teeth (Fig. 18-12), and eventual bony expansion.

RADIOLOGIC FEATURES

Radiographic findings are variable and reflect the tumor grade. Low-grade tumors appear expansive, destroying adjacent bone, but usually have a well-defined leading

edge with a lytic radiolucent tumor core. High-grade tumors create a more diffuse radiolucency with ragged destruction of bone and extension into soft tissue. When teeth are involved, a distinct triad of radiographic findings are seen, those being symmetrical widening of the periodontal ligament, elevation of the interdental alveolar cortical bone, and tooth resorption (Figs. 18-13, 18-14). Tumors producing significant mineralization have spotty calcifications with a ring-like pattern, specific for chondrosarcoma (Fig. 18-15). The borders of maxillary tumors are difficult to identify, as tumors frequently destroy maxillary indigenous bone, invading into the adjacent soft tissue, nasal cavity, and sinuses. CT and

CHONDROSARCOMA DISEASE FACT SHEET	
Definition	Second most common malignant tumor of the craniofacial bones characterized by malignant hyaline cartilage with diverse histology
Incidence and location	11% of all bone tumors, but 2% of malignant head and neck tumors
	Arising in central (54%), peripheral (38%), and juxtacortical (8%)
Gender, race, and age distribution	Male > Female (2 : 1)
	Peak in 3rd–6th decades (mean, 55 yr)
	Mesenchymal variant has younger mean age (30 yr)
Clinical features	75% present with bony expansion and pain present for a long duration
	Malocclusion with tooth movement and developing diastemas
Radiographic features	Mixed radiolucency with irregular opacities, central ossification and radiolucent peripheral margin
	Mottled and "moth-eaten"
	Widening of periodontal ligament
Prognosis and treatment	Wide en bloc resection with 2–3 cm margins
	Grade determine management and outcome:
	Grade 1, rare metastasis, 68%–89% 5-yr survival rate
	Grade 2, 33% metastatic rate
	Grade 3, 70% metastatic rate
	Mesenchymal chondrosarcoma: 55% 5-yr survival rate
	Pediatric patients have better prognosis
	Primary site of metastasis is the lungs

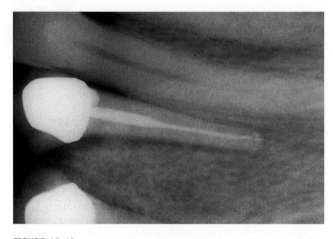

FIGURE 18-13
Radiographic appearance of chondrosarcoma is fine diffuse spiculation with increased alveolar height, splaying of teeth and widened periodontal ligament.

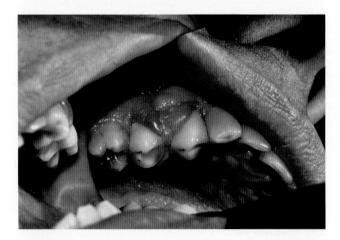

FIGURE 18-12
Chondrosarcoma creating alveolar expansion with separation of bicuspids and clinical malocclusion.

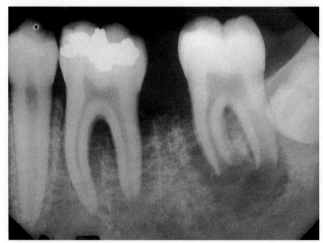

FIGURE 18-14
Chondrosarcoma of the mandible presenting a radiolucent lesion involving molars with resorption and expanded periodontal ligament.

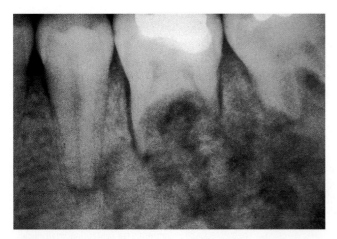

FIGURE 18-15
Chondrosarcoma with mixed radiolucent/radiopaque with "spotty-calcification" and tooth resorption.

CHONDROSARCOMA PATHOLOGIC FEATURES	
Gross findings	Cut surface opalescent blue to pearly white with gritty foci
	Translucent areas of hyaline cartilage and chalky calcifications
	Irregular tumor margin interface with central mucoid and cystic areas
Microscopic findings	Invasive into bone
	Lobules of cartilaginous matrix around atypical chondrocytes
	Increased cellularity
	Enlarged, atypical nuclei, and multinucleated cells
	Higher grade tumors have increased atypia, cellularity, less matrix, and mitotic figures
	Mesenchymal variant is a small cell neoplasm with scattered island of cartilage and "stag-horn" vascular pattern
Immunohistochemical features	Cartilage stains S-100 positive
	Mesenchymal chondrosarcoma: Sox 9, CD99, and Leu 7 positive
Pathologic differential diagnosis	Enchondroma, osteochondroma, chondroblastic osteosarcoma, odontogenic myxoma, small round cell malignant neoplasms

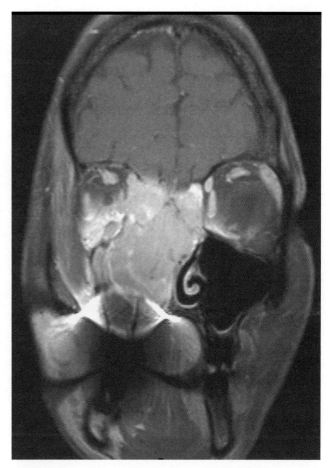

FIGURE 18-16
A T1-weighted MRI scan demonstrating an expansile tumor of the maxillary sinus, extending into the paranasal sinuses of this mesenchymal chondrosarcoma.

scattered areas of gritty calcifications. Foci of recognizable hyaline cartilage, myxomatous areas and lobules with chalky white calcification are commonly seen. High grade tumors have an irregular rough interface with native bone and areas of hemorrhage, and necrosis.

MICROSCOPIC FINDINGS

Chondrosarcomas have a wide breath of histologic character, ranging from bland tumors emulating an enchondroma to highly atypical cellular tumors with minimal matrix formation. The diagnosis of chondrosarcoma is made by the presence of invasive growth into bone, abnormal chondrocytes, increased cellularity, and the production of lobules of cartilage with an irregular maturation and mineralization pattern (Fig. 18-17). Malignant chondrocytes are identified by variability of vesicular cells exhibiting nuclear hyperchromasia and stellate, spindled, pleomorphic, and multinucleated nuclei (Fig. 18-18). Cartilaginous lobules are delineated by fibrous septa with peripheral ossification. Entrapment and resorption of native bony trabeculae is common; however, malignant osteoid or bone is not

MRI radiographic studies are helpful in determining the extent of less well-defined maxillary lesions (Fig. 18-16).

PATHOLOGIC FEATURES

GROSS FINDINGS

At resection, tumors have a variegated appearance with areas of translucent light blue to pearly white and

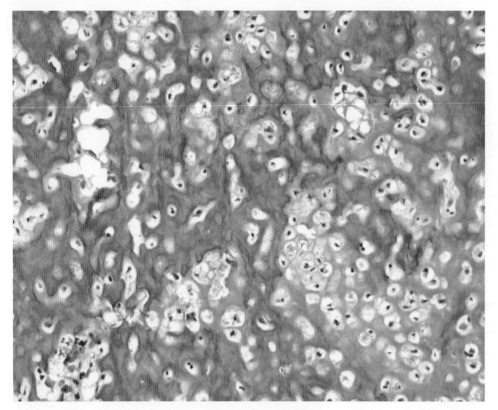

FIGURE 18-17
Low-grade chondrosarcoma (grade 1) with calcifying sheeted matrix with low cellularity with chondrocytes of uniform size containing small nuclei.

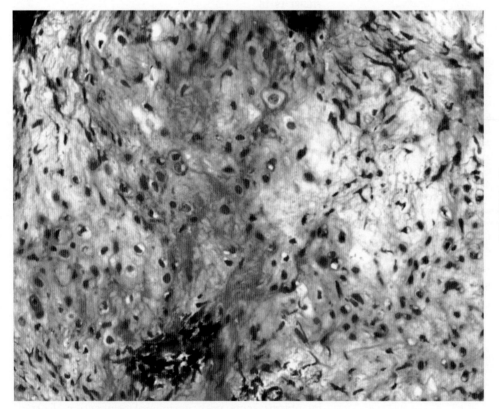

FIGURE 18-18
Grade 2 chondrosarcoma at high power showing irregular density of matrix, moderate cellularity, binucleation, pleomorphism, and nuclear atypia.

seen arising from malignant cellular stroma and if present supports a diagnosis of osteosarcoma (Fig. 18-19). Additional histologic variants of chondrosarcoma have been described, and include myxoid (Fig. 18-20), dedifferentiated, clear cell, and mesenchymal chon-drosarcoma. The jaw is a common site for mesenchymal chondrosarcoma which microscopically is a small cell malignant neoplasm consisting of undifferentiated oval cells with hyperchromatic nuclei and scattered islands of well-differentiated cartilage (Fig. 18-21). In addition,

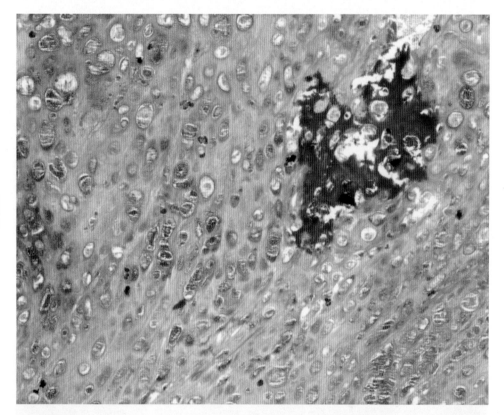

FIGURE 18-19

High-grade chondrosarcoma with ossification, high cellularity, and marked pleomorphism characterized primarily by nuclear atypia.

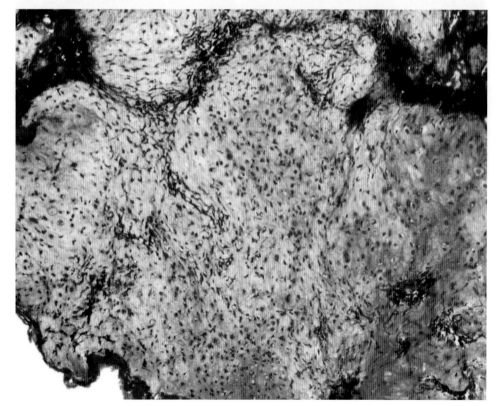

FIGURE 18-20

Low-power view of grade 2 chon-drosarcoma with myxoid features characterized by myxoid stroma, "string of pearls" architecture, and increased cellularity.

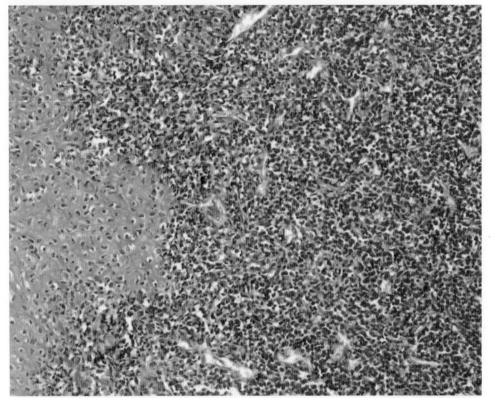

FIGURE 18-21
Low-power view of mesenchymal chondrosarcoma with neoplastic small round cell area merging into areas of chondroid formation.

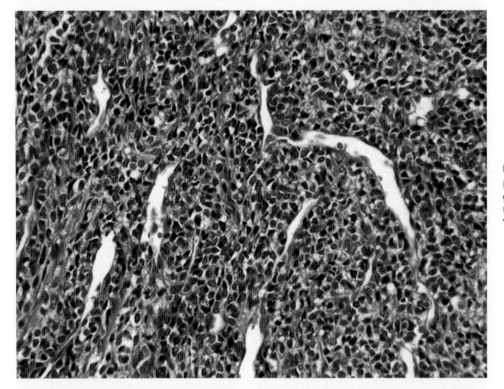

FIGURE 18-22
Hemangiopericytoma-like "stag-horn" growth is characteristic for a mesenchymal chondrosarcoma. No cartilage is visible in this field.

mesenchymal chondrosarcomas are characterized by stag-horn vascular spaces reminiscent of a hemangiopericytoma (Fig. 18-22).

Grading of chondrosarcoma is pertinent, as tumor grade dictates treatment and prognosis. Histologic grade is based primarily on the degree of cellularity, increas-ing nuclear pleomorphism, and mitotic activity, and necrosis. Grade 1 tumors represent 77% of gnathic tumors and histologically have increased cellularity, dominated by chondroid matrix with only scattered pleomorphic nuclei and bi-nucleate cells. Grade 2 tumors show moderate cellularity with easily identified enlarged atypical nuclei and lacunae containing multiple chondrocytes. The ratio of cartilaginous matrix to cell ratio is decreased with prominent myxoid areas. Grade 3 tumors are highly cellular with minimal matrix and abundant pleomorphic cells, multinucleation, and occasionally mitotic figures and liquefaction necrosis.

ANCILLARY STUDIES

FNA of chondrosarcoma is comprised of abundant, chondro-myxoid matrix material surrounding atypical chondrocytes (Fig. 18-23). The cells are usually enlarged with an increased nuclear to cytoplasmic ratio, vacuolated cytoplasm, and nuclear atypia. The matrix material is often difficult to appreciate on alcohol-fixed preparations, but the deep magenta, fibrillar chondroid matrix is characteristic in air-dried preparations. The degree of cellularity and presence of chondroid matrix varies as the grade of the tumor increases.

DIFFERENTIAL DIAGNOSIS

The histologic differential considerations for conventional chondrosarcoma is separating benign cartilaginous tumors from low-grade chondrosarcoma, and chondroblastic osteosarcoma from high-grade chondrosarcoma. Differentiation of low-grade chondrosarcoma from enchondromas and osteochondromas can be challenging; fortunately, benign cartilaginous tumors rarely, if ever, occur in the craniofacial bones. Separation from benign cartilaginous tumors is based on subtle atypia, increased cellularity, binucleated cells

and, most importantly, permeation and encroachment of cartilage around trabecular bone, seen only in chondrosarcomas.

Chondrosarcomas with a predominant myxoid matrix may be confused with an odontogenic myxoma; the latter is less cellular with more uniform distribution of cytologically normal cells and the presence of odontogenic epithelium. Separation of chondrosarcoma from chondroblastic osteosarcoma rests almost solely on the demonstration of malignant osteoid or bone arising from the cellular sarcomatous stroma in chondroblastic osteosarcomas. Mesenchymal chondrosarcoma may emulate other small cell malignant neoplasms, particularly when there is a paucity of chondroid matrix present. The majority of mesenchymal chondrosarcomas are CD99 and Sox 9 positive, which is useful in separating the tumor from other small round cell neoplasms. However, adequate sampling is probably the most important task, as the cartilage can be scant.

PROGNOSIS AND THERAPY

Chondrosarcomas of the jaws, although not highly aggressive, tend to be relentless tumors with frequent local recurrence, while demonstrating limited metastatic potential. The propensity for recurrence is likely related to the radiographic and clinical difficulty of defining the tumor margin. En bloc resection with a 2–3 cm margin of normal tissue is the recommended treatment, but this may be difficult to achieve in the anatomic confines of the jaws and sinuses. Histologic tumor grade is important prognostically: Grade 1 tumors seldom metastasize; grade 2 tumors metastasize 33 % of the time; while grade 3 tumors metastasize 70 % of the time. The vast majority of tumors are grade 1 and

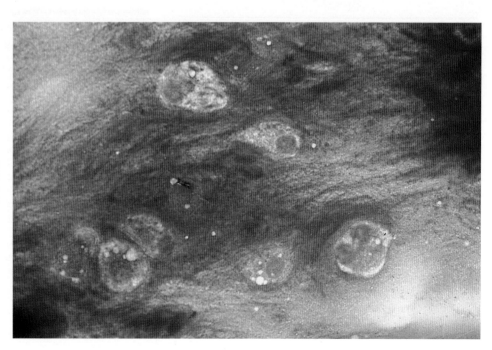

FIGURE 18-23
This low-grade chondrosarcoma has intensely magenta, fibrillar, chondroid matrix material with enlarged, binucleated cells within lacunar spaces (air-dried, MGG-stained FNA).

have an 89% 5-year survival rate and long-term rates approximating 50%. Mesenchymal chondrosarcomas have a worse prognosis with 42%–55% 5-year survival and 28% 10-year survival. Although rare in the pediatric population, craniofacial bone chondrosarcomas tend to have a better prognosis regardless of the tumor's histologic grade.

FIBROSARCOMA

CLINICAL FEATURES

Intraosseous fibrosarcoma of the gnathic arches arise de novo within bone, from periosteum or from odontogenic elements creating a combination tumor of benign odontogenic epithelium and fibrosarcoma (ameloblastic fibrosarcomas). Fibrosarcomas show an increased incidence after irradiation therapy, in Paget's disease, and preexisting benign tumors including desmoplastic fibroma, ameloblastic fibroma, and odontogenic myxoma. Fibrosarcomas in the jaws may occur at any age, but are most frequent in the 3rd decade, with males affected more commonly than females (2 : 1). There is a slight predilection for the mandible over the maxilla, except for those tumors of odontogenic origin which favor the mandible 3 : 1. Pain and swelling are the first signs of the tumor, with subsequent development of paresthesia, loosening of teeth, malocclusion, and proptosis in maxillary tumors.

RADIOLOGIC FEATURES

Radiographically intramedullary fibrosarcomas are nondescript, but obviously malignant tumors as portrayed by irregular diffuse radiolucencies with ill-defined borders (Fig. 18-24). The typical ubiquitous "moth-eaten" appearance of malignant bone tumors is commonly seen along with diffuse imperceptible margins (Fig. 18-25). Long-standing tumors may show a secondary osteoblastic periosteal reaction in tumors eroding into soft tissue. Fibrosarcomas are radiographically destructive with obliteration of cortical bone and resorption of teeth a frequent finding.

PATHOLOGIC FEATURES

GROSS FINDINGS

Gross specimens are unicentric lesions with an irregular peripheral border, feathering into the medullary and confining cortical bone. Low-grade tumors tend to be firm, white or tan, and have a fibrous appearance. Higher grade tumors are more likely to have a mottled character with areas of hemorrhage and necrosis.

MICROSCOPIC FINDINGS

Ameloblastic fibrosarcoma and fibrosarcomas lacking odontogenic elements share common mesenchymal features of sheeted, closely packed, spindled cells with minimal collagen production and the formation of interlacing fascicles (Fig. 18-26). A "herring bone" or "chevron" pattern histologically symbolizes the classic

FIBROSARCOMA DISEASE FACT SHEET	
Definition	A rare malignant, cellular, spindle cell neoplasm arising in bone or preexisting odontogenic tumor of the jaws
Incidence and location	Represents <5% of all bone tumors Rare in the jaws Slight predilection for mandible, although ameloblastic fibrosarcoma favors mandible 3 : 1
Gender, race, and age distribution	Slight male predilection Peak in 3rd–4th decades
Clinical features	Pain with swelling Loosening of teeth and malocclusion
Radiographic features	Ill-defined radiolucent tumor with irregular fuzzy borders Lytic central area with "moth-eaten" periphery
Prognosis and treatment	Prognosis is better in ameloblastic fibrosarcoma variant Radical resection with frequent local recurrence 5-yr survival rate: 27%–71%; 10-yr: as low as 17%

FIBROSARCOMA PATHOLOGIC FEATURES	
Gross findings	Firm fibrous white/tan tumor Irregular, shaggy interface with native bone High-grade tumor may have hemorrhage and necrosis
Microscopic findings	Cellular fibroblastic tumor with "herringbone" pattern Low grade: Cellular with mild atypia, and low mitotic rate High grade: High cellularity, marked atypia, high mitotic rate Minimal collagen formation with focal myxoid areas Ameloblastic fibrosarcoma variant has scattered benign epithelial islands
Pathologic differential diagnosis	Fibroblastic osteosarcoma, dedifferentiated chondrosarcoma, malignant fibrous histiocytoma, synovial sarcoma, melanoma

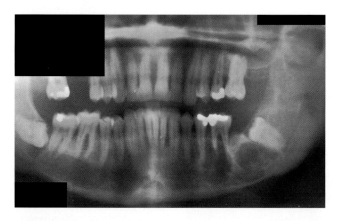

FIGURE 18-24

Radiograph of a fibrosarcoma presenting as biloculated tumor of mandible from anterior of left impacted molar to cuspid with mottled and speculated septal bone.

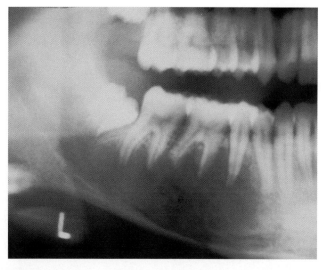

FIGURE 18-25

X-ray of a radiolucent fibrosarcoma with poorly defined margins extending from second molar to bicuspid with apical tooth root resorption.

FIGURE 18-26

A low-grade fibrosarcoma composed of sheets of fibrocytic cells with fusiform and oval nuclei forming a fascicular pattern.

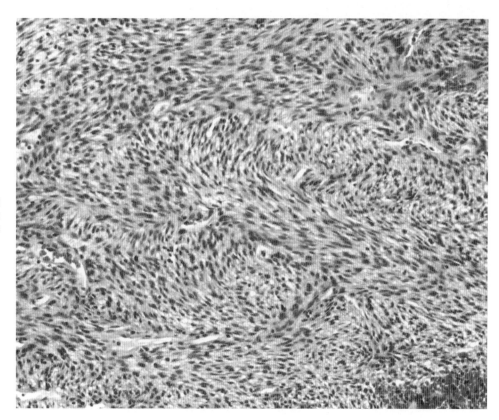

fibrosarcoma, with vague fasciculation and storiforming (Fig. 18-27). Ameloblastic fibrosarcomas may be identical to those without odontogenic islands; however, the malignant mesenchymal stroma tends to be looser and occasionally almost myxomatous (Fig. 18-28). The enclaved odontogenic islands are small benign nests, strands, and rosettes which are widely scattered and often require diligent searching. Rarely a preexisting ameloblastic fibroma is seen as the precursor lesion. Some pathologists favor tumors without odontogenic

elements to be fibroblastic osteosarcomas or malignant fibrous histiocytomas.

Fibrosarcomas are graded 1 to 3 with grade 1 tumors showing moderate cellularity, little cellular atypia, and few mitotic figures (Fig. 18-29). Grade 2 lesions are more cellular with scattered larger cells with prominent nucleoli, minimal cytoplasm, and noticeable mitotic figures. Grade 3 tumors are highly pleomorphic with numerous aberrant mitotic figures and occasional foci of necrosis and hemorrhage (Fig. 18-30).

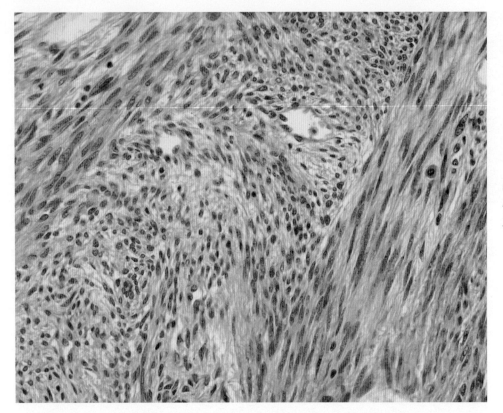

FIGURE 18-27
Abrupt junctions create a "herring bone" or "chevron" pattern seen in fibrosarcoma.

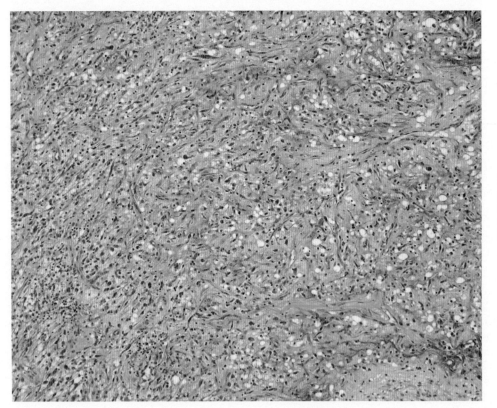

FIGURE 18-28
A maxilla and maxillary sinus fibrosarcoma demonstrates remarkable myxoid change, a frequent finding in ameloblastic fibrosarcomas.

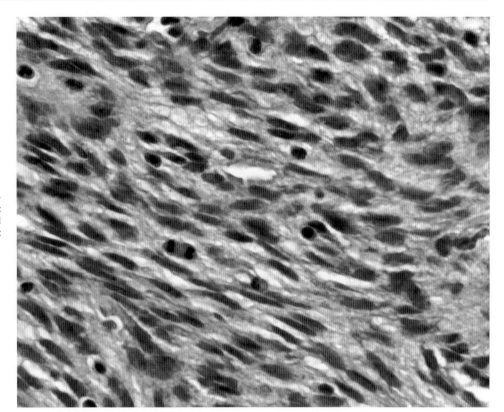

FIGURE 18-29

A low-grade fibrosarcoma is characterized by closely packed fibroblastic cells with nuclei showing blunted ends and single nucleoli. A mitotic figure is noted.

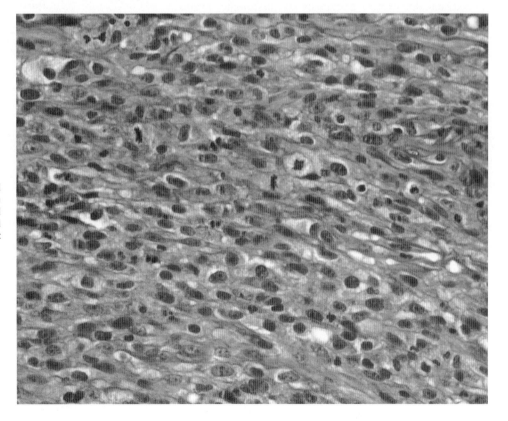

FIGURE 18-30

A high-grade fibrosarcoma composed of sheets of fibroblastic cells with sparse, fine collagen fibrils, and nuclei of varying sizes with dispersed to clumped chromatin. Mitotic figures are numerous and atypical.

DIFFERENTIAL DIAGNOSIS

Differentiating a low-grade fibrosarcoma from desmoplastic fibroma is accomplished by noting the lower cellularity and lack of mitotic activity in desmoplastic fibromas. High-grade tumors with less fasciculation raise the consideration of fibroblastic osteosarcoma, malignant fibrous histiocytoma, dedifferentiated chondrosarcoma, and melanoma. The absence of osteoid precludes a diagnosis of osteosarcoma. Dedifferentiated chondrosarcoma can be established by identifying foci of cartilage, highlighted by S-100 protein. MFH may have a "herring bone" pattern, but fascicular architecture is not seen in the whole tumor; tumor cells in MFH tend to be more epithelioid. Furthermore, MFH tends to have malignant tumor giant cells. Spindle cell melanoma may have pigment, intranuclear cytoplasmic inclusions, and prominent nucleoli, while also positive with S-100 protein, HMB45, and melan A, features not seen in fibrosarcomas.

PROGNOSIS AND THERAPY

Radical surgical resection is the proven therapy of choice, although adjuvant chemotherapy shows promise. Tumors are primarily locally aggressive with frequent recurrence, although lung and regional node metastasis do occur. Prognosis is histologic grade related. Most gnathic tumors are low grade, resulting in a better survival than extragnathic fibrosarcomas. The tumor is uncommon with only limited studies, yielding a wide range of survival data: 27%–71% 5-year survival. Ameloblastic fibrosarcomas appear to be only locally aggressive with little metastatic potential.

MULTIPLE MYELOMA

CLINICAL FEATURES

Multiple myeloma is a neoplasm of plasma cells disseminated in multiple intraosseous sites. Multiple myeloma of the craniofacial bones is manifested as multiple oval to round "punched out" radiolucencies. Approximately a third of patients with disseminated disease will have jaw lesions, and in 30% of cases mandibular lesions are the initial presentation. Solitary lesions (plasmacytoma of bone) are rare in the jaws (2%); however, 25% of solitary plasmacytomas progress to disseminated disease within 3 years. Patients may develop constitutional signs prior to development of bone lesions including anemia, fever, weight loss, hypercalcemia, renal failure, and proteinemia. Multiple myeloma rarely occurs before 40 years with the median age of onset at 70 years. Males are affected twice as often as females and blacks develop multiple myeloma twice as frequently as whites. The disease originates in hematopoietic marrow, favoring vertebrae, pelvis, skull, ribs, and the posterior mandible. Jaw lesions are initially painful with tooth mobility and lip paresthesia. Large lesions may lead to pathologic fractures. Laboratory confirmation of multiple myeloma may be achieved by identifying increased immunoglobulin light chains (Bence-Jones proteins) in the urine and by using serum electrophoresis to determine elevation of monoclonal immunoglobulin (Ig) levels. Elevated serum IgG and IgA are the most commonly identified, at 55% and 25% respectively.

RADIOLOGIC FEATURES

Multiple myeloma is radiographically distinctive with radiolucencies with sharp borders, ranging from 1–2 cm in the jaws (Fig. 18-31). The borders of the radiolucencies show no evidence of sclerosis, portraying a classic "punched out" appearance (Fig. 18-32). Multiple lesions may coalesce forming large, irregular radiolucencies with less distinct irregular borders (Fig. 18-33). Differential radiographic considerations include hyperparathyroidism and Langerhans cell histiocytosis.

MULTIPLE MYELOMA DISEASE FACT SHEET	
Definition	Multiple myeloma is a neoplasm of plasma cells disseminated in multiple intraosseous sites
Incidence and location	Most common tumor of bone in adults >40 yr
	Early lesions in vertebrae, pelvis, ribs, and skull
	Mandible involved in up to 30% of disseminated cases
Gender, race, and age distribution	Male > Female (2 : 1)
	Black > White (2 : 1)
	Most present in 6th–8th decades
Clinical features	Pain and paresthesia
	Loosening of teeth
	Swelling in later stages with pathologic fracture
Radiographic features	Multiple or single "punched out" round radiolucencies with sharp noncorticated borders
	Similar to Langerhans cell histiocytosis and hyperparathyroidism
Prognosis and treatment	Initial response of 70%, but <10% 10-yr survival rate
	Solitary tumors have better prognosis than multifocal tumors
	Solitary tumors can be managed with radiation
	Chemotherapy (alkylating agents with steroids or alpha-interferon)

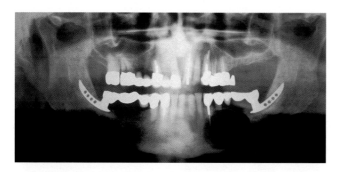

FIGURE 18-31

Solitary plasmacytoma of left mandible presenting as a large radiolucency with well-defined "punched out" peripheral margin.

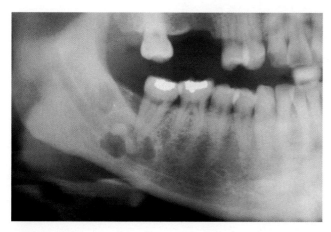

FIGURE 18-32

Multiple discrete oval radiolucencies of right posterior mandible at apex of second molar and in ascending ramus.

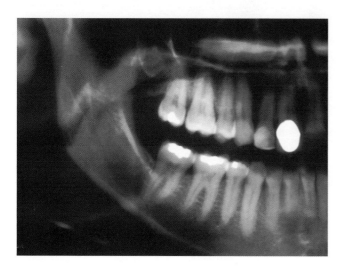

FIGURE 18-33

Multiple myeloma in right mandible with diffuse contiguous merging lesions and pathologic fracture at angle of mandible.

PATHOLOGIC FEATURES

GROSS FINDINGS

Fresh specimens appear similar to hematogenous bone marrow with red to gray mottled areas. The color and consistency of gross tumors has elicited the term "currant jelly." Some tumors have a whitish "fish flesh" appearance similar to lymphoma. The central portions of the lesions show little evidence of residual medullary bone spicules and are easily removed by curettage.

MICROSCOPIC FINDINGS

Myeloma is histologically exemplified by sheets of closely packed plasma and plasmacytoid cells (Fig. 18-34), displaying eccentric nuclei with "cartwheel" or "clock face" chromatin (Fig. 18-35). While most tumor cells closely resemble well-formed plasma cells with eosinophilic perinuclear halos, higher grade tumors may have binucleation, clumped chromatin, polygonal cells, macronucleoli, and atypical mitotic figures (Fig. 18-36). Accumulating among sheets of plasma cells may be amyloid and globules of amorphous eosinophilic immunoglobulin (Russell bodies). The proliferation of neoplastic plasma cells may not be obviously malignant, requiring immunohistochemistry to demonstrate monoclonal kappa (κ) or lambda (λ) immunoglobulin to establish the diagnosis of multiple myeloma (Fig. 18-37).

DIFFERENTIAL DIAGNOSIS

Common inflammatory jaw lesions are easily confused with multiple myeloma, as both are composed of

MULTIPLE MYELOMA PATHOLOGIC FEATURES	
Gross findings	Gray/red tumor intermixed with marrow
	"Currant jelly" appearance
	"Waxy" character when amyloid is present
Microscopic findings	Solid aggregations of neoplastic plasma cells
	Plasma cells vary from normal to anaplastic
	Eccentric nucleus with "cartwheel" appearance
	Higher grade tumors have atypical and binucleated plasmacytoid cells with irregular clumped chromatin
Immunohistochemical features	Monotypic expression for either kappa or lambda light-chain
	Positive with CD79a, CD56, CD58, CD138
Pathologic differential diagnosis	Reactive inflammatory plasmacytoid odontogenic lesions, immunoblastic lymphoma, Langerhans cell histiocytosis

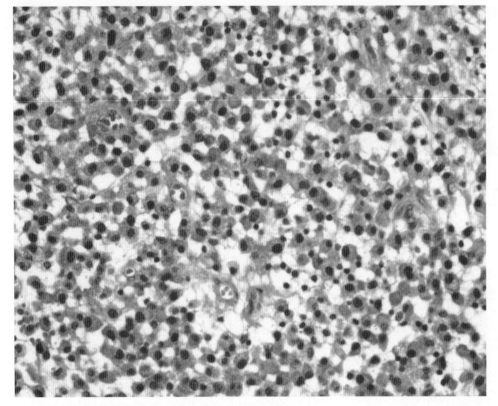

FIGURE 18-34
Medium power of well-differentiated myeloma characterized by sheets of plasma cells with eccentric nuclei in background of intermixed adipose cells with minimal stroma.

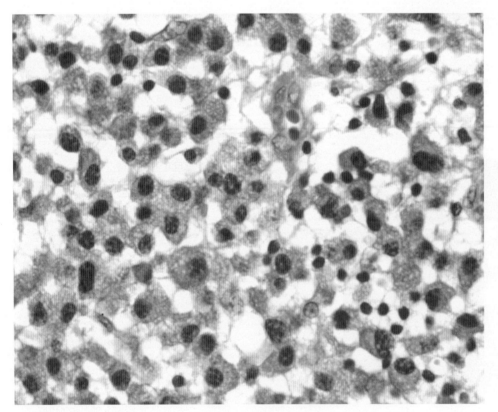

FIGURE 18-35
Well-differentiated myeloma at high power with characteristic plasmacytoid features of eccentric nuclei with peripheral and "cartwheel" chromatin patterns and abundant eosinophilic cytoplasm and distinct cell borders.

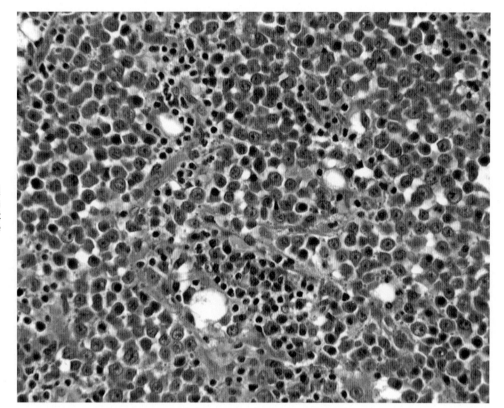

FIGURE 18-36

Moderate to poorly differentiated myeloma at medium power with closely packed oval cells reminiscent of plasma cells with variability in size and minimal background stoma.

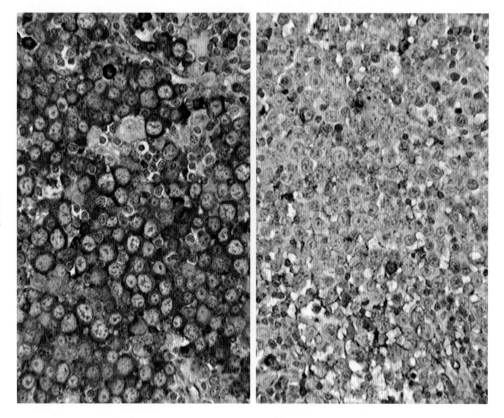

FIGURE 18-37

Immunohistochemistry shows a kappa (κ) light-chain restriction *(left)* in plasmacytoma *(right side* is lambda [λ]).

aggregated plasma cells. Periapical granuloma and chronic periodontitis have aggregated plasma cells and may be mistaken for multiple myeloma, requiring immunohistochemical separation by performing light-chain studies. Furthermore, myeloma cells react with natural killer antigen CD56/58 which is negative in reactive lesions. Anaplastic and plasmablastic myeloma may simulate a poorly differentiated carcinoma, but myeloma is keratin negative. Separation of B cell immunoblastic lymphoma from myeloma can be quite challenging due to considerable immunophenotypic overlap. Clinical evidence may be helpful, as multiple myeloma is seldom seen in lymph nodes. Lymphomas tend to be CD45RB positive, while myelomas are not. Langerhans cell histiocytosis, if morphologically considered, is CD1a positive, a finding not seen in myeloma.

PROGNOSIS AND THERAPY

Multiple myeloma is treated with chemotherapy, primarily alkylating agents, such as cyclophosphamide and melphalan, in combination with steroids or alpha-interferon. Although initial response rates approach 70%, long-term prognosis is poor with median survival less than 3 years and a 10-year survival rate of 10%. Higher grade and stage tumors with significant marrow replacement have a worse prognosis with shortened survival. Solitary tumors generally have a better prognosis and may be treated by irradiation, particularly when the tumor is surgically inaccessible.

METASTATIC NEOPLASMS

CLINICAL FEATURES

Development of a metastatic tumor in the craniofacial bones is rare, representing only 4% of metastatic carcinomas; carcinomas constitute the bulk of metastatic tumors. The mechanism of metastasis to the jaws is thought to occur via Batson's plexus, a low-pressure valveless system in the vertebral venous system. Metastatic tumors arise in medullary bone via the venous or arterial system; periosteal lymphatics play a role in periosteal tumors. Although uncommon in the jaws, when metastatic disease is seen, it indicates widespread disease and a poor prognosis. Interestingly, a pathologic fracture due to metastasis is the initial presentation of the primary tumor in up to 30% of cases.

Low-grade pain and progressive paresthesia are the initial symptoms, preceding any radiologic evidence of tumor. A soft tissue mass as extension of the bony metastasis is frequent (Fig. 18-38). Most metastatic tumors of the jaws occur in the 5th–8th decades (mean, 45 yr). Metastatic tumors affect males and females equally. The gender-specific order of frequency is as follows: female patients present with breast (42%), adrenal (9%), female genitalia (8%), and thyroid (6%); male patients present with lung (22%), prostate (12%), kidney (10%), and bone (9%). Of gnathic bones, the mandible is the most frequent site of metastatic disease (86%). About 5% affect both jaws simultaneously.

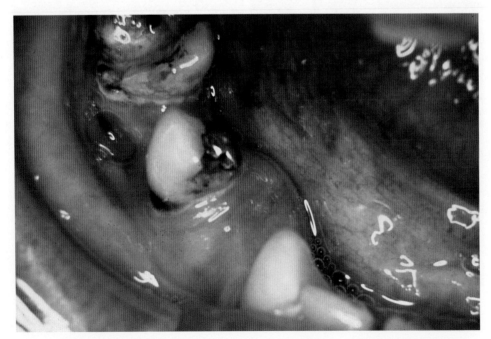

FIGURE 18-38

A metastatic carcinoma presenting as soft tissue swelling surrounding mandibular bicuspid with loosening and migration of teeth.

RADIOLOGIC FEATURES

Metastatic bone tumors may be osteoblastic, osteolytic or mixed and portray the primary tumor radiologic characteristics. The majority of metastatic tumors are carcinomas, which usually present as lytic radiolucent lesions (Fig. 18-39). Metastatic breast carcinoma usually produces lytic lesions, but additionally has the potential to produce osteoblastic radiopaque or mixed lesions (Fig. 18-40). Radiopaque osteoblastic lesions are produced by prostate carcinoma (Fig. 18-41), carcinoid tumors, and medulloblastomas. Almost all metastatic tumors of the jaws are lytic tumors with irregular borders, lacking a sclerotic border. Lesions reaching sufficient size to violate the cortical bone may produce a secondary "sun-burst" or "onion skin" appearance seen in about 40% of cases with multifocal disease. Metastatic tumors are initially subtle, indistinct radiopacities, frequently not appreciated on flat radiographic films. If metastatic disease is suspected, CT and MRI scans may be required.

PATHOLOGIC FEATURES

GROSS FINDINGS

Metastatic tumors on gross examination are nonspecific, often reflecting the gross features of the primary tumor. The majority of lesions are well demarcated and easily curetted from their bony crypts. Some tumors may predict the primary tumor origin as in osteoblastic tumors with calcified gritty foci, indicating possible prostate carcinoma and highly vascular tumors suggestive of kidney or thyroid primaries.

MICROSCOPIC FINDINGS

The histologic spectrum of metastatic tumors is diverse, usually replicating the primary site. When the

---

METASTATIC NEOPLASMS
DISEASE FACT SHEET

Definition	Metastasis of distant primary tumors to the craniofacial bones
Incidence and location	1% of all oral malignancies
	30% are first indication of metastatic disease
	80% are in posterior mandible
Morbidity and mortality	Dependent on the underlying tumor type
Gender, race, and age distribution	Nearly equal gender distribution
	Peak in 5th–8th decades (mean, 45 yr)
Clinical features	Pain and paresthesia early
Radiographic features	Bony expansion with cortical erosion late
	Lytic radiolucent lesion with ill-defined margins
Prognosis and treatment	Poor prognosis as jaw metastasis is usually a late event

---

METASTATIC NEOPLASMS
PATHOLOGIC FEATURES

Gross findings	Nodular intrabony foci with soft core and irregular bony wall
Microscopic findings	Tumor's histologic character is dependent on and usually similar to primary tumor
Immunohistochemical features	Immunologic studies appropriate for primary tumor
	Cytokeratin is useful as 2/3 of metastatic lesions are carcinomas
Pathologic differential diagnosis	Primary or metastatic carcinoma, sarcoma, lymphoma, melanoma

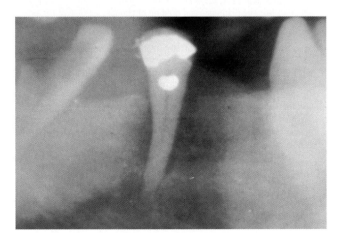

FIGURE 18-39
Radiographic presentation of metastatic carcinoma is elevation of soft tissue surrounding crown and midroot diffuse radiolucency.

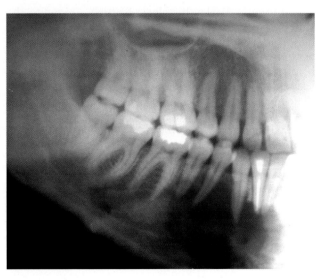

FIGURE 18-40
Solitary intrabony expansive lesion in body of mandible creating uniform radiolucency with indistinct borders and divergence of bicuspid roots in this metastatic breast carcinoma.

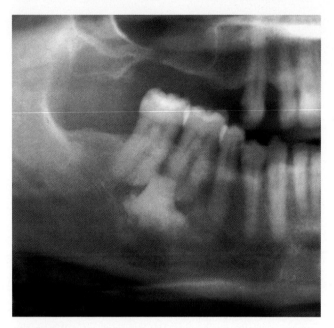

FIGURE 18-41
Metastatic prostate carcinoma of the right mandible characterized as a mixed radiolucent/radiopaque lesion with irregular peripheral radiolucent borders and central sclerotic radiopaque mass.

patient has a known primary tumor, histologic comparison with the original cytologic or histologic material is essential to rule out the possibility of a second primary tumor. Occasionally, dedifferentiation may make comparison difficult.

DIFFERENTIAL DIAGNOSIS

When tumors display histologic features unique to the site, additional investigation is required, including taking a thorough clinical history, reviewing radiographic studies, and performing immunohistochemical studies on the histologic material. As most metastatic lesions are carcinomas, cytokeratin is a good initial screen. Undifferentiated or mesenchymal tumors may have phenotypic infidelity and plasticity, resulting in a perplexing overlap. However, a pertinent battery of immunohistochemical stains will often resolve the diagnosis. Suffice it to say, not all tumors can be specifically categorized even with immunohistochemistry studies, ultrastructural, or genetic studies. Thorough clinical evaluation may be required to identify the primary tumor.

PROGNOSIS AND THERAPY

Treatment of metastatic disease is incumbent on first identifying the primary site with determination of the extent of metastatic spread. Prognosis varies with the type of tumor and the number of metastatic sites; however, presentation of a metastatic tumor in the jaws is often a late event and is likely the harbinger of incurable disease.

SUGGESTED READING

Osteosarcoma

1. Clark JL, Unni KK, Dahlin DC, Devine KD: Osteosarcoma of the jaw. Cancer 1983;51:2311–2316.
2. Davis AM, Bell RS, Goodwin PJ: Pronostic factors in osteosarcoma: a critical review. J Clin Oncol 1994;12:423–431.
3. Fechner RE, Mills SE: Tumors of the bones and joints. Atlas of Tumor Pathology. Third Series. Fascicle 8. Rosai J, Sobin LH, series ed. Bethesda: Armed Forces Institute of Pathology, 1993:38–67.
4. Gadwal SR, Gannon FH, Fanburg-Smith JC, et al.: Primary osteosarcoma of the head and neck in pediatric patients: a clinicopathologic study of 22 cases with a review of the literature. Cancer 2001;91:598–605.
5. Raymond AK, Ayala AG, Knuutila S: Conventional osteosarcoma. In: Fletcher CDM, Unni KK, Mertens F, eds. Pathology and Genetics of Tumours of Soft Tissue and Bone. Kleihues P, Sobin LH, series eds. World Health Organization Classification of Tumours. Lyon, France: IARC Press, 2002:264–270.
6. Sciubba JJ, Fantasia JE, Kahn LB: Tumors and cysts of the jaw. Altas of Tumor Pathology. Third Series. Fascicle 29. Rosai J, Sobin LH, series ed. Bethesda: Armed Forces Institute of Pathology, 2001:181–202.
7. Sundaram M, McGuire MH, Herbold DR: Magnetic resonance imaging of osteosarcoma. Skeletal Radiol 1987;16;23–29.

Chondrosarcoma

1. Bertoni F, Bacchini P, Hogendoorn PCW: Chondrosarcoma. In: Fletcher CDM, Unni KK, Mertens F, eds. Pathology and Genetics of Tumours of Soft Tissue and Bone. Kleihues P, Sobin LH, series eds. World Health Organization Classification of Tumours. Lyon, France: IARC Press, 2002:247–251.
2. Fechner RE, Mills SE: Tumours of the bones and joints. Atlas of Tumor Pathology. Third Series. Fascicle 8. Rosai J, Sobin LH, series ed. Bethesda: Armed Forces Institute of Pathology, 1993:101–121.
3. Gadwal SR, Fanburg-Smith JC, Gannon FH, Thompson LD: Primary chondrosarcoma of the head and neck in pediatric patients: a clinicopathologic study of 14 cases with a review of the literature. Cancer 2000;88:2181–2188.
4. Hackney FL, Aragon SB, Aufdemorte TB, et al.: Chondrosarcoma of the jaws: clinical findings, histopathology and treatment. Oral Surg Oral Med Oral Pathol 1991;71:139–143.
5. Sanerkin NG: The diagnosis and grading of chondrosarcoma of the bone: a combined cytologic and histologic approach. Cancer 1980;45:582–594.
6. Sciubba JJ, Fantasia JE, Kahn LB: Tumors and cysts of the jaw. Atlas of Tumor Pathology. Third Series. Fascicle 29. Rosai J, Sobin LH, series ed. Bethesda: Armed Forces Institute of Pathology, 2001:204–209.
7. Soderstrom M, Bohling T, Ekfors T, et al.: Molecular profiling of human chondrosarcomas for matrix production and cancer markers. Int J Cancer 2002:10:144–151.
8. Vencio EF, Reeve CM, Unni KK, Nascimento AG: Mesenchymal chondrosarcoma of the jaw bones: clinicopathologic study of 19 cases. Cancer 1998;82:2350–2355.

Fibrosarcoma

1. Fechner RE, Mills SE: Tumours of the bones and joints. Atlas of Tumor Pathology. Third Series. Fascicle 8. Rosai J, Sobin LH, series ed. Bethesda: Armed Forces Institute of Pathology, 1993:158–161.
2. Kahn LB, Vigorita V: Fibrosarcoma of bone. In: Fletcher CDM, Unni KK, Mertens F, eds. Pathology and Genetics of Tumours of Soft Tissue and Bone. Kleihues P, Sobin LH, series eds. World Health Organization Classification of Tumours. Lyon, France: IARC Press, 2002:289–290.

3. Marks KE, Bauer TW: Fibrous tumors of bone. Orthop Clin North Am 1989;20:377–393.
4. Sciubba JJ, Fantasia JE, Kahn LB: Tumors and cysts of the jaw. Atlas of Tumor Pathology. Third Series. Fascicle 29. Rosai J, Sobin LH, series ed. Bethesda: Armed Forces Institute of Pathology, 2001:212–215.
5. Sootweg PJ, Muller H: Fibrosarcoma of the jaws. A study of 7 cases. J Maxillofac Surg 1984;12:157–162.
6. Taconis WK, van Rijssel TG: Fibrosarcoma of the jaws. Skeletal Radiol 1986;15:10–13.

Multiple Myeloma

1. Brunning RD, McKenna RW: Benign odontogenic tumors. In: Rosai J, Sobin LH, eds. Tumors and Cyst of the Bone Marrow. Washington, DC: Armed Forces Institute of Pathology, 1994:323–351.
2. Epstein IB, Voss NJS, Stevenson-Moore P: Maxillofacial manifestations of multiple myeloma. Oral Surg Oral Med Oral Pathol 1984;51:267–271.
3. Furutani, M, Ohnishi M, Tanaka Y: Mandibular involvement in patients with multiple myeloma. J Oral Maxillofac Surg 1994;52:23–25.
4. Marick EL, Vencio EF, Inwards CY, et al.: Myeloma of the jaw bones: a clinicopathologic study of 33 cases. Head Neck 2003;25:373–381.
5. Martinez-Tello FJ, Calvo-Asensio M, Lorenzo-Roldan JC: Plasma cell myeloma. In: Fletcher CDM, Unni KK, Mertens F, eds. Pathology and Genetics of Tumours of Soft Tissue and Bone. Kleihues P, Sobin LH, series eds. World Health Organization Classification of Tumours. Lyon, France: IARC Press, 2002:302–305.
6. Neville, BW, Damm DD, Allen CM, Bouquot JE, eds: Oral and Maxillofacial Pathology. Philadelphia: WB Saunders, 1995:437–438.
7. Reinish EI, Raviv M, Srolovitz H, Gornitsky M: Tongue, primary amyloidosis, and multiple myeloma. Oral Surg Oral Med Oral Pathol 1994;77:121–125.
8. Sciubba JJ, Fantasia JE, Kahn LB: Tumors and cysts of the jaw. Atlas of Tumor Pathology. Third Series. Fascicle 29. Rosai J, Sobin LH, series ed. Bethesda: Armed Forces Institute of Pathology, 2001:220–224.

9. Witt C, Borges AC, Klein K, Neumann H: Radiographic manifestations of multiple myeloma in the mandible: a retrospective study of 77 patients. J Oral Maxillofac Surg 1997;55:450–453.

Metastatic Neoplasms

1. Bloom RA, Libson E, Husband JE, Stoker DJ: The periosteal sunburst reaction to bone metastases. A literature review and report of 20 additional cases. Skeletal Radiol 1987;16:629–634.
2. DeYoung BR, Wick MR: Immunologic evaluation of metastatic carcinomas of unknown origin: an algorithmic approach. Semin Diagn Pathol 2000;17:184–193.
3. Hirschberg A, Leibovich P, Buchner A: Metastatic tumors to the jawbones: analysis of 390 cases. J Oral Pathol Med 1994;23:337–341.
4. Jambhekar NA: Borges A: Metastases involving bone. In: Fletcher CDM, Unni KK, Mertens F, eds. Pathology and Genetics of Tumours of Soft Tissue and Bone. Kleihues P, Sobin LH, series eds. World Health Organization Classification of Tumours. Lyon, France: IARC Press, 2002:334–335.
5. Kyle RA: Diagnostic criteria of multiple myeloma. Hematol Oncol Clin North Am 1992;29:24–45.
6. Neville BW, Damm DD, Allen CM, Bouquot JE, eds: Oral and Maxillofacial Pathology. Philadelphia: WB Saunders, 1995:489–490.
7. Sciubba JJ, Fantasia JE, Kahn LB: Tumors and cysts of the jaw. Altas of Tumor Pathology. Third Series. Fascicle 29. Rosai J, Sobin LH, series ed. Bethesda: Armed Forces Institute of Pathology, 2001:263–265.
8. Stypulkowska J, Bartkowski S, Pana's M, Zaleska M: Metastatic tumors of the jaws and oral cavity. J Oral Surg 1979;37:805–808.

BRANCHIAL CLEFT ANOMALIES

Normally, when the name "branchial cyst" is used without further qualifications, one generally refers to a cyst of second branchial cleft origin (see Chapter 13). Of all branchial anomalies 80%–90% are associated with the second apparatus. Branchial cleft cysts constitute 17% of all congenital cervical cysts in children. Cysts of this apparatus are 3 times more common than sinuses.

CLINICAL FEATURES

Patients usually present with a painless nodule up to 6 cm located along the anterior border of the sternocleidomastoid muscle from the hyoid bone to the suprasternal notch. There is no gender difference, and 75% of patients are between 20–40 years at the time of diagnosis. The cysts are usually nontender masses, which may become secondarily inflamed or infected bringing them to clinical attention. They may be bilateral, especially in syndromic association.

RADIOLOGIC FEATURES

A well-circumscribed cystic mass with smooth cavity and a dense wall.

PATHOLOGIC FEATURES

GROSS FINDINGS

Grossly the cysts are unilocular, between 2 to 6 cm in diameter, containing clear to grumous material.

BRANCHIAL CLEFT ANOMALIES
DISEASE FACT SHEET

Definition	A lateral cervical cyst that results from congenital/developmental defects arising from the primitive 2nd branchial apparatus
Incidence and location	17% of all congenital cervical cysts
	Lateral neck, with most near the mandibular angle
Gender, race, and age distribution	Equal gender distribution
	75% patients between 20–40 yr
	Only 1% occur in patients >50 yr
Clinical features	Mass along the anterior border of the sternocleidomastoid muscle
	Painless mass of long duration
	May become secondarily infected, which will bring to clinical attention
Prognosis and treatment	Complete excision
	Recurrence rate 2.7%

BRANCHIAL CLEFT ANOMALIES
PATHOLOGIC FEATURES

Gross findings	Cystic mass containing fluid up to 6 cm
Microscopic findings	Cysts lined by squamous epithelium (90%), respiratory (8%), or both (2%)
	Keratinaceous debris
	Lymphoid tissue nodular or diffuse (90%)
	Fibrosis and secondary changes
Fine needle aspiration	Mature squamous epithelium
	Anucleate squames
	Debris, including macrophages
	Lymphoid infiltrate
Immunohistochemical features	Keratin positive, type dependant on lining
Pathologic differential diagnosis	Metastatic cystic squamous carcinoma, thymic cyst, bronchial cyst, thyroglossal duct cyst

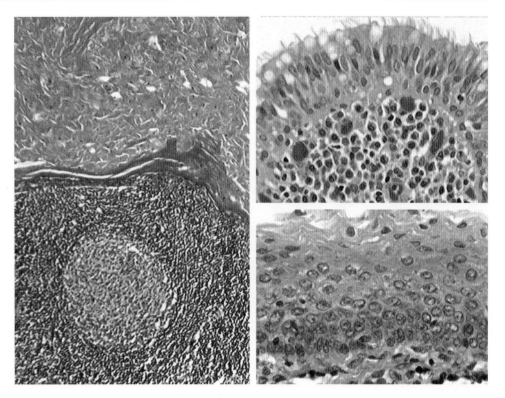

FIGURE 19-1

Branchial cleft cyst is often filled with keratinaceous debris. The cyst can be lined by stratified columnar epithelium (*right upper*) or squamous epithelium (*right lower*).

MICROSCOPIC FINDINGS

A branchial cleft cyst is lined by stratified squamous epithelium (90 %), respiratory epithelium (8 %), or both (2 %) (Fig. 19-1). Keratinaceous debris is present within the cavity. Lymphoid aggregates with or without reactive germinal centers beneath the epithelial lining are found in about 70 %–85 % of the cysts (Fig. 19-2). While germinal center formation is frequently seen in the lymphoid component, no true lymph node architecture with sinus formation, medullary region, or interfollicular zones are seen. Acute and chronic inflammation, foreign body giant cell reaction, and fibrosis are secondary changes in the wall of the cyst. Exceptionally salivary gland tissue may be found in the wall.

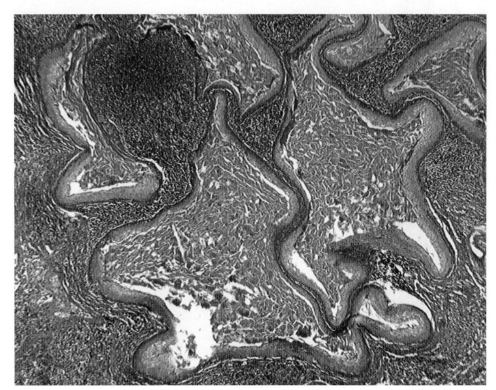

FIGURE 19-2

The epithelial lining is subtended by a rich inflammatory infiltrate, with lymphoid germinal center formation.

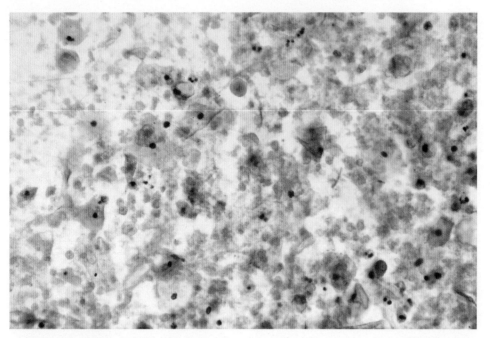

FIGURE 19-3
Keratinaceous debris with inflammatory cells are diagnostic for a branchial cleft cyst in this fine needle aspiration smear, as long as there is no atypia in the epithelial component (Papanicolau stain).

ANCILLARY STUDIES

IMMUNOHISTOCHEMICAL FEATURES

The epithelial lining expresses cytokeratin of different types depending on the type of lining—pseudostratified respiratory, transitional, stratified keratinizing, or nonkeratinizing.

FINE NEEDLE ASPIRATION

Fine needle aspiration (FNA) of a branchial cleft cyst will yield a thick, yellow, pus-like material which microscopically is composed of mature squamous epithelium, although sometimes columnar respiratory epithelium may be noted. There are numerous ancleate squames, a background of amorphous debris along with macrophages, and a variable lymphoid infiltrate composed

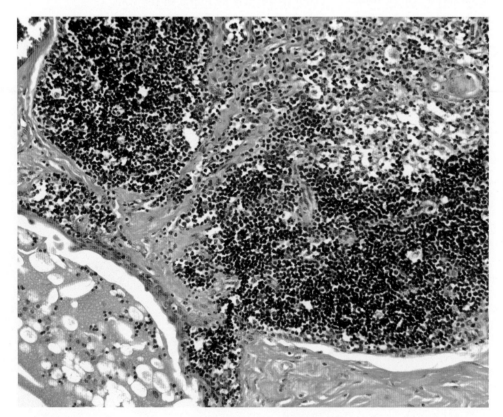

FIGURE 19-4
A wall of a thymic cyst contains lymphoid aggregates, fat, and Hassall's corpuscle which may sometimes mimic a branchial cleft cyst.

of mature lymphocytes and occasional plasma cells (Fig. 19-3). There is not epithelial atypia to suggest malignancy.

DIFFERENTIAL DIAGNOSIS

Thymic cysts contain thymic tissue in the wall, with Hassall's corpuscles (Fig. 19-4). A thyroglossal duct cyst occurs in the midline; is associated with the hyoid bone and contains thyroid tissue. Bronchial cysts are more common in the subcutaneous tissue of the supraclavicular region and are lined by respiratory mucosa; smooth muscle and bronchial glands may be found in the wall. A malignant lining of the cyst distinguishes metastatic cystic squamous cell carcinoma from branchial cleft cyst.

PROGNOSIS AND THERAPY

The recurrence rate is 2.7% for cases with no history of infection or prior surgery; 14% and 21%, respectively, with history of infection or prior attempts at surgical removal. A complete excision of the cyst is indicated.

CAT SCRATCH DISEASE (GRANULOMATOUS INFLAMMATION)

Many infectious agents can affect the neck, including the skin, soft tissues, and lymph nodes. Rather than cover an exhaustive litany of all infectious agents, cat scratch disease will be highlighted as a single example. Cat scratch disease (CSD) is a zoonotic infection caused by any one of a group of rickettsial microorganisms of the alpha-2 subgroup of alpha-protobacteria, specifically *Bartonella henselae*, with some taxonomic overlap with *Afipia felis* and *B. quintana*. CSD is worldwide and most common in autumn and winter, and found especially in dwellings where cats are kept as pets.

CLINICAL FEATURES

The characteristic clinical syndrome consists of an initial lesion that develops at the site of inoculation followed by enlargement of regional lymph nodes. The primary lesion may go unnoticed or it may persist and

CAT SCRATCH DISEASE (GRANULOMATOUS INFLAMMATION) DISEASE FACT SHEET	
Definition	A zoonotic infection caused by a group of gram-negative rickettsial bacillus organisms, specifically *Bartonella henselae, Afipia felis,* and *B. quintana*
Incidence and location	Worldwide, most common in autumn and winter
	Found specially in dwellings where cats are kept as pets
Morbidity and mortality	No mortality unless patients is immunosuppressed
Gender, race, and age distribution	Equal gender distribution
	Children and young adults between 3–21 yr (majority <18 yr)
Clinical features	Usually associated with a cat scratch or bite
	Solitary, tender lymphadenopathy
	Constitutional symptoms including low-grade fever, malaise, and headaches
Prognosis and treatment	Excellent prognosis
	Supportive therapy is adequate, although ciprofloxacin has been advocated by a few

be slightly painful. The primary lesion usually appears 3–5 days after the scratch, with lymphadenopathy developing up to 3 weeks after the primary insult. The affected nodes are those that drain the primary lesion. Lymphadenopathy involves only one node region in about 85% of patients. The nodes are enlarged, tender, and occasionally drain to the surface, forming a fistula. Constitutional symptoms may be present and include a low-grade fever, headaches, and malaise. Most infections are in children and young adults usually <21 years.

PATHOLOGIC FEATURES

GROSS FINDINGS

The lymph nodes are soft, swollen, and have foci of necrosis on the cut surface.

MICROSCOPIC FINDINGS

The histology can be divided into three stages of progression, the findings dependent on which stage the lesion is at the time of biopsy. Histologically, early lesions show foci of swollen capillaries, which have a pink hyaline appearance and are associated with lymphoid follicular hyperplasia. As the foci of suppuration grow, they coalesce to form stellate abscesses (Fig. 19-5), which become surrounded by histiocytes,

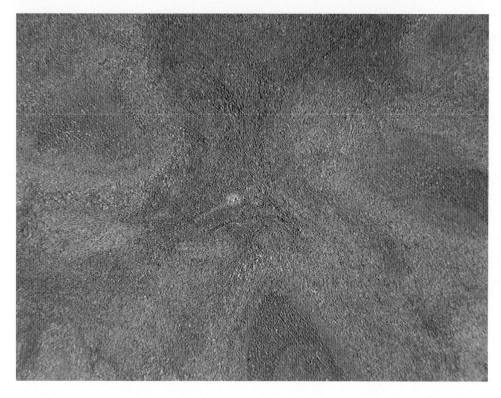

FIGURE 19-5
The characteristic stellate abscess with central necrosis surrounded by granulomatous reaction and inflammatory cells in this case of cat scratch disease.

epithelioid cells, and occasionally giant cells (Fig. 19-6). Eventually, a granulomatous perimeter surrounding a central area of caseation remains. The casseous center, however, unlike the center of tuberculosis lesions, is rarely calcified. Obviously, these changes are nonspecific, requiring additional studies to document the causative agent.

ANCILLARY STUDIES

HISTOCHEMISTRY

Tissue Gram stain will demonstrate the bacillus, but a Warthin-Starry silver impregnation technique stains

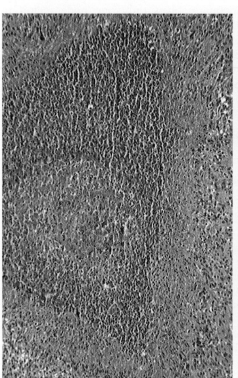

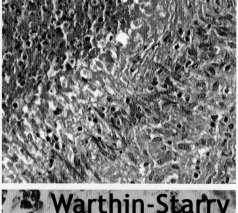

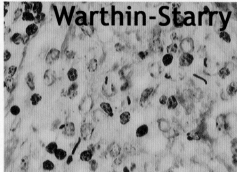

FIGURE 19-6
Left: Caseating necrosis with central degeneration. *Right upper:* Epithelioid histiocytes palisaded around the periphery. *Right lower:* Black, rod-shaped organisms accentuated with the Warthin-Starry silver impregnation stain.

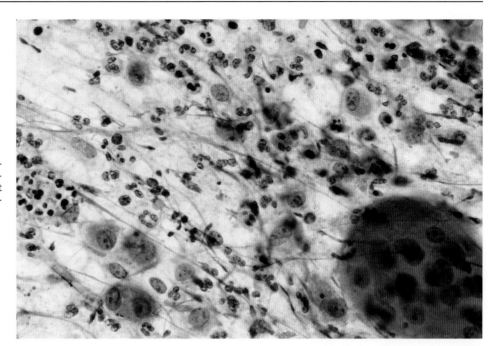

FIGURE 19-7

A fine needle aspiration usually demonstrates granulomatous-type inflammation with epithelioid histiocytes, giant cells, and mixed inflammation (Papanicolau stain).

the bacteria black, highlighting the organisms in the wall of the vessels in the early stages and in the suppurative areas in the latter stages (Fig. 19-6).

FINE NEEDLE ASPIRATION

The features on FNA are those of a granulomatous inflammation and are nonspecific. Epithelioid histiocytes, Langhans-type giant cells, inflammatory cells, and debris are present to a variable degree depending on

stage (Figs. 19-7, 19-8). However, additional studies, including culture and/or special studies, are necessary to confirm the diagnosis.

IMMUNOHISTOCHEMICAL FEATURES

An indirect immunoperoxidase stain has been developed to demonstrate the organisms, but is capricious, requiring a volume of cases to achieve reproducible results.

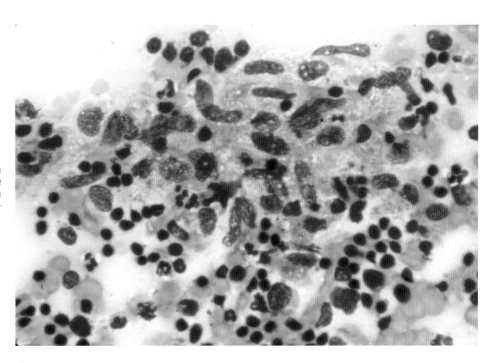

FIGURE 19-8

Inflammatory cells are noted with epithelioid histiocytes in this example of granulomatous inflammation from a patient with cat scratch disease (air-dried, MGG stain).

CAT SCRATCH DISEASE (GRANULOMATOUS INFLAMMATION) PATHOLOGIC FEATURES	
Gross findings	Enlarged, swollen lymph nodes with areas of necrosis
Microscopic findings	Three stages of progression are generally identified:
	Early shows follicular hyperplasia
	Stellate abscess surrounded by histiocytes, epithelioid cells, and occasionally giant cells
	Late stage granulomas with central caseation
Fine needle aspiration	Granulomatous inflammation with epithelioid histiocytes and occasional giant cells
	Lymphoid infiltrate
	Necrotic debris, depending on stage
Special techniques	Warthin Starry stain for rod-shaped organisms
	Immunoperoxidase stain
	DNA primer for use with polymerase chain reaction
	Culture using brain–heart agar at 32°C
Pathologic differential diagnosis	Infectious agents, including brucellosis, tuberculosis, lymphogranuloma venereum

ADDITIONAL STUDIES

DNA primers have been developed for use with a polymerase chain reaction for evaluation of CSD. The organisms may be cultured using brain–heart infusion agar with incubation at 32°C.

DIFFERENTIAL DIAGNOSIS

Stellate abscesses, characteristic of CSD, are also seen in lymphogranuloma venereum as well as in other rare infections such as tularemia and brucellosis. Most helpful in diagnosing CSD is the clinical setting and the demonstration of the bacilli by silver impregnation or by culture.

PROGNOSIS AND THERAPY

The prognosis is excellent with supportive treatment alone. Antibiotics are generally not required to relieve symptoms, but ciprofloxacin has been advocated by a few.

NODULAR FASCIITIS

Nodular fasciitis is a mass-forming fibroblastic proliferation that usually occurs in the subcutaneous tissue, and typically displays a tissue culture-like growth pattern. Cranial fasciitis and intravascular fasciitis are histologically related lesions. Nearly 30% of nodular fasciitis will develop in the head and neck.

CLINICAL FEATURES

Most patients give a history of a rapidly growing mass present for only a short duration (up to 3 wk). It usually measures <3 cm and almost always <5 cm. Nodular fasciitis is almost always subcutaneous, although occasional cases are intramuscular. The upper extremities and head and neck are the most frequently affected regions. In the latter, it has been reported in the neck, face, orbit, oral cavity, and ear. Nodular fasciitis is more common in children and young adults up to 35 years. It is rare in adults older than 60 years. There is no sex predilection. It is interesting that trauma is considered an etiologic factor, although the trauma may be slight or of a limited degree (seat belt pushing against the neck; cotton-tipped applicator inserted into the external auditory canal).

RADIOLOGIC FEATURES

Most of the lesions show moderate to strong enhancement on computed tomography and magnetic resonance imaging with preservation of smooth margins.

NODULAR FASCIITIS DISEASE FACT SHEET	
Definition	A mass-forming myofibrillastic proliferation, usually within subcutaneous tissues
Incidence and location	Most common in upper extremities and head and neck
Gender, race, and age distribution	Equal gender distribution
	Up to 35 yr most commonly
Clinical features	Rapidly growing mass of up to 3-wk duration
	Usually <3 cm mass
	Neck, orbit, and ear
	Trauma may play an etiologic role
Prognosis and treatment	Excellent prognosis with <2% recurrence rate
	Complete surgical excision

PATHOLOGIC FEATURES

GROSS FINDINGS

The lesion consists of a round to oval, nodular nonencapsulated mass, usually measuring <3 cm in greatest dimension. There is often attachment to the fascia. The cut surfaces may be firm, gray-white, or may be soft and gelatinous. Areas of cystic change are frequent.

MICROSCOPIC FINDINGS

Nodular fasciitis is poorly circumscribed and often assumes an irregular stellate appearance. It consists of plump immature fibroblasts, resembling the fibroblasts found in tissue culture or granulation tissue, with areas of central degeneration (Fig. 19-9). The fibroblasts vary little in size and shape and have oval, pale staining nuclei with prominent nucleoli. The fibroblasts are arranged in short irregular bundles and storiform fascicles (Fig. 19-10). Extravasated erythrocytes and keloid-like collagen are common (Fig. 19-11). Mitotic figures are common, but atypical mitoses are never seen (Fig. 19-11). Chronic inflammatory cells and giant cells are variably present. The collagen deposition increases

NODULAR FASCIITIS PATHOLOGIC FEATURES	
Gross findings	Solid to cystic, nonencapsulated mass Usually <3 cm
Microscopic findings	Plump, immature fibroblasts resembling tissue culture Cystic spaces or areas of degeneration common Mitosis are abundant but not atypical Extravasated erythrocytes, inflammatory cells, keloid-like collagen, and giant cells often present
Fine needle aspiration	Cellular smears Plump, spindled fibroblasts with wispy cytoplasmic extensions Binucleated forms may be seen Finely dispersed chromatin without atypia Blood, giant cells, and bundles of collagen occasionally present
Immunohistochemical features	Not necessary for diagnosis, but actins are positive CD68 positive histiocytes Negative for keratin and S-100 protein
Pathologic differential diagnosis	Fibrosarcoma, rhabdomyosarcoma, fibromatosis, fibrous histiocytoma, fetal rhabdomyoma

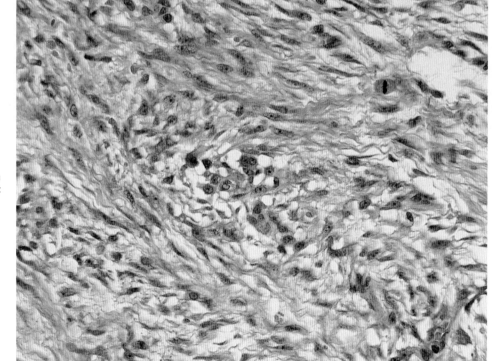

FIGURE 19-9

Tissue culture-like growth with myxoid degeneration and mitotic figure.

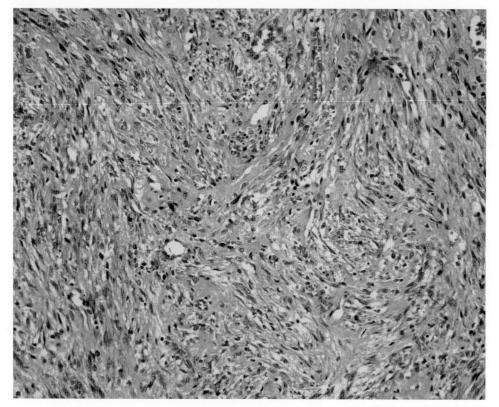

FIGURE 19-10

Tissue culture-like growth with collagen deposition and extravasated erythrocytes. A storiform growth is typical.

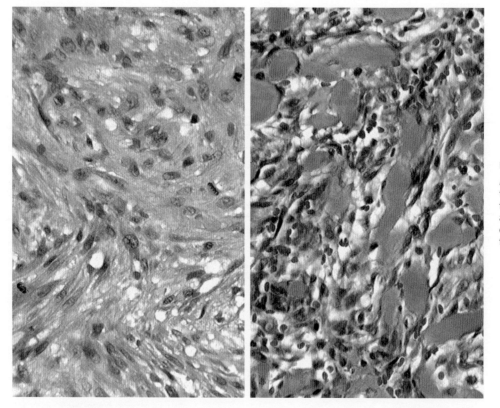

FIGURE 19-11

Left: Short irregular bundles of fibroblasts with increased mitotic figures. *Right:* Keloid-like collagen and increased fibroblasts with extravasated erythrocytes in nodular fasciitis.

with time, such that an extensive amount of keloid-like collagen is often present in the later stages of the reaction (Fig. 19-11).

ANCILLARY STUDIES

ULTRASTRUCTURAL FEATURES

The elongated, bipolar fibroblastic cells have abundant rough endoplasmic reticulum and have cisternae with granular, electron-dense material. There is a fine distribution of the nuclear chromatin. Intracytoplasmic bundles of microfilaments are seen. Collagen fibers are seen in the background.

IMMUNOHISTOCHEMICAL FEATURES

Immunohistochemistry is usually unnecessary for the diagnosis, although the fibroblasts are positive with the actins, while the histiocytes will be CD68 reactive. Desmin may rarely be positive. Keratin and S-100 protein are typically negative.

FINE NEEDLE ASPIRATION

FNA will typically demonstrate a cellular smear composed of short, plump, spindled fibroblasts in a slightly myxoid background (Fig. 19-12). The cells

may be binucleated with eccentric nuclear placement. Blood and giant cells are present, and occasionally collagen may be present. The plump spindle cells are not atypical; mitotic figures are common.

DIFFERENTIAL DIAGNOSIS

Nodular fasciitis is often clinically worrisome, yielding a neoplastic differential diagnosis. Histologically, the reaction is often misdiagnosed as a sarcoma. The cells in fibrosarcoma are densely packed without stroma and are arranged in short, tight "herringbone" or "chevron" bundles. The individual cells differ in size and shape with numerous atypical mitosis. Rhabdomyosarcoma may occasionally have spindle-shaped cells, but tends to have pleomorphic cells, increased mitotic figures, and a unique immunohistochemical and molecular profile. Fibromatosis is less circumscribed, usually larger, and often "invasive," characterized by slender spindle-shaped fibroblasts that are arranged in long, sweeping fascicles separated by abundant, dense collagen. Fibrous histiocytoma is made up of more rounded cells that are arranged in a storiform pattern. Fetal rhabdomyoma has a gradient of cellularity with large cells showing cross-striation set in a cellular background (Fig. 19-13).

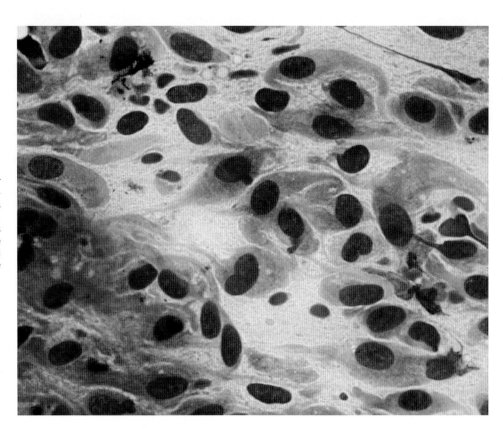

FIGURE 19-12

A fine needle aspiration of nodular fasciitis shows a cellular smear composed of single, spindle, bipolar cells in a background of myxoid material. Slightly vacuolated cytoplasm is wispy and "tadpole"-like, while the nuclear chromatin is delicate and evenly distribution. Nucleoli are prominent (air-dried, MGG stain).

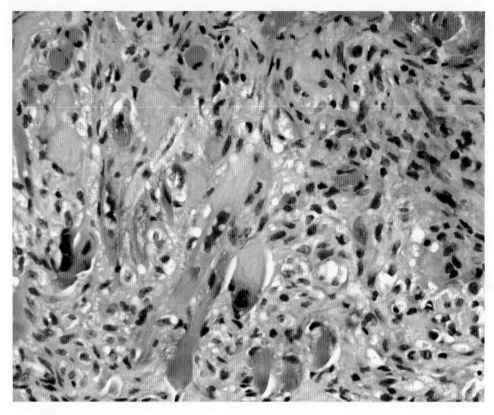

FIGURE 19-13
A fetal rhabdomyoma has large, strap-like cells with cross-striations set in a cellular stroma of benign-appearing cells. There is often a gradient of cellularity.

PROGNOSIS AND THERAPY

Complete excision is the treatment of choice. Recurrences occur in about 2% of cases, and may represent a "reaction" to the trauma of surgery. Recurrences usually develop shortly after surgery.

SUGGESTED READING

Branchial Cleft Anomalies

1. Deane SA, Telander RL: Surgery for thyroglossal duct and branchial cleft anomalies. Am J Surg 1978;136:348–353.
2. Mandell DL: Head and neck anomalies related to the branchial apparatus. Otolaryngol Clin North Am 2000;33:1309–1332.
3. Rea PA, Hartley BE, Bailey CM: Third and fourth branchial pouch anomalies. J Laryngol Otol 2004;118:19–24.
4. Regauer S, Gogg-Kamerer, Braum H, et al.: Lateral neck cyst, the branchial cleft theory revisited. A critical review and clinicopathologic study of 97 cases with special emphasis on cytokeratin expression. APMIS 1997;105:623–630.
5. Triglia JM, Nicollas R, Ducroz V, et al.: First branchial cleft anomalies. A study of 39 cases and a review of the literature. Arch Otolaryngol Head Neck Surg 1998;124:291–295.

Cat Scratch Disease (Granulomatous Inflammation)

1. Adal KA, Cockerell CJ, Petri WA Jr.: Cat scratch disease, bacillary angiomatosis, and other infections due to *Rochalimaea*. N Engl J Med 1994;330:1509–1515.
2. Bruijnesteijn Van Coppenraest ES, Lindebbom JA, Pins JM: Real-time PCR assay using fine-needle aspirates and tissue biopsy specimens for rapid diagnosis of mycobacterial lymphadenitis in children. J Clin Microbiol 2004;42:2644–2650.
3. Carithers HA: Cat scratch disease. An overview based on a study of 1,200 patients. Am J Dis Chil 1985;139:1124–1133.
4. Lamps LW, Scott MA. Cat scratch disease: historic, clinical and pathologic perspectives. Am J Clin Pathol 2004;121:S71–S80.
5. Tsuneoka H, Umeda A, Tsukahara M, et al.: Evaluation of indirect fluorescence antibody assay for detection of Bartonella clarridgeiae and seroprevalence of B. clarridgeiae among patients suspected cat scratch disease. J Clin Microbiol 2004;42:3346–3349.

Nodular Fasciitis

1. Bernstein KE, Lattes R: Nodular (pseudosarcomatous) fasciitis, a non-recurrent lesion: clinicopathologic study of 134 cases. Cancer 1982;49: 1668–1678.
2. Montgomery EA, Meis JM: Nodular fasciitis its morphologic spectrum and immunohistochemical profile. Am J Surg Pathol 1991;15:942–948.
3. Thompson LDR, Fanburg-Smith JC, Wenig BM: Nodular fasciitis of the external ear region: a clinicopathologic study of 50 cases. Ann Diagn Pathol 2001;5:191–198.
4. Weibolt VM, Buresh CJ, Roberts CA, et al.: Involvement of 3q21 in nodular fasciitis. Cancer Genet Cytogenet 1998;106:177–179.
5. Weiss SW, Goldblum JR: Benign fibrous tissue tumors. In: Weiss SW, Goldblum JR, eds. Enzinger and Weiss's soft tissue tumors, 4th ed. St. Louis: Mosby, 2001:247–307.

20 Benign Neoplasms of the Neck
Mario A. Luna • Lester D. R. Thompson

LYMPHANGIOMA (CYSTIC HYGROMA)

Lymphangiomas are rare congenital malformations, with up to 70% reported in the head and neck. They are separated into three types: capillary, cavernous, and cystic (cystic hygroma). Lymphangiomas comprise about 25% of all vascular neoplasms in children and adolescents and about 25% of cervical cysts are lymphangiomas.

CLINICAL FEATURES

Approximately two-thirds of lymphangiomas are noted shortly after birth, and 95% are present by the end of the 2nd year of life. Cystic hygroma may also be detected in utero by ultrasonography. Cystic hygroma is commonly associated with fetal hydrops and Turner syndrome. In general, symptoms relate to pressure caused by the enlarging mass in the posterior neck, although it may extend into the anterior compartment, upward into the cheek, or down into the mediastinum or axilla. When located superior to the hyoid bone, they may cause dysphagia or airway compression. Cystic hygromas vary from a single soft mass with a pseudo contour to lobulated multicystic masses.

Cavernous lymphangioma is found in the tongue, cheek, floor of mouth, and lips, but is uncommon in the soft tissues; it forms an ill-defined, spongy, and compressible mass. Capillary lymphangioma is clinically the least significant of the three types and is usually confined to the skin.

PATHOLOGIC FEATURES

Lymphangiomas (cystic type specifically) consist of dilated thin-walled spaces filled with eosinophilic, proteinaceous fluid, and lined by flat endothelial cells (Fig. 20-1). The intervening stroma contains scattered lymphoid aggregates and wisps of smooth muscle fibers (Fig. 20-2). Fibrosis may be increased in lesions which have been present for a long duration.

LYMPHANGIOMA (CYSTIC HYGROMA) DISEASE FACT SHEET

Definition	A benign cystic lesion composed of dilated lymph vessels
Incidence and location	Represents 25% of congenital cervical cysts
	Up to 70% of lymphangiomas occur in the head and neck
Morbidity and mortality	Mortality 5%–7%
Gender, race, and age distribution	No significant gender difference
	Most present shortly after birth and 95% by the 2nd year
Clinical features	Slowly enlarging painless mass
	May produce pressure symptoms due to size
	Associated with fetal hydrops and Turner syndrome
Prognosis and treatment	Up to 50% recurrence depending on size and site of lesion
	May become secondarily infected
	Surgery; sclerosing agents and laser can be used

LYMPHANGIOMA (CYSTIC HYGROMA) PATHOLOGIC FEATURES

Gross findings	Sponge-like cystic mass
Microscopic findings	Dilated, thin-walled spaces filled with proteinaceous fluid
	Lined by flat endothelial cells
	Lymphoid aggregates in stroma
	Wisps of smooth muscle in the wall
Immunohistochemical features	Positive with FVIII-RAg, CD 31, CD 34, *ulex europaeus*
	CD9 and podoplanin may be lymph vessel specific
Pathologic differential diagnosis	Cavernous hemangioma, metastatic papillary carcinoma

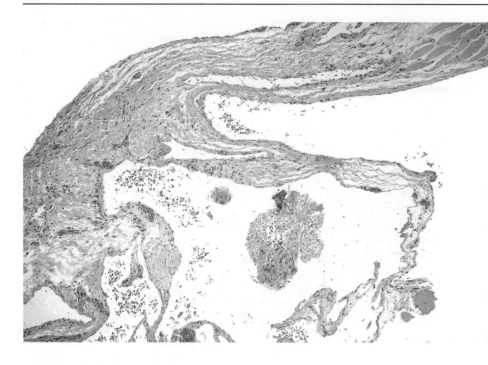

FIGURE 20-1
Cystic lymphangioma showing dilated lymphatic spaces.

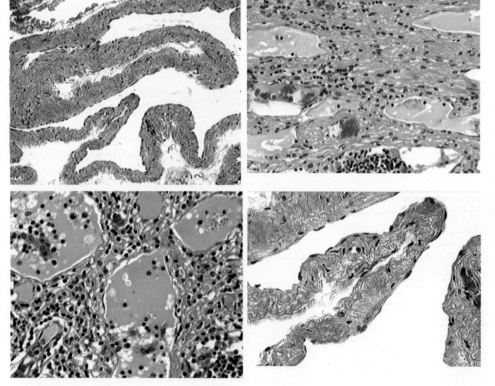

FIGURE 20-2
Left upper: Lymphatic spaces subtended by smooth muscle. *Right upper:* Lymphoid cells and proteinaceous fluid. *Left lower:* Lymphoid elements with serum fluid. *Right lower:* Flat, attenuated endothelial cells line the cavity.

ANCILLARY STUDIES

Endothelial markers (FVIII-RAg, CD31, CD34, and *ulex europaeus*) can be expressed by endothelial cells in both hemangiomas and lymphangiomas. It has been claimed that CD9 and podoplanin are specific markers for lymphatic endothelial cells.

DIFFERENTIAL DIAGNOSIS

The most common differential diagnosis is with cavernous hemangioma. Lymphangioma contains proteinaceous fluid, and the surrounding tissues are usually infiltrated by lymphocytes, whereas cavernous hemangiomas are filled with red blood cells and lack valve structures. Metastatic papillary carcinoma of the thyroid may have flattened cells along the spaces, but TTF-1 or thyroglobulin will be positive. Furthermore, a lymph node architecture should be seen.

PROGNOSIS AND THERAPY

Recurrence rates range from 15%–50%. Mortality rates are between 3%–7%, specifically related to pressure destruction of vital structures of the neck. Lymphangiomas may occasionally become infected. Surgery is the treatment of choice, while laser treatment or injected sclerosing agents are alternative therapies.

TERATOMA

Teratomas are neoplasms composed of elements from each of the three germ cell layers (ectoderm, endoderm, and mesoderm). In the head and neck, the most common locations are neck, oropharynx, nasopharynx, and orbit. Cervical teratomas represent <3% of all teratomas and represent <1% of all neck masses in children. Teratomas are separated into mature or immature and benign or malignant depending on the degree of tissue maturation histologically. In general, teratomas of the neck in neonates or infants are clinically benign, although they may be histologically mature or immature, while those of adults are more likely to be clinically malignant and histologically immature.

CLINICAL FEATURES

More than 90% of cervical teratomas occur in neonates or infants and are rare in patients older than 1 year. They occur with similar frequency in males and females. In addition to a neck mass, severe respiratory distress is notable in neonates, frequently leading to airway compromise and requiring immediate surgery. If detected prenatally by ultrasonographic examination, surgical planning may yield a better outcome. Polyhydramnios and other malformations may be seen in about 20% of patients. Failure of midline structure development may result in fetal demise, even though the lesion is histologically benign. Cervical teratomas in adults are extremely rare, with patients reporting a rapidly enlarging neck mass.

PATHOLOGIC FEATURES

GROSS FINDINGS

Grossly, the tumors are encapsulated, lobulated, and usually cystic, but they can be solid or multiloculated. They measure up to 12 cm in greatest diameter.

MICROSCOPIC FINDINGS

Histologically, the tumors are composed of an assemblage of mature or immature tissues from the three embryonic germ cell layers: ectoderm, endoderm, mesoderm (Fig. 20-3). The most common finding is neural tissue, arranged in islands, tubules, and rosette-like for-

TERATOMA DISEASE FACT SHEET	
Definition	Neoplasm composed of mature or immature elements from ectoderm, endoderm, and mesoderm
Incidence and location	Cervical teratomas represent 3% of all teratomas
	<1% of pediatric neck masses
Morbidity and mortality	High morbidity, but low mortality in neonates and infants
	High mortality in older children and adults
Gender, race, and age distribution	Equal gender distribution
	>90% occur in neonates or infants
Clinical features	Neck mass
	Respiratory distress
	Frequent association with congenital malformations
	Polyhydramnios seen in 20% of neonatal lesions
Prognosis and treatment	Prognosis is very good in neonates and infants, but guarded in older children and adults
	Surgery

TERATOMA PATHOLOGIC FEATURES	
Gross findings	Cystic, solid, or multilocular lobulated mass
Microscopic findings	Mature or immature tissues from all germ cell layers
	Squamous, respiratory, glandular and cuboidal epithelium
	Organ differentiation may be seen
	Neural tissues, including glial elements, choroid plexus, immature neuroblastema and pigmented retinal anlage
	Bone, cartilage, muscle, and fat
Immunohistochemical features	Alpha-fetoprotein and human chorionic gonadotropin if endodermal sinus tumor and choriocarcinoma are present
Pathologic differential diagnosis	Hamartoma, neuroblastoma, metastatic testicular teratoma

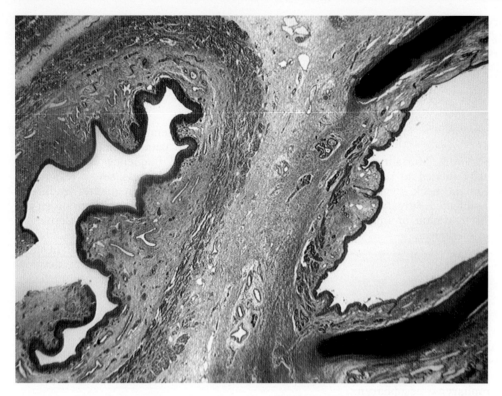

FIGURE 20-3
This benign mature teratoma contains a primitive esophagus adjacent to a primitive trachea. Other germ cell layers were noted elsewhere.

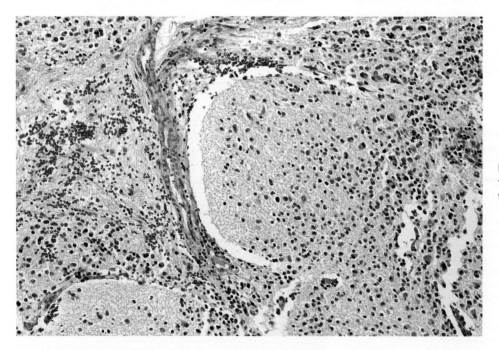

FIGURE 20-4
Teratoma containing mature glial tissue.

mations of immature neuroepithelium or mature glial tissue (Fig. 20-4), including retinal anlage epithelium (Fig. 20-5). A variety of epithelia are seen, including squamous, respiratory and enteric-type mucosa, with solid organ tissues occasionally noted (pancreas, liver, thyroid) (Fig. 20-5). The epithelium may line a cyst, with sebaceous units and hair frequently identified. Nodules of cartilage, fat, and muscle blend with the sur-

rounding epithelial or glial tissues. The tissue may be mature or immature (embryonic), with the volume of immature tissues determining the overall grade of the tumor. *Benign mature* is used for tumors containing only mature elements; *benign immature* is used if there are foci of immature elements within a tumor that has a majority of mature elements; *malignant* is used if the majority of the tumor is comprised of immature

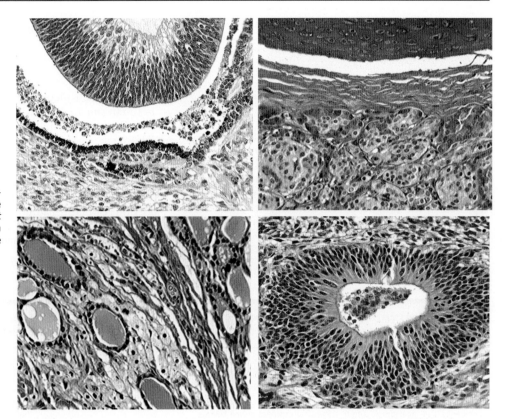

FIGURE 20-5

Left upper: Retinal anlage epithelium. *Right upper:* Mature cartilage adjacent to pancreatic tissue. *Left lower:* Thyroid parenchyma with immature fat. *Right lower:* A rosette of immature glial tissue.

elements. Foci of malignant germ cell tumor (such as endodermal sinus tumor, embryonal carcinoma, or choriocarcinoma), while uncommon, automatically place the tumor in the malignant category.

ANCILLARY STUDIES

Immunohistochemical stains with alpha-fetoprotein and human chorionic gonadotropin may be of help in findings islands of endodermal sinus tumor or choriocarcinoma, respectively, in malignant teratomas. However, immunohistochemistry is generally not necessary for diagnosis.

DIFFERENTIAL DIAGNOSIS

A broad differential diagnosis exists with these tumors when initially evaluated on small biopsies. Hamartoma, choristoma, ectopia, neuroblastoma, and malignant germ cell tumors are considered in the differential. Attention to the nondescript mesenchymal background and heterogeneity of elements provide clues to the diagnosis. Tissues that are not indigenous to the location and have an immature appearance rule out hamartoma. Depending on the age, cervical metastasis from a gonadal teratoma should also be considered in the differential diagnosis.

PROGNOSIS AND THERAPY

The prognosis of cervical teratoma in newborns and infants is excellent, although teratomas of the neck may cause significant morbidity despite their favorable histology. Death does occur as a result of associated developmental malformations of the vital structures of the neck. Therefore, surgery should be instituted without delay because the preoperative mortality is significant. Many advocate the use of intrauterine surgery to yield the best possible outcome.

In adults, when there is a malignant histology, a more aggressive biologic behavior with lethal consequences is to be expected. Metastasis to lymph nodes and lung are common. Surgery with adjuvant chemotherapy and radiation is advocated, although often with mixed results.

SPINDLE CELL LIPOMA/PLEOMORPHIC LIPOMA

Spindle cell and pleomorphic lipomas are distinctive types of lipoma histologically on a continuum and characterized by replacement of mature fat cells by bland spindle cells, hyperchromatic round cells, and multinucleated giant cells associated with ropey collagen. They account for approximately 1.5% of all adipose tissue neoplasms.

CLINICAL FEATURES

Over 90% of spindle cell/pleomorphic lipomas occur in men (mean age, 60 yr). Almost all of the tumors are located in the subcutaneous tissue of the posterior neck, upper back, and shoulders. Patients present with a painless, mobile, subcutaneous mass. Rarely, cases are reported in the tongue, cheek, and larynx. Characteristically the tumors are solitary, although rarely they may be familial and multiple.

PATHOLOGIC FEATURES

GROSS FINDINGS

Spindle cell/pleomorphic lipomas range in size from 1–13 cm (mean, 3.5 cm). Grossly, they resemble an ordinary lipoma, although the deep tumors may be myxoid.

MICROSCOPIC FINDINGS

Microscopically, at one end at the histological spectrum, spindle cell lipoma is composed of varying proportions of mature adipocytes and spindle cells admixed with wire- or rope-like collagen fibers, and myxoid stroma (Fig. 20-6). Mast cells are frequently numerous.

SPINDLE CELL LIPOMA/PLEOMORPHIC LIPOMA DISEASE FACT SHEET

Definition	A distinct group of lipomas composed of spindle cells, adipocytes, and multinucleated giant cells associated with ropey collagen
Incidence and location	About 1.5% of all adipose tissue tumors
Gender, race, and age distribution	Male >>> Female (9 : 1) Mean age, 58 yr
Clinical features	Painless, subcutaneous, mobile mass Posterior neck, upper back, shoulders Seldom multiple
Prognosis and treatment	Excellent, although isolated reports of recurrence Surgery

---

SPINDLE CELL LIPOMA/PLEOMORPHIC LIPOMA PATHOLOGIC FEATURES

Gross findings	Yellow to grey-white circumscribed mass Mean, 3.5 cm (range, 1–13 cm)
Microscopic findings	Mixture of bland spindle cells arranged in parallel, adipocytes, and multinucleated giant cells ("floret-like") Bands of mature, rope-like collagen fibers Mast cells may be numerous
Ancillary studies	Spindle cells of both types of lipoma express CD34 Negative for S-100 protein Loss of 13q and/or 16q
Pathologic differential diagnosis	Sclerosing and spindle cell liposarcoma, neurofibroma, nuchal fibroma

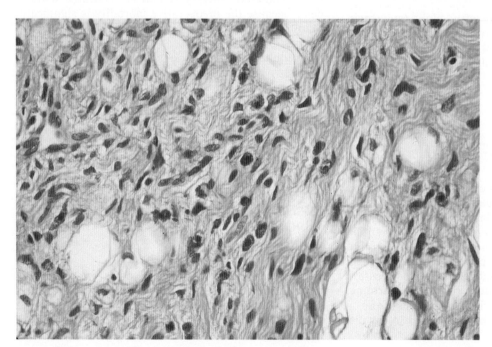

FIGURE 20-6

Spindle cell lipoma with bland spindle cells in a background of thick, ropy collagen fibers. Adipocytes are scattered throughout.

At the opposite end of the spectrum, pleomorphic lipoma is characterized by small, round hyperchromatic cells with multinucleated giant cells with radially arranged ("floret-like") nuclei, like petals of a flower (Fig. 20-7). Cases with mixed features of spindle cell and pleomorphic lipoma occur quite often. By definition, no lipoblasts are present.

ANCILLARY STUDIES

ULTRASTRUCTURAL FEATURES

Electron microscopic studies revealed spindle cells thought to represent fibroblasts or fibroblast-like cells analogous to the stellate mesenchymal cells seen in primitive fat lobules.

IMMUNOHISTOCHEMICAL FEATURES

Immunohistochemically, the spindle cells in spindle/pleomorphic lipomas express CD34, but are negative for S-100 protein (unlike ordinary lipocytes).

GENETIC STUDIES

Loss of chromosomes 13q and/or 16q are characteristic of this family of lipomas.

DIFFERENTIAL DIAGNOSIS

The differential diagnosis is with liposarcoma and neurofibroma, while nuchal fibroma is occasionally a consideration. The uniformity of the spindle cells, association with mature collagen fibers, the absence of lipoblasts, characteristic location, patient age, and overall circumscription support the diagnosis of spindle lipoma instead of liposarcoma. Neurofibroma tends to be infiltrative, contains spindle cells which are more randomly arranged, and may contain characteristic Wagner-Meissner bodies. Moreover, the spindle cells express S-100 protein in neurofibroma but are CD34 positive in lipoma. A nuchal fibroma has fat, but has a much heavier collagen deposition and has entrapped nerves (Fig. 20-8).

PROGNOSIS AND THERAPY

Complete local excision is curative in both lipomas.

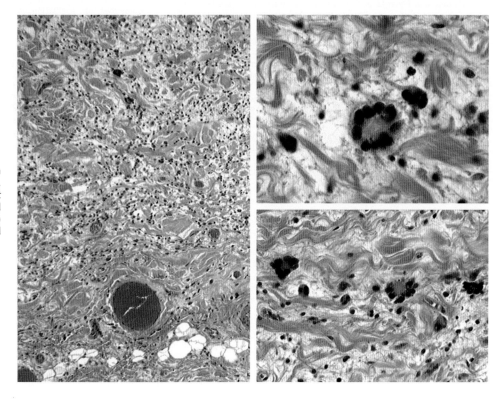

FIGURE 20-7

Left: Hyperchromatic nuclei are seen in cells separated by dense collagen. There are a few adipocytes. *Right upper:* A floret-like multinucleated cell. *Right lower:* Floret-like ("petal") multinucleated giant cells associated with mast cells.

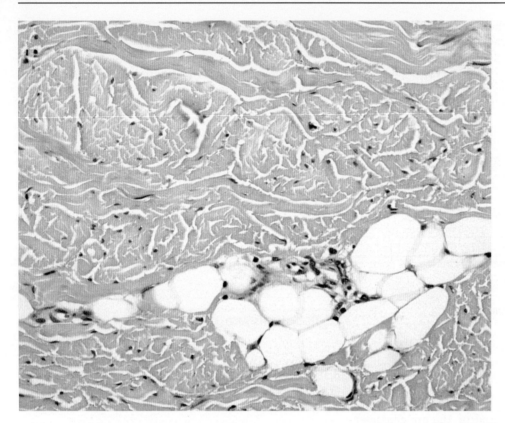

FIGURE 20-8
A nuchal fibroma has very heavy, dense collagen deposition with small islands of adipocytes and nerve twigs. There are no spindled tumor cells and no floret-like giant cells.

SUGGESTED READING

Lymphangioma (Cystic Hygroma)

1. Beham A: Lymphangioma. In: Fletcher CDM, Unni KK, Mertens F, eds. Pathology and Genetics of Tumours of Soft Tissue and Bone. Kleihues P, Sobin LH, series eds. World Health Organization Classification of Tumours. Lyon, France: IARC Press, 2002:162–163.
2. Chervenak FA, Issacson G, Blakemore KJ, et al.: Fetal cystic hygroma. Cause and history. N Engl J Med 1983;309:822–825.
3. Coffin CM, Dehner LP: Vascular tumors in children and adolescents: a clinicopathologic study of 228 tumors in 222 patients. Pathol Annu 1993;28:97–120.
4. Erovic BM, Neuchrist C, Kandustsch S, et al.: CD9 expression in lymphatic vessels in head and neck mucosa. Mod Pathol 2003;16:1 028–1034.
5. Hsieh YY, Hsueh S, Hsueh C, et al.: Pathologic analysis of congenital cervical cysts in children: 20 years of experience at Chang Gung Memorial Hospital. Chang Gung Med J 2003;26:107–113.
6. Weiss SW, Goldblum JR: Tumors of lymph vessels. In: Weiss SW, Goldblum JR, eds. Enzinger and Weiss's soft tissue tumors, 4th ed. St. Louis: Mosby, 2001:955–983.

Teratoma

1. Azizkhan RG, Haase GM, Applebaum H, et al.: Diagnosis, management, and outcome of cervicofacial teratomas in neonates: a Children's Cancer Group study. J Pediatr Surg 1995;30:312–316.
2. Batsakis JG, El Naggar AK, Luna MA, et al.: Teratomas of the head and neck with emphasis on malignancy. Ann Otol Rhinol Laryngol 1995;104: 456–500.

3. Berge SJ, von Lidern JJ, Appel T, et al.: Diagnosis and management of cervical teratoma. Br J Oral Maxillofac Surg 2004;42:41–45.
4. Jordan RB, Gauderer MW: Cervical teratomas: an analysis, literature review and proposed classification. J Pediatr Surg 1988;23:583–591.
5. Torsigliori AJ Jr, Tom IWC, Ross AJ III, et al.: Pediatric neck masses guidelines for evaluation Int J Pediatr Otorhinolaryngol 1988;16: 199–210.

Spindle Cell Lipoma/Pleomorphic Lipoma

1. Del Cin P, Sciot R, Polito P, et al.: Lesions of 13q may occur independently of deletions of 16q in spindle cell/pleomorphic lipomas. Histopathology 1997;31:222–225.
2. Domaniski HH, Carlen B, Jonsson K, et al.: Distinct cytologic features of spindle cell lipoma. A cytologic-histologic study with clinical, radiologic, electron microscopic and cytogenetic correlation. Cancer 2001;93:381–389.
3. Enzinger FM, Harvey DA: Spindle cell lipoma. Cancer 1975;36: 1852–1859.
4. Miettinen MM, Mandahl N: Spindle cell lipoma/pleomorphic lipoma. In: Fletcher CDM, Unni KK, Mertens F, eds. Pathology and Genetics of Tumours of Soft Tissue and Bone. Kleihues P, Sobin LH, series eds. World Health Organization Classification of Tumours. Lyon, France: IARC Press, 2005:31–32.
5. Shmookler BM, Enzinger FM: Pleomorphic lipoma. A benign tumor simulating liposarcoma. A clinicopathologic analysis of 48 cases. Cancer 1981;47:126–133.
6. Weiss SW, Goldblum JR: Benign lipomatous tumors. In: Weiss SW, Goldblum JR, eds. Enzinger and Weiss's soft tissue tumors, 4th ed. St. Louis: Mosby, 2001:571–639.

21 Malignant Neoplasms of the Neck
Mario A. Luna • Lester D. R. Thompson

SYNOVIAL SARCOMA

Synovial sarcoma accounts for 7%–11% of all soft tissue sarcomas. While there is a predilection for the extremities, approximately 10% occur in the head and neck, usually in the neck, oropharynx, or hypopharynx. A juxta-articular location is unnecessary, as it is postulated synovial sarcoma develops from a pluripotential mesenchymal cell through abnormal differentiation into synovial neoplasms.

SYNOVIAL SARCOMA DISEASE FACT SHEET	
Definition	A malignant tumor with variable epithelial differentiation and a specific chromosomal translocation t(X:18) (p11;q11)
Incidence and location	Represents about 10% of all soft issue sarcomas
	About 10% occur in the head and neck
Morbidity and mortality	About one-third die with tumor
Gender, race, and age distribution	Male > Female (3:1)
	Median age, 25 yr
Clinical features	Painless, solitary mass in neck or hypopharynx
	Hoarseness, upper respiratory distress or dysphagia may occur
Radiographic features	Soft tissue mass on CT
	Calcifications within the tumor may help with diagnosis
Prognosis and treatment	About 25% develop recurrence
	About 25% have metastatic disease
	About 30% die from disease, usually <4 years from diagnosis
	Clear surgical margins and calcifications portend a better prognosis
	Wide surgical excision with adjuvant multimodality therapy

CLINICAL FEATURES

Although all age groups may be affected, most patients are young, with a median age of 25 years. Males tend to be affected more commonly than females (3 : 1). Typically, the symptoms are nonspecific, manifesting as a solitary, painless mass. Occasionally, hoarseness, upper respiratory distress, and dysphagia may be present.

RADIOLOGIC FEATURES

A soft tissue mass is seen on radiographic studies in most patients, with computed tomography (CT) scan providing valuable information about the site of origin and the extent of the tumor. Irregular calcifications may be present (~20% of cases), a finding which may suggest a better prognosis.

PATHOLOGIC FEATURES

GROSS FINDINGS

Head and neck synovial sarcomas range in size from 1–12 cm. The tumors are partially encapsulated and variably circumscribed, solid to cystic masses. The cut surface is yellow, gray-white with a firm, gritty and friable, to soft, boggy and rubbery consistency. The cut surface is whorled, with areas of cyst formation, and mucoid or hemorrhagic degeneration.

MICROSCOPIC FINDINGS

Tumors are separated into biphasic (both epithelial and spindled; Fig. 21-1), monophasic spindle or monophasic epithelial, and poorly differentiated. The monophasic spindled type is most common, while the biphasic is second. The biphasic type contains a mesenchymal spindle and a glandular epithelioid component (Fig. 21-2). The spindle cells are arranged in orderly, densely packed, short interlacing fascicles of

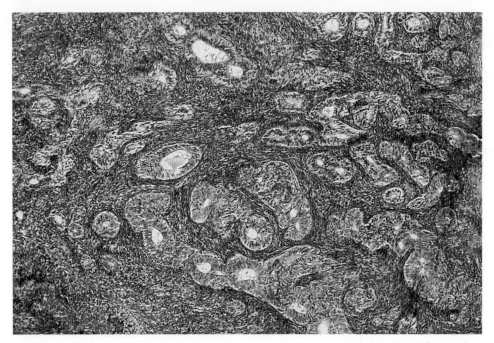

FIGURE 21-1

This is a predominantly glandular synovial sarcoma, although the spindle cell component is easily identified.

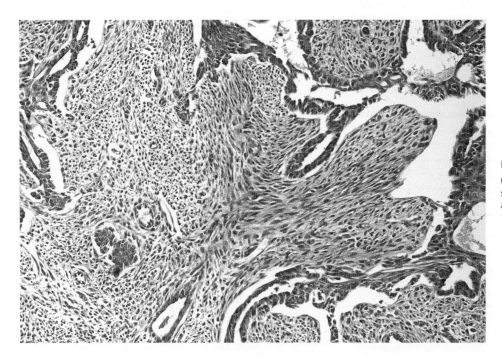

FIGURE 21-2

Glands and spindle cells in a biphasic synovial sarcoma. The spindle cells are arranged in fascicles.

plump cells with oval to spindle, vesicular to hyperchromatic nuclei, and scant cytoplasm with indistinct cellular boundaries, often resembling fibrosarcoma (Fig. 21-3). The glandular component is comprised by cuboidal or columnar epithelial cells arranged in cords, nests, whorls, or pseudoglandular spaces, with round to oval vesicular nuclei encompassed by abundant pale or clear cytoplasm (Fig. 21-3). The monophasic synovial sarcoma can be purely spindle or purely epithelial (Fig.

21-4). The former is composed of spindled elements arranged in whorls and fascicles of closely packed tumor cells. Mitotic activity is easily identified, although not excessive. The latter has numerous cuboidal or columnar cells arranged in glands. Mast cells and exceptional calcifications can be seen in the spindle cell regions, more easily recognized in hypocellular foci or in areas of myxoid change or necrosis. A rich vascularity is often present. There is usually little collagen deposition.

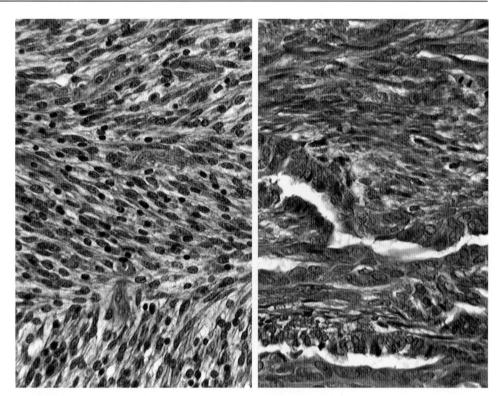

FIGURE 21-3

Left: Monophasic synovial sarcoma is usually spindled, composed of relatively bland cells. Mast cells are present. *Right:* High power of a biphasic tumor shows intimate association of glands and spindle cells. A mitotic figure is noted in the stroma.

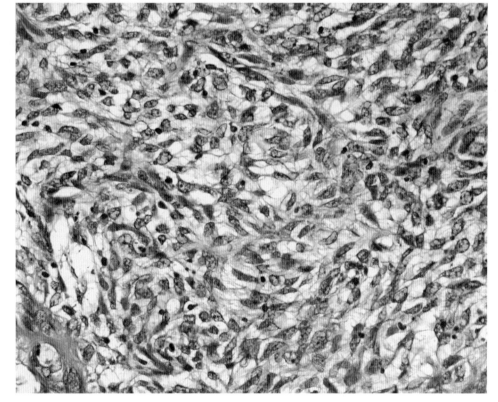

FIGURE 21-4

An epithelioid variant of synovial sarcoma still has a vaguely "spindled" appearance to the epithelioid cells. A myxoid stroma is noted.

SYNOVIAL SARCOMA PATHOLOGIC FEATURES

Gross findings	Solid or multicystic mass with calcifications
	Partially encapsulated with variable circumscription
	Cut surface is yellow, gray-white
	Firm, gritty to soft and boggy
	Mucoid and hemorrhagic degeneration may be present
Microscopic findings	Biphasic has epithelial/glandular and mesenchymal spindle cell components
	Spindle cells are arranged in short, interlacing fascicles of plumb cells with oval nuclei with indistinct cell borders
	Epithelioid component is glandular with cuboidal to columnar epithelial cells arranged in cords, nests, and pseudoglandular spaces
	Mitotic activity is easy to identify
	Mast cells and calcifications may be present
	Monophasic is either spindled or epithelioid
Special studies	Ultrastructure shows hemidesmosomes, microvilli and intercellular junctions in the epithelioid component
	Histochemistry will show mucicarminophilic material in the cytoplasm and lumens, while mesenchymal, alcian blue (hyaluronidase-sensitive) mucin is seen in mesenchymal areas
	Keratin and EMA positive epithelial and spindle cells, while vimentin only positive spindle cells
	Characteristic molecular t(X;18)(p11.2;q11.2) translocation
Pathologic differential diagnosis	Hemangiopericytoma, fibrous histiocytoma, spindle cell carcinoma, malignant peripheral nerve sheath tumors, fibrosarcoma, leiomyosarcoma, malignant melanoma, epithelioid sarcoma, metastatic adenocarcinoma

ANCILLARY STUDIES

ULTRASTRUCTURAL FEATURES

The epithelial elements exhibit hemidesmosomes, microvilli, intercellular junctions, tonofilaments, and an intact basal lamina. The spindle cells demonstrate poorly formed rudimentary cellular junctions, non-branching cytoplasm, intermediate filaments, and perhaps focal short-cell processes surrounded by an external lamina.

HISTOCHEMICAL FEATURES

Mucicarmine positive and diastase-resistant PAS-positive *epithelial* mucin can be seen within the cyto-plasm of the epithelial cells, within the glandular lumens and in intracellular areas, while hyaluronidase-sensitive alcian blue and colloidal iron *mesenchymal* mucin can be identified in the spindle cell and myxoid areas.

IMMUNOHISTOCHEMICAL FEATURES

The epithelial and the spindle cells may express low- and high-molecular weight cytokeratin and epithelial membrane antigen. Only the spindle cells are vimentin and bcl-2 positive. The spindle cell staining with epithelial markers may be focal, weak, or absent. Due to vagaries of reactivity, both epithelial markers should be performed.

GENETIC STUDIES

By use of reverse transcriptase polymerase chain reaction or fluorescence in situ hybridization, the characteristic balanced, reciprocal translocation between chromosome X and 18 can be identified: t(X;18)(p11.2;q11.2).

DIFFERENTIAL DIAGNOSIS

Biphasic synovial sarcoma presents a unique differential diagnosis, although monophasic synovial sarcoma is more challenging. The neoplasms included in the differential are hemangiopericytoma, fibrous histiocytoma, spindle cell squamous cell carcinoma, malignant peripheral nerve sheath tumors, fibrosarcoma, leiomyosarcoma, malignant melanoma, and epithelioid sarcoma, while metastatic adenocarcinoma may also be considered. In general, patient's age, specific anatomic site, unique histologic appearance, immunoprofile, and characteristic translocation will yield a definitive separation. An immunohistochemical panel may need to include keratin, epithelial membrane antigen (EMA), vimentin, S-100 protein, HMB45, CD34, desmin, and actins. A caveat must be kept in mind: recurrent or metastatic foci may have a different histologic appearance than the primary.

PROGNOSIS AND THERAPY

Local recurrence develops in about 25% of patients, with about 25% also demonstrating metastatic disease (usually to lung). About one-third of patients die from their disease, usually doing so within 4 years of the diagnosis. Interestingly, there is a suggestion that patients with calcifications in their tumors have a better prognosis than those without calcifications. Surgery with multimodality therapy (radiation and chemotherapy) is usually employed. Meticulous attention to surgical margins will achieve locoregional control and thereby successful therapy.

CHORDOMA

Chordomas are low- to intermediate grade malignant tumors that recapitulate the notochord. They are divided into three broad categories: sacrococcygeal (60%), spheno-occipital (25%), and vertebral (15%). About 10% of all tumors are cervical.

CLINICAL FEATURES

Chordomas account for approximately 4% of malignant bone tumors. The age of patients with chordoma is quite broad, from children to the elderly, although vertebral/neck chordomas occur most frequently in the 5th–6th decades. In the cervical region, there is no gender difference, a feature unique from other anatomic sites. The most common symptoms in the neck include neurological symptoms (nerve impingement) and progressive pain, while headaches may develop if the lesion encroaches on the skull base. A parapharyngeal mass may occur in cervical lesions, as the mass protrudes forward.

RADIOLOGIC FEATURES

Chordomas are typically solitary, central, lytic, and destructive lesions. They frequently produce an extraosseous soft tissue mass. Matrix calcification is radiographically evident in up to 70% of cases.

PATHOLOGIC FEATURES

GROSS FINDINGS

Chordomas are expansive, lobulated tumors with a neural appearance. A myxoid and slippery appearance is described. Tumors of the neck, involve the vertebral column, almost always destroying the vertebral disc space, with extension into the surrounding tissues. Tumors range in size from 1–10 cm (mean, 5 cm).

MICROSCOPIC FINDINGS

Three types of chordomas can be histologically identified: classic, chondroid, and dedifferentiated. The classic microscopic appearance of chordoma is a lobulated growth of cords and islands of polygonal tumors cells suspended in a myxoid-mucus background. The constituent cells are elongate epithelioid cells and large mucus-containing physaliphorous cells (Fig. 21-5). The nuclei are round and uniform, but may exhibit considerable pleomorphism (Fig. 21-6). The cytoplasm is abundant and eosinophilic, and at times clear. Vacuolated cells (physaliferous cells) are present to a variable degree. About 5% of cervical chordomas contain islands of hyaline-type chondroid or cartilaginous tissue, invoking the term "chondroid chordomas" (Fig. 21-7). In <5% of chordomas, there is an association with a high-grade sarcoma (often after radiation) where the term "dedifferentiated" is applied.

CHORDOMA
DISEASE FACT SHEET

Definition	A malignant tumor of notochord origin
Incidence and location	Represents about 4% of malignant bone tumors
	Cervical account for about 10%
Morbidity and mortality	65% 5-yr survival
Gender, race, and age distribution	Male > Female (2:1), but not in the cervical region
	Mean age, 56 yr
Clinical features	Neurological symptoms referable to nerve roots
	Progressive pain
	Parapharyngeal mass if it protrudes forward
Prognosis and treatment	Recurrences rates up to 60%
	Approximately 65% 5-yr survival, but in the cervical lesions, about 60% ultimately die of disease
	Chondroid chordomas have better prognosis
	Radical, complete surgical removal yields best outcome
	Radiotherapy may be used if nonresectable

CHORDOMA
PATHOLOGIC FEATURES

Gross findings	Expansive, lobulated, glistening mass with a neural/mucoid appearance
Microscopic findings	Lobulated neoplasm
	Cords and island of tumors cells lying in mesenchymal mucus
	Epithelioid cells with remarkable nuclear pleomorphism
	Physaliphorous cells with "bubbly," vacuolated cytoplasm
	Island of hyaline chondroid tissue may be seen
Immunohistochemical features	Express keratin, EMA, and S-100 protein
Pathologic differential diagnosis	Chondrosarcoma, pleomorphic adenoma, carcinoma ex-pleomorphic adenoma, metastatic carcinoma

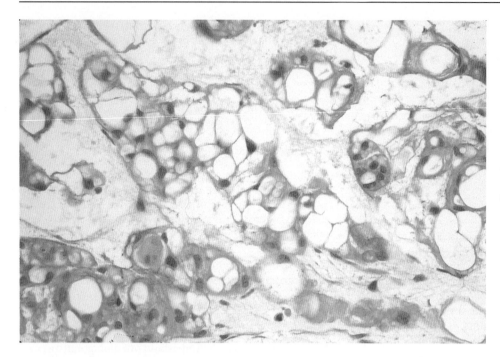

FIGURE 21-5
Physaliphorous cells in a conventional chordoma show vacuolated cytoplasm.

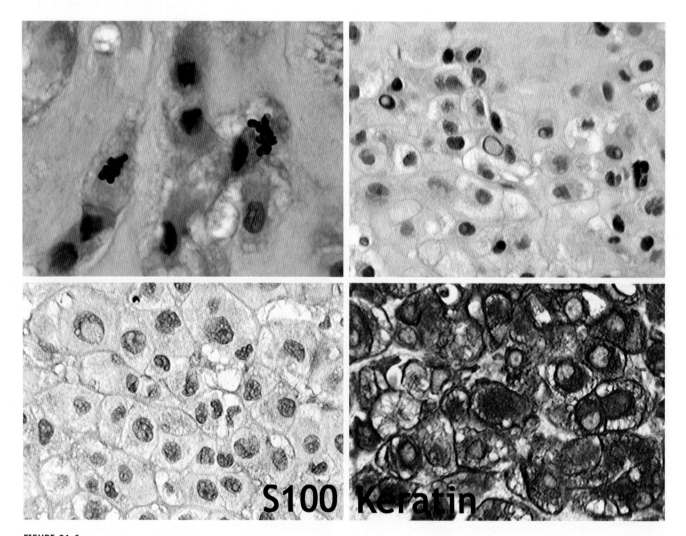

FIGURE 21-6
Left upper: Cords of atypical epithelial cells. Mitotic figures are easily identified. *Right upper:* Nests of epithelial cells with distinct cellular borders. Intranuclear cytoplasmic inclusions are present. *Left lower:* S-100 protein stains the nucleus and cytoplasm. *Right lower:* There is heavy, strong keratin immunoreactivity in the neoplastic cells.

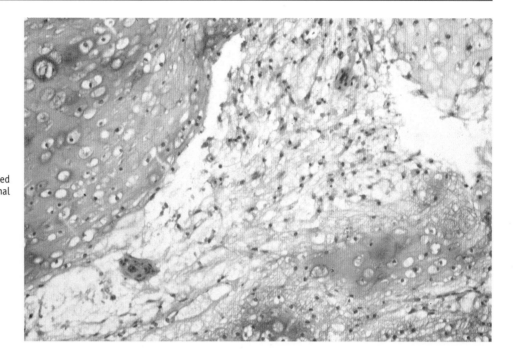

FIGURE 21-7

Islands of hyaline cartilage are noted in the background of a conventional chordoma.

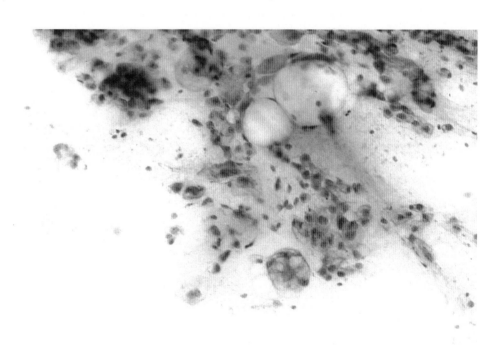

FIGURE 21-8

A cellular preparation with epithelioid cells in a delicate background of myxoid material. There is a finely vacuolated "physaliphorous" cell in the lower center (H&E stained FNA).

ANCILLARY STUDIES

IMMUNOHISTOCHEMICAL FEATURES

Chordomas are immunoreactive with vimentin, keratin, EMA, and S-100 protein (Fig. 21-6). The staining can be variable, with heavy and intense staining to light and focal reactivity.

FINE NEEDLE ASPIRATION

The smears of chordoma are usually cellular with abundant, myxoid background matrix substance, which often encircles the neoplastic cells (Fig. 21-8). The cells are arranged in small clusters and short cords of epithelioid cells, while larger cells with abundant, bubbly cytoplasm (physaliphorous cells) are sprinkled throughout (Fig. 21-9). The physaliphorous cells are usually more

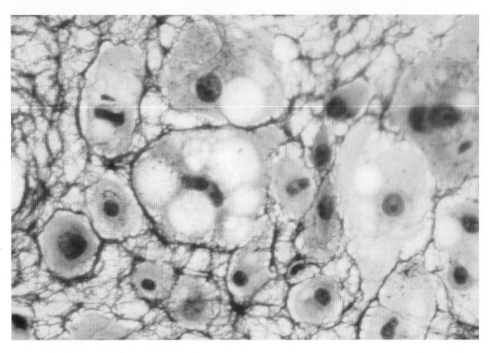

FIGURE 21-9
Epithelioid cells arranged in a magenta background of myxoid material. The center shows a physaliphorous cell (air-dried, Wright stained FNA).

easily identified on alcohol-fixed preparations. The epithelioid cells may be pleomorphic in size and shape, but generally the chromatin distribution is even and regular.

GENETIC STUDIES

Cytogenetic studies have shown abnormalities of chromosome 21, including loss or structural rearrangement of 21(q22). However, chordomas have been shown to lose chromosomes 3, 4, 10, and 13, while also showing other chromosomal deletions and or additions.

DIFFERENTIAL DIAGNOSIS

In the neck, the main differential diagnoses are epithelial neoplasms (such as mucinous carcinoma, salivary gland tumors, poorly differentiated carcinoma) and chondrosarcoma, along with benign notochord tumors. The lobulation, physaliferous cells, and diffuse, strong S-100 protein immunoreactivity distinguish chordoma from carcinoma. Chondrosarcoma is negative for cytokeratin. Benign notochord tumors lack intercellular myxoid matrix and bone destruction. The presence of ductal structures and the immunoreactivity to myoepithelial markers and glial fibrillary acidic protein distinguishes pleomorphic adenoma and carcinoma ex-pleomorphic adenomas from chordoma.

PROGNOSIS AND THERAPY

Chordoma is a low-grade tumor and distant metastases are rare. However, it is an indolent tumor with a 65% 5-year survival, although nearly 60% of patients ultimately die from tumor. The chondroid variant may have a better prognosis. Radical, complete surgical removal of the chordoma is associated with longer survival and delayed recurrences, but is often difficult to achieve in the anatomic confines of the neck. For these and unresectable tumors, adjuvant radiotherapy is employed.

METASTATIC CYSTIC SQUAMOUS CELL CARCINOMA

Predominantly cystic, metastatic, squamous cell carcinoma in the neck often presents without a clinically apparent primary, and therefore are frequently incorrectly considered to be of branchial cleft origin. About one-third of patients who have metastatic squamous cell carcinoma in the neck have exclusively cystic metastases. Due to the rich lymphatic plexus of Waldeyer's ring, primaries are often small and clinically unapparent, but result in early metastasis via the jugulodigastric lymph node chain. As there is a difference in management, identifying this type of metastasis is important.

CLINICAL FEATURES

Patients most frequently present with short history (<6 mo) of a painless mass in the upper neck involving the jugulodigastric lymph nodes. Patients may have bilateral disease (10%). There is frequently a smoking and alcohol abuse history. Most patients are in the 6th

METASTATIC CYSTIC SQUAMOUS CELL CARCINOMA DISEASE FACT SHEET

Definition	A predominantly cystic metastatic squamous carcinoma to cervical lymph nodes
Incidence and location	About one-third of cervical metastatic squamous cell carcinomas are cystic
	When typical histology is present, nearly 80% are from Waldeyer's ring
Morbidity and mortality	Radiation mucositis
	About 30% mortality at 5 yr
Gender, race, and age distribution	Male >> Female (4:1)
	Mean presentation in 6th decade
Clinical features	Painless mass involving jugulodigastric lymph nodes
	Usually short duration (<6 mo)
	May have bilateral disease
	Often have smoking and alcohol abuse history
	Once metastatic disease is diagnosed, nearly 70% will have primary in Waldeyer's ring
Prognosis and treatment	70%–80% 5-yr survival
	Identification of the primary may require extensive examination under anesthesia, pan-endoscopy, high-resolution radiographic studies, and/or ipsilateral tonsillectomy
	Selected lymphadenectomy (used to make diagnosis) followed by focused radiation therapy (targeted to primary or Waldeyer's ring if no primary is identified)

METASTATIC CYSTIC SQUAMOUS CELL CARCINOMA PATHOLOGIC FEATURES

Gross findings	Well-circumscribed, thickly encapsulated cystic mass
	Thick, tenacious, purulent, yellow-brown fluid
	Mean of 4 cm
Microscopic findings	Thick, desmoplastic fibrous connective tissue capsule
	Cystic spaces lined by ribbon-like growth
	Uniformly thick epithelium composed of bland epithelium, lacking maturation, demonstrating loss of polarity, cells with high nuclear to cytoplasmic ratio and mitotic figures
	Usually lacks keratinization and profound pleomorphism
Immunohistochemical features	Keratins positive, but usually not necessary for diagnosis
Fine needle aspiration features	Cellular smears
	Anucleate squames and debris
	Atypical squamous cells with dyskeratosis, irregular nuclear contours, nuclear hyperchromasia, and increased nuclear to cytoplasmic ratio
Pathologic differential diagnosis	Branchial cleft cyst, thymopharyngeal cyst, thymic cyst, bronchial cyst

decade of life, with a strong male predilection (4 : 1). Once the diagnosis of metastatic cystic squamous cell carcinoma is established, a primary tumor is discovered in about 70% of patients usually involving Waldeyer's ring area (base of the tongue, lingual or faucial tonsils). Other sites include the nasopharynx, esophagus, and laryngotracheal region. In about 30% of patients, a primary is never discovered, even though aggressively sought.

RADIOLOGIC FEATURES

CT or magnetic resonance imaging (MRI) show a cystic or multilocular mass with thick capsule in the region of the jugulodigastric lymph nodes.

PATHOLOGIC FEATURES

GROSS FINDINGS

The neck mass ranges in size from 1.5–12 cm, with an average size of about 4 cm. Macroscopically there is

a thick, fibrotic capsule defining the well-circumscribed lymph node border (Fig. 21-10). The cut surface is uni- or multilocular, with the cyst(s) filled with grumous, granular, thick, tenacious, and purulent yellow, brown to hemorrhagic fluid.

MICROSCOPIC FINDINGS

Histologically, the lesion is predominantly cystic, the contents generally washed away in processing. A dense, fibrous connective tissue capsule is often present, a response by the lymph node capsule to the metastatic tumor. The spaces are lined by a ribbon-like growth of transitional type epithelium, generally of a uniform thickness (Fig. 21-11). In some areas the lining has an endophytic growth pattern, budding into the lymphoid stroma, while in other areas it is papillary. The overall histologic appearance in many areas is remarkably bland, recapitulating the normal squamous to transitional-type epithelium identified in the tonsillar crypts (Fig. 21-12). The cells are enlarged with a high nuclear-to-cytoplasm ratio, no appreciable degree of surface maturation, and limited (if any) keratinization. Sometimes, an abrupt transition to remarkably atypical epithelium can be seen, but this is not a common finding (Fig. 21-13). Suffice it to say that the epithelium is often quite bland on initial review and requires careful examination to make the correct diagnosis.

The primary tumors are usually small and located deep in the crypts demonstrating a histologic appearance

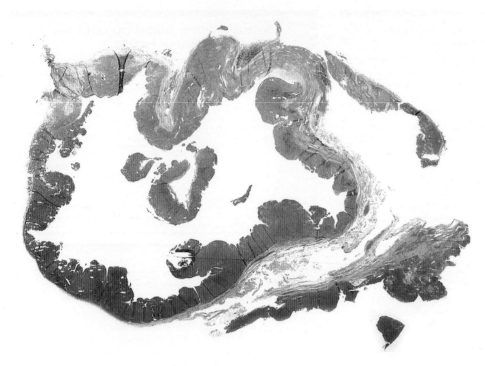

FIGURE 21-10
There is a thicken capsule at the periphery of this lymph node which is replaced by a thin ribbon of epithelial cells around the periphery. The cyst contents were removed in processing.

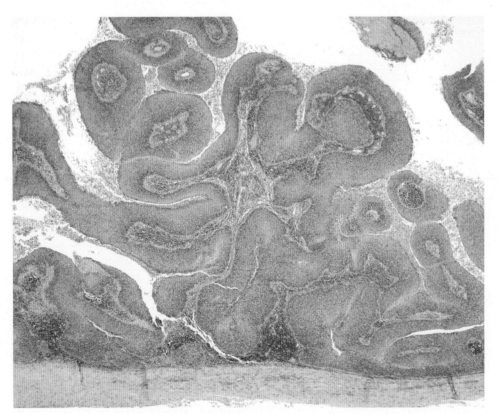

FIGURE 21-11
Ribbon-like arrangement of the metastatic squamous epithelium creates papillary infoldings into the cystic spaces of the replaced lymph node.

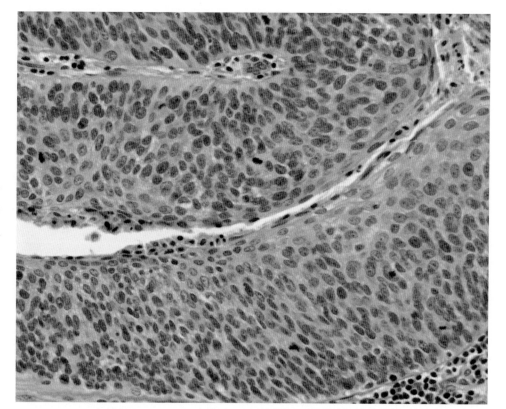

FIGURE 21-12

There is a subtle loss of polarity, a disorganization to the growth, increased mitotic figures, and an overall mild nuclear pleomorphism in this metastatic cystic squamous cell carcinoma.

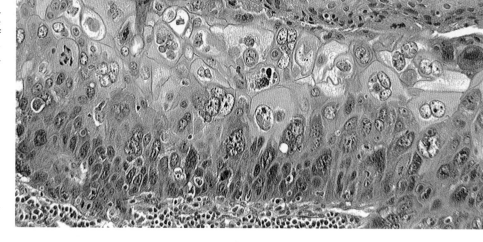

FIGURE 21-13

A monotonous, albeit atypical epithelium is seen at the top of the field, while the opposite ribbon of epithelium shows remarkable anaplasia in this cystic squamous cell carcinoma.

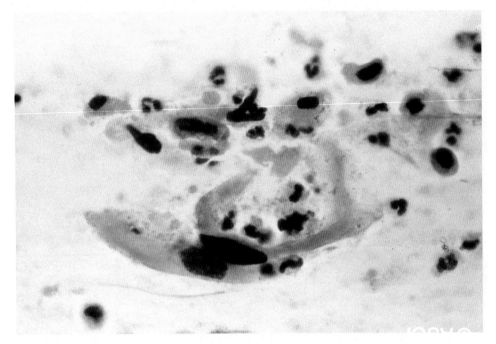

FIGURE 21-14
Atypical squamous cells with "tadpole"-like cytoplasmic extension, nuclear hyperchromasia and contour irregularity are helpful features on FNA for the diagnosis of squamous cell carcinoma (alcohol-fixed FNA).

similar to that of the metastatic foci described above. It is important to realize that this type of "lymphoepithelial carcinoma" has a transitional appearance, and that ordinary, keratinizing squamous cell carcinoma can also be seen in the Waldeyer's ring region.

ANCILLARY STUDIES

IMMUNOHISTOCHEMICAL FEATURES

Immunohistochemistry is not necessary for the diagnosis, as it is a histologic one in most cases. However, the cells are positive with a variety of keratins (AE1, AE3, CK1, CK8, CK14, and CK19), although usually not with CK7.

FINE NEEDLE ASPIRATION

The smears are often quite cellular and in many cases dominated by anucleate squamous and debris from the cystic area of the tumor. However, fragments of atypical squamous epithelium is found or individual atypical keratinocytes are noted (Fig. 21-14). Nuclear atypia, cellular pleomorphism, increased nuclear to cytoplasm ratio, and mitotic figures all help confirm the diagnosis of carcinoma.

DIFFERENTIAL DIAGNOSIS

Cystic, metastatic squamous carcinoma must be distinguished from a branchial cleft cyst, while thymic cyst, bronchial cyst and thymopharyngeal cysts are rarely encountered. Brachial cleft cysts have benign epithe-

lium, maturing toward the cystic cavity, may have keratinization, and usually does not have a thickened or "desmoplastic" fibrous capsule. For all intents and purposes in clinical management of patients, a primary branchial cleft carcinoma does not exist.

PROGNOSIS AND THERAPY

Once the cystic metastasis is accurately classified, efforts toward identifying the primary should include extensive physical examination under anesthesia, pan-endoscopy (nasopharynx, larynx, esophagus, nasal cavity), and detailed, high-resolution CT or MRI studies of the greater Waldeyer's ring area. If these studies do not provide evidence of the primary, then prophylactic lingual and faucial tonsillectomy, specifically on the ipsilateral side, should be performed, with complete embedding of the tonsils and thorough sectioning. Still, an occasional patient will defy attempts at identifying the primary tumor. In any event, focused radiation therapy on the region of Waldeyer's ring, after the selected lymphadenectomy, will yield a good long-term clinical outcome of 70%–80% at 5 years. Overall, this type of carcinoma appears to be more indolent than conventional squamous cell carcinoma of the tonsil (survival rates of <35% at 5 yr).

METASTATIC NEOPLASM OF UNKNOWN PRIMARY

The term "occult primary tumor" means a primary neoplasm that has not been found in a patient with neck metastasis, even after a thorough clinical evaluation. This evaluation includes a systematic and often systemic approach, usually before a lymph node biopsy, although a fine needle aspiration (FNA) is frequently the initial procedure. Evaluation protocols are well established and include pan-endoscopy, radiographic studies, and serologic markers. The neck metastasis may represent disease from regional or distant primary neoplasm. Despite aggressive assessment, in about 10% of patients, a primary tumor will not be identified. While axiomatic, lymphomas must always be excluded if there is a poorly differentiated neoplasm in the lymph node, as their management is unique from that of metastatic disease.

CLINICAL FEATURES

The most common symptom is a painless mass in the neck. The most frequent sites of adenopathy are upper jugular-digastric (70%), midjugular (22%), supraclavicular (18%), and posterior cervical lymph nodes (12%), with more than one site affected. The masses may be present for quite some time, and are often slowly enlarging. The mean age at presentation is in the 6th decade, although it depends on the primary tumor type.

METASTATIC NEOPLASM OF UNKNOWN PRIMARY DISEASE FACT SHEET

Definition	An unidentified primary neoplasm with cervical metastasis
Incidence and location	Neck lymph node metastasis is frequent, although only about 10% of patients have unknown primaries
	Upper jugular lymph nodes account for most metastatic tumors (70%)
Morbidity and mortality	Mortality depends on primary tumor
Gender, race, and age distribution	For upper aerodigestive tract primaries, Male >> Female (4:1)
	Usually adults, with a mean presentation in the 6th decade
	Other primaries are gender and age specific
Clinical features	Painless cervical mass
	Slow growing over several months
	Primary sites include Waldeyer's ring, nasopharynx, larynx, and esophagus, while lung, gastrointestinal tract, breast, pancreas and prostate account for carcinomas outside of the head and neck region
	Melanoma and sarcoma also present as metastatic tumors
Prognosis and treatment	Prognosis is determined by the underlying primary, but is usually poor as metastatic disease is already present
	Initial FNA evaluation guides therapy, which includes lymph node dissection and radiation

When the primaries are from the upper aerodigestive system, men are affected more commonly than women (4 : 1), with many patients reporting heavy smoking and drinking. Non head and neck carcinoma primary sites (gender dependent) include lung, gastrointestinal tract, breast, pancreas, and prostate, while melanoma and sarcomas round out the list.

PATHOLOGIC FEATURES

GROSS FINDINGS

The lymph nodes may be solid, uni- or multicystic, white, gray to dark, and hemorrhagic. The size ranges up to 10 cm in size (mean, ~3 cm). The primary tumor type will frequently dictate the lymph node appearance.

MICROSCOPIC FINDINGS

Spatial constraints limit the discussion, as nearly every known malignancy may at some time result in metastatic deposits in cervical lymph nodes. However, the most common metastatic primary sites in the cervical lymph nodes are squamous cell carcinoma (60%), adenocarcinoma (20%; Fig. 21-15), undifferentiated carcinoma (12%), melanoma (5%; Fig. 21-16), and others (3%). Adenocarcinomas, undifferentiated carcinoma, and thyroid carcinomas are more common in the supraclavicular and scalene lymph nodes.

ANCILLARY STUDIES

HISTOCHEMICAL AND IMMUNOHISTOCHEMICAL STUDIES

Histochemical studies, such as mucicarmine (Fig. 21-17), may help to confirm the diagnosis. In many cases,

METASTATIC NEOPLASM OF UNKNOWN PRIMARY PATHOLOGIC FEATURES

Gross findings	Solid or cystic mass
	Up to 10 cm in size (mean, ~3 cm)
Microscopic findings	Tumor type determines the lymph node appearance
	Squamous cell carcinoma, adenocarcinoma, undifferentiated carcinoma, melanoma, sarcoma, and lymphoma are all considerations, with carcinomas most common
Special studies	Variable depending on the histologic type
	Screening panel to include keratin, CD45RB, S-100 protein, HMB45, actin, and desmin with follow-on targeted antibodies
Pathologic differential diagnosis	Developmental cysts, lymphoma, ectopic nests in the lymph node

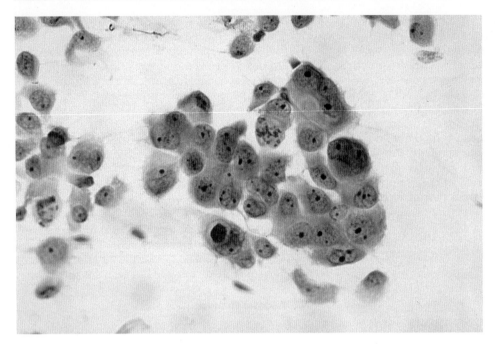

FIGURE 21-15

A metastatic adenocarcinoma from the breast demonstrates small intracytoplasmic vacuoles of mucin. Nucleoli are also easily identified (air-dried, Diff Quick stained FNA).

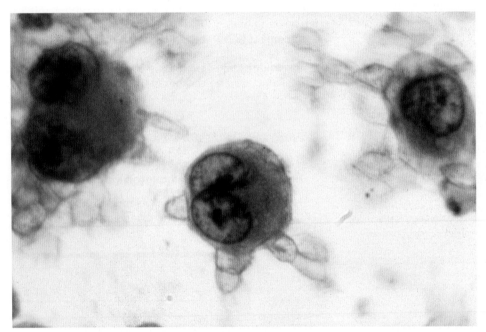

FIGURE 21-16

Large, binucleated atypical individual cells raise the differential diagnosis of a melanoma, sarcoma or Hodgkin lymphoma. This case represented metastatic melanoma, but without cytoplasmic pigmentation, immunohistochemical analysis would be necessary, along with the clinical history (alcohol-fixed, Papanicolau stained FNA).

a targeted immunohistochemical panel may help to suggest a primary site. Keratin, CD45RB, S-100 protein, HMB45, actin, and desmin are initial screening studies which can then narrow the selection of additional antibodies as suggested by gender, age, physical examination, laboratory studies, and histologic results.

FINE NEEDLE ASPIRATION

Fine needle aspiration is an excellent screening study which is a rapid, inexpensive, and safe procedure that can be performed at the time of the patient's initial presentation. When it comes to metastatic tumors, separation can usually be made between squamous and adenocarcinoma, with additional histochemical or immunohistochemical studies performed on the smears as directed by the cytologic findings. A diagnosis of lymphoma, carcinoma, melanoma, or sarcoma as major categories, can then direct the search in a specific direction, eliminating the need for more invasive and costly procedures while also enhancing treatment planning.

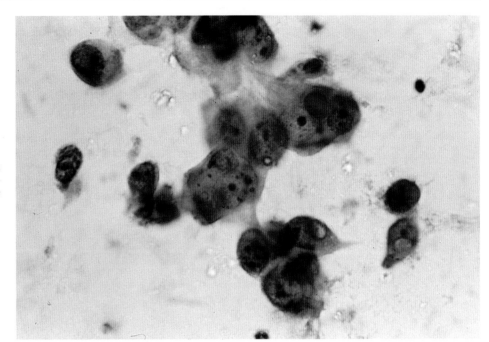

FIGURE 21-17
A mucicarmine stain highlights the intracellular mucin in this metastatic adenocarcinoma (mucicarmine stained FNA).

DIFFERENTIAL DIAGNOSIS

The differential diagnosis usually encompasses benign and reactive versus neoplastic lesions; however, given the lymph node location, other than lymphoma, neoplasms are assumed to be malignant. Branchial cleft cysts, developmental cysts, infections, and reactive inflammatory lymphoid hyperplasias are also in the differential and can usually be easily separated.

PROGNOSIS AND THERAPY

The prognosis is determined by the underlying primary, and by dint of metastatic disease, the prognosis is usually poor, although exceptions occur. Lymph node dissection and radiation can often palliate tumor progression.

SUGGESTED READING

Synovial Sarcoma

1. Bertolini F, Bianchi B, Pizzigallo A, et al.: Synovial sarcoma of the neck. Cases report and review of the literature. Acta Otorhinolaryngol Ital 2003;23:391–395.
2. Bilgic B, Mete O, Ozturk SA, et al.: Synovial sarcoma: a rare laryngeal tumor. Pathol Oncol Res 2003;9:242–245.
3. Coindre JM, Pelmus M, Hostein I, et al.: Should molecular testing be required for diagnosing synovial sarcoma? A prospective study of 204 cases. Cancer 2003;98:2700–2707.
4. Fisher C, de Bruijn DRH, Geurts van Kessel A: Synovial sarcoma. In: Fletcher CDM, Unni KK, Mertens F, eds. Pathology and Genetics of Tumours of Soft Tissue and Bone. Kleihues P, Sobin LH, series eds. World Health Organization Classification of Tumours. Lyon, France: IARC Press, 2002:200–204.
5. Kartha SS, Bumpous JM: Synovial sarcoma: diagnosis, treatment, and outcomes. Laryngoscope 2002;112:1979–1982.
6. Weiss SW, Goldblum JR: Malignant soft tissue tumors of uncertain type. In: Weiss SW, Goldblum JR, eds. Enzinger and Weiss's Soft Tissue Tumors, 4th ed. St. Louis: Mosby, 2001:1483–1509.

Chordoma

1. Coffin CM, Swanson PE, Wick MR, et al.: An immunohistochemical comparison of chordoma with renal cell carcinoma, colorectal adenocarcinoma, myxopapillary ependymoma: a potential diagnostic dilemma in the diminutive biopsy. Mod Pathol 1993;6:531–538.
2. Mirra JM, Nelson SD, Della Rocca C, Mertens F: Chordoma. In: Fletcher CDM, Unni KK, Mertens F, eds. Pathology and Genetics of Tumours of Soft Tissue and Bone. Kleihues P, Sobin LH, series eds. World Health Organization Classification of Tumours. Lyon, France: IARC Press, 2002:316–317.
3. Scolyer RA, Bonar SF, Palmer AA, et al.: Parachordoma is not distinguishable from axial chordoma using immunohistochemistry. Pathol Int 2004;54:364–370.
4. Tallini G, Dorfman H, Brys P, et al.: Correlation between clinicopathological features and karyotypes in 100 consecutive cartilaginous and chordoid tumors. A report from the Chromosome and Morphology (CHAMP) Collaborative Study Group. J Pathol 2002;196:194–203.
5. Yamasuchi T, Suzuki S, Ishiiwa H, et al.: Benign notochordal cell tumor: a comparative histological study of benign notochordal cell tumor, classic chordoma, and notochordal vestiges of fetal intervetebral discs. Am J Surg Pathol 2004;28:756–761.

Metastatic Cystic Squamous Cell Carcinoma

1. Micheau C, Klijanienko I, Luboinski B, et al.: So-called branchiogenic carcinoma is actually cystic metastases in the neck from a tonsillar primary. Laryngoscope 1990;100:878–883.
2. Regauer S, Mannweller S, Anderhuber W, et al.: Cystic lymph node metastases of squamous carcinoma of Waldeyer's ring. Brit J Cancer 1999;79:1437–1442.
3. Regauer S, Beham A, Mannweller S, et al.: CK7 expression in carcinoma of the Waldeyer's ring area. Hum Pathol 2000;31:1096–1101.

4. Thompson LDR, Heffner DK: The clinical importance of cystic squamous cell carcinoma in the neck. A study of 136 cases. Cancer 1998;82: 944–956.

Metastatic Neoplasm of Unknown Primary

1. Ansari-Lari MA, Westra WH: The prevalence and significance of clinically unsuspected neoplasms in cervical lymph nodes. Head Neck 2003;25:841–847.
2. Califano J, Westra WH, Koch W, et al.: Unknown primary head and neck squamous cell carcinoma molecular identification of the site of origin. J Natl Cancer Inst 1999;91:599–604.
3. Eisele DW, Sherman ME, Koch WM: Utility of immediate on-site cytopathologic procurement and evaluation in fine needle aspiration biopsy of head and neck masses. Laryngoscope 1992;102:1328–1330.
4. el Hag IA, Chiedozi LC, al Reyees FA, et al.: Fine needle aspiration cytology of head and neck masses. Seven years experience in a secondary care hospital. Acta Cytol 2003;47:387–392.
5. Koivunen P, Laranne J, Jakobsen J, et al.: Cervical metastasis of unknown origin: a series of 72 patients. Acta Otolaryngol 2002;122: 569–574.
6. Luna MA, Pfaltz M: Cysts of the neck, unknown primary tumor, and neck dissection. In: Gnepp DR, ed. Diagnostic Surgical Pathology of the Head and Neck. Philadelphia: WB Saunders, 2001:650–680.
7. Talmi YP, Hoffman HT, Horowitz Z, et al.: Patterns of metastases to the upper jugular lymph nodes (the "submuscular recess"). Head Neck 1998;20:682–686.
8. Tong CC, Luk MY, Chow SM, et al.: Cervical nodal metastases from occult primary: undifferentiated carcinoma versus squamous cell carcinoma. Head Neck 2002;24:361–369.
9. Werner JA, Dunne AA, Myers JN: Functional anatomy of the lymphatic drainage system of the upper aerodigestive tract and its role in metastasis of squamous cell carcinoma. Head Neck 2003;25:322–332.

22 Diseases of the Paraganglia System
Jennifer L. Hunt

PARAGANGLIOMA

Extra-adrenal paragangliomas arise from paraganglia distributed along the paravertebral sympathetic and parasympathetic chains, and include carotid body, jugulotympanic, orbital, nasopharynx, vagal, laryngeal, paraspinal (aortico-sympathetic and visceral-autonomic), urinary bladder, and the organ of Zuckerkandl tumors. While the most common site of paraganglioma is within the adrenal gland (referred to as pheochromocytoma), discussion will be limited to head and neck sites.

The pathogenesis of paraganglioma is not entirely understood. The best-studied tumor is the carotid body tumor, which is derived from the oxygen-sensing chemoreceptive organ at the bifurcation of the carotid artery. In people who live at high altitudes, this organ can become hyperplastic, presumably secondary to chronic hypoxia. The oxygen sensing activity in the carotid body led investigators to the germline mutations associated with hereditary paragangliomatosis. These mutations are located in several genes encoding the various subunits of the succinate-ubiquinone oxidoreductase gene (SDH), which is an enzyme in the mitochondrial respiratory chain complex II. These genes include PGL1, which encodes SDH subunit D (on 11q23), PGL2 mapping to 11q13; PGL3, which encodes SDH subunit C (on 1q21), and PLG4, which encodes the SDH subunit B (on 1p36). Interestingly, point mutations and/or deletion mutations in these genes can also be identified in up to 20% of patients with presumed spontaneous paragangliomas.

CLINICAL FEATURES

Normal paraganglia are located throughout the body, and consequently paragangliomas have been described in nearly every anatomical location. The head and neck are the most common locations for extra-adrenal paragangliomas, accounting for up to 70% of these tumors, with the most common subsites being carotid body tumors at the bifurcation of the internal and external carotid arteries, glomus tympanicum or glomus jugulare

in the middle ear, and glomus vagale. In the head and neck, the normal paraganglia are associated with the parasympathetic nervous system, adjacent to cranial nerves or to the arterial vasculature. It must be stressed that cervical or thoracic sympathetic paragangliomas are separated from parasympathetic paragangliomas arising in nearby locations. Cervical sympathetic paragangliomas are separate from the carotid body and other structures, and are vanishingly rare.

PARAGANGLIOMA DISEASE FACT SHEET	
Definition	Tumors arising from the paraganglia along the parasympathetic or sympathetic nerves
Incidence and location	Rare (incidence estimate of 0.2–1/ 100,000 population)
	Carotid body, vagal body, middle ear (jugulotympanic), organ of Zuckerkandl, aortico-pulmonary, larynx,
Morbidity and mortality	Infiltrative growth and local recurrence can lead to death
	<10% are malignant
Gender, race, and age distribution	Equal gender distribution (Female > Male at high altitude for carotid body tumors)
	5th–6th decades
Clinical features	Slow growing, painless mass
	Ear lesions may produce tinnitus, hearing loss and nerve dysfunction
	Occasionally may be a pulsatile lesion
	Headache, perspiration, palpitation, pallor, and hypertension for abdominal cavity lesions
	About 10% are bilateral, multiple, familial, and malignant
Radiographic findings	CT shows enhancing mass in characteristic location
	Hyperintense T2-weighted MRI
	Angiography shows splaying of the internal and external carotid arteries with a tumor blush
	^{123}I-MIBG localizes tumor(s)
Prognosis and treatment	Good prognosis if completely resected, although may be indolent and recur/ metastasize years later
	Surgery with preoperative adrenergic blockage and/or embolization

Most patients with head and neck paragangliomas are in the 4th–5th decades without any gender differences, although females predominate in patients living at high altitude. Patients present with a slow growing, painless mass and may have related symptoms. These symptoms commonly include tinnitus, hearing loss, or cranial nerve dysfunction depending on the location of the tumor. Only rare head and neck paragangliomas are biochemically active (up to 4%). In superficial locations, paragangliomas are often described clinically as a pulsatile mass. In the middle ear, for instance, examination of the ear may demonstrate a reddish-purple mass behind the tympanic membrane. About 10%–15% of tumors are bilateral, multiple, familial, and malignant.

In the abdomen (nonadrenal), the neoplasms are most often associated with the sympathetic nervous system. Tumors in the abdomen are more often functional, and patients can present with clinical symptoms secondary to the secretion of catecholamines, such as headache, perspiration, palpitations, pallor, and hypertension. Abdominal paraganglioma (organ of Zuckerkandl accounts for the majority of extra-adrenal sympathetic paragangliomas) may be discovered incidentally when radiologic surveys are performed for other reasons. Paragangliomas can be associated with hereditary paragangliomatosis. Tumors arising in patients with a genetic syndrome are more likely to be multiple and bilateral (Table 22-1). Pheochromocytomas are more commonly syndrome associated.

RADIOLOGIC FEATURES

The most common studies used to assess paragangliomas are angiography, computed tomography (CT), magnetic resonance imaging (MRI), and iodinated metaiodobenzylguanidine (^{123}I-MIBG) scans. Contrast-enhanced CT scans will demonstrate an enhancing mass in characteristic locations (Fig. 22-1). Contrast-enhanced MRI is also characteristic, showing a hyperintense T2-weighted image, and a salt and pepper vascularity within the tumor.

Angiography is often used for patients who are undergoing operative resection and this type of imaging will demonstrate the characteristic pronounced tumor vascularity. In carotid body paragangliomas, the tumor will splay the internal and external carotid arteries, which is a diagnostic feature of paraganglioma (Fig. 22-2). In some cases, ultrasound may be helpful in localizing superficial paragangliomas. ^{123}I-MIBG scans have been reported to aid in localization of paragangliomas.

PATHOLOGIC FEATURES

GROSS FINDINGS

Most paragangliomas are resected en bloc, although the surgery is often bloody and difficult. The resected specimen will consist of a round to oval mass lesion with a smooth, encapsulated or well circumscribed periphery (Fig. 22-3). Carotid body tumors average about 4 cm, but can grow to 10 cm. Tumors of the middle ear tend to be small. The tumors are firm and vary from light tan to dark reddish-brown, the latter correlating with the hemorrhage or congestion within these highly vascular tumors. The risk of recurrence due to incompletely resected tumors makes a comment about inked margins vital in the final report.

TABLE 22-1
Genetic Syndromes Associated with Paraganglioma and Pheochromocytoma

Syndrome	Gene Locus	Gene	Paraganglia Tumor	Other Abnormalities
Von Hippel-Lindau	3p26	VHL	Pheochromocytoma in 10%–20%	Renal cysts and renal cell carcinoma Visceral organ cysts Hemangioblastomas
Hereditary paragangliomatosis	11q23 11q13 1q21 1p36	PGL1 PGL2 PGL3 PGL4	Multiple paragangliomas (100%)	
Neurofibromatosis type 1 (von Recklinghausen disease)	17q11.2	Neuro-fibroma	Pheochromocytoma in 1%–5%	Neurofibromas Schwannomas CNS gliomas
MEN 2A	10q11.2	RET	Pheochromocytoma in 50%–70%	Parathyroid hyperplasia Medullary thyroid carcinoma
MEN 2B	10q11.2	RET	Pheochromocytoma in 50%–70%	Medullary thyroid carcinoma Mucosal neuromas Skeletal abnormalities

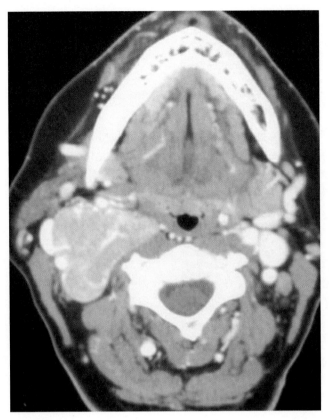

FIGURE 22-1

Contrast-enhanced CT demonstrates a large enhancing mass at the bifurcation of the carotid artery on the left.

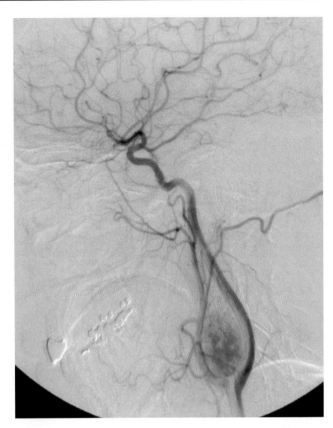

FIGURE 22-2

Angiography demonstrates splaying of the internal and external carotid arteries by a well-vascularized tumor.

PARAGANGLIOMA PATHOLOGIC FEATURES	
Gross findings	Gray to hemorrhagic mass lesion with fibrous pseudocapsule
Microscopic findings	Nests of various sizes
	Polygonal cells with granular, basophilic to eosinophilic cytoplasm
	Hyperchromatic nuclei with possible pleomorphism
	Network of fibrovascular septae
Immunohistochemical features	Chief cells positive with chromogranin, synaptophysin, NSE, CD56
	S-100 protein positive sustentacular cells
Pathologic differential diagnosis	Neuroendocrine adenoma of the middle ear, ceruminous adenoma, meningioma, schwannoma, hyalinizing trabecular adenoma of thyroid, metastatic renal cell carcinoma, carcinoid, atypical carcinoid, medullary thyroid carcinoma

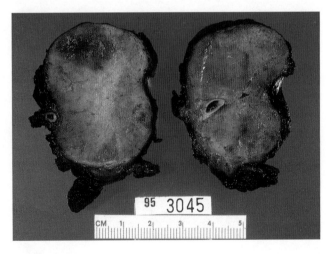

FIGURE 22-3

Gross image of a carotid body paraganglioma with a pseudocapsule and congested cut surface. (Courtesy of Dr. J. A. Ohara.)

MICROSCOPIC FINDINGS

A fibrous pseudocapsule that can be incomplete on histologic sections will most often surround paragangliomas. The periphery of the tumor should be examined for clear margins of resection. In some cases, capsular penetration and vascular invasion may be found, but these features are not indicative of malignancy. Architecturally, the tumor cells are arranged in round to oval nests that can vary in size, the so-called Zellballen pattern (Fig. 22-4). Sometimes, fibrosis may obscure the classic nested pattern (Fig. 22-5). Rarely, other types of patterns can predominate, such as trabecular, angioma-like, or spindled growth.

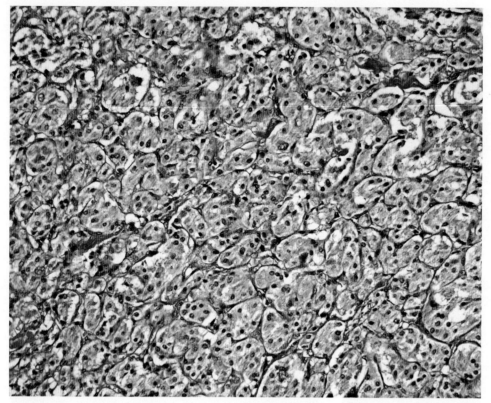

FIGURE 22-4
A paraganglioma showing the nested growth (Zellballen) with delicate fibrovascular septae.

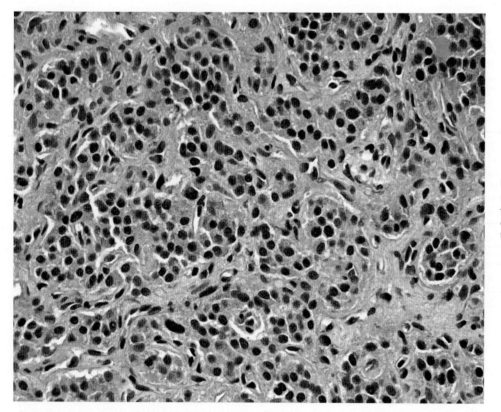

FIGURE 22-5
Fibrosis separates the islands of tumor cells which have eosinophilic cytoplasm and the centrally placed round, hyperchromatic nuclei.

Hemorrhage may be present in these tumors, but frank necrosis is not a common feature. Paragangliomas may be embolized before surgery. In these cases, the tumor may be infracted or hemorrhagic, and may contain foreign material in the vascular channels secondary to the embolization (Fig. 22-6). This should not be mistaken for tumor necrosis.

The cytomorphology of paraganglioma tumor cells varies. The main cell type is the chief cell (type I cells, chemoreceptive cells). These cells are neuroectodermal in origin. The cytoplasm can vary from a finely granular eosinophilic appearance, to deeply basophilic, or even clear cytoplasm in some cases (Fig. 22-7). Similarly, the nuclear features can vary from small, round, and inconspicuous to large and vesicular with bizarre random pleomorphism. Mitoses are sparse and they should not be atypical.

A characteristic feature in paragangliomas is the supporting network of stromal cells and vessels that surround the nests of neoplastic cells. These supporting cells are called sustentacular cells. They are histologically and ultrastructurally nondistinct, but are highlighted with S-100 protein immunohistochemistry.

Middle ear and laryngeal paraganglioma deserve special mention, as the histologic features can be somewhat confusing in these locations. Jugulotympanic paragangliomas are often fragmented and tend to be comprised of smaller nests of cells and higher vascularity (Fig. 22-8), which can lead to confusion with other tumors in the middle ear. Laryngeal paragangliomas are extremely rare and must not be confused with neu-

roendocrine tumors of the larynx (atypical carcinoid and neuroendocrine carcinoma). Occasionally, paragangliomas can be pigmented (postulated to be neuromelanin), may contain amyloid, and may occasionally have eosinophilic cytoplasmic globules (Fig. 22-9). None of these features alter prognosis, but may be a pitfall for appropriate diagnosis.

ANCILLARY STUDIES

ULTRASTRUCTURAL FEATURES

Electron microscopy is not used often, but shows characteristic dense-core neurosecretory granules. The granules can vary in number and in morphology, often correlating with the secretory characteristics.

IMMUNOHISTOCHEMICAL FEATURES

The "nonchromaffin" cells of paragangliomas will invariably stain for neuroendocrine immunohistochemical markers, including chromogranin, synaptophysin, neuron-specific enolase (NSE), CD56, leu-7, S-100 protein, and a variety of specialized neuropeptides in a smaller subset of tumors (i.e., somatostatin, substance P, ACTC, and calcitonin). The supporting sustentacular cells have a unique staining pattern in that they are uniformly S-100 protein positive, highlighting the periphery of the tumor (Fig. 22-10).

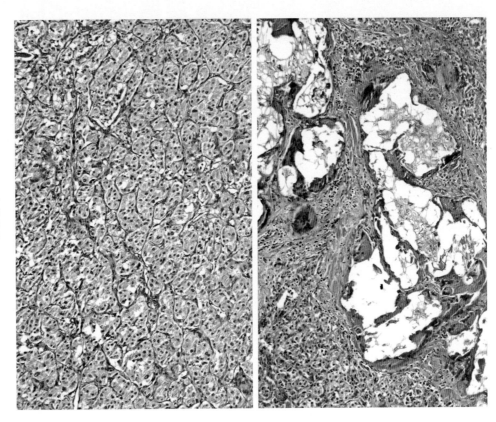

FIGURE 22-6

Portions of the tumor show the characteristic nested pattern (*left*), while embolic material associated with foreign-body giant cells is noted in this embolized neoplasm (*right*).

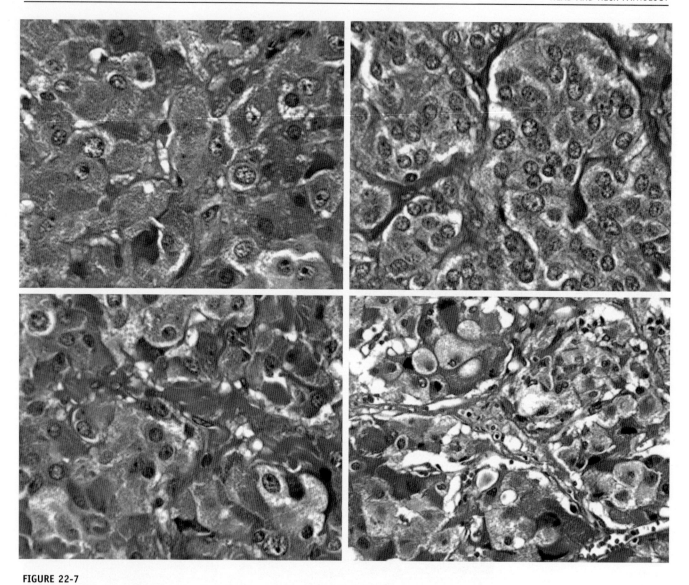

FIGURE 22-7

The various cytomorphologic features include basophilic cytoplasm (*left upper*), a syncytial architecture (*right upper*), granular cytoplasm with fibrosis (*left lower*), and focal clearing in cells that are moderately pleomorphic (*right lower*).

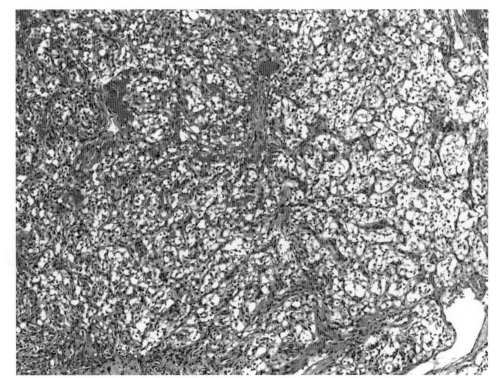

FIGURE 22-8

A jugulotympanic paraganglioma showing small nests and high vascularity.

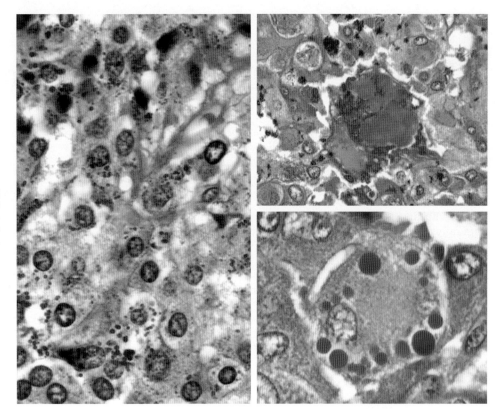

FIGURE 22-9

Left: Melanin pigment may be found in paraganglioma. *Right upper:* Amyloid deposition in a paraganglioma. *Right lower:* Eosinophilic cytoplasmic globules in a paraganglioma.

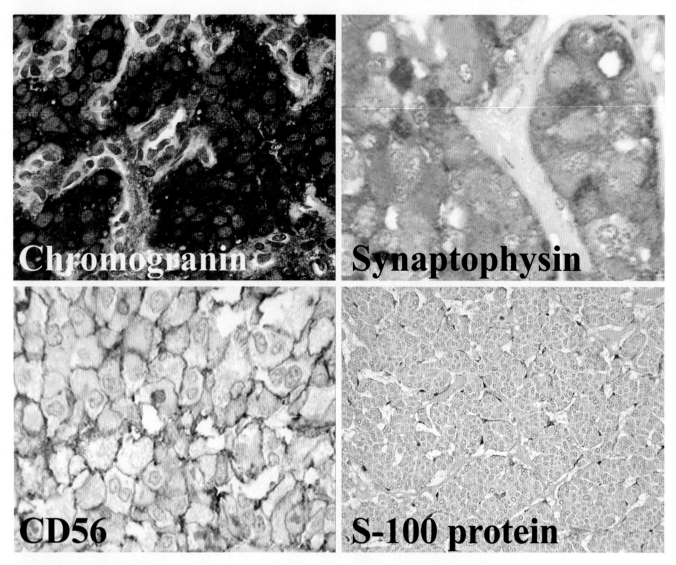

FIGURE 22-10
The paraganglia cells will be positive with chromogranin (*upper left*, ×150), synaptophysin (*right upper*, ×300), and CD56 (*lower left*, ×300); S-100 protein highlights the sustentacular cells (*right lower*, ×50).

FINE NEEDLE ASPIRATION

Fine needle aspiration (FNA) of paraganglioma is generally not recommended as it may result in significant hemorrhage and manipulation of a functional tumor can produce hypertensive crisis. However, in unsuspected cases, the FNA specimens are usually hypercellular, demonstrating single cells or small groups arranged in a "pseudorosette" pattern (Fig. 22-11). Small to moderate sized polygonal cells have wispy, pale cytoplasm with variably sized and shaped nuclei. Binucleated or multinucleated cells are noted (Fig. 22-12).

DIFFERENTIAL DIAGNOSIS

The differential diagnosis for paraganglioma depends on the location of the tumor.

JUGULOTYMPANIC PARAGANGLIOMA

Paraganglioma may be difficult to separate from other tumors when biopsies are small and may be crushed. Tumors include middle ear adenoma, ceruminous adenoma, meningioma, schwannoma, and metastatic renal cell carcinoma. Morphologic overlap can usually resolve the diagnosis with a pertinent panel of immunohistochemistry studies (Table 22-2). Paraganglioma is not reactive with keratin or epithelial membrane antigen, while these markers can help separate between a number of these tumors.

LARYNGEAL PARAGANGLIOMA

Laryngeal paraganglioma is very uncommon. Carcinoid, atypical carcinoid, small cell neuroendocrine carcinomas, and other neuroendocrine tumors that can secondarily involve the larynx, such as medullary

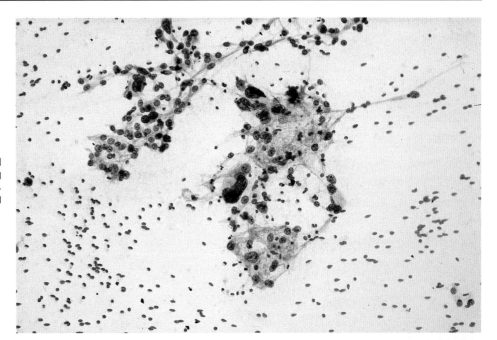

FIGURE 22-11

A Papanicolau stained, alcohol-fixed smear of a paraganglioma showing small "rosette" of cells with variable, hyperchromatic nuclei. Focal spindling is noted.

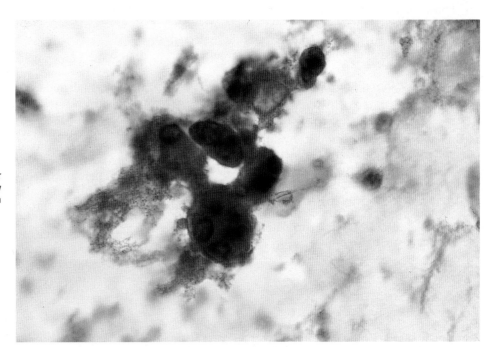

FIGURE 22-12

An alcohol-fixed, H&E stained smear shows a multinucleated cell with wispy cytoplasm and nuclear variability in this paraganglioma.

TABLE 22-2

Immunohistochemical Separation of Ear Tumors

Stain	Paraganglioma	Neuroendocrine Adenoma of the Middle Ear	Metastatic Renal Cell CA	Meningioma
Chromogranin	+	+	−	−
Synaptophysin	+	+	−	−
S-100 protein	+ (sustentacular)	−	−	−/+ (rare)
Cytokeratin	−	+	+	−/+ (rare)
EMA	−	+	+	+
CD10	Unknown	Unknown	+	Unknown

TABLE 22-3

Immunohistochemical Separation of Neck Paraganglioma

Stain	Paraganglioma	Medullary Thyroid Carcinoma	Larynx Neuroendocrine Carcinoma	Metastatic Neuroendocrine Carcinoma
Chromogranin	+	+	+	+
Synaptophysin	+	+	+	+
S-100 protein	+ (sustentacular)	−	−	−
Cytokeratin	−	+	+	+
CEA	−	+	+	+
Calcitonin	−	+	+/−	+/−
TTF-1	−	+	−	+/−

thyroid carcinoma or metastases from other locations are raised in the differential. However, different patterns of growth, increased nuclear pleomorphism, necrosis, increased mitoses, and a carefully selected immunostaining panel will help in this differential.

VAGAL AND CAROTID BODY TUMORS

In this location, paraganglioma must be differentiated from other neuroendocrine tumors, including medullary thyroid carcinoma, hyalinizing trabecular adenoma of the thyroid, and neuroendocrine carcinoma. Medullary thyroid carcinoma will be positive for calcitonin, TTF-1, and carcinoembryonic antigen. Neuroendocrine carcinomas will be positive for cytokeratins, as well as the typical neuroendocrine markers (Table 22-3). Clinical and radiographic correlation will also be of use in separating these tumors.

PROGNOSIS AND THERAPY

Paragangliomas are indolent tumors, without very well-established histologic criteria for malignancy. Therefore, even though the tumors are histologically benign in appearance, life-long clinical (including biochemical and/or radiographic studies) follow-up is necessary to exclude potential recurrence or metastasis (regional lymph node or distant sites). Local symptoms may persist due to mass effect, or if the tumor was functional, catecholamine excess can be debilitating and dangerous. For the most part, if recurrence or metastasis does develop, an overall >90% 5-year survival will decrease substantially (10% 5-yr survival).

Surgery is the treatment of choice, with preoperative treatment with alpha and beta-blockers and/or embolization. Gamma knife radiation has been used with mixed results.

MALIGNANT PARAGANGLIOMA

Malignant paragangliomas are relatively uncommon, although in some studies of extra-adrenal paragangliomas, malignancy rates are 50%. Regrettably, the pathologist is rarely able to make the diagnosis of malignancy in the primary tumor, as there are no reproducible, reliable, and well-accepted histologic criteria for malignancy. Multifocal, multiple, and bilateral tumors can make the determination of metastatic disease a challenge. Therefore, malignancy is narrowly defined as the presence of metastatic disease in sites not normally known to have chromaffin tissue. The most common sites for diagnosis of true metastatic disease are regional lymph nodes, bone, and lungs. The clinical course is indolent and prolonged in many patients, despite known metastatic disease. Functional tumors may make the determination of recurrence a little easier.

CLINICAL FEATURES

The clinical parameters are indistinguishable, although patients tend to be slightly older and are more likely to be symptomatic than patients with benign tumors.

RADIOLOGIC FEATURES

The principle role of radiographic studies is to define the extent of disease and presence of multifocal or metastatic deposits preoperatively to allow for appropriate intervention. Metastatic deposits can be FDG-avid, suggesting PET scanning may be useful. ^{123}I-MIBG

MALIGNANT PARAGANGLIOMA DISEASE FACT SHEET

Definition	Malignant tumor arising from the paraganglia along the parasympathetic or sympathetic nerves
Incidence and location	Very rare
	Most malignant paragangliomas are abdominal
Morbidity and mortality	Protracted clinical course with late recurrences
	Functional tumors have symptomatic recurrences
Gender, race, and age distribution	Equal gender distribution
	5th–7th decades
Clinical features	May be larger than benign tumors
	More likely to be functional (catecholamine secretion)
Prognosis and treatment	<50% 10-yr survival
	Recurrences and metastases in about 50%, often late
	Surgery (debulking), with radiolabeled analogues showing promise

MALIGNANT PARAGANGLIOMA PATHOLOGIC FEATURES

Gross findings	Usually larger tumors with hemorrhage and necrosis
Microscopic findings	Widely invasive lesions (capsule, vessel, into surrounding parenchyma/soft tissue)
	Confluent necrosis
	Large nests or diffuse growth
	Profound pleomorphism
	Increased mitotic figures and atypical forms
Immunohistochemical features	*Decreased* S-100 protein positive sustentacular cells suggests malignancy
	Increased Ki-67 labeling index suggests malignancy
Pathologic differential diagnosis	Benign paraganglioma, atypical carcinoid, neuroendocrine carcinoma, medullary thyroid carcinoma

PATHOLOGIC FEATURES

GROSS FINDINGS

Malignant paragangliomas tend to be large, demonstrating areas of confluent necrosis and hemorrhage. Extensive and significant gross capsular and/or vascular invasion may be noted.

MICROSCOPIC FINDINGS

While no features are absolute, a few histologic features are correlated with metastatic potential: extensive capsular or vascular invasion, confluent necrosis, increased cellularity, large nests or diffuse growth, profound pleomorphism, increased mitoses (>3/10 HPF), and atypical mitotic figures. These features are uncommon in head and neck locations, making it difficult to prospectively predict outcome.

ANCILLARY STUDIES

There are no currently available histochemical, immunohistochemical, ploidy, or molecular/genetic markers which accurately predict a malignant paraganglioma. However, malignancy is suggested when there is a *loss* of S-100 protein positive sustentacular cells, cor-

studies or a labeled dopamine analog tracer may be useful for imaging as well as therapy.

relating with a diffuse growth or large nest pattern, and if there is an increased proliferation index (Ki-67). Additional techniques show promise, but require validation.

DIFFERENTIAL DIAGNOSIS

Separation between benign and malignant paraganglioma causes the most difficulty and may be impossible to accurately diagnose. Paragangliomatosis may sometimes be mistaken for metastatic tumor. Malignant paraganglioma may mimic other neuroendocrine tumors, such as medullary thyroid carcinoma. These tumors can usually be eliminated with immunohistochemistry studies.

PROGNOSIS AND THERAPY

The tumors are indolent, but progressive, resulting in <50% 10-year survival for malignant paraganglioma overall. When metastasis develops, lymph node, bone, liver, and lung are the most common sites. Without accepted histologic criteria for malignancy, all patients with paraganglioma will need life-long clinical follow-up for any evidence of metastatic or recurrent disease. Surgery, especially debulking procedures, is the treatment of choice, with symptomatic management of the excess catecholamines (α-blockade and β-blockade). Radio-labeled analogues may be used in functional tumors, but chemotherapy and radiation do not seem to impact survival.

SUGGESTED READING

Paraganglioma

1. Ali-el-Dein B, el-Sobky E, el-Baz M, Shaaban AA: Abdominal and pelvic extra-adrenal paraganglioma: a review of literature and a report on 7 cases. In Vivo 2002;16:249–254.
2. Barnes L, Tse LLY, Hunt JL: Carotid body paraganglioma. In: Barnes EL, Eveson JW, Reichart P, Sidransky D, eds. Pathology and Genetics of Head and Neck Tumours. Kleihues P, Sobin LH, series eds. World Health Organization Classification of Tumours. Lyon, France: IARC Press, 2005:364–365.
3. Barnes L, Tse LLy, Hunt JL: Vagal paraganglioma. In: Barnes EL, Eveson JW, Reichart P, Sidransky D, eds. Pathology and Genetics of Head and Neck Tumours. Kleihues P, Sobin LH, series eds. World Health Organization Classification of Tumours. Lyon, France: IARC Press, 2005:368–369.
4. Bauters C, Vantyghem MC, Leteurtre E, et al.: Hereditary phaeochromocytomas and paragangliomas: a study of five susceptibility genes. J Med Genet 2003;40:e75.
5. Baysal BE, Myers EN: Etiopathogenesis and clinical presentation of carotid body tumors. Microsc Res Tech 2002;59:256–261.
6. Bikhazi PH, Messina L, Mhatre AN, et al.: Molecular pathogenesis in sporadic head and neck paraganglioma. Laryngoscope 2000;110:1346–1348.
7. Edstrom Elder E, Hjelm Skog AL, Hoog A, Hamberger B: The management of benign and malignant pheochromocytoma and abdominal paraganglioma. Eur J Surg Oncol 2003;29:278–283.
8. Erickson D, Kudva YC, Ebersold MJ, et al.: Benign paragangliomas: clinical presentation and treatment outcomes in 236 patients. J Clin Endo Metabol 2001;86:5210–5216.
9. Ferlito A, Barnes L, Wenig BM: Identification, classification, treatment, and prognosis of laryngeal paraganglioma. Review of the literature and eight new cases. Ann Otol Rhinol Laryngol 1994;103:525–536.
10. Kimura N, Capella C, De Krijger RR, T et al.: Extra-adrenal sympathetic paraganglioma: superior and inferior paraaortic paraganglioma. In: DeLellis RA, Lloyd R, LiVolsi VA, Eng C, eds. Pathology and Genetics of Tumours of the Endocrine Organs and Paraganglia. Kleihues P, Sobin LH, series eds. World Health Organization Classification of Tumours. Lyon, France: IARC Press, 2004:164–165.
11. Kimura N, Chetty R, Capella C, et al.: Extra-adrenal paraganglioma: carotid body, jugulotympanic, vagal, laryngeal, aortico-pulmonary. In: DeLellis RA, Lloyd R, LiVolsi VA, Eng C, eds. Pathology and Genetics of Tumours of the Endocrine Organs and Paraganglia. Kleihues P, Sobin LH, series eds. World Health Organization Classification of Tumours. Lyon, France: IARC Press, 2004:159–161.
12. Koch CA, Vortmeyer AO, Zhuang Z, et al.: New insights into the genetics of familial chromaffin cell tumors. Ann N Y Acad Sci 2002;970:11–28.
13. Lack EE, Lloyd RV, Carney JA, Woodruff JM: Association of Directors of Anatomic and Surgical Pathology: recommendations for reporting of extra-adrenal paragangliomas. Mod Pathol 2003;16:833–835.
14. Maher ER, Eng C: The pressure rises: update on the genetics of phaeochromocytoma. Hum Mole Genet 2002;11:2347–2354.
15. McCaffrey TV, Meyer FB, Michels VV, et al.: Familial paragangliomas of the head and neck. Arch Otolaryngol Head Neck Surg 1994;120:1211–1216.

16. McNichol AM: Differential diagnosis of pheochromocytomas and paragangliomas. Endocr Pathol 2001;12:407–415.
17. Michaels L, Soucek S, Beale T, Sandison A: Jugulotympanic paraganglioma. In: Barnes EL, Eveson JW, Reichart P, Sidransky D, eds. Pathology and Genetics of Head and Neck Tumours. Kleihues P, Sobin LH, series eds. World Health Organization Classification of Tumours. Lyon, France: IARC Press, 2005:366–367.
18. Milroy CM, Ferlito A: Immunohistochemical markers in the diagnosis of neuroendocrine neoplasms of the head and neck. Ann Otol Rhinol Laryngol 1995;104:413–418.
19. Moran CA, Albores-Saavedra J, Wenig BM, Mena H: Pigmented extraadrenal paragangliomas: a clinicopathology and immunohistochemical study of five cases. Cancer 1997;79:398–402.
20. Pellitteri PK, Rinaldo A, Myssiorek D, et al.: Paragangliomas of the head and neck. Oral Oncol 2004;40:563–575.
21. Plukker JT, Brongers EP, Vermey A, et al.: Outcome of surgical treatment for carotid body paraganglioma. Br J Surg 2001;88:1382–1386.
22. Rao AB, Koeller KK, Adair CF: From the archives of the AFIP. Paragangliomas of the head and neck: radiologic–pathologic correlation. Radiographics 1999;19:1605–1632.
23. Tischler AS, Komminoth P: Extra-adrenal sympathetic paraganglioma: cervical paravertebral, intrathoracic and urinoary bladder. In: DeLellis RA, Lloyd R, LiVolsi VA, Eng C, eds. Pathology and Genetics of Tumours of the Endocrine Organs and Paraganglia. Kleihues P, Sobin LH, series eds. World Health Organization Classification of Tumours. Lyon, France: IARC Press, 2004:165–166.
24. van der Mey AG, Jansen JC, van Baalen JM: Management of carotid body tumors. Otolaryngol Clin North Am 2001;34:907–924.
25. Wasserman PG, Savargaonkar P: Paragangliomas: classification, pathology, and differential diagnosis. Otolaryngol Clin North Am 2001;34:845–862, v–vi.
26. Weber PC, Patel S: Jugulotympanic paragangliomas. Otolaryngol Clin North Am 2001;34:1231–1240.
27. Whiteman ML, Serafini AN, Telischi FF, et al.: [111]In octreotide scintigraphy in the evaluation of head and neck lesions. AJNR Am J Neuroradiol 1073;18:1073–1080.

Malignant Paraganglioma

1. Argiris A, Mellott A, Spies S: PET scan assessment of chemotherapy response in metastatic paraganglioma. Am J Clin Oncol 2003;26:563–566.
2. Brown HM, Komorowski RA, Wilson SD, et al.: Predicting metastasis of pheochromocytomas using DNA flow cytometry and immunohistochemical markers of cell proliferation: a positive correlation between MIB-1 staining and malignant tumor behavior. Cancer 1999;86:1583–1589.
3. Edstrom Elder E, Hjelm Skog AL, Hoog A, Hamberger B: The management of benign and malignant pheochromocytoma and abdominal paraganglioma. Eur J Surg Oncol 2003;29:278–283.
4. Shah MJ, Karelia NH, Patel SM, et al.: Flow cytometric DNA analysis for determination of malignant potential in adrenal pheochromocytoma or paraganglioma: an Indian experience. Ann Surg Oncol 2003;10:426–431.
5. Thompson LD: Pheochromocytoma of the Adrenal Gland Scaled Score (PASS) to separate benign from malignant neoplasms: a clinicopathologic and immunophenotypic study of 100 cases. Am J Surg Pathol 2002;26:551–566.

Anatomy, Embryology, and Histology
Jason C. Fowler

INTRODUCTION

Nowhere in the human body is the embryology and anatomy more complex than in the head and neck. The purpose of this appendix is to provide a brief reference to the major anatomic subsites often encountered in routine surgical pathology of the head and neck. This section will serve as a beginning reference only, with the interested reader referred to the suggested reading for a more comprehensive discussion on the anatomy, embryology, and histology. The following anatomic sites will be discussed: larynx, nasal cavity, paranasal sinuses, nasopharynx, oral cavity (including tongue), salivary gland, ear and temporal bone, mandible and teeth, and neck, with a specific presentation of the embryology, anatomy, and histology.

LARYNX

The larynx can be a very challenging specimen to orient and dissect, with a multitude of anatomic structures intricately associated in a complex arrangement to achieve functionality. The larynx is composed of all three germ layers and starts to develop during the 3rd week as an outcropping from the pharynx. The specific anatomy of the larynx develops from the third to sixth arches (see neck section).

The laryngeal skeleton is composed of nine cartilages attached by ligaments (three single and three paired) and the hyoid bone. The three unpaired cartilages are the thyroid, cricoid, and epiglottic. The thyroid cartilage is the largest laryngeal cartilage and forms from two lamina fused anteriorly, giving it the shape of a V. The point of the "V" is referred to as the laryngeal prominence or "Adam's apple." Superiorly, the thyroid cartilage is attached to the hyoid bone and inferiorly it articulates with the cricoid cartilage (Fig. A-1). The cricoid cartilage is the strongest of all laryngeal cartilages and is the only cartilage in the entire airway that forms a complete ring. The cricoid cartilage is also shaped like a signet ring with the narrowest portion of the ring lying

anteriorly where the cartilage attaches to the thyroid cartilage via the cricothyroid membrane (Fig. A-2). The cricoid cartilage is attached to the tracheal rings inferiorly. The epiglottic cartilage is uniquely composed of flexible fibroelastic cartilage. The epiglottic cartilage is somewhat heart-shaped and attaches inferiorly to the thyroid cartilage near the level of the anterior commissure (Fig. A-3). The epiglottic cartilage functions to close off the airway during swallowing. The paired cartilages are the arytenoid, corniculate, and cuneiform, with the arytenoids considered the only cartilages of pathologic significance. The arytenoid cartilages are somewhat pyramidal in shape and are located atop the posterior aspect of the cricoid cartilage bilaterally (Fig. A-4). The arytenoids function during phonation by acting as a lever to which the true vocal cords (vocalis muscles) are attached. The hyoid bone is directly superior to the

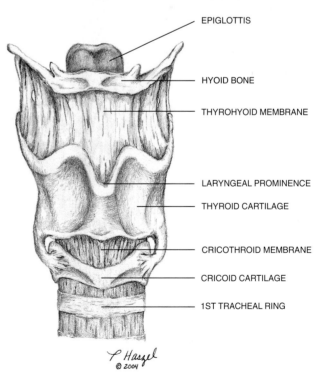

FIGURE A-1

Surface anatomy of the anterior aspect of the larynx. Reprinted by permission of Trisha Haszel, Des Moines, IA.

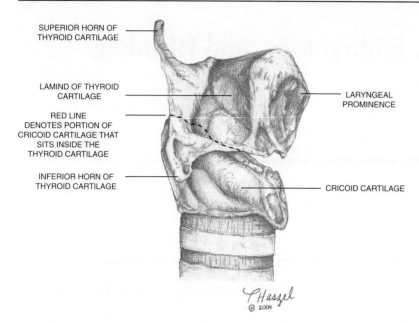

SUPERIOR HORN OF
THYROID CARTILAGE

LAMIND OF THYROID
CARTILAGE

LARYNGEAL
PROMINENCE

RED LINE
DENOTES PORTION OF
CRICOID CARTILAGE THAT
SITS INSIDE THE
THYROID CARTILAGE

INFERIOR HORN OF
THYROID CARTILAGE

CRICOID CARTILAGE

FIGURE A-2

A lateral view of the laryngeal skeleton showing the relationship of the cricoid and thyroid cartilages. It is important to remember that the cricoid cartilage is the only complete ring in the entire human airway and that it sits inside of the thyroid cartilage. Reprinted by permission of Trisha Haszel, Des Moines, IA.

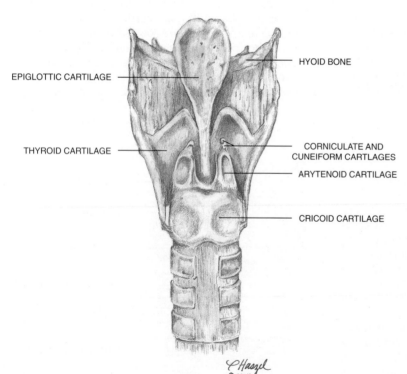

EPIGLOTTIC CARTILAGE

HYOID BONE

THYROID CARTILAGE

CORNICULATE AND
CUNEIFORM CARTLAGES

ARYTENOID CARTILAGE

CRICOID CARTILAGE

FIGURE A-3

Surface anatomy of the cartilages of the posterior aspect of the larynx. Reprinted by permission of Trisha Haszel, Des Moines, IA.

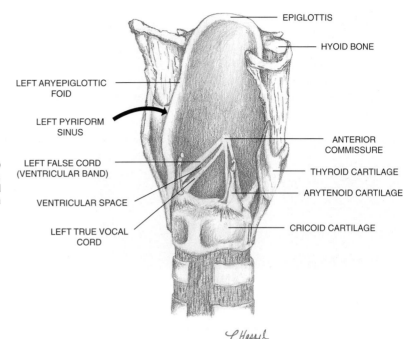

FIGURE A-4

A cut-away of the posterior larynx shows the relationship of the vocal cords to the rest of the laryngeal anatomy, specifically the spaces created by the ligaments and muscles of the larynx. Reprinted by permission of Trisha Haszel, Des Moines, IA.

thyroid cartilage and is attached via the thyrohyoid membrane. The area directly superior to the hyoid bone and anterior to the epiglottis is referred to as the base of tongue or vallecula.

While beyond the scope of this text, a number of the various muscular, ligamentous, and membranous attachments of the laryngeal skeletal parts are important to pathology staging and surgical dissection. The laryngeal musculature is divided into extrinsic (move the larynx as a whole) and intrinsic (function specifically in speech). The epiglottis is connected to the arytenoids via the aryepiglottic folds. Just lateral to each of these folds is the pyriform sinus or pyriform recess. Both of these anatomic locations are significant to the staging of supraglottic and pharyngeal tumors. The arytenoids are also attached to the vocalis muscles, which create the bulk of the true vocal cord on either side of the larynx. The true vocal cords are bordered superiorly by the false vocal cords. The space in between the true and false cords is commonly referred to as the ventricle or ventricular space (Fig. A-5). Depending on individual variation, the ventricle often extends laterally and superiorly to create a space known as the saccule of the larynx. The true vocal cords meet anteriorly and posteriorly to form the anterior and posterior commissures, respectively.

In accordance with the American Joint Committee on Cancer (AJCC), the larynx is broken down into three anatomic subsites based on location of tumor occurrence. These three subsites are supraglottis, glottis, and subglottis. The specific relationships of these subsites will be discussed further in Appendix B, although suffice it to say it is extremely important to have a sound understanding of laryngeal anatomy in order to adequately dissect and stage a laryngeal malignancy. Table A-1 demonstrates the specific anatomic landmarks

within each of these laryngeal subsites that are pertinent to the staging of epithelial malignancies.

At birth, the larynx is composed primarily of respiratory epithelium, with the exception of the true vocal cords, which are covered in stratified squamous epithelium. In time, some of the respiratory epithelium is replaced by squamous mucosa, particularly in the location of the false vocal cords and the epiglottis. With the exception of the true cords, the lamina propria tends to contain numerous mucoserous glands. The false cords tend to be the area with the most abundant number of mucoserous glands (Fig. A-6). The true vocal cords are significant for the presence of the vocalis muscle and the vocal ligament. Invasion of the vocalis muscle by carci-

---

TABLE A-1

Laryngeal Landmarks Specific to AJCC Staging

Location	Specific Anatomy
Supraglottis	Suprahyoid epiglottis Infrahyoid epiglottis Aryepiglottic folds Arytenoids Ventricular bands (false vocal cords)
Glottis	True vocal cords Anterior commissure Posterior commissure
Subglottis	Anything 1 cm or more below the true vocal cords

Note: Pyriform sinus malignancies are staged as pharynx lesions.

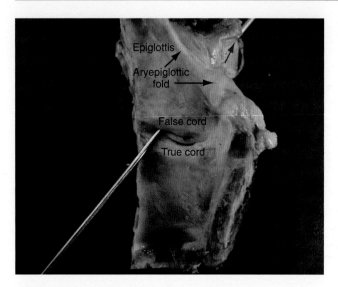

FIGURE A-5

A total laryngectomy specimen demonstrating surface anatomy of the internal larynx. The specimen has been bisected vertically along the midsagittal plane through the anterior commissure, and the metal probe is located within the ventricular space. There is a laryngopyocele protruding from the right pyriform sinus (location of probe exiting the specimen; *red arrow*).

nomas of the larynx can have prognostic implications by affecting the stage of the tumor.

NASAL CAVITY, PARANASAL SINUSES, AND NASOPHARYNX

The complexity of the embryological development of the nasal cavity and paranasal sinuses is beyond the scope of this text. In brief, the nose and nasal passages form from invaginations of ectoderm overlying mesenchyme, with the nasal placodes forming nasal pits which gradually grow deeper until they form nasal sacs. Formation of these passages begins at roughly the 4th week of fetal development. The communication between the oral and nasal cavities is separated by the formation of the oronasal membrane with the choanae formed in this region. The nasal septum results from a merged medial nasal prominence (Fig. A-7). The paranasal sinuses are outgrowths of the nasal cavity, but do not necessarily aerate and fully develop until post-fetal life (frontal and sphenoid sinuses, specifically). The sinuses are named for the bones in which they are located (maxillary, sphenoid, ethmoid, and frontal; Fig. A-8).

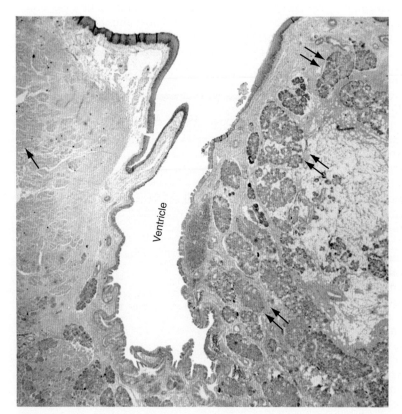

FIGURE A-6

A midsagittal section shows both the true and false vocal cords. The true cord is identified by the location of the vocalis muscle (*arrow*), whereas the false cord is identified by the presence of the numerous minor salivary glands (*double arrows*).

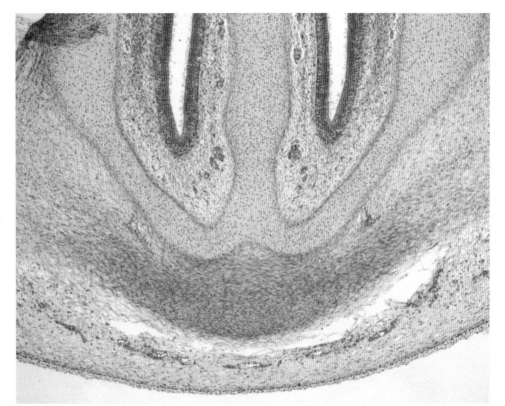

FIGURE A-7

The embryologic development of the nasal cavity with immature cartilage separating primitive respiratory epithelium.

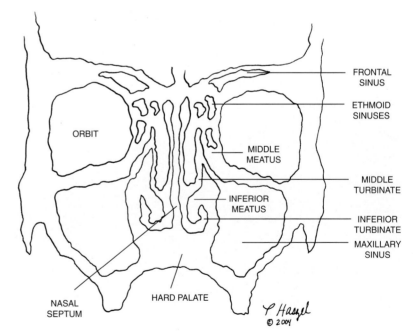

FIGURE A-8

A coronal view of the nasal cavity and paranasal sinuses. Reprinted by permission of Trisha Haszel, Des Moines, IA.

The nose projects from the face and is supported mainly by a cartilaginous skeleton. The nares (nostrils) are separated by the nasal septum and bordered laterally by the nasal alae. The external nose is covered with thick skin containing abundant sebaceous glands. The skin covers the internal portion of the nares (nasal vestibule) where numerous hairs are present. The skin meets the mucosa of the nasal cavity beyond this hair-bearing portion of skin. The nasal cavity is separated in the midline by a continuation of the nasal septum, which forms the medial wall of each cavity. Each cavity is pear-pyramidal shape and is bordered superiorly by the cribriform plate of the ethmoid bone. The hard palate forms the floor of the nasal cavity. The lateral wall contains the opening for the paranasal sinuses and the nasal turbinates. The turbinates, or concha, are posteriorly oriented projections of bone covered with highly vascularized mucosa that extend on either side of each cavity. Typically there are three turbinates on either side: inferior, middle, and superior (Fig. A-9). A fourth turbinate may also be identified (roughly 60% of patients) and is commonly called the supreme turbinate.

The space directly inferior and lateral to each turbinate is known as the meatus. The majority of the nasal septum is formed from septal cartilage anteriorly and the perpendicular plate of the ethmoid bone posteriorly.

The nose functions to humidify and cleanse inspired air. The mucosa of the nasal cavities is composed of highly vascularized pseudostratified, ciliated columnar epithelium. There is also an abundance of both serous and mucus glands, particularly near the opening of the paranasal sinuses (Fig. A-10). It should be mentioned that the mucosa of the nasal cavity is also often termed "Schneiderian mucosa" because of its embryonic origins. The mucosa of the superior nasal cavity (cribriform plate) is slightly different due to a lesser degree of vascularity and the presence of olfactory fibers.

The paranasal sinuses consist of the frontal, ethmoid, sphenoid, and maxillary sinuses. All of the sinuses originate as invaginations from the nasal fossae during fetal development and all are covered with the same Schneiderian mucosa as the nasal cavity. The frontal sinuses are the most superior of the paranasal sinuses, are located within the frontal bone, and will typically drain into the frontal recess via the nasofrontal duct. The ethmoid sinuses or ethmoid complex are comprised of numerous air cells with considerable variation (Fig. A-11). This complex collection of air cells lies medial to the orbits and is connected in the midline by the cribriform plate of the ethmoid bone. The lateral wall is formed from the thin lamina papyracea, which forms the medial orbital wall, an important landmark in staging sinonasal

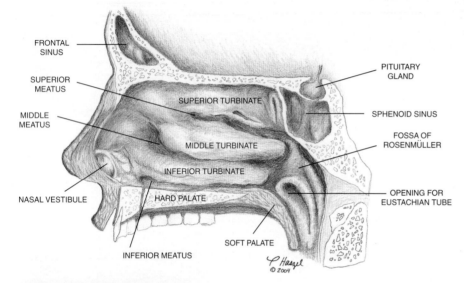

FIGURE A-9

Sagittal view of the nasal cavity and nasopharynx. Reprinted by permission of Trisha Haszel, Des Moines, IA.

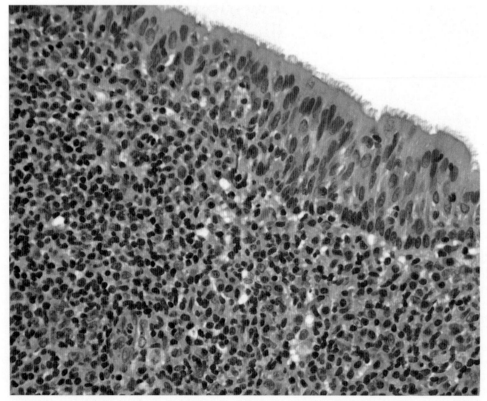

FIGURE A-10

A high-power micrograph of pseudostratified, columnar epithelium with small mucus globules at the surface and heavy inflammatory cells within the stroma.

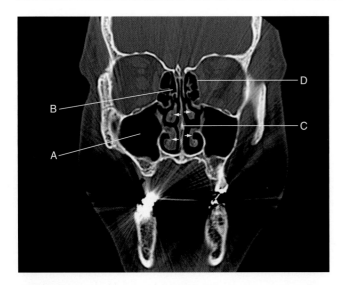

FIGURE A-11

A computed tomography coronal scan of the nasal sinuses demonstrating the maxillary (A) and ethmoid sinuses (B), as well as the nasal septum (C) and turbinates (*arrows*). The lamina papyracea is easily identified (D). (Courtesy of Dr. G. Marano.)

neoplasms. The medial aspect of the ethmoid complex is formed from the thin bony aspects of the middle and superior turbinates. The sphenoid sinuses are the most posterior of the paranasal sinuses and invaginate from the developing nasal cavity into the sphenoid bone. The roof of the sphenoid sinus forms the floor of the sella turcica and the lateral wall is formed from the orbital apex, which contains the optic nerve and cavernous sinus. The cavernous sinus contains the internal carotid artery and cranial nerves III, IV, V (V^1 and V^2), and VI. Posterior to the sphenoid sinus are the clivus, pons, and basilar artery. The roof of the nasopharynx forms the

inferior aspect of the sphenoid sinus. The maxillary sinuses are the largest of all the paranasal sinuses, located within the body of the maxillary bone. The roof of the maxillary sinus forms the floor of the orbit; the medial wall is formed by the lateral aspect of the nasal cavity; the posterolateral aspect separates the maxillary sinus from the infratemporal fossa; and the floor of the maxillary sinus usually overlies the premolars and first molar teeth. The maxillary ostia are located on the superior aspect of the medial wall and drain into the nasal fossa through the ethmoidal infundibulum.

The nasopharynx develops from the foregut and the branchial arches and pouches, containing the tonsils and containing the tubotympanic recess which develops into the eustachian tube. The nasopharynx is located just posterior to but continuous with the nasal cavity. The nasopharynx extends inferiorly and posteriorly where it becomes continuous with the posterior wall of the pharynx. The superior border is formed by the sphenoid bone and clivus. The floor of the nasopharynx is the junction with the soft palate where it becomes continuous with the oropharynx. The lateral walls of the nasopharynx are formed from the pterygoid plates and the pharyngobasilar soft tissue. The eustachian tubes enter the nasopharynx just posterior to the medial pterygoid plates. Just posterior to the location of the eustachian tubes is the lateral recess of the nasopharynx, the superior portion of which is known as the fossa of Rosenmüller (Fig. A-9).

In infants the nasopharynx is lined by respiratory epithelium, while in adults metaplastic stratified squamous mucosa is present. The superior and lateral walls of the nasopharynx contain ciliated, squamous, and transitional mucosa. The adenoids are portions of lymphoid tissue within the nasopharynx, the superior portion of Waldeyer's ring, a collection of lymphoid tissue within the oro- and nasopharynx (Fig. A-12).

FIGURE A-12

The typical mucosal lining of the nasopharynx with pseudostratified columnar epithelium and lymphoid follicles that comprise part of the adenoids.

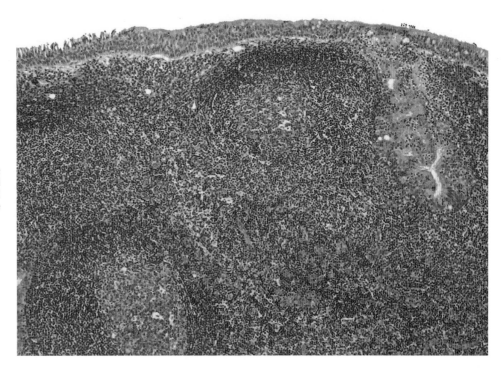

ORAL CAVITY AND TONGUE

The primitive oral cavity, or stomodeum, is an ectodermal recess that starts to form as early as the 3rd–4th week of gestation in association with the endodermally derived foregut. The roof of the oral cavity, or primary palate, forms when the oronasal membranes separating the oral cavity (stomodeum) and nasal sacs break down and ossification of the maxilla takes place. This typically happens during the 7th–10th weeks. The epithelium is ectodermally derived and is stratified nonkeratinizing squamous epithelium. The muscles of mastication are derived from the first branchial arch, while the various nerves supplying the oral cavity are derived from the first through fourth branchial arches. A complex vascular supply and lymphatic drainage make specific lymph nodes more likely to be involved by tumors of specific anatomic structures.

The oral cavity functions in respiration, digestion, swallowing, and taste. The oral apparatus can be separated into an external and an internal portion. The external portion (oral vestibule) includes the lips (with vermillion border and central philtrum), cheeks, and buccal mucosa. The nasolabial fold separates the nose and lips. Various muscles of facial expression (that are too numerous for inclusion here) are what determine the size and shape of the mouth. The internal portion is bordered by the maxillary and mandibular arches (teeth) anteriorly and laterally, and the palate superiorly. The inferior aspect of the oral cavity is completely occupied by the tongue and its associated musculature. Posteriorly, the oral cavity communicates with the oropharynx. The palate forms the roof of the oral cavity and is composed of both a hard and a soft portion (Fig. A-13). The hard palate makes up the anterior two-thirds

and is formed from the maxillary and palatine bones. The posterior soft palate is suspended from the posterior aspect of the hard palate by a muscular aponeurosis that attaches it to both the tongue and the pharynx. The uvula is an appendage suspended from the posterior soft palate and contains abundant mucoserous glands. The palatine tonsils are lateral and somewhat inferior to the uvula within the tonsillar fossa. They are bordered anteriorly by the palatoglossal folds and posteriorly by the glossopharyngeal folds. The gingiva is the fibrous tissue covered with nonkeratinizing squamous epithelium that attaches the teeth to the jaws.

The entire oral cavity is covered with a mucus membrane often referred to as oral mucosa (Fig. A-14). Keratinization may be present in areas of friction, such as the palate. The underlying stroma consists primarily of dense, collagenous tissue. This supporting framework of collagen can be loosely attached to muscle and soft tissue, but can also be tightly bound to the periosteum where it overlies bone (i.e., near the teeth). The submucosa of the oral cavity is also notable for numerous mucoserous glands.

The tongue is a highly specialized organ that resides partly in the oral cavity and partly within the pharynx. The tongue is involved in a variety of functions including mastication and taste and cleansing of the oral cavity. The primary functions of the tongue, however, are manipulation of speech and assisting in swallowing by forcing food into the pharynx.

As with nearly all other head and neck structures, the tongue develops from the pharyngeal arches and associated mesoderm. Specifically, arches 1–4 are the most involved. The initial structures that make up the tongue begin to appear during the 5th–6th weeks of development when the lateral lingual swellings form from the first pharyngeal arch. These swellings will eventually form the anterior two-thirds of the tongue in

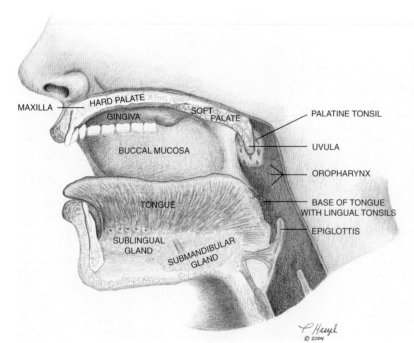

FIGURE A-13

A sagittal view of the oral cavity demonstrates a number of anatomic structures. Reprinted by permission of Trisha Haszel, Des Moines, IA.

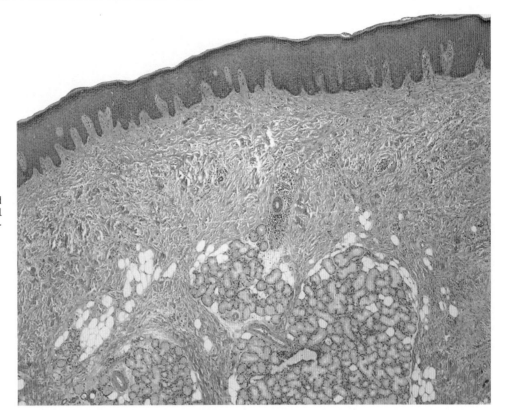

FIGURE A-14

A medium-power shows stratified squamous epithelium of the oral cavity (palate), subtended by numerous mucoserous glands.

conjunction with the median tongue bud (tuberculum impar). The posterior one-third of the tongue forms mainly from the third pharyngeal arch with a small amount being contributed from the fourth arch.

The tongue is a very unique organ composed of a body, a base (or root), a dorsal surface, a ventral surface, and an apex (or tip). The majority of the tongue musculature is anchored to both the hyoid bone and the mandible, with the styloid process also serving as a focus of attachment. The dorsal surface of the tongue is remarkable for the presence of the sulcus terminalis and numerous specialized papillae. The sulcus terminalis separates the anterior and posterior portions of the tongue and points posteriorly to the foramen cecum, a remnant of the embryologic thyroglossal tract (Fig. A-15). The numerous papillae on the dorsal tongue include vallate (circumvallate), foliate, filiform, and fungiform. With the exception of the foliate, which are sparse in humans, nearly all papilla contain specialized receptors for taste and hence are collectively called "taste buds." The base of the tongue is continuous with the epiglottis and also has lymphoid follicles often referred to as lingual tonsil. The lingual tonsil, combined with the palatine tonsils and the adenoids of the nasopharynx collectively make up what is referred to as "Waldeyer's ring." The lymphatic drainage of the tongue is topographically regional and segmental with varying degrees of crossover.

The tongue is composed mainly of bulky skeletal muscle covered with specialized oral mucosa. The mucosa is firmly attached to the epimysium of the muscle with a thick fibrous lamina propria. The mucosal epithelium demonstrates various papillae, of which the

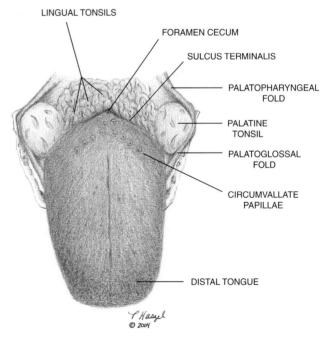

FIGURE A-15

An anterior view of the tongue and the tonsillar fossa. Reprinted by permission of Trisha Haszel, Des Moines, IA.

fungiform and circumvallate are most notable (Fig. A-16). The circumvallate are notable for the presence of serous glands that aid in the initial digestion of food and are also known as von Ebner's glands. The fungiform have a thin nonkeratinized epithelium with a highly vascular stroma.

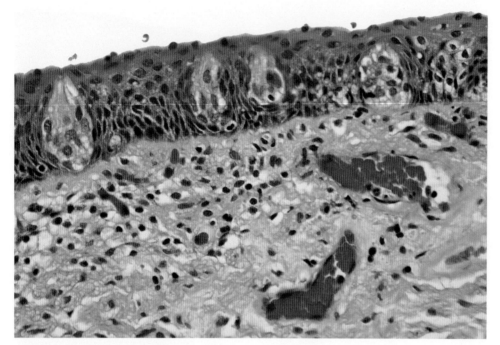

FIGURE A-16

This high-power micrograph show the dorsal surface of the tongue with specialized "taste buds" within the mucosa.

SALIVARY GLAND

The salivary glands arise from buds of the stomodeum during the 5th–7th weeks of gestation. The parotid glands form first, with an ectodermal epithelium and a mesodermal mesenchymal component. During early gland development, lymph nodes will often become entrapped in the parotid parenchyma. The submandibular and sublingual glands develop slightly later, arising from the floor of the stomodeum and paralingual sulcus, respectively, and are endodermally derived. The glands are composed of ducts, acini, and stroma (Fig. A-17). The salivary glands are responsible for the production and secretion of saliva. Humans have three pairs of major salivary glands (parotid, submandibular, and sublingual) in addition to approximately 1,000 minor salivary glands.

The parotid gland is the largest salivary gland, located anterior to the ear, and divided into superficial and deep lobes. The superficial lobe is covered by skin and superficial fascia and overlies the ramus of the mandible, whereas the deep lobe is located medial and posterior to the mandibular ramus. The facial nerve exits the stylomastoid foramen and courses between the two lobes of the parotid with great variance in its distribution. The secretory ducts of the parotid gland eventually empty into a main duct (Stenson's duct) that pierces the buccinator muscle and enters the oral cavity via the parotid papilla. Histologically, the parotid is composed primarily of serous acini (Fig. A-18).

The submandibular gland is much smaller than the parotid and is located within the submandibular triangle of the neck. Like the parotid, the submandibular gland is also lobulated and covered with a dense, fibrous capsule. The submandibular gland is located just medial

and slightly inferior to the body of the mandible and rests atop the bellies of the digastric muscle and inferior to the mylohyoid muscle. The submandibular duct (Wharton's duct) forms from many smaller ducts and emerges in the anterior floor of mouth directly lateral to the lingual frenulum. Histologically, the submandibular gland demonstrates both serous and mucus acini in a relatively equal distribution (Fig. A-19).

The sublingual glands are nonencapsulated and lie directly under the floor of the mouth atop the mylohyoid muscle. The sublingual glands are composed primarily of mucinous acini.

The functional unit of all salivary glands is the acinar-ductal apparatus (Fig. A-20). Acini are composed either of serous or mucus glands or a combination of the two. Serous acini consist of somewhat ovoid-shaped epithelial cells with a prominent basement membrane. The epithelial cells of serous acini have dense cytoplasm packed with basophilic secretory granules. Mucinous acini tend to be larger than serous acini and somewhat haphazard in their arrangement. The hallmark of mucinous acini is secretory cells filled with clear mucoid substances of varying concentrations. Mixed acini demonstrate mucoid cells surrounded by a rim of serous cells arranged in a crescent shape, referred to as a serous demilune. Acini are subtended by myoepithelial cells, often difficult to appreciate on standard histology.

Terminal acini empty into a duct system subdivided into secretory and excretory components. The first two portions of the ductal system are secretory and are known as the intercalated and striated ducts, respectively. The remaining ducts are excretory. The striated and intercalated ducts are *intra*lobular, whereas the excretory portions are *inter*lobular. The intercalated ducts are lined by a single layer of cuboidal epithelium with adjacent myoepithelial cells. The parotid gland has the longest intercalated ducts while they are virtually

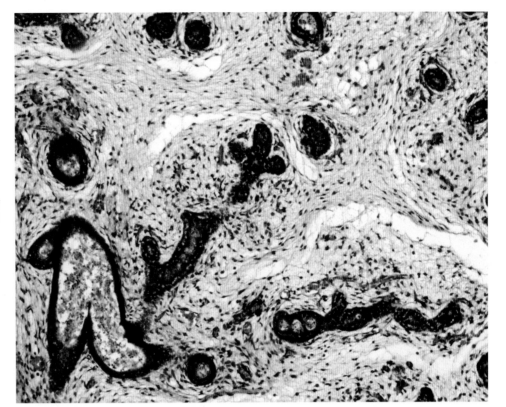

FIGURE A-17

An early embryonic development of salivary gland tissue with small ducts and their surrounding mesenchyme.

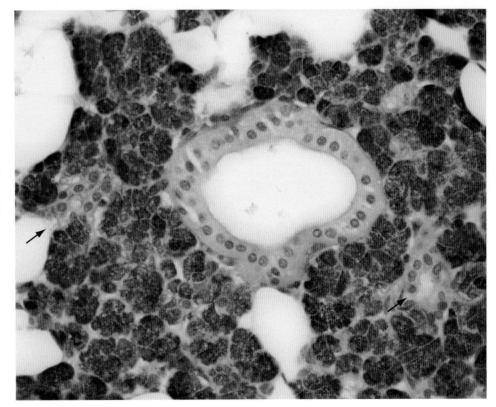

FIGURE A-18

The parotid gland is composed of predominantly serous glands interspersed with adipose tissue. The larger duct at the center of the figure is a striated duct, while the smaller ducts immediately adjacent are intercalated duct.

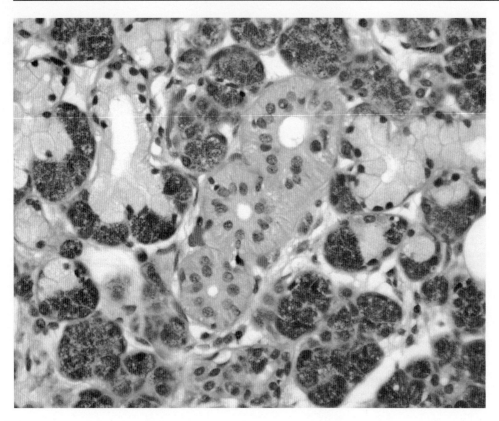

FIGURE A-19

The submandibular gland has ducts interspersed between serous glands and mucus glands. Note the numerous serous demilunes at the termination of the acinus.

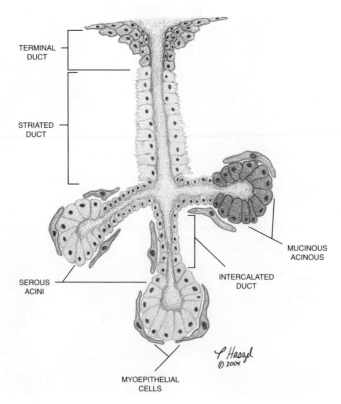

TERMINAL DUCT

STRIATED DUCT

MUCINOUS ACINOUS

SEROUS ACINI

INTERCALATED DUCT

MYOEPITHELIAL CELLS

FIGURE A-20

The normal histology of the salivary gland functional unit. Reprinted by permission of Trisha Haszel, Des Moines, IA.

nonexistent in the sublingual gland. Striated ducts are lined by a single layer of columnar epithelium; however, they demonstrate invaginations on their basal side that form parallel striations that are quite visible on routine H&E sections. The striated ducts then connect with the interlobular excretory ducts that transition from pseudostratified columnar to stratified squamous near the opening into the oral cavity.

EAR AND TEMPORAL BONE

The embryology of the ear and temporal bone is extremely complex. The ear forms as an integration of all three germ layers, and forms three distinctly different parts: external ear, middle ear, and internal ear. These anatomical units function in hearing and equilibrium. The first branchial arch serves as the backbone by which all structures in the ear will form (Tables A-2 and A-3). The ear begins to develop as a thickening of the surface ectoderm on the side of the rhombencephalon. These otic placodes invaginate to form the three otic vesicles which give rise to the saccule, cochlear duct, utricle, semicircular canals, and the endolymphatic duct—all referred to as the membranous labyrinth. A full description is well beyond the scope of this text, but briefly, the inner ear develops further to form the scala vestibuli, scala tympani, and spiral liga-

ment with inner and outer hair cells. The middle ear, comprised of the tympanic cavity, eustachian tube, and ossicles are formed from the first branchial pouch and arch, considered of endodermal origin. The external ear (auditory meatus, tympanic membrane, and auricle) develop from ectodermal epithelium and endodermal tissues, all from the first branchial apparatus (Fig. A-21).

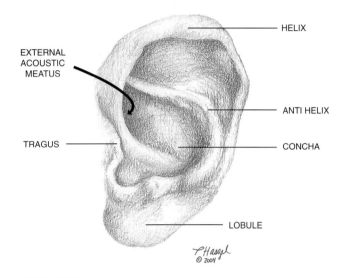

FIGURE A-21

Surface anatomy of the external ear. Reprinted by permission of Trisha Haszel, Des Moines, IA.

TABLE A-2

Anatomic Derivatives of the Pharyngeal (Branchial) Arches

Pharyngeal Arch	Cranial Nerve	Anatomic Structures Derived from Arch
1	V (Trigeminal)	Muscles of mastication, tensor veli palatini muscle, tensor tympani muscle, anterior belly of digastric muscle, mylohyoid muscle, mandibular process, malleus, sphenomandibular ligament, incus
2	VII (Facial)	Muscles of the face, stapedius muscle, stylohyoid muscle, posterior belly of digastric muscle, stapes, styloid process, stylohyoid ligament, hyoid bone (portion of body)
3	IX (Glossopharyngeal)	Stylopharyngeus muscle, greater cornu and body of hyoid bone
4	X (Vagus)	Cricothyroid and constrictor muscles of the pharynx, laryngeal cartilages
6	X (Vagus)	Laryngeal muscles, laryngeal cartilages

TABLE A-3

Anatomic Derivatives of the Pharyngeal (Branchial) Pouches (Clefts)

Cleft (Pouch)	Cleft Derivative (External)	Pouch Derivative (Internal)
1	External acoustic meatus (Work type I & II fistulas)	Middle ear cavity and auditory tube
2	Cervical fistula (abnormal)	Palatine tonsil
3	Cervical fistula (abnormal)	Thymus, inferior parathyroid gland
4	Pyriform sinus fistula (abnormal)	Superior parathyroid gland
5	N/A	Ultimobranchial body of the thyroid

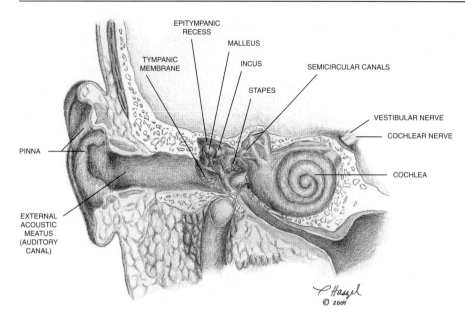

FIGURE A-22

The anatomy of the middle and internal ear shown by a coronal cut away. Reprinted by permission of Trisha Haszel, Des Moines, IA.

The ear and temporal bone anatomy can be subdivided into three distinct areas: the external ear and auditory canal, the middle ear, and the inner ear. The major anatomic structures found in each of these areas are detailed in Table A-4. The surface anatomy of the ear appendage (also known as auricle or pinna) is frequently encountered in specimens resected for skin lesions. In fact, the majority of ear disorders occur on either the pinna or within the external canal. The external auditory canal is S shaped and functions to conduct sound toward the middle and inner ear. The external third is composed of skin, cartilage, and ceruminous glands, whereas the inner two-thirds is epithelial lined and composed of bone and cartilage. The middle ear is located within the petrous portion of the temporal bone and contains the tympanic membrane and the epitympanic recess (Fig. A-22). The tympanic membrane separates the ear canal from the middle ear and vibrates in response to sound. The epitympanic recess contains the three auditory ossicles, a chain of small bones that

TABLE A-4
Anatomic Structures of the Ear

Location	Specific Anatomy
External ear and external auditory canal	Auricle or pinna
	External 1/3 of canal—skin and cartilage
	Internal 2/3 of canal—bone and cartilage
Middle ear	Tympanic membrane
	Stapedius muscle
	Epitympanic recess
	Tensor tympani muscle
	Chorda tympani nerve
	Auditory ossicles (malleus, incus, stapes)
Inner ear	Semicircular canal
	Cochlea (cochlear duct)
	Endolymphatic sac
	Ampulla
	Vestibule of bony labyrinth
	Auditory tube (Eustachion tube)
	Utricle
	Saccule

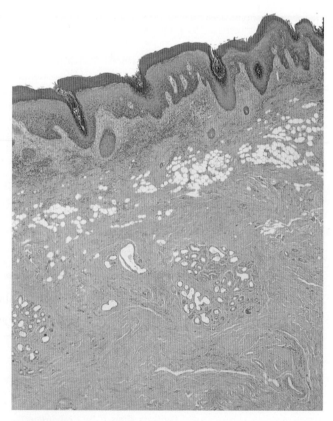

FIGURE A-23

A medium-powered micrograph of the epithelium of the external auditory canal with ceruminal glands deep in the stroma.

conduct sound to the inner ear. The three ossicles are the malleus, incus, and stapes, considered the smallest bones in the human body. The epitympanic recess opens into the eustachian (auditory) tube, which connects to the nasopharynx. The inner ear contains the vestibulocochlear apparatus, which is responsible for hearing and balance.

The epithelium of the external ear and the outer one-third of the external auditory canal is keratinized, stratified squamous epithelium with adnexal structures similar to those found elsewhere in the body (hair follicles, sebaceous glands, ceruminous glands; Fig. A-23). Ceruminal glands combine their secretions with those of sebaceous glands to form cerumen ("earwax"). The

subcutaneous tissue of the external ear is composed primarily of loose connective tissue, fat, and fibrocartilage, giving flexibility to the external ear. The innermost portion of the canal is devoid of ceruminal glands or other adnexal structures.

MANDIBLE AND TEETH

The jaws are U-shaped structures which develop as part of the face and branchial arches. The mandible arises from the mandibular arch (first pharyngeal arch) carti-

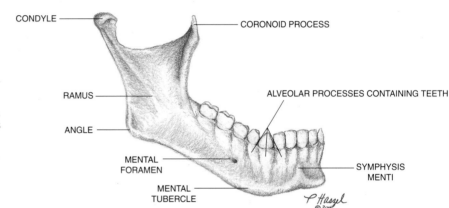

FIGURE A-24

Anatomic landmarks of the mandible. Reprinted by permission of Trisha Haszel, Des Moines, IA.

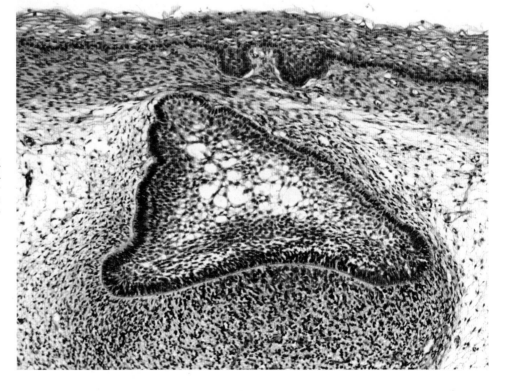

FIGURE A-25

The oral epithelium shows two small dental buds at the surface. The bell stage of tooth development demonstrates dental pulp at the base with odontoblasts, ameloblasts, and stellate reticulum.

lage (often referred to as Meckel's cartilage). The maxillary process gives rise to the maxilla. The mandible articulates with the skull via the temporomandibular joint. It is the strongest of the jaws and contains the alveolar processes for the mandibular teeth. The posterior aspect of each side of the mandible where the gingiva of the last molar meets the buccal mucosa and the base of the tongue is referred to as the retromolar trigone (Fig. A-24).

At about 6 weeks, a C-shaped dental lamina forms along the basal lining of the oral cavity. Approximately 10 buds form from this lamina on each jaw and form the primordia of the tooth. The deep surface invaginates to form the cap stage with an inner and outer dental epithelium and a central core of stellate reticulum with dental papilla below. The bell stage forms when the mesenchymal cells of the dental papilla differentiate into odontoblasts (Fig. A-25). Odontoblasts form dentin at a later stage of development, while the outer dental epithelium differentiates into ameloblasts. The root of the tooth develops from the mesenchyme; cementoblasts outside of the tooth develop to produce cementum—the outer layer of which gives rise to the periodontal ligament. These 20 teeth are referred to as deciduous teeth. A number of these have permanent tooth buds associated with them, giving rise to 32 teeth in adults: incisors (8), canines (4), premolars (8), and molars (12). The teeth are attached to the jaws via "sockets" called

alveolar processes. Each tooth socket contains the tooth root and associated vessels and nerves.

NECK

Much of head and neck embryology centers around the pharyngeal (branchial) arches, pouches, and clefts. The branchial apparatus is responsible for a vast majority of the development of structures in the head and neck (Fig. A-26). The branchial arches arise as swellings of mesenchyme along the sidewalls of the developing gut tube. There are five arches that arise, although the fifth arch is vestigial and eventually disappears, but not before giving rise to the ultimobranchial body. Each branchial arch is supplied by its own cranial nerve and blood supply. Each of the arches is separated by depressions on the inside of the pharynx known as pouches and depressions on the outside known as clefts. There are total of four pouches and four clefts between the five arches. Each arch gives rise to specific anatomic structures in the head and neck (Tables A-2 and A-3), with the interplay of the ectoderm, mesoderm, and endoderm layers too complicated to describe in detail here.

The neck, for anatomy purposes, is broken down into triangles, each of which contains specific structures. The sternocleidomastoid (SCM) muscle divides each

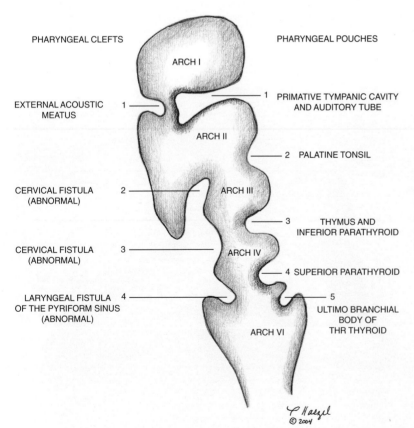

FIGURE A-26

The five pharyngeal arches and the anatomic structures (or abnormalities) resulting from the pouches (internal) and clefts (external). Virtually all structures in the head and neck are derived from the pharyngeal (branchial) arches and pouches. Reprinted by permission of Trisha Haszel, Des Moines, IA.

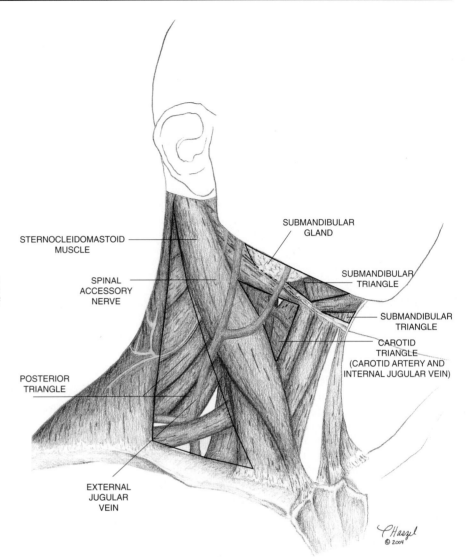

FIGURE A-27

The triangles on the right side of the neck and the major anatomic structures relative to each triangle. Reprinted by permission of Trisha Haszel, Des Moines, IA.

STERNOCLEIDOMASTOID MUSCLE

SPINAL ACCESSORY NERVE

POSTERIOR TRIANGLE

EXTERNAL JUGULAR VEIN

SUBMANDIBULAR GLAND

SUBMANDIBULAR TRIANGLE

SUBMANDIBULAR TRIANGLE

CAROTID TRIANGLE (CAROTID ARTERY AND INTERNAL JUGULAR VEIN)

side of the neck into anterior and posterior triangles (Fig. A-27). The posterior triangle contains the spinal accessory nerve (CN XI), as well as a number of lymph nodes. The anterior triangle can be further broken down into submental, submandibular, and carotid triangles, each with their respective lymph nodes, draining specific anatomic sites. The carotid triangle is extremely important as it contains the internal carotid artery and the internal jugular vein. The internal jugular vein courses deep to the SCM and is usually attached to radical neck dissection specimens. The submandibular gland is within its own triangle, commonly resected during modified and radical neck dissections.

ACKNOWLEDGMENT

The author would like to express his sincerest gratitude to Ms. Trisha Haszel of Des Moines, Iowa, for her superb artwork and illustrations.

SUGGESTED READING

1. Agur AM, Lee MJ: Grant's Atlas of Anatomy, 10th ed. Lippincott Williams & Wilkins, Philadelphia, 1999.
2. Cochard LR: Netter's Atlas of Human Embryology. Teterboro, NJ: Icon Learning Systems LLC, 2002.
3. Dalley AF, Moore KL: Clinically Oriented Anatomy, 4th ed. Lippincott Williams & Wilkins, Philadelphia, 1999.
4. Heath JW, Young B: Wheater's Functional Histology: A Text and Color Atlas, 4th ed. London: Churchill Livingstone, 2000.
5. Langman J: Medical Embryology, 4th ed. Baltimore: Williams & Wilkins, 1981.
6. Larsen WJ: Human Embryology, 3rd ed. Philadelphia: Churchill-Livingstone, 2001.
7. Moore KL: The Developing Human: Clinically Oriented Embryology, 7th ed. Philadelphia: WB Saunders, 2003.
8. Netter FH: Atlas of Human Anatomy, 3rd ed. Los Angeles: Icon Learning Systems, 2002.
9. Sadler TW: Langman's Medical Embryology, 7th ed. Baltimore: Williams & Wilkins, 1995.
10. Sternberg SS: Histology for Pathologists, 2nd ed. Philadelphia: Lippincott-Raven, 1997.

Intraoperative Consultation and Grossing Techniques

Jason C. Fowler • Melissa H. Fowler

INTRAOPERATIVE CONSULTATION

Intraoperative consultations (whether frozen sections, crush preparations, smears, touch preparations, or gross examinations) are widely accepted as an efficient tool for patient management. The pathologist often plays a crucial role in determining the surgical outcome of patients undergoing resections for diseases of the head and neck and endocrine organs. There are a number of scenarios for which surgeons will request an intraoperative consultation, but most of the time the aim is to obtain accurate diagnostic information that will either determine or alter the course of surgical treatment. Five areas result in possible errors: inaccurate communication, indications for intraoperative assessment, inadequate sampling (by surgeon or pathologist), incorrect interpretation, and technical difficulties.

COMMUNICATION

It is imperative that clear, open, and effective communication is achieved among all parties during intraoperative consultation: surgeons, pathologists, operating room (OR) staff, and pathologist's assistants. Physical presence in either the operating room or the gross laboratory by the pathologist and/or surgeon, respectively, is often critical to achieve proper orientation and to identify specific areas of interest or concern. Furthermore, interaction is necessary for building confidence and teamwork. While axiomatic, the pathologist is ultimately responsible for appropriate specimen handling.

Specimens submitted for intraoperative consultation should be received fresh, but kept moist with a small amount of saline, optimally wrapped in a portion of sterile, saline-soaked gauze. Specimens for intraoperative consultation should never be submitted in formalin or other fixatives. Ideally, specimens should be submitted to the frozen section suite as they are removed to

facilitate decision making in real time. Education and training of operating room and grossing room staff in correct specimen handling, labeling, and transportation is essential to achieving error-free specimen processing.

INDICATIONS AND CONTRAINDICATIONS FOR INTRAOPERATIVE CONSULTATION

There are only a selected number of instances in which samples in head and neck and endocrine pathology need to have a frozen section performed. These include: (a) determination of specimen adequacy for special procedures such as cultures, immunophenotypic analysis, molecular studies, ultrastructural examination, or flow cytometry; (b) a different definitive therapy would be conducted based on the diagnosis (extent of disease determinations); (c) numerous previous attempts at diagnosis have been unsuccessful; and (d) assessment of adequate surgical margins of resection. In specimen adequacy determinations, only a portion of the tissue should be initially evaluated in order to triage the material and maintain tissue integrity for the specific studies chosen.

The vast majority of frozen sections requested during head and neck surgery are for the assessment of surgical margins, as >90 % of neoplasms are epithelial in origin. When assessing margins of resection, specimens should be taken (after appropriate inking and orientation) to include the closest margin as well as other mucosal margins (proximal, distal, superior, inferior, medial, lateral, anterior, deep as indicated; Fig. B-1). Margins should be routinely examined on all head and neck carcinoma resections, ideally on the main specimen, rather than small biopsies sent separately. However, if sent separately, no more than 2 cm of margin should be submitted to reduce sampling errors. The number and location of frozen sections depends on the confidence level and skill of the surgeon. A tumor is usually removed en bloc with a rim of normal mucosa and supporting tissue. A shave (en face) margin or a radial (perpendicular)

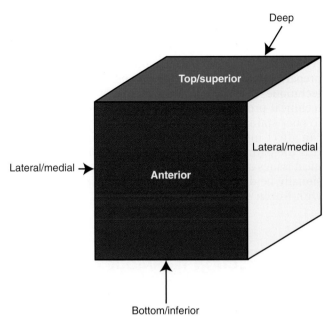

FIGURE B-1

A basic three-dimensional diagram by which all complex specimens should be approached. For most composite resections, there will be six margins of resection.

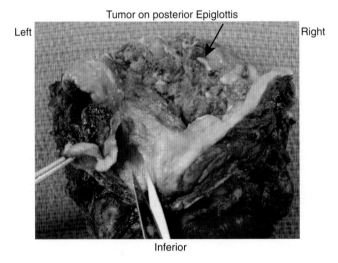

FIGURE B-2

A supraglottic laryngectomy with the left false cord mucosal margin being removed for intraoperative consultation. A shave or enface mucosal margin includes both the inked margin and the adjacent mucosal surface. The arrow denotes the large, exophytic tumor obliterating the epiglottis.

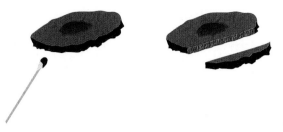

FIGURE B-3

Diagram of correct technique for taking a shave or en face margin from a specimen with multiple margins (i.e., wide resection). It is important to note that the true margin (with ink) must be embedded "up" for frozen sectioning and "down" in a histologic cassette for permanent sections. This preserves the true orientation of the margin.

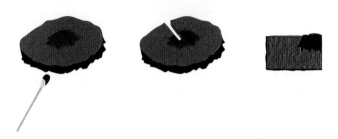

FIGURE B-4

The correct technique for taking a radial (perpendicular margin) on a surgical specimen. The principle of this margin is to demonstrate both tumor and margin in the same section so as to ascertain how close the tumor is to the margin.

tive consultation, specifically frozen section, should ***never*** be performed just for intellectual or academic curiosity, gamesmanship, family reassurance, financial gain, or rote examination; and should be discouraged when the tissue is heavily calcified, predominantly fat, if the specimen is exceptionally small, and for lesions suspected of being unique or unusual, requiring a number of additional studies (such as cultures, flow cytometry, immunofluorescence, ultrastructural examination). Levelheaded, direct communication with the surgeons on a regular basis, particularly during tumor board conferences, should help to avoid unnecessary requests for intraoperative consultation.

SAMPLING

While sampling errors cannot be completely eliminated, they can be avoided to an extent by thoroughly examining the specimen(s) submitted for intraoperative consultation while communicating directly with the surgeon about specific area(s) in question. The use of sutures or a tissue pen to orient the margins of the specimen is crucial (Fig. B-5). Sampling errors may also be avoided by taking multiple sections from the main specimen. This is particularly the case with thyroid neoplasms. Proper orientation is extremely important, especially when trying to assess mucosal margins. These

margin can be performed depending on whether a distance to the closest margin is to be assessed (radial) or if a large surface is to be assessed (en face) (Figs. B-2, B-3, B-4).

While intraoperative consultations are an invaluable tool, they are also frequently misused. An intraopera-

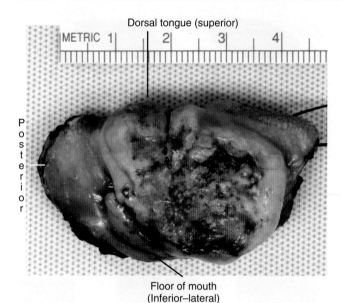

FIGURE B-5

Right hemiglossectomy for a squamous cell carcinoma arising in the lateral tongue and extending to the inferior floor of mouth margin. The suture denotes the right anterior tip of the tongue.

samples should be placed in frozen section media such that both the epithelium and submucosal soft tissues are seen on the slide. Margins submitted by the surgeon should be marked with either ink or cautery so that the "true margin" is the one represented on the slide for diagnosis.

INTERPRETATION

There are a number of factors that can lead to a pathologist misinterpreting an intraoperative consultation. The most problematic area of histopathologic interpretation on frozen section diagnosis rests with epithelial lesions, especially epithelial hyperplasia, pseudoepitheliomatous hyperplasia, radiation changes, and squamous cell carcinoma (verrucous and spindle cell types). Mesenchymal and inflammatory lesions usually present with the problem of insufficient sampling, as the diagnostic material often rests in the submucosal deep tissue. Of particular importance is the clinical history, as previous radiation, chemotherapy, and/or surgery can alter the tissue architecture. Of course, communication errors are often only realized after the fact. While a personal bias, it is better to err on the side of benignancy and delay definitive therapy rather than perform a radical surgery for a benign disease. According to Dr. Lauren Ackerman, frozen section should be performed by a person "rich in experience, conservative in attitude, and most important, he [/she] must have judgment."

TECHNICAL PROBLEMS

A variety of commercial preparations are available for preparing and cutting the specimens, without a specific technique or product better than another. However, technical problems can result from cryostat difficulties to poor staining quality. Any type of technical problem can affect interpretation and the subsequent diagnosis. It is the pathologist's responsibility to correct any technical issues as they arise. Although diagnoses may occasionally be deferred, there is a high degree of accuracy with frozen section techniques.

FROZEN SECTION TECHNIQUE

The wide array of equipment and stains available precludes recommending a particular protocol by which intraoperative consultations be performed. However, a few points are considered universal in achieving technically high quality frozen sections. Assign a unique identifier to the specimen after delivery time stamp. A thorough macroscopic examination will determine the proper sample for evaluation. If a frozen section is to be performed, make certain the sample is taken perpendicular to the mucosa (for most head and neck cancers) which has been inked appropriately, and that it is oriented correctly in the mounting media. The optimal freezing temperature is at least −20°C, with sections cut at 5–6 μm intervals. Multiple levels (ribbons) should be obtained during the initial evaluation. Results should be orally communicated to the surgeon in a timely fashion; the College of American Pathologists recommends that 90% or greater of all frozen sections be reported within 20 minutes. A permanent record of the frozen section request and diagnosis should be maintained in the patient's record and in the pathology suite (electronically as allowed by governing bodies), with the slide retained indefinitely along with the permanent H&E (hematoxylin and eosin) sections.

GROSSING TECHNIQUES

INITIAL EVALUATION

Every specimen prior to evaluation must have accurate patient identification and a unique identifier associated with it. Pertinent clinical history is imperative, including symptoms, past treatment, radiographic findings, and clinical suspicion. Specific specimen identification, including exact anatomic site is essential, including laterality (right or left). Any specific or special requests should be noted, including cultures, ultrastructural examination, immunofluorescence, immunohistochemistry, flow cytometry, molecular/genetic studies, and/or chain of custody requirements.

ORIENTATION

The complexity of many head and neck resections is further compounded by lack of distinct anatomic landmarks. Orientation is easily maintained and preserved through the use of suture and tissue marking pens, although ideally direct communication with the surgeon to orient the sample is paramount. Sometimes, a small drawing on the requisition can serve to orient the specimen.

GROSSING PROCEDURES AND TECHNIQUES

The importance of a thorough gross description cannot be stressed enough! The aim of each dissection is to answer questions that will lead to an accurate pathologic diagnosis and pathologic staging if a tumor is present. The macroscopic description must include the patient name and identifier, surgeon, specific specimen(s), and procedure performed (biopsy, lymph node dissection, radical resection, etc.). It is also important to note whether the specimen was received fresh, in formalin or in another fixative.

All anatomic structures present must be measured and described, specifically paying attention to recognized landmarks which will later aid in staging. Measuring the whole specimen (in centimeters), along with including measurements of specific structures included in the sample are important, to say nothing of measuring the lesion (tumor) itself. Giving distances from the tumor to margins or extent of involvement into adjacent structures is imperative. Weights are usually included for parathyroid, thyroid, and pituitary samples, using an ultra sensitive scale for parathyroid and pituitary gland specifically.

The application of indelible (permanent) inks as an aid to recognizing specimen margins on histologic slides is vital for margin assessment. In most cases, a single color is sufficient; however there are many instances when multiple colors are necessary to accurately identify specific margins of resection (Fig. B-6). While pedantic, the authors prefer to use blue—superior (the sky is up); green—inferior (the grass is down); yellow—lateral (two "l's" in yellow and lateral); orange—medial; anterior—red; posterior—black. The ink should be "fixed" to the tissue by the use of a mordant such as 95% ethyl alcohol, 10% glacial acetic acid, or Bouin's. It is imperative that the ink is completely dry before sectioning to prevent ink tracking, seepage, and spilling from creating a false-positive margin.

The main lesion/tumor must be accurately described in terms of size, location, appearance, growth pattern, color, structures involved, and distance from margins.

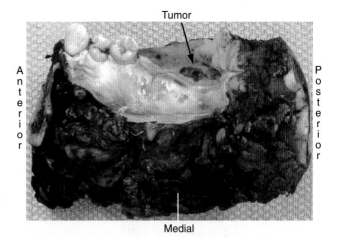

FIGURE B-6

Right hemimandibulectomy for a retromolar trigone tumor (*arrow*). Note the multiple ink colors used to retain the orientation.

Prior to any sectioning, the margins must be assessed and submitted as necessary. For the vast majority of complex specimens, there are numerous margins, both mucosal and soft tissue. As an example, a left partial hemimandibulectomy is shown (Fig. B-7). Serial sections will result in cross sections, each of which shows multiple margins and their relationship to the tumor (Fig. B-8). Decalcification may be required (as in this example), but multiple inks will preserve histologic orientation. Shave margins may be preferred in cases with bone, while radial margins can be submitted for other specimens.

Most specimens will need to be sectioned in order to determine the extent of disease and routes of infiltration. If the sample is a biopsy, the description should include the number and size of the fragments, all of which should be completely embedded. The mucosal surface needs to be sectioned on edge. If the sample of tissue is >4 mm, the specimen should be bisected. When the tissue is <4 mm, multiple serial cuts should be requested at the time of the initial sectioning to avoid loss of diagnostic material in subsequent recut requests. If needed, alternate levels can be stained with H&E, with the unstained (or positively charged) slides held for additional studies as needed. Developing a routine or standard approach is suggested, with minor alterations implemented for each unique specimen/sample as necessary to try to demonstrate the relationship of the "lesion" or "tumor" to the surrounding structures histologically.

Although perhaps slightly out of sequential order, proper and adequate fixation of all specimens is unconditionally required to obtain high quality histologic sections. Depending on tissue type and size of the resection, 6–8 hours of fixation in 10% formalin is minimum, with 24 hours considered ideal. Specimens which contain a substantial component of bone should be fixed with a mixture of formalin and decalcifying solution for at least 48 hours. Clearing agents may aid in lymph node dissections by removing the fat. When faced with turnaround time constraints, the authors

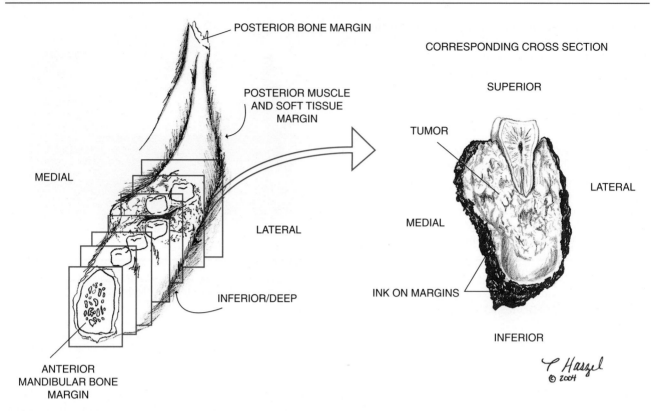

POSTERIOR BONE MARGIN

CORRESPONDING CROSS SECTION

POSTERIOR MUSCLE
AND SOFT TISSUE
MARGIN

SUPERIOR

MEDIAL

TUMOR

LATERAL

LATERAL

MEDIAL

INFERIOR/DEEP

INK ON MARGINS

INFERIOR

ANTERIOR
MANDIBULAR BONE
MARGIN

FIGURE B-7

A left hemimandibulectomy and the standard approach for sectioning a specimen of this nature. The anterior and posterior bone margins should be removed first, and then the specimen serially sectioned from anterior to posterior. Reprinted by permission of Trisha Haszel, Des Moines, IA.

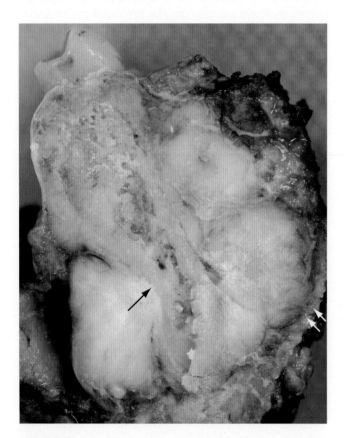

FIGURE B-8

Cross-section of a retromolar trigone tumor. Note the focal invasion of the mandibular bone (*arrow*) and the extension of tumor close to the lateral soft tissue margin (*double arrow*).

suggest that a correct diagnosis made in 3 days on a well-fixed and grossed specimen is always superior to an inaccurate diagnosis rendered the following day on hastily grossed and insufficiently fixed material.

The histologic sections submitted depend on the anatomic site and the lesion in question. Trying to demonstrate normal or uninvolved in relation to the lesion/tumor is vital in making an accurate diagnosis. Thin sections (<2 mm thick) that are well fixed will yield the best histologic slides. Sections with bone are often best obtained by using a striker or hand saw rather than a band saw. Decalcification can then follow on the already cut sample.

GROSSING TECHNIQUES FOR SELECTED SPECIFIC ANATOMIC SITES

LARYNX

Laryngeal specimens can be most challenging, requiring a solid understanding of anatomy. A brief description of cordectomy, hemilaryngectomy, and total laryngectomy will be presented.

CORDECTOMY

Vocal cordectomies or "stripping" are extremely small specimens more akin to a biopsy than a resection.

Most cordectomies include the mucosa of the true cord, and in some cases, underlying soft tissue and vocalis muscle. Surgical margins are of great importance, hence orientation is essential. Ink is applied with each shaved margin submitted in an individual cassette.

HEMILARYNGECTOMY

For small, localized tumors, surgeons will often opt for a voice-sparing, partial or hemilaryngectomy. The more common hemilaryngectomy will consist of the true and false vocal cords from one side of the larynx, as well as the underlying soft tissue and lamina of the thyroid cartilage (Fig. B-9). The specimen will usually extend from the anterior commissure to the posterior commissure and the lateral aspect of the thyroid cartilage will have been skeletonized. It is imperative to demonstrate whether the tumor involves the anterior and posterior commissures, as well as the other mucosal and soft tissue margins. While the thyroid cartilage is technically a margin, it is less significant than the anterior and posterior commissure margins whose connective tissue is a barrier to cancer spread. After measuring and describing the specimen, it should be sectioned vertically at 3–4 mm intervals from anterior to posterior, noting the exact location, size, extent, depth of invasion, and appearance of the uninvolved mucosa. The sections are submitted from anterior to posterior, so as to preserve orientation (Fig. B-10). It is important to state whether the specimen is from right or left.

TOTAL LARYNGECTOMY

A total laryngectomy specimen will generally contain the hyoid bone, epiglottis, glottis (true and false vocal cords) and subglottis down to the first 3 or 4 tracheal rings. The mucosal borders will generally include the base of tongue or vallecula, the pyriform sinuses, the posterior pharyngeal mucosa (esophageal inlet), and

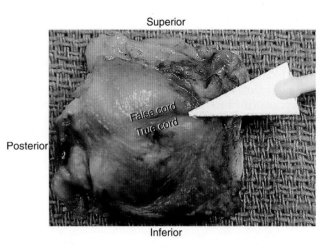

FIGURE B-9

A left vertical hemilaryngectomy for a T1 true vocal cord lesion in a patient that is status postradiation therapy. Note the absence of the ventricular space and adhesion of the true and false cords as a result of the radiation treatment (*pointer*).

FIGURE B-10

A dissection protocol for a vertical hemilaryngectomy specimen. Once the margins are inked, the specimen should be serially sectioned from anterior to posterior, sections made in the superior/inferior plane, with each block demonstrating true cord, false cord, and the underlying thyroid cartilage. Reprinted by permission of Trisha Haszel, Des Moines, IA.

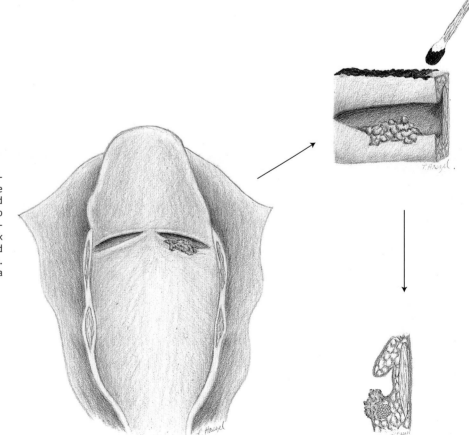

the inferior tracheal ring mucosa. The thyroid gland may also be included. Selective or radical neck dissections are also common and will most often consist of levels 2 through 4 and include the SCM, jugular vein, and even carotid artery. Based on lymphatic drainage and consequently staging, the larynx is divided into three anatomic subsites: Supraglottis: epiglottis (suprahyoid and infrahyoid), aryepiglottic folds, arytenoids and the false cords (ventricular bands); Glottis: true vocal cords, anterior and posterior commissures; and Subglottis: defined as ≥1 cm below the level of the true vocal cords (Fig. B-11). Transglottic is used to describe lesions that cross the ventricle to involve both the true and false cords (Fig. B-12).

The larynx should be separated from the radical neck dissection (if present). It is important to preserve soft tissue relationships if the tumor extends into the soft tissue from the larynx. If the thyroid gland is included,

dissect it away from the larynx, "bread-loaf" at 3-mm intervals, and embed any abnormal areas, or submit a section from each lobe if there are no abnormalities. Parathyroid glands should be sought along the posterior surface of the thyroid, and also embedded.

The larynx should be opened posteriorly down the midline, sectioning through the posterior commissure. A description of the tumor, including the color, growth pattern (endophytic, exophytic), mucosal or submucosal location, surface ulceration, tumor necrosis, hemorrhage, or degeneration should be given along with the specific location of the tumor (Fig. B-13). A statement about the involvement of the true or false vocal cords, whether glottic, supra-, trans-, or subglottic, and whether unilateral or extending across the midline. Distances from the tumor to the tracheal margin and the mucosal margins (base of tongue, epiglottic fold, and aryepiglottic fold) should be documented. The mucosal

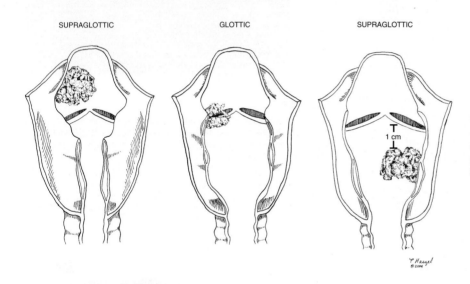

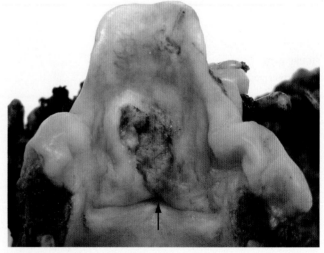

FIGURE B-11

Examples of epithelial tumors of the three anatomic subsites of the larynx: supraglottic, glottic, and subglottic. Reprinted by permission of Trisha Haszel, Des Moines, IA.

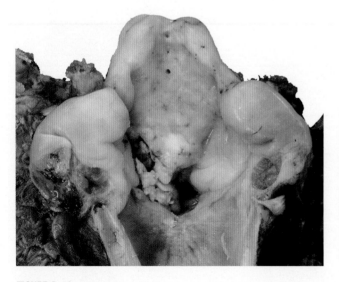

FIGURE B-12

This tumor is transglottic because it involves both the true and false vocal cords. It is important to note the extent (distance) of tumor spread into the subglottis, as glottic cancers with >1 cm of subglottic spread are associated with a worse prognosis.

FIGURE B-13

A midline supraglottic tumor confined to the infrahyoid epiglottis and false vocal cords. The tumor approaches the anterior commissure (*arrow*), but does not cross the ventricle to involve the true cords.

FIGURE B-14

Sectioning in the vertical plane through a total laryngectomy specimen with each slice should include both true and false cord with underlying soft tissue and cartilage. Sections are taken vertically to demonstrate relationship of the tumor to the true and false cords, the anterior commisure, and the underlying cartilage.

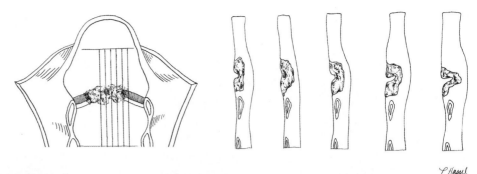

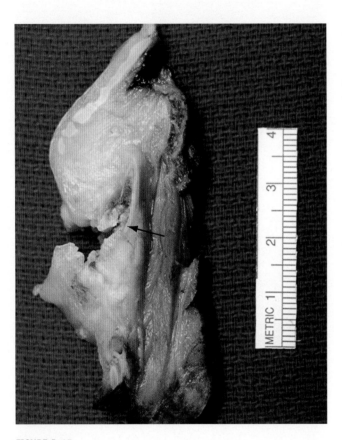

FIGURE B-15

Vertical section of a tumor through the left true and false vocal cords. Note the obvious invasion of the thyroid cartilage (*arrow*).

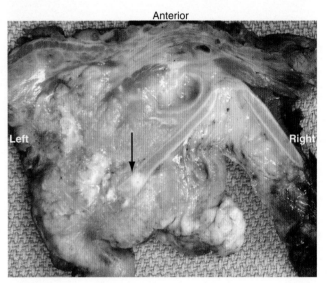

FIGURE B-16

Horizontal cross section of a large left-sided pyriform sinus tumor showing extensive soft tissue involvement and necrosis of the anterior neck. Also note the subtle thyroid cartilage invasion on the left side (*arrow*).

margins are inked and photographs taken if desired. The specimen must be fixed for several hours or preferably overnight to obtain the best sections when cutting through the tumor.

Vertical or horizontal sections can be used to serially section the specimen (Fig. B-14). Modifications can be implemented depending on the exact site. Vertical sections through glottic tumors allow for the entire ventricle to be seen, showing the relationship of the tumor to the true and false cords. After cutting vertically through the tumor, describe the size, shape, color, and consistency of the tumor, noting specifically the depth of invasion and extension to or through the laryngeal cartilages. At least two to three vertical sections through the tumor at the deepest point of invasion and in an area which will demonstrate the tumor's relationship to sur-

rounding structures should be submitted and divided into several blocks, as necessary (Fig. B-15). If there is only scar tissue remaining post-radiotherapy, take an adequate number of sections from the abnormal areas. If the carcinoma involves only one side of the larynx, a section from the anterior commissure (to document bilateral or unilateral involvement) and the middle of the other vocal cord should be submitted, taken vertically and including the soft tissue up to, but not including the cartilage. If the cartilage or bone is involved, separately submit these sections for decalcification. If the tumor does not involve the bone or cartilage, no sections of these structures is necessary. If the tumor is nonlaryngeal, a section of both cords, as described above, should be embedded. A section of the epiglottis, including the anterior mucosal margin should also be included.

Horizontal sectioning allows for slightly easier sectioning because the sample is easier to hold, and it gives the prosector a view of the thyroid cartilage in relation to the cricoid cartilage. This method also allows for a better representation of the cartilages and cricothyroid space as a result of the increased area of examination (Fig. B-16). Care should be taken to make a cut through

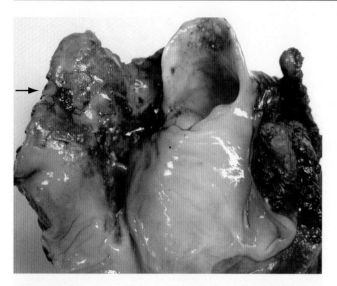

FIGURE B-17

A large left-sided pyriform sinus lesion involving the aryepiglottic fold with extension to the left lateral pharyngeal wall (*arrow*).

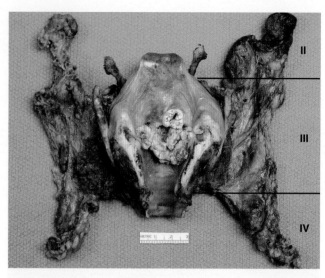

FIGURE B-18

Total laryngectomy with bilateral selective neck dissections, consisting of jugular lymph node changes from levels 2–4: level 2 is superior to the level of the hyoid bone and level 4 is directly below the inferior border of the cricoid cartilage.

the ventricle to preserve orientation of the true and false cords and allow sections of these structures to be taken. Furthermore, the epiglottis should still be sectioned vertically to demonstrate the base of tongue margin.

When tumors involve the pyriform sinus and hypopharynx, these tumors are staged as primary pharyngeal tumors, although sectioning is similar to laryngeal samples. However, care must to be taken to note invasion into adjacent structures which can significantly alter the stage (Fig. B-17).

NECK DISSECTION

If a neck dissection was attached, the zones of dissection can be determined based on the anatomy of the laryngeal sample. Usually, they are comprised of zones 2, 3, and 4: zone 2 is located superior to the hyoid bone and level 4 is below the inferior border of the cricoid cartilage, with zone 3 in between (Fig. B-18). See section on neck dissection evaluation below.

MAXILLECTOMY

Most radical maxillectomy specimens are removed for biopsy proven neoplasms, with squamous cell carcinoma comprising the majority. Partial maxillectomy resections are generally performed for localized lesions limited to the inferior aspects of the maxilla. Orientation can usually be achieved by identifying structures such as the palate, alveolar processes, orbital floor, and lateral nasal wall (Fig. B-19), although if orientation is unclear, particularly in smaller resections, orientation by the surgeon

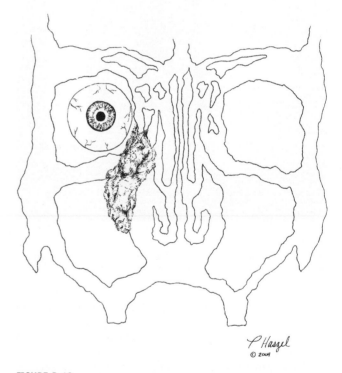

FIGURE B-19

A tumor arises from the medial wall of the maxillary sinus and involves the right lateral nasal wall and medial aspect of the orbital floor. Reprinted by permission of Trisha Haszel, Des Moines, IA.

is critical. Radical maxillectomy specimens will usually include an entire side of the maxilla, portions of the zygomatic bone, portions of the orbital wall, and in some cases the entire orbit (termed radical maxillectomy with orbital exenteration; Figs. B-20, B-21).

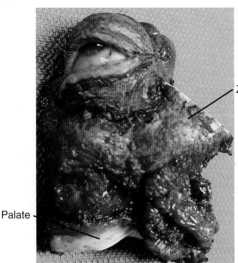

FIGURE B-20
Radical maxillectomy with orbital exenteration (anterior–lateral view).

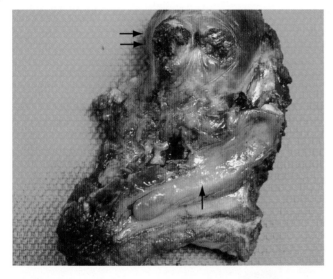

FIGURE B-21
Posterior view of the radical maxillectomy in Fig. B-20. The inferior turbinate (*arrow*) is an anatomic landmark. Note the posterior optic nerve margin (*double arrow*).

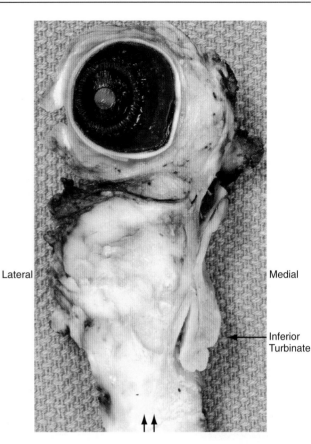

FIGURE B-22
Cross-section of a left-radical maxillectomy with orbital exenteration for a squamous cell carcinoma arising in the maxillary sinus. This posterior view shows the inferior turbinate on the right side of the image (*arrow*), and the extensive tumor involving the entire maxillary sinus with invasion into the palate (*double arrow*).

After orientation, it is important to identify the surgical margins, which are both mucosal and bony. These may include *anterior:* mucosa and soft tissue of the alveolar ridge (may also include skin if resection is anterior); *lateral:* zygomatic arch which may include bone, soft tissue, and in rare cases, skin; *medial:* palate, maxillary bone, nasal septum, and turbinates; *superior:* orbital floor or contents of orbit; *posterior:* pterygoid musculature and optic nerve margin; *inferior:* usually palate, however, the alveolar ridge mucosa and even bone at the anterior/inferior aspect may be the true margin (Fig. B-22). It is important in the gross description to include all structures removed (maxilla, inferior turbinate, orbital floor, zygomatic bone, etc.), tumor size, location, and presence of invasion of adjacent structures, including bone and/or cartilage. After taking anterior and posterior margins, the specimen should be sectioned in the coronal plane from anterior to posterior and laid out from left to right like a book. Sections should be made at 3–4 mm, where possible, so as to provide the best histologic appearance of the tumor.

HEMIGLOSSECTOMY

Tongue resections have easy to recognize anatomic landmarks, making dissection a little easier. As surgical margins are of utmost importance, marking the mucosal and soft tissue margins should be one of the first steps in handling such a specimen (Fig. B-23). Once this is accomplished, histologic sections of all suspicious margins should be submitted, as well as sections demonstrating the extent of tumor invasion. The macroscopic description must include the size and type of specimen (partial glossectomy, composite resection with mandible, etc.), size and location of tumor, appearance

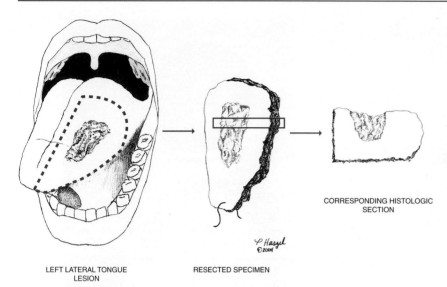

CORRESPONDING HISTOLOGIC
SECTION

FIGURE B-23

Sectioning of a hemiglossectomy specimen can include many of the margins in the same histologic section. Dotted line denotes course of resection. Reprinted by permission of Trisha Haszel, Des Moines, IA.

of tumor (ulcerated, necrotic, firm, etc.), extent of tumor invasion, proximity of tumor to margins, and if there is involvement of adjacent structures (see Fig. B-5).

PAROTID RESECTIONS

SUPERFICIAL PAROTIDECTOMY

Parotid resections for benign tumors (pleomorphic adenoma) are quite common, with the overwhelming majority of benign parotid lesions developing within the superficial lobe. Superficial parotidectomy involves

removal of the superficial lobe while painstakingly separating the lobe from the facial nerve. Resected specimens, if unoriented, can usually be identified according to their superficial and deep surfaces. The superficial aspect of a parotidectomy is generally smooth and fibrous where the investing fascia was separated from the overlying skin, whereas the deep aspect tends to be irregular and coarse where it was dissected off the facial nerve. Even though possibly removed for benign disease, the external surface must be inked (Fig. B-24), with different ink colors for the superficial and deep aspects if possible. After external description, the specimen should be bivalved in the anterior-posterior direction, thus separating the specimen into superficial and deep portions. The location and size of any lesions should be

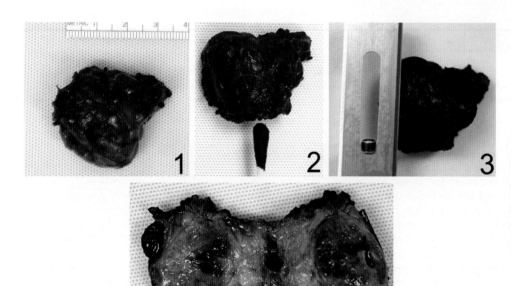

FIGURE B-24

Cross dissection of a superficial parotidectomy specimen. The entire external surface is marked with India ink and the specimen is then bivalved. Sections would then be taken vertically through the entire lesion (both sides) and the entire lesion with inked capsule submitted. (This is a Warthin tumor.)

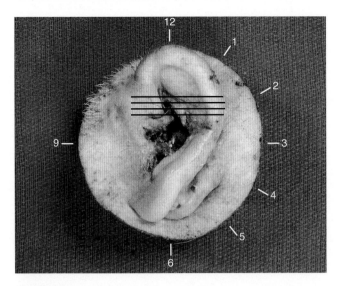

FIGURE B-25

Composite resection of a primary parotid cancer that has invaded the cartilaginous ear canal. The peripheral margins in this case would be extremely important. The best way to submit these margins would be en face like a clock face. Once the margins are taken, then the specimen would be serially sectioned from anterior to posterior (see section lines).

recorded, as well as any obvious invasion (capsular or other). By bivalving the specimen, you are able to view a large surface area of parotid parenchyma in relation to any lesions present. Each half should then be serially sectioned from anterior to posterior and histologic sections submitted accordingly. For most parotid lesions, the entire tumor should be submitted with overlying capsule and adjacent normal tissue.

RADICAL PAROTID RESECTIONS

Occasionally, large malignant tumors will require radical resection of the entire parotid gland, the facial nerve, overlying skin, and even the ear canal and mastoid (Fig. B-25). Such composite resections should be viewed as a clock face, with the peripheral skin and soft tissue margins being the numbers on the clock. The deep margins, including bone and cartilage, would be submitted separately (Fig. B-26). As with all complex resections, assessment of margins and evaluation of the extent of tumor involvement are crucial to an adequate gross dissection. Review of the normal anatomy is generally a good idea prior to approaching this type of specimen.

MANDIBLE

The size and type of resection for a mandibular tumor can vary from a small segmental resection to such radical procedures as a total mandibulectomy or composite resection. Viewing the specimen as a six-sided cube aids in determining margins. The anterior margin will usually consist of a bone margin, and likewise

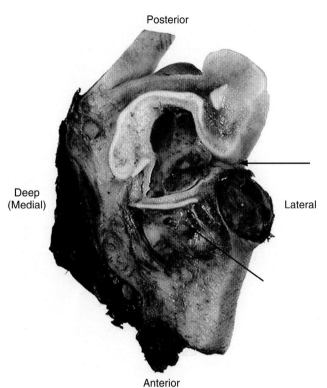

FIGURE B-26

Cross-section (axial) of a true malignant mixed tumor arising in the parotid gland and erupting through the skin anterior to the external acoustic meatus. Note the complete replacement of the cartilaginous ear canal by the tumor (*arrows*).

the posterior margin will also consist of bone. In cases where the mandibular condyle and coronoid are resected, then the pterygoid musculature and adjacent soft tissue would be considered true margin and not the bone. The medial and lateral margins will generally consist of oral cavity mucosa; however, extensive tumors may also invade soft tissue (both floor of mouth and lateral) and even skin, in which case those structures would also be considered as margins (Fig. B-27). Sectioning should be approached in the same manner as maxillectomy specimens, with the anterior/posterior margins being removed and the specimen sectioned in a coronal plane from anterior to posterior. Histologic sections should include: bone and soft tissue margins, tumor with adjacent soft tissue and mucosa, tumor with bone and extent of bony invasion, and tumor with closest margin(s). Needless to say, taking pertinent and sensible sections which will allow for an accurate determination of the tumor will remove some of the difficulty associated with complex specimens.

NECK DISSECTIONS

Neck dissections are performed to either evaluate a patient's lymph node status or to resect obvious clinical disease. For clinical and pathologic staging purposes, the

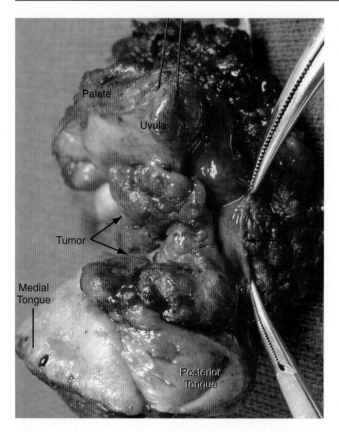

FIGURE B-27

Posterior view of a composite mandibulectomy including the tongue and palate (surgical suture attached to the palate). Note the close proximity of the tumor to the posterior mucosal margin (*arrow*) held by clamps.

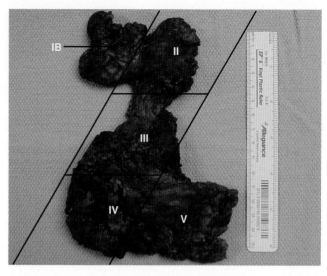

FIGURE B-28

Left-sided neck dissection showing the representative lymphatic zones. With the exception of level Ia (submental), there are two corresponding zones, one for each side of the neck. Level Ib (submandibular); levels II–IV (jugular chain); level V (posterior triangle); P (parotid); and R (retroauricular).

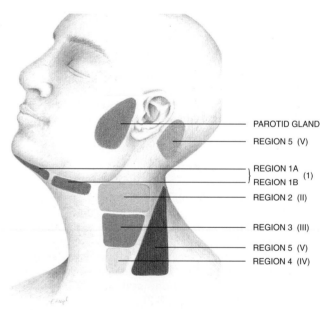

FIGURE B-29

Layout of a comprehensive left neck dissection including levels 1b–5. Courtesy of Trisha Haszel.

neck is broken down in lymphatic zones. With the exception of zone Ia (submental), each zone is paired on either side of the neck. Specific zones are identified, with particular attention to the jugular chain (Fig. B-28).

Neck dissections can be done on a limited basis where only the lymph nodes and soft tissue are removed (selective neck dissection), or they can be quite extensive and involve removal of many structures within the neck (modified-radical neck dissection). Selective neck dissections generally tend to include levels 2–4, although level 1 and level 5 nodes may also be removed. Removal of the submandibular gland (level 1b) is also quite frequent. A truly radical neck dissection involves removal of the internal jugular vein, the SCM, and the spinal accessory nerve in addition to the lymph nodes and associated soft tissue (Fig. B-29). A modified-radical dissection would include preservation of any one of the three aforementioned structures. Extended neck dissections would include any structures not previously mentioned (paratracheal nodes, carotid artery, etc.).

Lymph nodes should be separated out from their respective levels or zones, and sections submitted accordingly for histology. All identified lymph nodes must be submitted. For larger lymph nodes, if the entire node is submitted, it is imperative to note in your gross dictation if a single cassette contains multiple sections of a single lymph node. Otherwise, the total lymph node

count could be affected and possibly have an adverse impact on the patient's adjuvant therapy.

ACKNOWLEDGMENT

The authors would like to express their sincerest gratitude to Ms. Trisha Haszel for her superb artwork and illustrations.

SUGGESTED READING

1. Ackerman LV, Ramirez GA: The indications for and limitations of frozen section diagnosis. A review of 1269 consecutive frozen section diagnoses. Br J Surg 1959;46:336–350.

2. Barnes EL: Surgical Pathology of the Head and Neck, 2nd ed. New York: Marcel Dekker, 2001.

3. Barnes L, Johnson JT: Pathologic and clinical considerations in the evaluation of major head and neck specimens resected for cancer. Part 1. In: Sommers SC, Rosen PP, Fechner RE, eds. Pathology Annual. Vol. 21, part 1. Norwalk, CT: Appleton-Century-Crofts, 1986.

4. Fu Y, Abemayor E, Wenig BM, et al.: Head and Neck Pathology with Clinical Correlations. Philadelphia: Churchill-Livingstone, 2001.

5. Gandour-Edwards RF, Donald PJ, Lie JT: Clinical utility of intraoperative frozen section diagnosis in head and neck surgery: a quality assurance perspective. Head Neck 1993;15:373–376.

6. Gnepp DR: Uses, abuses and pitfalls of frozen section diagnoses. In: Ferlito A, ed. Surgical Pathology of Laryngeal Neoplasms. London: Chapman Hall, 1996.

7. Holaday WJ, Assor D: Ten thousand consecutive frozen sections. A retrospective study focusing on accuracy and quality control. Am J Clin Pathol 1974;61:769–777.

8. Kirchner JA: Pathways and pitfalls in partial laryngectomy. Ann Otol Rhinol Laryngol 1984;93:301–305.

9. Lester S: Manual of Surgical Pathology. Philadelphia: Churchill-Livingstone, 2001.

10. Michaels L: Examination of specimens of the larynx. J Clin Pathol 1990;43:792–795.

11. Saltzstein SL, Nahum AM: Frozen section diagnosis: accuracy and errors; uses and abuses. Laryngoscope 1973;83:1128–1143.

12. Slootweg PJ, de Groot J: Surgical pathological anatomy of head and neck specimens: a manual for the dissection of surgical specimens from the upper aerodigestive tract. London: Springer-Verlag, 1999.

13. Spiro RH, Guillamondegui O Jr, Paulino AF, Huvos AG: Pattern of invasion and margin assessment in patients with oral tongue cancer. Head Neck 1999;21:408–413.

14. Westra WH, Hruban RH, Phelps TH, Isacson C: Surgical Pathology Dissection: An Illustrated Guide, 2nd ed. London: Springer-Verlag, 2003.

15. Wong DS: Frozen section during parotid surgery revisited: efficacy of its applications and changing trend of indications. Head Neck 2002;24:191–197.

TNM Classification and Consensus Reporting of Head and Neck Tumors

Leslie H. Sobin • Lester D. R. Thompson

INTRODUCTION

This section presents the current UICC/AJCC TNM classifications for head and neck carcinomas (1,2). They are found in many of the following tables, although the UICC/AJCC does not classify a number of unique entities in the head and neck (olfactory neuroblastoma, nasopharyngeal angiofibroma, nasal, paranasal, and nasopharyngeal melanomas), for which proposed staging systems have been presented (Tables C-3, C-4, C-6). The following introduction contains a general discussion of TNM principles and a summary of the major changes in the TNM classifications that occurred from the previous (5th) to the present (6th) edition.

The TNM classification describes the anatomic extent of cancer. It is based on the fact that the choice of treatment and the chance of survival are related to the extent of the tumor at the primary site (T), the presence or absence of tumor in regional lymph nodes (N), and the presence or absence of metastasis beyond the regional lymph nodes (M). Tumors are classified prior to treatment, i.e., clinical or cTNM, and after resection, i.e., pathological or pTNM. T is usually divided into four major parts (T1–T4), expressing increasing size or spread of the primary tumor. N and M comprise at least two categories each (0 and 1—absence or presence of tumor). A number of sites have subcategories. The criteria for cTNM and pTNM are identical for head and neck tumors. Note: A help desk for specific questions about the TNM classification is available at http://uicc.org/tnm.

STAGE GROUPING

Classification by TNM achieves a reasonably precise description of and system for recording the apparent anatomical extent of disease. However, a tumor with four T, three N, and two M categories will have 24 possible TNM categories. For purposes of tabulation and analysis, except in very large series, it is necessary to condense these categories into a more convenient number of TNM stages. This aims to ensure that each stage group is more or less homogeneous in respect to survival and management, and that the survival rates of these groups for each cancer site are distinctive, e.g., patients with stage I tumors usually survive their disease; those with stage IV usually succumb to the disease.

OBJECTIVES

TNM's objectives are to: (a) aid the clinician in the planning of treatment; (b) give some indication of prognosis; (c) assist in the evaluation of the results of treatment; (d) facilitate the exchange of information; and (e) TNM can also serve as a means of assessing the management of patients and as a yardstick to measure early detection (screening) efforts.

The 6th edition TNM classification of the International Union Against Cancer (UICC) (1) and American Joint Committee on Cancer (AJCC) (2) was introduced in January 2003. Although relatively unchanged for most cancer sites, the head and neck sections of the classification underwent substantial revision in the 6th edition. The major changes that occurred between the 5th and 6th TNM editions are summarized below, with a detailed description and discussion of the changes in the head and neck sections of the 6th edition prepared by O'Sullivan and Shah. (3). Much of the following text is based on their excellent work.

T4

The fundamental composition and content of the head and neck TNM classification has not changed in decades. However, with evolution in treatment approaches over the past decade, a simple description of the primary tumor beyond the site of origin to characterize locally "advanced" disease is no longer adequate for this group of patients. Therefore, the 6th edition introduced a subdivision of T4 across all head and neck sites into T4a and T4b based on the principle of a reasonable opportunity for disease control in T4a, compared to the virtual certainty of poor outcome in T4b.

SPECIAL SYMBOLS

Developments in multimodality therapy have increased the importance of the "y" symbol (designating tumors that are classified after radiation or chemotherapy) and the "r" symbol (residual tumor) classification. New surgical techniques have resulted in the elaboration of the "sn" (sentinel node) symbol. Immunohistochemistry has brought about the classification of "itc" (isolated tumor cells) and their distinction from micrometastasis (1,2).

MODIFICATIONS IN THE 6TH EDITION TNM FOR HEAD AND NECK SITES (3)

GENERAL ISSUES

a. Stage IVA is classified as T4a N0-N1, or any N2 lesion without T4b.
b. T-category and N-category allocation remains the same for stages I, II, III, and IVC as in the 5th edition.
c. T4 lesions have been divided into T4a (lower risk) and T4b (higher risk), facilitating a division of stage IV into stage IVA, stage IVB, and stage IVC.
d. Excepting thyroid, stage IVB is N3 disease, or T4b with any other N category (excepting nasopharynx).

SPECIFIC ISSUES

a. Larynx
   T3 lesions (glottic and supraglottic) include paraglottic space invasion, and specify minor erosion of the thyroid cartilage in addition to the features in the 5th edition (Table C-1).

b. Nasal cavity and paranasal sinuses
   i. A new site has been added for inclusion into the staging system. In addition to maxillary sinus, the nasoethmoid complex is described as a second site with two regions within this site: nasal cavity and ethmoid sinuses (Table C-2).
   ii. The nasal cavity region is further divided into four subsites: septum, floor, lateral wall, and vestibule.
   iii. The ethmoid sinus region is divided into two subsites: right and left.
   iv. The T categories for ethmoid lesions have been revised to reflect nasoethmoid tumors, and appropriate description of their T categories has been added. For T4a and T4b, see Table C-2.
   v. Minor rewording of T1-T3 maxillary antrum.
c. Pharynx
   i. Code C10.3 (Posterior wall of oropharynx) was inadvertently excluded from 6th edition AJCC.
   ii. For nasopharynx, rewording to permit other soft issue extensions outside nasopharynx to be classified as T2 even if parapharynx not involved (Table C-5). Stage groupings for nasopharynx same as in 5th edition.
d. Major salivary gland sites
   For consistency of T categories across all sites, the description for T3 has been revised. In addition to tumors having extraparenchymal extension, all tumors larger than 4 cm are considered T3 unless they have criteria for T4a and T4b (Table C-9). T3N1 is stage III in 6th edition instead of stage IV (5th edition).

REFERENCES

1. International Union Against Cancer (UICC): TNM classification of malignant tumors, 6th ed. Sobin LH, Wittekind CH, eds. New York: Wiley, 2002.
2. AJCC Cancer Staging Manual, 6th ed. Greene FL, Page D, Morrow M, et al., eds. New York: Springer, 2002.
3. O'Sullivan B, Shah J: New TNM staging criteria for head and neck tumors. Semin Surg Oncol 2003;21:30–42.
4. Kadish S, Goodman M, Wang CC: Olfactory neuroblastoma. A clinical analysis of 17 cases. Cancer 1976;37:1571–1576.
5. Thompson LDR, Wieneke JA, Miettinen M: Sinonasal tract and nasopharyngeal melanomas: a clinicopathologic study of 115 cases with a proposed staging system. Am J Surg Pathol 2003;2:594–611.
6. Thompson LDR, Fanburg-Smith JC: Nasopharyngeal angiofibroma. In: Barnes EL, Eveson JW, Reichart P, Sidransky D, eds. Pathology and Genetics of Head and Neck Tumours. Kleihues P, Sobin LH, series eds. World Health Organization Classification of Tumours. Lyon, France: IARC Press, 2005:102–103.
7. Wittekind CH, Henson DE, Hutter RVP, Sobin LH (eds): TNM supplement: a commentary on uniform use. New York: Wiley, 2003:130–131.

TABLE C-1

TNM Classification of Carcinomas of the Larynx[1,2]

TNM

T—PRIMARY TUMOR

TX	Primary tumor cannot be assessed
T0	No evidence of primary tumor
Tis	Carcinoma in situ

Supraglottis

T1	Tumor limited to one subsite of supraglottis with normal vocal cord mobility
T2	Tumor invades mucosa of more than one adjacent subsite of supraglottis or glottis or region outside the supraglottis (e.g., mucosa of base of tongue, vallecula, medial wall of pyriform sinus) without fixation of the larynx
T3	Tumor limited to larynx with vocal cord fixation and/or invades any of the following: postcricoid area, pre-epiglottic tissues, paraglottic space, and/or with minor thyroid cartilage erosion (e.g., inner cortex)
T4a	Tumor invades through the thyroid cartilage and/or invades tissues beyond the larynx, e.g., trachea, soft tissues of neck including deep/extrinsic muscle of tongue (genioglossus, hyoglossus, palatoglossus, and styloglossus), strap muscles, thyroid, esophagus
T4b	Tumor invades prevertebral space, mediastinal structures, or encases carotid artery

Glottis

T1	Tumor limited to vocal cord(s) (may involve anterior or posterior commissure) with normal mobility
T1a	Tumor limited to one vocal cord
T1b	Tumor involves both vocal cords
T2	Tumor extends to supraglottis and/or subglottis, and/or with impaired vocal cord mobility
T3	Tumor limited to larynx with vocal cord fixation and/or invades paraglottic space, and/or with minor thyroid cartilage erosion (e.g., inner cortex)
T4a	Tumor invades through the thyroid cartilage, or invades tissues beyond the larynx, e.g., trachea, soft tissues of neck including deep/extrinsic muscle of tongue (genioglossus, hyoglossus, palatoglossus, and styloglossus), strap muscles, thyroid, esophagus
T4b	Tumor invades prevertebral space, mediastinal structures, or encases carotid artery

Subglottis

T1	Tumor limited to subglottis
T2	Tumor extends to vocal cord(s) with normal or impaired mobility
T3	Tumor limited to larynx with vocal cord fixation
T4a	Tumor invades through cricoid or thyroid cartilage and/or invades tissues beyond the larynx, e.g., trachea, soft tissues of neck including deep/extrinsic muscle of tongue (genioglossus, hyoglossus, palatoglossus, and styloglossus), strap muscles, thyroid, esophagus
T4b	Tumor invades prevertebral space, mediastinal structures, or encases carotid artery

N—REGIONAL LYMPH NODES (THE REGIONAL LYMPH NODES ARE THE CERVICAL NODES)*

NX	Regional lymph nodes cannot be assessed
N0	No regional lymph node metastasis
N1	Metastasis in a single ipsilateral lymph node, <3 cm in greatest dimension
N2	Metastasis as specified in N2a, 2b, 2c below
N2a	Metastasis in a single ipsilateral lymph node, >3 cm but ≤6 cm in greatest dimension
N2b	Metastasis in multiple ipsilateral lymph nodes, ≤6 cm in greatest dimension
N2c	Metastasis in bilateral or contralateral lymph nodes, ≤6 cm in greatest dimension
N3	Metastasis in a lymph node >6 cm in greatest dimension

M—DISTANT METASTASIS

MX	Distant metastasis cannot be assessed
M0	No distant metastasis
M1	Distant metastasis

Stage Definitions

Stage 0	Tis	N0	M0
Stage I	T1	N0	M0
Stage II	T2	N0	M0
Stage III	T1, T2	N1	M0
	T3	N0, N1	M0
Stage IVA	T1, T2, T3	N2	M0
	T4a	N0, N1, N2	M0
Stage IVB	T4b	Any N	M0
	Any T	N3	M0
Stage IVC	Any T	Any N	M1

*Midline nodes are considered ipsilateral nodes.

TABLE C-2

TNM Classification of Carcinomas of the Nasal Cavity and Paranasal Sinuses[1,2]

	TNM

T—Primary Tumor

TX	Primary tumor cannot be assessed
T0	No evidence of primary tumor
Tis	Carcinoma in situ

Maxillary Sinus

T1	Tumor limited to the antral mucosa with no erosion or destruction of bone
T2	Tumor causing bone erosion or destruction, including extension into hard palate and/or middle nasal meatus, except extension to posterior antral wall of maxillary sinus and pterygoid plates
T3	Tumor invades any of the following: bone of posterior wall of maxillary sinus, subcutaneous tissues, floor or medial wall of orbit, pterygoid fossa, ethmoid sinuses
T4a	Tumor invades any of the following: anterior orbital contents, skin of cheek, pterygoid plates, infratemporal fossa, cribriform plate, sphenoid or frontal sinuses
T4b	Tumor invades any of the following: orbital apex, dura, brain, middle cranial fossa, cranial nerves other than maxillary division of trigeminal nerve V^2, nasopharynx, clivus

Nasal Cavity and Ethmoid Sinus

T1	Tumor restricted to one subsite of nasal cavity or ethmoid sinus, with or without bony invasion
T2	Tumor involves two subsites in a single site or extends to involve an adjacent site within the nasoethmoid complex, with or without bony invasion
T3	Tumor extends to invade the medial wall or floor of the orbit, maxillary sinus, palate, or cribriform plate
T4a	Tumor invades any of the following: anterior orbital contents, skin of nose or cheek, minimal extension to anterior cranial fossa, pterygoid plates, sphenoid or frontal sinuses
T4b	Tumor invades any of the following: orbital apex, dura, brain, middle cranial fossa, cranial nerves other than V^2, nasopharynx, clivus

N—Regional Lymph Nodes (The regional lymph nodes are the cervical nodes)*

NX	Regional lymph nodes cannot be assessed
N0	No regional lymph node metastasis
N1	Metastasis in a single ipsilateral lymph node, <3 cm in greatest dimension
N2	Metastasis as specified in N2a, 2b, 2c below
N2a	Metastasis in a single ipsilateral lymph node, >3 cm but ≤6 cm in greatest dimension
N2b	Metastasis in multiple ipsilateral lymph nodes, ≤6 cm in greatest dimension
N2c	Metastasis in bilateral or contralateral lymph nodes, ≤6 cm in greatest dimension
N3	Metastasis in a lymph node >6 cm in greatest dimension

M—Distant Metastasis

MX	Distant metastasis cannot be assessed
M0	No distant metastasis
M1	Distant metastasis

Stage Definitions

Stage 0	Tis	N0	M0
Stage I	T1	N0	M0
Stage II	T2	N0	M0
Stage III	T1, T2	N1	M0
	T3	N0, N1	M0
Stage IVA	T1, T2, T3	N2	M0
	T4a	N0, N1, N2	M0
Stage IVB	T4b	Any N	M0
	Any T	N3	M0
Stage IVC	Any T	Any N	M1

*Midline nodes are considered ipsilateral nodes.

TABLE C-3

Staging of Olfactory Neuroblastoma

The following classification is not an official TNM classification, i.e., not approved or published by the UICC and AJCC. However, the Kadish clinical staging system is well accepted as the staging system for olfactory neuroblastoma.[4]

Stage	Extent of Tumor	5-Year Survival
A	Tumor confined to nasal cavity	75%–91%
B	Tumor involves the nasal cavity plus one or more paranasal sinuses	68%–71%
C	Extension of tumor beyond the sinonasal cavities	41%–47%

TABLE C-4

Proposed Staging for Malignant Melanoma of the Nasal Cavity, Paranasal Sinuses, and Nasopharynx[5]

The following classification is not an official TNM classification, i.e., not approved or published by the UICC and AJCC. It is a proposal based on a study of 115 cases.[5] It is presented here for testing. Publication of results is encouraged.

TNM

T—PRIMARY TUMOR

TX	Primary tumor cannot be assessed
T0	No evidence of primary tumor
Tis	Melanoma in situ
T1	Tumor limited to a single anatomic site, namely: nasal cavity, maxillary sinus, frontal sinus, ethmoid sinus, sphenoid sinus, nasopharynx
T2	Tumor involving more than one anatomic site, as cited above, including extension into any of the following: subcutaneous tissues, skin, palate, pterygoid plate, floor, wall, or apex of the orbit, cribriform plate, infratemporal fossa, dura, brain, middle cranial fossa, cranial nerves, clivus

N—REGIONAL LYMPH NODES (THE REGIONAL LYMPH NODES ARE THE CERVICAL NODES)

NX	Regional lymph nodes cannot be assessed
N0	No regional lymph node metastasis
N1	Metastasis in regional lymph node(s) of any size, whether ipsilateral, bilateral, or contralateral (midline nodes are considered ipsilateral nodes)

M—DISTANT METASTASIS

MX	Distant metastasis cannot be assessed
M0	No distant metastasis
M1	Distant metastasis

Stage Definitions

Stage	T	N	M
Stage 0	Tis	N0	M0
Stage I	T1	N0	M0
Stage II	T2	N0	M0
Stage III	Any T	N1	M0
Stage IV	Any T	Any N	M1

TABLE C-5

TNM Classification of Carcinomas Nasopharynx[1,2]

[It is important to note that lymphomas are not considered in this classification.]

TNM

T—PRIMARY TUMOR

TX	Primary tumor cannot be assessed
T0	No evidence of primary tumor
Tis	Carcinoma in situ
T1	Tumor confined to nasopharynx
T2	Tumor extends to soft tissues
T2a	Tumor extends to oropharynx and/or nasal cavity without parapharyngeal extension*
T2b	Tumor with parapharyngeal extension*
T3	Tumor invades bony structures and/or paranasal sinuses
T4	Tumor with intracranial extension and/or involvement of cranial nerves, infratemporal fossa, hypopharynx, orbit, or masticator space

N—REGIONAL LYMPH NODES (THE REGIONAL LYMPH NODES ARE THE CERVICAL NODES)

NX	Regional lymph nodes cannot be assessed
N0	No regional lymph node metastasis
N1	Unilateral metastasis, in lymph node(s), ≤6 cm in greatest dimension, above the supraclavicular fossa[†]
N2	Bilateral metastasis in lymph node(s), ≤6 cm in greatest dimension, above the supraclavicular fossa[†]
N3	Metastasis in lymph node(s) >6 cm in dimension or in the supraclavicular fossa[†]
N3a	>6 cm in dimension
N3b	In the supraclavicular fossa[†]

M—DISTANT METASTASIS

MX	Distant metastasis cannot be assessed
M0	No distant metastasis
M1	Distant metastasis

Stage Definitions

Stage 0	Tis	N0	M0
Stage I	T1	N0	M0
Stage IIA	T2a	N0	M0
Stage IIB	T1	N1	M0
	T2a	N1	M0
	T2b	N0, N1	M0
Stage III	T1	N2	M0
	T2a, T2b	N2	M0
	T3	N0, N1, N2	M0
Stage IVA	T4	N0, N1, N2	M0
Stage IVB	Any T	N3	M0
Stage IVC	Any T	Any N	M1

*Parapharyngeal extension denotes posterolateral infiltration of tumor beyond the pharyngobasilar fascia.
[†]The supraclavicular fossa is the triangular region defined by three points: (1) the superior margin of the sternal end of the clavicle; (2) the superior margin of the lateral end of the clavicle; (3) the point where the neck meets the shoulder. This includes caudal portions of levels IV and V.
Note: Midline nodes are considered ipsilateral nodes.

TABLE C-6

System for Staging Nasopharyngeal Angiofibroma[6]

The following classification is not an official TNM classification, i.e., not approved or published by the UICC and AJCC. It is a proposal based on the World Health Organization Classification of Tumours modification of a number of systems.[6] It is presented here for testing. Publication of results is encouraged.

Stage	Extent of Tumor
Stage I	Tumor limited to the nasopharynx with no bone destruction
Stage II	Tumor invading the nasal cavity, maxillary, ethmoid, and sphenoid sinuses with no bone destruction
Stage III	Tumor invading the pterygopalatine fossa, infra-temporal fossa, orbit and parasellar region
Stage IV	Tumor with massive invasion of the cranial cavity, cavernous sinus, optic chiasm, or pituitary fossa

TABLE C-7

TNM Classification of Carcinomas of the Oropharynx[1,2]

	TNM

T—PRIMARY TUMOR

TX	Primary tumor cannot be assessed
T0	No evidence of primary tumor
Tis	Carcinoma in situ
T1	Tumor <2 cm in greatest dimension
T2	Tumor >2 cm but ≤4 cm in greatest dimension
T3	Tumor >4 cm in greatest dimension
T4a	Tumor invades the larynx, deep/extrinsic muscle of tongue (genioglossus, hyoglossus, palatoglossus, and styloglossus), medial pterygoid, hard palate, and mandible
T4b	Tumor invades lateral pterygoid muscle, pterygoid plates, lateral nasopharynx, skull base or encases the carotid artery

N—REGIONAL LYMPH NODES (THE REGIONAL LYMPH NODES ARE THE CERVICAL NODES)*

NX	Regional lymph nodes cannot be assessed
N0	No regional lymph node metastasis
N1	Metastasis in a single ipsilateral lymph node, ≤3 cm in greatest dimension
N2	Metastasis in a single ipsilateral lymph node, >3 cm but ≤6 cm in greatest dimension, or in multiple ipsilateral lymph nodes, ≤6 cm in greatest dimension, or in bilateral or contralateral lymph nodes, ≤6 cm in greatest dimension
N2a	Metastasis in a single ipsilateral lymph node >3 cm but ≤6 cm in greatest dimension
N2b	Metastasis in multiple ipsilateral lymph nodes, ≤6 cm in greatest dimension
N2c	Metastasis in bilateral or contralateral lymph nodes, ≤6 cm in greatest dimension
N3	Metastasis in a lymph node >6 cm in greatest dimension

M—DISTANT METASTASIS

MX	Distant metastasis cannot be assessed
M0	No distant metastasis
M1	Distant metastasis

Stage Definitions

Stage 0	Tis	N0	M0
Stage I	T1	N0	M0
Stage II	T2	N0	M0
Stage III	T3	N0	M0
	T1	N1	M0
	T2	N1	M0
	T3	N1	M0
Stage IVA	T4a	N0	M0
	T4a	N1	M0
	T1	N2	M0
	T2	N2	M0
	T3	N2	M0
	T4a	N2	M0
Stage IVB	T4b	Any N	M0
	Any T	N3	M0
Stage IVC	Any T	Any N	M1

*Midline nodes are considered ipsilateral nodes.

TABLE C-8
TNM Classification of Carcinomas of the Lip and Oral Cavity[1,2]

	TNM
T—PRIMARY TUMOR	
TX	Primary tumor cannot be assessed
T0	No evidence of primary tumor
Tis	Carcinoma in situ
T1	Tumor <2 cm in greatest dimension
T2	Tumor >2 cm but ≤4 cm in greatest dimension
T3	Tumor >4 cm in greatest dimension
T4a (lip)	Tumor invades through cortical bone, inferior alveolar nerve, floor of mouth, or skin (chin or nose)
T4a (oral cavity)	Tumor invades through cortical bone, into deep/extrinsic muscle of tongue (genioglossus, hyoglossus, palatoglossus, and styloglossus), maxillary sinus, or skin of face
T4b (lip and oral cavity)	Tumor invades masticator space, pterygoid plates, or skull base, or encases internal carotid artery
N—REGIONAL LYMPH NODES (THE REGIONAL LYMPH NODES ARE THE CERVICAL NODES)*	
NX	Regional lymph nodes cannot be assessed
N0	No regional lymph node metastasis
N1	Metastasis in a single ipsilateral lymph node, <3 cm in greatest dimension
N2	Metastasis as specified in N2a, 2b, 2c below
N2a	Metastasis in a single ipsilateral lymph node, >3 cm but ≤6 cm in greatest dimension
N2b	Metastasis in multiple ipsilateral lymph nodes, ≤6 cm in greatest dimension
N2c	Metastasis in bilateral or contralateral lymph nodes, ≤6 cm in greatest dimension
N3	Metastasis in a lymph node >6 cm in greatest dimension
M—DISTANT METASTASIS	
MX	Distant metastasis cannot be assessed
M0	No distant metastasis
M1	Distant metastasis

Stage Definitions			
Stage 0	Tis	N0	M0
Stage I	T1	N0	M0
Stage II	T2	N0	M0
Stage III	T1, T2	N1	M0
	T3	N0, N1	M0
Stage IVA	T1, T2, T3	N2	M0
	T4a	N0, N1, N2	M0
Stage IVB	T4b	Any N	M0
	Any T	N3	M0
Stage IVC	Any T	Any N	M1

*Midline nodes are considered ipsilateral nodes.
Note: Superficial erosion alone of bone/tooth socket by gingival primary is not sufficient to classify a tumor as T4.

TABLE C-9

TNM Classification of Carcinomas of Salivary Glands[1,2]

[Tumors arising in minor salivary glands localized to the mucous membrane of the upper aerodigestive tract are classified according to the rules for tumors of their respective locations.]

TNM

T—Primary Tumor

TX	Primary tumor cannot be assessed
T0	No evidence of primary tumor
T1	Tumor <2 cm in greatest dimension without extraparenchymal extension*
T2	Tumor >2 cm but ≤4 cm in greatest dimension without extraparenchymal extension*
T3	Tumor >4 cm and/or tumor with extraparenchymal extension*
T4a	Tumor invades skin, mandible, ear canal, or facial nerve
T4b	Tumor invades base of skull, pterygoid plates, or encases carotid artery

N—Regional Lymph Nodes (The regional lymph nodes are the cervical nodes)[†]

NX	Regional lymph nodes cannot be assessed
N0	No regional lymph node metastasis
N1	Metastasis in a single ipsilateral lymph node, <3 cm in greatest dimension
N2	Metastasis as specified in N2a, 2b, 2c below
N2a	Metastasis in a single ipsilateral lymph node, >3 cm but ≤6 cm in greatest dimension
N2b	Metastasis in multiple ipsilateral lymph nodes, more than ≤6 cm in greatest dimension
N2c	Metastasis in bilateral or contralateral lymph nodes, ≤6 cm in greatest dimension
N3	Metastasis in a lymph node >6 cm in greatest dimension

M—Distant Metastasis

MX	Distant metastasis cannot be assessed
M0	No distant metastasis
M1	Distant metastasis

Stage Definitions

Stage I	T1	N0	M0
Stage II	T2	N0	M0
Stage III	T3	N0	M0
	T1, T2, T3	N1	M0
Stage IVA	T1, T2, T3	N2	M0
	T4a	N0, N1, N2	M0
Stage IVB	T4b	Any N	M0
	Any T	N3	M0
Stage IVC	Any T	Any N	M1

*Extraparenchymal extension is clinical or macroscopic evidence of invasion of soft tissues or nerve, except those listed under T4a and 4b. Microscopic evidence alone does not constitute extraparenchymal extension for classification purposes.
[†]Midline nodes are considered ipsilateral nodes.

TABLE C-10

TNM Classification of Carcinomas of the External Ear[1,2]

[Rhabdomyosarcomas are staged according to the Intergroup Rhabdomyosarcoma Study Group, while middle ear and temporal bone tumors are not classified by this system.]

TNM

T—PRIMARY TUMOR

TX	Primary tumor cannot be assessed
T0	No evidence of primary tumor
Tis	Carcinoma in situ
T1	Tumor <2 cm in greatest dimension
T2	Tumor >2 cm but ≤5 cm in greatest dimension
T3	Tumor >5 cm in greatest dimension
T4	Tumor invades deep extradermal structures, i.e., cartilage, skeletal muscle, orbone

N—REGIONAL LYMPH NODES (THE REGIONAL LYMPH NODES ARE THE CERVICAL NODES)

NX	Regional lymph nodes cannot be assessed
N0	No regional lymph node metastasis
N1	Regional lymph node metastasis

M—DISTANT METASTASIS

MX	Distant metastasis cannot be assessed
M0	No distant metastasis
M1	Distant metastasis

Stage Definitions

Stage 0	Tis	N0	M0
Stage I	T1	N0	M0
Stage II	T2, T3	N0	M0
Stage III	T4	N0	M0
	Any T	N1	M0
Stage IV	Any T	Any N	M1

Note: In the case of multiple simultaneous tumor, the tumor with the highest T category is classified and the number of separate tumor is indicated in parentheses, e.g., T2(5), or by (m).

Page numbers followed by *f* indicate a figure; those followed by *t* indicate tabular material.

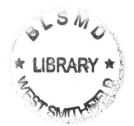